Hematopoietic Growth Factors in Oncology

CANCER DRUG DISCOVERY AND DEVELOPMENT

Beverly A. Teicher, Series Editor

Proteasome Inhibitors in Cancer Therapy, edited by *Julian Adams, 2004*
Nucleic Acid Theapeutics in Cancer, edited by *Alan M. Gewirtz, 2004*
Cancer Chemoprevention, Volume 1: *Promising Cancer Chemopreventive Agents,* edited by *Gary J. Kelloff, Ernest T. Hawk, and Caroline C. Sigman,* 2004
DNA Repair in Cancer Therapy, edited by *Lawrence C. Panasci and Moulay A. Alaoui-Jamali,* 2004
Hematopoietic Growth Factors in Oncology: *Basic Science and Clinical Therapeutics,* edited by *George Morstyn, MaryAnn Foote, and Graham J. Lieschke,* 2004
Handbook of Anticancer Pharmacokinetics and Pharmacodynamics, edited by *William D. Figg and Howard L. McLeod,* 2004
Anticancer Drug Development Guide: *Preclinical Screening, Clinical Trials, and Approval, Second Edition,* edited by *Beverly A. Teicher and Paul A. Andrews,* 2004
Handbook of Cancer Vaccines, edited by *Michael A. Morse, Timothy M. Clay, and Kim H. Lyerly, 2004*
Drug Delivery Systems in Cancer Therapy, edited by *Dennis M. Brown, 2003*
Oncogene-Directed Therapies, edited by *Janusz Rak,* 2003
Cell Cycle Inhibitors in Cancer Therapy: *Current Strategies,* edited by *Antonio Giordano and Kenneth J. Soprano,* 2003
Chemoradiation in Cancer Therapy, edited by *Hak Choy,* 2003
Fluoropyrimidines in Cancer Therapy, edited by *Youcef M. Rustum,* 2003
Targets for Cancer Chemotherapy: *Transcription Factors and Other Nuclear Proteins,* edited by *Nicholas B. La Thangue and Lan R. Bandara, 2002*
Tumor Targeting in Cancer Therapy, edited by *Michel Pagé,* 2002
Hormone Therapy in Breast and Prostate Cancer, edited by *V. Craig Jordan and Barrington J. A. Furr,* 2002
Tumor Models in Cancer Research, edited by *Beverly A. Teicher,* 2002
Tumor Suppressor Genes in Human Cancer, edited by *David E. Fisher,* 2001
Matrix Metalloproteinase Inhibitors in Cancer Therapy, edited by *Neil J. Clendeninn and Krzysztof Appelt,* 2001
Farnesyltransferase Inhibitors in Cancer, edited by *Saïd M. Sebti and Andrew D. Hamilton,* 2001
Platinum-Based Drugs in Cancer Therapy, edited by *Lloyd R. Kelland and Nicholas P. Farrell,* 2000
Apoptosis and Cancer Chemotherapy, edited by *John A. Hickman and Caroline Dive,* 1999
Signaling Networks and Cell Cycle Control: *The Molecular Basis of Cancer and Other Diseases,* edited by *J. Silvio Gutkind,* 1999
Antifolate Drugs in Cancer Therapy, edited by *Ann L. Jackman,* 1999
Antiangiogenic Agents in Cancer Therapy, edited by *Beverly A. Teicher,* 1999
Anticancer Drug Development Guide: ***Preclinical Screening, Clinical Trials, and Approval,*** edited by *Beverly A. Teicher,* 1997
Cancer Therapeutics: ***Experimental and Clinical Agents,*** edited by *Beverly A. Teicher,* 1997

Hematopoietic Growth Factors in Oncology

Basic Science and Clinical Therapeutics

Edited by

George Morstyn, MBBS, PhD, FRACP

Amgen, Australia, Pty. Ltd.
Monash University, Victoria, Australia

MaryAnn Foote, PhD

Amgen Inc., Thousand Oaks, CA

Graham J. Lieschke, MBBS, PhD, FRACP

Ludwig Institute for Cancer Research, Royal Melbourne Hospital
Melbourne, Australia

Humana Press
Totowa, New Jersey

Softcover reprint of the hardcover 1st edition 2004
999 Riverview Drive, Suite 208
Totowa, New Jersey 07512

www.humanapress.com

Cover design by Patricia F. Cleary.

Production Editor: J. Morgan

This publication is printed on acid-free paper. ∞

ANSI Z39.48-1984 (American National Standards Institute) Permanence of Paper for Printed Library Materials

For additional copies, pricing for bulk purchases, and/or information about other Humana titles, contact Humana at the above address or at any of the following numbers: Tel.: 973-256-1699; Fax: 973-256-8341; Email: humana@humanapr.com; or visit our Website: http://www.humanapress.com.

ISBN 978-1-4684-9847-9 ISBN 978-1-59259-747-5 (eBook)
DOI 10.1007/978-1-59259-747-5

Library of Congress Cataloging-in-Publication Data
Hematopoietic growth factors in oncology basic science and clinical therapeutics / edited by George Morstyn, MaryAnn Foote, Graham J. Lieschke.
p. ; cm. -- (Cancer drug discovery and development)
Includes bibliographical references and index.
ISBN 978-1-4684-9847-9
1. Hematopoietic growth factors--Therapeutic use. 2. Hematopoietic growth factors--Mechanism of action. 3. Cancer--Chemotherapy.
[DNLM: 1. Hematopoietic Cell Growth Factors--therapeutic use. 2.
Hematopoietic Cell Growth Factors--pharmacology. 3.
Neoplasms--therapy. WH 140 H487383 2004] I. Morstyn, George, 1950- II.
Foote, MaryAnn. III. Lieschke, Graham J. IV. Series.
RC271.H43H45 2004
616.99'4061--dc22

2003017466

PREFACE

Several hematopoietic growth factors (HGFs) have achieved widespread clinical application. In the United States alone, more than US $5 billion per year of the health care budget is spent on these factors. The first patients were treated with recombinant human erythropoietin (rHuEPO, epoetin alfa, Epogen®) in 1985 and the first patients received recombinant methionyl human granulocyte colony-stimulating factor (r-metHuG-CSF, filgrastim, Neupogen®) or recombinant human granulocyte-macrophage colony-stimulating factor (rHuGM-CSF, sargramostim, Leukine® or Prokine®) in 1986. The first agent promoting platelet recovery was formally approved in 1997 (recombinant human interleukin-11 [rHuIL-11], oprelvekin, Neumega®). In 2002, sustained-duration derivative r-metHuG-CSF (pegfilgrastim, Neulasta®) was formally approved for clinical use. Likewise in 2002, a new erythropoietic protein (darbepoetin alfa, Aranesp®) with a longer serum half-life and increased biologic activity compared with rHuEPO was formally approved for clinical use. Pharmaceutical forms of several other agents have been assessed in clinical studies but are yet to find a widespread clinical utility or niche (e.g., stem cell factor, thrombopoietin, interleukin-3, colony-stimulating factor-1 [macrophage colony-stimulating factor]). The efficacy of the marketed agents to ameliorate the complications of cancer and the side effects of chemotherapy has led to their broad clinical application; however, their cost has led to efforts to ensure that their use is focused onto clinically appropriate indications. *Hematopoietic Growth Factors in Oncology: Basic Science and Clinical Therapeutics* is a further contribution to this endeavor.

HGFs are produced in the bone marrow, kidney, brain, and fetal liver by a wide variety of cells, and they exhibit exquisite selectivity of action dependent on the expression of specific receptors by target cells. The factors stimulate proliferation and differentiation, have antiapoptotic effects, and enhance the function of mature cells.

Hematopoietic Growth Factors in Oncology: Basic Science and Clinical Therapeutics introduces the molecular basis for the activity of HGFs and discusses their specific role in the treatment of various malignancies. The clinical application of these agents continues to expand because of their benefits and relative lack of side effects. Chemotherapy remains a mainstay of cancer treatment despite the introduction of newer therapeutic approaches, and so there remains a need to optimize chemotherapy-related supportive care. In the chapters presented from a systematic oncology perspective, we hope to help oncologists treating patients with particular tumor types to make informed evidence-based decisions about adjunctive HGF therapy within disease-focused treatment regimens. The volume also describes progress in various areas of basic science that may lead to further advances in hemopoietic cell regulation. There are also sections on the utility of growth factors in infectious disease settings such as AIDS.

Some notes about the preparation of the book are in order. Because of the nature of scientific inquiry, the editors have allowed overlap in chapter topics and varying opinions. We encouraged the authors to be comprehensive regarding the available HGFs, and we actively sought chapters covering the currently available agents. The opinions expressed are not necessarily the opinions of the editors or the publisher. Great care has been taken to ensure the integrity of the references and drug doses, but the package inserts of any drug should always be consulted before administration.

Readers will realize that many scientists and clinicians worldwide have worked and continue to work in the fields of basic and applied research of HGFs. We would, however, like to recognize one of our colleagues, Dr. Dora M. Menchaca. Dora joined Amgen in July 1991 as a clinical manager and was a close colleague of MaryAnn Foote and George Morstyn. She was involved in the design and conduct of many clinical trials, including the use of filgrastim in the setting of acute myeloid leukemia and myelodysplastic syndromes; the use of stem cell factor in many clinical settings; the use of megakaryocyte growth and development factor for the treatment of thrombocytopenia and for harvesting peripheral blood progenitor cells; and several other molecules. Dora was an advocate for patients enrolled in clinical trials and worked diligently to help get new therapeutic molecules registered and marketed to help patients worldwide. Dora was returning on an early morning flight after a meeting with the FDA and was on American Airlines flight 77 that was hijacked and crashed into the US Pentagon on September 11, 2001. We still mourn the loss of this dedicated scientist and continue to miss her enthusiasm, her intelligence, her warm and caring personality, and her infectious smile and laughing eyes. We dedicate this book to Dora.

George Morstyn, *MBBS, PhD, FRACP*
MaryAnn Foote, *PhD*
Graham J. Lieschke, *MBBS, PhD, FRACP*

Contents

CONTRIBUTORS

C. GLENN BEGLEY, MBBS, PhD, FRACP, FRCPath, FRCPA • *Senior Director, Basic Research in Hematology, Amgen Inc., Thousand Oaks, CA*

BEN A. CROKER, BSc • *Cancer and Hematology Division, The Walter and Eliza Hall Institute of Medical Research, Victoria, Australia*

DAVID C. DALE, MD • *Professor, Department of Medicine, University of Washington, Seattle, WA*

CHRISTOPHE A. DOOMS, MD • *Respiratory Oncology Unit (Pulmonology), University Hospital Gasthuisberg, Leuven, Belgium*

STEVEN ELLIOTT, PhD • *Fellow, Hematology Department, Amgen Inc., Thousand Oaks, CA*

ANN M. FARESE, MS, MT (ASCP) • *Greenebaum Cancer Center, University of Maryland, Baltimore, Maryland*

MARYANN FOOTE, PhD • *Director, Medical Writing, Amgen Inc., Thousand Oaks, CA*

RICHARD M. FOX, MB, PhD, FRACP • *Department of Medical Oncology, Royal Melbourne Hospital, Melbourne, Australia*

BARBARA C. GOOD, PhD • *Director, Scientific Publications, National Surgical Adjuvant Breast and Bowel Project, Pittsburgh, PA*

LAWRENCE T. GOODNOUGH, MD • *Professor, Departments of Medicine and Pathology and Immunology, Washington University School of Medicine, St. Louis, MO*

JASON GOTLIB, MD • *Clinical Research Fellow, Hematology Division, Stanford University Medical Center, Stanford, CA*

PETER L. GREENBERG, MD • *Professor, Department of Medicine, Stanford University Medical Center, Stanford, CA; Head, Hematology, VA Palo Alto Health Care System, Palo Alto, CA*

ANNE C. HEATHERINGTON, PhD • *Research Scientist, Department of Pharmacokinetics and Drug Metabolism, Amgen Inc., Thousand Oaks, CA*

TIMOTHY R. HERCUS, PhD • *Cytokine Receptor Laboratory, Hanson Institute, Adelaide, Australia*

FRANKIE ANN HOLMES, MD, FACP • *US Oncology; Texas Oncology, Houston, TX*

NICOLE M. KUDERER, MD • *James P. Wilmot Cancer Center, University of Rochester Medical Center, Rochester, NY*

DAVID J. KUTER, MD, DPhil • *Chief of Hematology, Massachusetts General Hospital, and Associate Professor of Medicine, Harvard Medical School, Boston, MA*

ELLEN G. LABER, PhD • *Senior Medical Writer, Medical Writing, Amgen Inc., Thousand Oaks, CA*

KEITH E. LANGLEY, PhD • *Principal Medical Writer, Medical Writing, Amgen Inc., Thousand Oaks, CA*

GRAHAM J. LIESCHKE, MBBS, PhD, FRACP • *Assistant Member and Laboratory Head, Cytokine Biology Laboratory, Ludwig Institute for Cancer Research, Melbourne Tumour Biology Branch, Parkville, Victoria, Australia; Clinical Hematologist, Department of Clinical Hematology and Medical Oncology, The Royal Melbourne Hospital, Parkville, Victoria, Australia*

CAROL ANN LONG, PhD • *Newbury Park, CA*

ANGEL F. LOPEZ, MD, PhD • *Cytokine Receptor Laboratory, Hanson Institute, Adelaide, Australia*

GARY H. LYMAN, MD, MPH, FRCP • *James P. Wilmot Cancer Center, University of Rochester Medical Center, Rochester, NY*

THOMAS J. MACVITTIE, PhD • *Greenebaum Cancer Center, University of Maryland, Baltimore, MD*

ERIC D. MININBERG, MD • *MD Anderson Cancer Center, University of Texas, Houston, TX*

GRAHAM MOLINEUX, PhD • *Associate Director, Hematology Department, Amgen Inc., Thousand Oaks, CA*

GEORGE MORSTYN, MBBS, PhD, FRACP • *Special Advisor, Development, Amgen Inc., Thousand Oaks, CA; Department of Microbiology, Monash University, Clayton, Victoria, Australia*

NICOS A. NICOLA, PhD • *Professor, Molecular Hematology, and Assistant Director, The Walter and Eliza Hall Institute of Medical Research, Parkville, Victoria, Australia*

IAN N. OLVER, MD, PhD • *Clinical Director, Royal Adelaide Hospital Cancer Center, Adelaide, Australia*

HAYLEY S. RAMSHAW, PhD • *Cytokine Receptor Laboratory, Hanson Institute, Adelaide, Australia*

ROY E. SMITH, MD • *Director, Medical Affairs and Medical Oversight, National Surgical Adjuvant Breast and Bowel Project, Pittsburgh, PA*

MARCIE R. TOMBLYN, MD • *Fellow, Division of Hematology/Oncology, Feinberg School of Medicine, Northwestern University; Robert H. Lurie Comprehensive Cancer Center, Chicago, IL*

JOHAN F. VANSTEENKISTE, MD, PhD • *Respiratory Oncology Unit (Pulmonology), University Hospital Gasthuisberg, Leuven, Belgium*

KARL WELTE, MD, PhD • *Professor of Pediatrics, Hannover Medical School; Head, Department of Pediatric Hematology and Oncology, Children Hospital, Hannover, Germany*

JANE N. WINTER, MD • *Professor of Medicine, Division of Hematology/Oncology, Feinberg School of Medicine, Northwestern University; Robert H. Lurie Comprehensive Cancer Center, Chicago, IL*

I BASIC RESEARCH

1 Introduction to Hematopoietic Growth Factors

A General Overview

George Morstyn, MBBS, PhD, FRACP
and MaryAnn Foote, PhD

CONTENTS

1. INTRODUCTION

A complex, inter-related, and multistep process called hematopoiesis controls the production and development of specific bone marrow cells from immature precursor cells to functional mature blood cells. The earliest cells are stem cells and are multipotential and able to self-renew. Up to 10^{11} blood cells are produced in an adult human each day. The proliferation of precursor cells, the commitment to one lineage, the maturation of these cells into mature cells, and the survival of hematopoietic cells require the presence of specific growth factors, which act individually and in various combinations in complex feedback mechanisms. The hematopoietic growth factors (HGFs) stimulate cell division, differentiation, maturation, and survival, convert the dividing cells into a population of terminally differentiated functional cells (Fig. 1), and in some cases also activate their mature functions *(1–4)*. Because the literature concerning every aspect of HGF discovery, cloning, function, and clinical use is burgeoning, in this chapter, we mention only a few of the most significant works and cite general references where possible.

These factors are important for both maintaining the steady state and mediating responses to infection. More than 20 HGFs have been identified. The properties of some are described in Table 1. The structure and function of these growth factors have been characterized and the gene that encodes for each factor identified and cloned. Several HGFs are commercially available as recombinant human forms, and they have utility in

From: *Cancer Drug Discovery and Development*
Hematopoietic Growth Factors in Oncology: Basic Science and Clinical Therapeutics
Edited by: G. Morstyn, M. A. Foote, and G. J. Lieschke © Humana Press Inc., Totowa, NJ

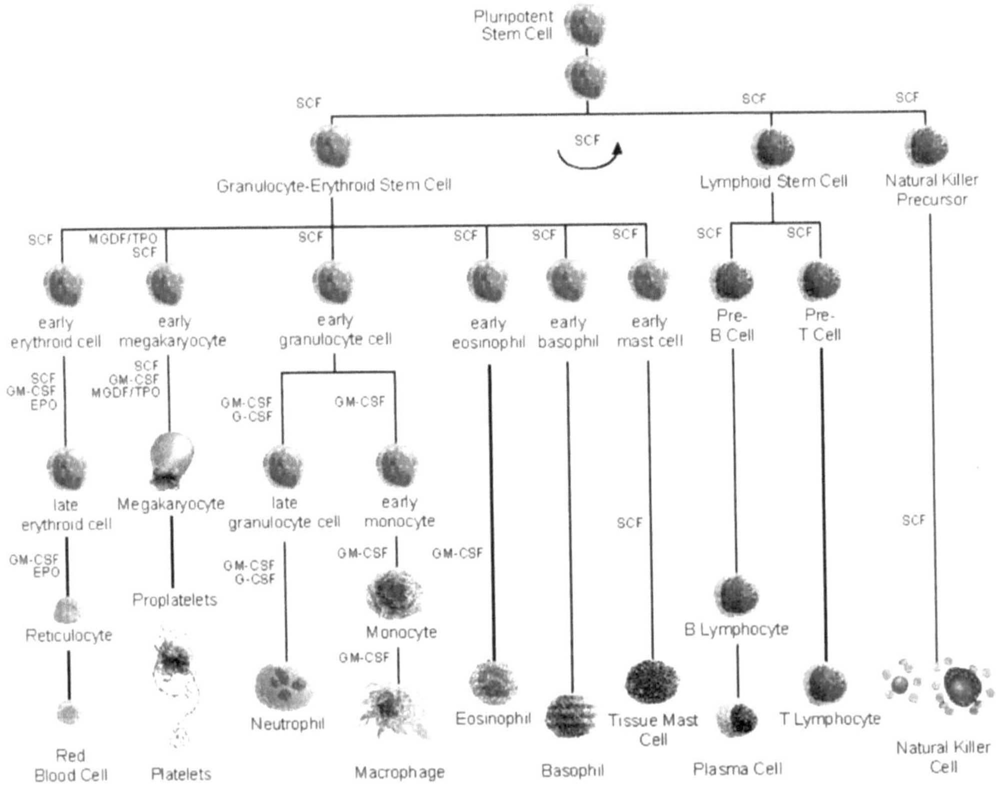

Fig. 1. Hematopoietic tree. EPO, erythropoietin; G-CSF, granulocyte colony-stimulating factor; GM-CSF, granulocyte-macrophage colony-stimulating factor; mGDF, megakaryocyte growth and development factor; SCF, stem cell factor; TPO, thrombopoietin. (Courtesy of Amgen, Thousand Oaks, CA.)

clinical practice. These factors include the recombinant forms of two myeloid hematopoietic growth factors, granulocyte colony-stimulating factor (G-CSF) and granulocyte-macrophage colony-stimulating factor (GM-CSF); erythropoietin (EPO), the red cell factor; stem cell factor (SCF), an early-acting HGF; and thrombopoietin (TPO) and interleukin-11 (IL-11), platelet factors. T lymphocytes, monocytes/macrophages, fibroblasts, and endothelial cells are the important cellular sources of most HGFs, excluding EPO and TPO *(5,6)*. EPO is produced primarily by the adult kidney *(7–9)*, and TPO is produced in the liver and in the kidney *(10–12)*.

G-CSF (recombinant products: filgrastim, lenograstim, pegfilgrastim) maintains neutrophil production during steady-state conditions and increases production of neutrophils during acute situations, such as infections *(13)*. Recombinant human G-CSF (rHuG-CSF) reduces neutrophil maturation time from 5 d to 1 d, leading to the rapid release of mature neutrophils from the bone marrow into the blood *(14)*. rHuG-CSF also increases the circulating half-life of neutrophils and enhances chemotaxis and superoxide production *(15)*. Pegfilgrastim is a sustained-duration formulation of rHuG-CSF that has been developed by covalent attachment of a polyethylene glycol molecule to the filgrastim molecule *(16)*.

GM-CSF (recombinant products: molgramostim, sargramostim) is locally active and remains at the site of infection to recruit and activate neutrophils *(13)*. Like G-CSF,

Table 1
Hematopoietic Growth Factors and Their Activities

Factor	*MW (kDa)*	*Abbreviation*	*Target cell*	*Actions*
Erythropoietin	34–39	EPO	Erythoid progenitors (BFU-E, CFU-E)	Increase red blood count
Granulocyte colony-stimulating factor	18	G-CSF	Granulocyte progenitors; mature neutrophils (G-CFC)	Increase ANC
Granulocyte-macrophage colony-stimulating factor	14–35	GM-CSF	Granulocyte, macrophage progenitors (GM-CFC) eosinophil progenitors	Increase neutrophil, eosinophil, and monocyte count
Interleukin-3	28	IL-3	Multipotential progenitor cells	Increase hematopoietic and lymphoid cells
Interleukin-5	40–50	IL-5	Eosinophil progenitor cells	Increase eosinophils
Interleukin-7	25	IL-7	Early B and T cells	Stimulate B and T cells
Interleukin-11	23	IL 11	Early hemopoietic progenitors, megakaryocytes	Increase platelet count
Monocyte colony-stimulating factor	40–70	M-CSF	Monocyte progenitor cells	Increase monocytes; but decrease in platelet count
Thrombopoietin	35	TPO	Stem cells, megakaryocyte and erythroid progenitors	Increase platelet count

ABBREVIATIONS: ANC, absolute neutrophil count; BFU-E, blast-forming unit-erythroid; CFU-E, colony-forming unit-erythroid; G-CFC, granulocyte colony-forming cell; GM-CFC, granulocyte-macrophage colony forming cells

GM-CSF and rHuGM-CSFs stimulate the proliferation, differentiation, and activation of mature neutrophils and enhance superoxide production, phagocytosis, and intracellular killing *(17–19)*. GM-CSF and rHuGM-CSF, unlike G-CSF, stimulate the proliferation, differentiation, and activation of mature monocytes/macrophages *(18)*.

Erythropoietic factors (recombinant products: epoetin alfa, epoetin beta, darbepoetin alfa) increase red blood cell counts by causing committed erythroid progenitor cells to proliferate and differentiate into normoblasts, nucleated precursors in the erythropoietic lineage *(20–22)*. Tissue hypoxia resulting from anemia induces the kidney to increase its production of EPO by a magnitude of a 100-fold or more. EPO stimulates the production of erythroid precursor cells and therefore increases the red blood cell content and oxygen-carrying capacity of blood. Anemia in patients with cancer can be owing to direct or indirect effects of the malignancy on the marrow, or as a complication of myelotoxic chemotherapy or radiotherapy. The onset is often insidious, and some of the clinical effects of anemia have in the past been wrongly attributed to the underlying malignancy. Darbepoetin alfa is another erythropoietic factor that has an extended half-life owing to its increased number of sialic acid-containing carbohydrate molecules *(20–21)*.

SCF (recombinant product: ancestim) is an early-acting hematopoietic growth factor that stimulates the proliferation of primitive hematopoietic and nonhematopoietic cells *(2,23)*. In vitro, SCF has minimal effect on hematopoietic progenitor cells, but it synergistically increases the activity of other HGFs, such as G-CSF, GM-CSF, and EPO. SCF and recombinant human (rHu)SCF stimulate generation of dendritic cells in vitro and mast cells in vivo, and rHuSCF has been used in combination with rHuG-CSF to increase progenitor cell mobilization *(24)*.

Thrombopoietic factors (recombinant products: rHuTPO, pegylated megakaryocyte growth and development factor [PEG-rHuMGDF], and rHuIL-11 [oprelvekin]) stimulate the production of megakaryocyte precursors, megakaryocytes, and platelets *(10,25,26)*. IL-11 has many effects on multiple tissues and can interact with IL-3, TPO, or SCF. Endogeous TPO values are increased in patients with thrombocytopenia; it is very effective at increasing the platelet count. TPO is thought to be the major regulator of platelet production.

2. DISCOVERY OF HEMATOPOIETIC GROWTH FACTORS

The study of hematopoiesis was greatly facilitated in the mid-1960s when techniques for studying hematopoietic stem cells and progenitor cells in vivo *(27)* and in clonal culture *(28,29)* were developed. It was clear that the proliferation and development of these cells was dependent on growth factors. In cultures, these growth factors were provided by serum, conditioned medium, or cell underlayers. The growth factors present in these sources were called colony-stimulating factors (CSFs) *(30)*.

In the 1970s and early 1980s, many of the growth factors were purified. It was recognized that several growth factors acted on the granulocyte lineage, including G-CSF, GM-CSF, and IL-3. At the time, it was a great challenge to achieve purity because these factors were present at very low concentrations. By the mid-1980s, it was apparent that the criterion for purity was when a single protein sequence could be obtained from the pure preparation and the gene encoding this sequence could be cloned and expressed to produce the same protein.

Once recombinant human forms of HGF were produced by recombinant DNA technology in large amounts, the focus shifted to studying the pharmacology and clinical effects. The focus of laboratory research changed from identifying additional growth factors to studying their mode of action. Site-directed mutagenesis and other techniques allowed the structure of the growth factors, their binding to receptors, and their intracellular signaling to be defined in detail. The study of HGFs in vivo was greatly facilitated by gene knockout as well as by gene overexpression studies. These areas are reviewed in later chapters of this book.

When the clinical development of recombinant human forms of HGF was initiated, a common belief was that since they were natural regulators of hematopoiesis, they would be well tolerated. Laboratory studies indicated redundancy in the effects of these HGF and also showed that their maximal effects were produced when they were used in combination with each other. Clinical studies appeared to indicate that the factors most selective on one cell lineage (such as recombinant forms of G-CSF, EPO, and TPO) were better tolerated than broadly acting factors. Combinations of recombinant growth factors in the clinic were not extensively tested, but combinations of rHuG-CSF and rHuEPO, rHuG-CSF and rHuGM-CSF, and rHuSCF and rHuG-CSF have been studied, with beneficial effects reported in some cases, for example, rHuG-CSF and rHuSCF for progenitor cell mobilization *(31)*.

Other chapters in this volume review the pharmacology of HGF in normal and special populations, as well as in relation to some of the most common cancers. The use of HGF in the oncology sector revolutionized the treatment of patients. Further work should offer more innovative methods for the treatment of patients with cancer.

3. CLINICAL DEVELOPMENT OF HEMATOPOIETIC GROWTH FACTORS

The clinical development of recombinant forms of HGF were directed by an extensive understanding of the biologic effects of these factors. The human gene encoding EPO was cloned in 1983 *(22)*, and clinical development of epoetin alfa began soon after. Initial studies were focused on patients with an endogenous EPO deficiency, such as patients with severe chronic renal failure receiving dialysis. The effects of epoetin alfa were apparent in the first dose levels with an increase in hemoglobin concentration and hematocrit. A reduction in the requirement for red blood cell transfusions was ultimately proved in the pivotal phase 3 trial. Further studies focused on defining a safe rate of rise in hemoglobin and an appropriate target; however, a conservative target rather than normalization of hematocrit was initially approved in the dialysis setting. In patients with underlying heart disease, the safety and benefits of correction to a normal hematocrit are still under investigation almost 20 years after the initiation of clinical studies *(32,33)*.

For the development of rHuEPO in the setting of cancer, a major challenge was to recognize the benefits of maintaining hematocrits at higher volumes than had been the previous practice when only blood transfusions were available. A second challenge was to obtain sufficient information on the reduction in the need for transfusions and improvement in quality of life to justify the cost of therapy with rHuEPO. Recent guidelines developed by the American Society of Clinical Oncology (ASCO) and the American Society of Hematology (ASH) address the optimum use of rHuEPO. They do not yet evaluate the impact of darbepoetin alfa on this field.

Another set of blood factors studied were the factors stimulating the platelet lineage. The development of factors stimulating platelets was impaired by several observations. The first was that the factors available, rHuIL-11 and rHuTPO, act on increasing the number and ploidy of megakaryoctes but do not stimulate platelet shedding. Therefore, the increase in platelet counts is slow. Second, IL-11 was pleiotropic and was associated with significant adverse events. The recombinant thrombopoietins (rHuTPO, PEG-rHuMGDF) tested in the clinic induced antibodies that inhibited their own activity and the activity of TPO, leading to prolonged thrombocytopenia.

HGFs such as SCF and flt3 ligand were also tested for activity on multipotential stem cells. rHuSCF enhanced progenitor cell mobilization induced by rHuG-CSF. The problems of severe stem cell deficiency states such as aplastic anemia remain unsolved, and rHuSCF was associated with side effects related to mast cell activation. Nevertheless, rHuSCF received marketing approval in Australia, New Zealand, and Canada.

4. FUTURE DIRECTIONS

A number of chapters in this volume focus on current research that could lead to future clinical applications. Croker and Nicola review the pathways of cytokine signaling. These pathways when aberrant could be involved in oncogenesis, and thus an understanding of signaling may lead to new targets for the development of therapeutics. It is also possible that for some applications, targeting of the intracellular signaling pathway will lead to more selective and orally active stimulants of hematopoietic cells. It may be possible to stimulate selectively early cells, mature cells, or mature cell function. Identifying more effective ways of reconstituting the marrow of patients with severe aplastic anemia or other forms of aplasia or dysplasia, would also be an important clinical objective. The development of antagonists for the treatment of inflammatory states or some types of leukemia may prove valuable.

An important area for future development arises from structure and function analyses of HGF. For example, at one time, it was not considered possible to modify the protein backbone of the HGF and thereby improve their pharmacologic properties, because of the risk of a loss of efficacy or the induction of immunogenicity. The recent regulatory approval of darbepoetin alfa, however, shows that changing the amino acid sequence of rHuEPO to produce a hyperglycosylated molecule results in prolonged half-life and maintained efficacy without inducing neutralizing antibodies. It is likely that further modifications will be explored.

We are currently able to stimulate the neutrophil and erythroid lineage effectively; however, Kuter reviews the data demonstrating that although recombinant TPO is effective in preclinical and clinical studies to increase platelet counts, it does not work rapidly enough to prevent platelet transfusions now that the trigger for these is as low as 10×10^9/L. In addition, the immunogenicity of the first-generation molecules needs to be overcome. Much work needs to be done to define better both the clinical need, and the optimal properties of a platelet stimulant.

Although in retrospect the clinical success of recombinant human HGF may seem to have been easily achieved, the chapter by Farese and MacVittie describes preclinical studies of chimeric growth factor receptor agonists that have not transitioned successfully to the clinic.

New anticancer agents are continually being developed, and these need to be integrated with current chemotherapy and radiotherapy regimens and hematologic support. A major area of investigation discussed by Fox and by Lyman and Kuderer is the effect on cost of introducing new agents. A positive development has been the objective review of data and the production of treatment guidelines by societies such as ASCO and ASH. Although such guidelines need to be updated, they have become an objective standard by which to define therapy for individual patients. The field of HGF has developed in 40 years from an in vitro cell culture phenomenon to an established field providing benefit to patients. The specificity of the late-acting factors and the ability to measure blood cell counts as surrogate endpoints greatly facilitated dose finding and clinical development.

Science now moves more quickly, and there is an expectation that basic discoveries can be applied clinically in 2–3 years. Perhaps an understanding of how the biologic effects of HGF were applied clinically will be useful for the successful development of other areas of translational medicine.

REFERENCES

1. Colgan SP, Gasper PW, Thrall MA, Boone TC, Blancquaert AMB, Bruyninckx WJ. Neutrophil function in normal and Chédiak-Higashi syndrome cats following administration of recombinant canine granulocyte colony-stimulating factor. *Exp Hematol* 1992; 20:1229–1234.
2. Langley KE, Bennett LG, Wypych J, et al. Soluble stem cell factor in human serum. *Blood* 1993; 81:656–660.

3. Lieschke GJ, Grail D, Hodgson G, et al. Mice lacking granolocyte colony-stimulating factor have chronic neutropenia, granulocyte and macrophage progenitor cell deficiency, and impaired neutrophil mobilization. *Blood* 1994; 84:1737–1746.
4. Du XX, Williams DA. Interleukin-11: review of molecular, cell biology, and clinical use. *Blood* 1997; 89:3897–3908.
5. Vellenga E, Rambaldi A, Ernst TJ, Ostapovicz D, Griffin JD. Independent regulation of M-CSF and G-CSF gene expression in human monocytes. *Blood* 1988; 71:1529–1532.
6. Groopman JE, Molina JM, Scadden DT. Hematopoietic growth factors. Biology and clinical applications. *N Engl J Med* 1989; 321:1449–1459.
7. Jacobson LO, Goldwasser E, Fried W, et al. Role of the kidney in erythropoiesis. *Nature* 1957; 179:633–634.
8. Mirand EA, Prentice TC. Presence of plasma erythropoietin in hypoxic rats with and without kidneys or spleen. *Proc Soc Exp Biol Med* 1957; 96:49–51.
9. Erslev AJ. Erythropoietin. *N Engl J Med* 1991; 324:1339–1344.
10. Bartley TD, Bogenberger J, Hunt P, et al. Identification and cloning of a megakaryocyte growth and development factor that is a ligand for the cytokine receptor Mpl. *Cell* 1994; 77:1117–1124.
11. de Sauvage FJ, Hass PE, Spencer SD, et al. Stimulation of megakaryocytopoiesis and thrombopoiesis by the c-Mpl ligand. *Nature* 1994; 369:533–538.
12. Foster DC, Sprecher CA, Grant FJ, et al. Human thrombopoietin: gene structure, cDNA sequence, expression, and chromosomal localization. *Proc Natl Acad Sci USA* 1994; 91:13023–13027.
13. Cebon J, Layton JE, Maher D, Morstyn G. Endogenous haemopoietic growth factors in neutropenia and infection. *Br J Haematol* 1994; 86:265–274.
14. Lord BI, Bronchud MH, Owens S, et al. The kinetics of human granulopoiesis following treatment with granulocyte colony-stimulating factor in vivo. *Proc Natl Acad Sci USA* 1989; 86:9499–9503.
15. Welte K, Gabrilove J, Bronchud MH, Platzer E, Morstyn G. Filgrastim (r-met Hu G-CSF): the first 10 years. *Blood* 1996; 88:1907–1929.
16. Molineux G, Kinstler O, Briddell B, et al. A new form of filgrastim with sustained duration in vivo and enhanced ability to mobilize PBPC in both mice and humans. *Exp Hematol* 1999; 27:1724–1734.
17. Nemunaitis J, Rabinowe SN, Singer JW, et al. Recombinant granulocyte-macrophage colony-stimulating factor after autologous bone marrow transplantation for lymphoid cancer. *N Engl J Med* 1991; 324:1773–1778.
18. Armitage JO. Emerging applications of recombinant human granulocyte-macrophage colony stimulating factor. *Blood* 1998; 92:4491–4508.
19. Angel JB, High K, Rhame F, et al. Phase III study of granulocyte-macrophage colony-stimulating factor in advanced HIV disease: effect on infections, CD4 cell counts and HIV suppression. *AIDS* 2000; 14:387–395.
20. Egrie JC, Dwyer E, Browne JK, Hitz A, Lykos MA. Darbepoetin alfa has a longer circulating half-life and greater in vivo potency than recombinant human erythropoietin. *Exp Hematol* 2003; 31:290–299.
21. Elliott S, Lorenzini T, Asher S, Aoki K, et al. Enhancement of therapeutic protein in vivo activities through glycoengineering. *Nat Biotechnol* 2003; 21:414–421.
22. Lin FK, Suggs S, Lin CH, et al. Cloning and expression of the human erythropoietin gene. *Proc Natl Acad Sci USA* 1985; 82:7580–7584.
23. Martin FH, Suggs SV, Langley KE, et al. Primary structure and functional expression of rat and human stem cell factor DNAs. *Cell* 1990; 63:203–211.
24. Broudy VC. Stem cell factor and hematopoiesis. *Blood* 1997; 90:1345–1364.
25. Lok S, Kaushansky K, Holly RD, et al. Cloning and expression of murine thrombopoietin CDNA and stimulation of platelet production in vivo. *Nature* 1994; 369:565–568.
26. Isaacs C, Robert NJ, Bailey FA, et al. Randomized placebo-controlled study of recombinant human interleukin 11 to prevent chemotherapy-induced thrombocytopenia in patients with breast cancer receiving dose-intensive cylclophosphamide and doxorubicin. *J Clin Oncol* 1997; 15:3368–3377.
27. Till JE, McCulloch EA. A direct measurement of the radiation sensitivity of normal mouse bone marrow cells. *Radiat Res* 1961; 14:213–222.
28. Bradley TR, Metcalf D. The growth of mouse bone marrow cells in vitro. *Aust J Exp Biol Med Sci* 1966; 44:287–299.
29. Pluznik DH, Sachs L. The induction of clones of normal mast cells by a substance from conditioned medium. *Exp Cell Res* 1966; 43:553–563.
30. Metcalf D. The colony-stimulating factors. Discovery, development, and clinical applications. *Cancer* 1990; 65:2185–2195.

31. Stiff P, Gingrich R, Luger S, et al. A randomized phase II study of PBPC mobilization by stem cell factor and filgrastim in heavily pretreated patients with Hodgkin's disease on non-Hodgkin's lymphoma. *Bone Marrow Transplant* 2000; 26:471–481.
32. Besarab A, Bolton WK, Browne JK, et al. The effects of normal as compared with low hematocrit values in patients with cardiac disease who are receiving hemodialysis and epoetin. *N Engl J Med* 1998; 339:584–590.
33. Strippoli GF, Manno C, Schena FP, Craig JC, et al. Haemoglobin and haematocrit targets for the anaemia of chronic renal failure. *Cochrane Database Syst Rev* 2003; CD003967.
34. American Society of Clinical Oncology. Update of recommendations for the use of hematopoietic colony-stimulating factors: evidence-based clinical practice guidelines. *J Clin Oncol* 2000; 18:3558–3585.

2 Animal Models of Hematopoietic Growth Factor Perturbations in Physiology and Pathology

Graham J. Lieschke, MBBS, PhD, FRACP

CONTENTS

1. INTRODUCTION

The clinical use of hematopoietic growth factors (HGFs) is built on nearly 20 years of in vitro studies followed by preclinical animal studies. These laboratory and animal studies, undertaken before first use in humans, provided the basis for expectations of what the biologic effects in humans would be.

Reflecting the available technologies, the initial animal studies primarily evaluated the in vivo effects of factor excess after administration of factors to various animal species and included transgenic models, particularly when the supply of factor itself was limiting or issues of chronic factor exposure were to be addressed. With the development of genetic technologies to disrupt genes in mice selectively, animal models of

From: *Cancer Drug Discovery and Development*
Hematopoietic Growth Factors in Oncology: Basic Science and Clinical Therapeutics
Edited by: G. Morstyn, M. A. Foote, and G. J. Lieschke © Humana Press Inc., Totowa, NJ

factor deficiency were developed in the 1990s. These models were particularly useful for defining the indispensable and physiologic roles of factors and their multicomponent receptors. Increasing sophistication of the technologies for transgenesis and targeted gene modification enabled generation of animal models with inducible and tissue-specific genetic modifications that included not only gene disruptions but also truncations, point mutations, and gene replacement. Animal models incorporating these latter changes were usually generated to test hypotheses regarding the role of specific lesions in gene function or disease pathogenesis. This range of approaches collectively contributes to the preclinical evaluation of new biologic agents or to the modeling of particular disease processes so that pathogenic mechanisms can be better understood and therapeutic strategies can be assessed.

This chapter presents a descriptive overview of animal models of perturbed amounts of HGF, with a particular emphasis on genetic models, and focuses on those factors in clinical use: erythropoietin (EPO), granulocyte colony-stimulating factor (G-CSF), granulocyte-macrophage colony-stimulating factor (GM-CSF), and interleukin (IL)-11. Since diseases are often acquired and not infrequently present somatic rather than germline genetic lesions, animal models with acquired rather than congenital perturbations of HGF concentrations and signaling are also described.

2. ANIMAL MODELS OF HEMATOPOIETIC GROWTH FACTOR DEFICIENCY

Early models of induced factor deficiency relied on immunologic mechanisms to neutralize factor activity. The ability to disrupt individual genes selectively by gene targeting provided a powerful method of generating mice with deficiencies of either selected ligands, receptors, or downstream-signaling molecules. Such engineered deficiencies have usually been designed to be absolute and are life-long, providing insight into the cumulative effects of nonredundant roles of the absent gene product. This genetic approach has been pre-eminent in defining the essential physiologic role of various factors. However, animal models with less-than-total factor deficiency have been generated using other methodologies, both before the gene targeting era and more recently. These models offer several advantages: although they may not result in absolute factor deficiency, they offer flexibilities including inducibility, reversibility, and nonlethality. A new approach, not yet applied to studying HGF, is the use of RNA interference *(1)*. Various experimental approaches to factor ablation are listed in Table 1 with some comparative relative advantages and disadvantages.

2.1. Spontaneously Arising Mutants With Hematopoietic Factor Deficiency

The first durable models of HGF deficiency resulted fortuitously from spontaneously arising or induced mutations in the genes encoding growth factors or their receptors. The two examples of this are mutants deficient in stem cell factor (SCF) and colony-stimulating factor-1 (CSF-1; also known as macrophage colony-stimulating factor [M-CSF]). These models presented prototypes for the models of other factor deficiencies generated by gene targeting.

The *steel (Sl)* mutation arose in 1956 *(2)*. In its most severe form, animals homozygous for the original *Sl* allele die before birth with macrocytic anemia, absent germ cell

Table 1
Comparison of Various Approaches to Impair Hematopoietic Growth Factor Action or Reduce Factor Production

Method of factor deficiency or impairment	Durability *Degree of impairment*	*Applicable for use*		*Technical difficulty and issues*	*Comments*
		In vitro	*In vivo*		
Neutralization by antibody	Transient *Incomplete*	Yes	Yes	If antibody available, straightforward	Standard approach to demonstrate specificity of factor effects in vitro; systemic administration may not achieve neutralization in all body compartments and local sites
Antisense RNA from transfected construct	Transient *Incomplete*	Yes	No	Oligonucleotide stability and potential toxicity	Specificity must be demonstrated
Antisense RNA from stable transgene	Permanent *Incomplete*	Yes	Yes	Similar to other transgenic projects	Expression of transgene may be variable in different tissues leading to variable degrees of factor impairment
Administration of antagonist	Transient *Incomplete*	Yes	Yes	Specific antagonist must be developed and validated	Antagonism at level of receptor most appropriate to study factor physiology
Induced innate autoimmunity to factor	Transient in long term *Incomplete*	No	Yes	Requires immunogenic form of factor	No control over induced immune response, which may be nonspecific or nonneutralizing
Natural or randomly-induced mutation	Permanent *Complete or incomplete*	No	Yes	Capricious and unreliable	Structure of disrupted allele must be characterized; may involve several adjacent or separate loci.
Targeted gene disruption	Permanent *Complete*	Yes	Yes	Difficult multistage process requiring several mouse generations	Total factor deficiency must still be formally proven at the protein level
Targeted gene modification or inducible disruption	Under experimental control *Incomplete*	Yes	Yes	Difficult multistage process requiring several mouse generations	More flexible than germline gene disruption—can be controlled in both time and anatomical location
RNA interference	Depends on methodology *Incomplete*	Yes	Yes	Techniques still under development in mammalian systems	Not yet applied to growth factor models

development, and defective skin pigment cell development *(2,3)*. Heterozygous *Sl*/+ animals have diluted hair pigment and mild macrocytic anemia and are fertile. Other alleles were noted that resulted in less severe phenotypes in homozygous animals, e.g., Sl^d (steel-Dickie), for which homozygotes are viable but have severe anemia, sterility, and a black-eyed/white-coated phenotype. A full list of characterized *Sl* alleles is found in Peters et al. *(4)*, and an overview of the major phenotypic subtleties is described in Russell *(5)*. When in 1990 the ligand for the cellular proto-oncogene c-*kit* was cloned by several groups *(6–8)*, it was shown to be the product of the *steel* locus on mouse chromosome 10 *(7,8)*. The *steel* gene product was a previously unknown growth factor that, among other functions, acts as a hematopoietic CSF in vitro *(8,9)* and was designated variously as kit-ligand, steel factor, mast cell growth factor, or stem cell factor.

Table 2
Animal Models of Reduced Eythropoietin Levels or Signaling

Animal	*Method of reduced erythropoietin signaling*	*Major phenotypic consequences*	*Reference*
Rabbit	Passive immunization with serum containing presumed anti-EPO antibodies	Anemia	*26, 27*
Mice	Passive immunization with serum containing presumed anti-EPO antibodies	Anemia	*25*
Monkey	Immunization during GM-CSF EPO hybrid protein administration resulting in anti-EPO antibodies crossreacting with simian EPO	Anemia	*28*
Mice	Targeted disruption of EPOR gene	Death *in utero* at E13.5 Ventricular hypoplasia Vascular abnormalities	*29, 30*
Mice	Targeted disruption of EPOR receptor gene	Death *in utero* at E13.5 Ventricular hypoplasia Vascular abnormalities Haploinsufficiency	*29, 30*

ABBREVIATIONS: E, embryonic day; EPO, erythropoietin; EPOR, EPO receptor; GM-CSF, granulocyte-macrophage colony-stimulating factor.

Mice with spontaneously arising mutations at the dominant spotting *W* locus have long been known *(10,11)*; this locus was only relatively recently molecularly characterized as being the SCF receptor c-*kit (12)*.

The *osteopetrosis (op)* mutant arose in 1970 and was characterized in 1976 *(13)*. The mutation was characterized as a base insertion generating a premature stop codon in the *Csfm* (M-CSF) gene on mouse chromosome 3 *(14)*. *op/op* mice have severe osteopetrosis with disordered bone remodeling and osteoclast deficiency *(13,15)*, marked but not absolute monocyte and tissue macrophage deficiency *(16–21)*, impaired female fertility *(22)*, a lactation defect *(23)*, and reduced survival *(13)*. Mice lacking the CSF-1 receptor were generated by gene targeting that largely replicate the ligand-deficiency phenotype *(24)*.

A challenge in interpreting the phenotype of naturally occurring mutations is to know whether the factor deficiency is absolute or partial. This question can be addressed by combining knowledge of necessary functional domains, gene expression analysis, and determination of amounts of bioactive and immunoreactive protein. Comparison of mice lacking ligand with those lacking the corresponding receptor can be helpful. Some spontaneous mutations involve deletions, which may potentially encompass several genes, thus potentially confounding the phenotype.

2.2. Erythropoietin

Early studies used serum from rabbits immunized with concentrated EPO-containing urine to achieve neutralization of endogenous EPO in recipient rabbits *(25–27)*. Passively immunized rabbits and mice developed anemia. In a more recent study involving active rather than passive immunization, monkeys treated with a human (Hu)GM-CSF-EPO fusion moiety developed anti-EPO (but not anti-GM-CSF) antibodies (Ab), with resultant anemia *(28)* (Table 2).

Mice with targeted disruption of the *EPO* gene or EPO receptor (EPOR) gene develop similar phenotypes. $EPO^{-/-}$ and $EPOR^{-/-}$ embryos die *in utero* at d 13.5 with failure of fetal liver erythropoiesis *(29)* and with cardiac defects including ventricular hypoplasia and epicardial and vascular abnormalities *(30)*. Although the $EPO^{-/-}$ and $EPOR^{-/-}$ mice had erythropoietic failure, fetal liver erythroid blast-forming units (BFU-E) and erythroid-colony-forming units (CFU-E) progenitor cells were isolated and capable of terminal differentiation in vitro, implicating EPO in the terminal proliferation and survival of erythroid lineage cells *(29)*. Comprehensive analysis of $EPOR^{+/-}$ mice showed evidence of haploinsufficiency, with lower hematocrits and reduced CFU-E frequencies in both bone marrow and spleen *(31)*.

A human EPO mutant in which Arg103 is replaced by Ala [Epo(R103A)] acts as a competitive inhibitor of EPO in vitro in human EPO signaling systems; its effects in vivo and in murine systems have not been reported, although an intent to study the molecule in animal models was foreshadowed *(32)*.

2.3. Granulocyte Colony-Stimulating Factor

Neutralizing polyclonal *(33)* and monoclonal *(34)* antibodies (MAbs) to HuG-CSF have been available; they formed the basis for determination of immunoreactive HuG-CSF levels and for showing specificity in HuG-CSF bioassays *(35)*. A polyclonal neutralizing antiserum to murine (Mu)G-CSF has been used for G-CSF neutralization in vitro *(36)*. Despite the availability of these reagents, no attempts to neutralize endogenous MuG-CSF in vivo were reported. One experiment in rats involved passive immunization with a rabbit anti-G-CSF Ab 2 h before pulmonary challenge with *Pseudomonas aeruginosa (37)*. Anti-G-CSF Ab pretreatment reduced pulmonary neutrophil recruitment and intrapulmonary bactericidal activity at 4 h after infection without affecting the number of circulating neutrophils, suggesting that a local pulmonary G-CSF response to the infection had been impaired.

The hematologic consequences of neutralization of endogenous G-CSF were first observed in dogs, resulting from Ab induced to HuG-CSF crossreacting against canine G-CSF *(38)* (Table 3). Dogs administered HuG-CSF developed an initial neutrophilia, but with ongoing HuG-CSF administration, neutropenia supervened. On cessation of HuG-CSF administration, neutrophil counts slowly returned to normal, but after a nontreatment interval, neutropenia rapidly recurred upon retreatment with HuG-CSF. Anti-HuG-CSF Abs in serum were seen, and passive immunization of dogs by plasma infusion was achieved.

Induction of autoimmunity to murine MuG-CSF required the use of immunostimulatory MuG-CSF conjugates *(39)*. Immunized mice developed neutropenia coincident with an IgG autoantibody response, without effect on other peripheral blood parameters or on the number of marrow progenitor cells. The neutropenia was sustained for >9 mo. Hematologically, these mice phenocopied mice with absolute G-CSF deficiency owing to disruption of either the G-CSF ligand *(40)* or receptor *(41)* genes.

Mice with absolute G-CSF deficiency induced by targeted disruption of either the G-CSF or G-CSF receptor (G-CSFR) gene have similar hematologic phenotypes *(40,41)*. $G\text{-}CSF^{-/-}$ mice display chronic neutropenia, reduced marrow granulopoiesis, and impaired G-CSF-provoked neutrophil mobilization *(40)*. Kinetic analysis of granulopoiesis revealed a reduced transit time through the mitotic compartment of $G\text{-}CSF^{-/-}$ mice, a normal transit time through the postmitotic compart-

Table 3
Animal Models of Reduced G-CSF Levels or Signaling

Animal	*Method of reduced G-CSF signaling*	*Major phenotypic consequences*	*Reference*
Dog	Immunization during HuG-CSF administration resulting in anti-HuG-CSF antibodies crossreacting with canine G-CSF	Transient neutropenia Rapid neutropenia on rechallenge	*38*
Rat	Passive immunization with anti-MuCSF antibodies	↓ Local response to pulmonary bacterial infection	*37*
Mouse	Active immunization with MuG-CSF-conjugates resulting in anti-MuG-CSF autoantibodies	Prolonged neutropenia	*39*
Mouse	Targeted disruption of G-CSF gene	Chronic neutropenia ↓ marrow granulopoiesis Pathogen susceptibility ↑ neutrophil apoptosis Haploinsufficiency	*40*
Mouse	Targeted disruption of G-CSF receptor gene	Chronic neutropenia ↓ marrow granulopoiesis ↓ progenitor cell and neutrophil mobilization ↓ neutrophil chemotaxis Haploinsufficiency	*41*

ABBREVIATIONS: G-CSF, granulocyte colony-stimulating factor; Hu, human; ↑, increased; ↓, decreased.

ment, and an increase in the proportion of Gr-1+ cells that have initiated apoptosis as detected by mercocyanine 540 staining *(42)*. G-CSF deficiency results in increased susceptibility to pathogens including *Listeria monocytogenes* and *Candida albicans* *(43)*. Surprisingly, despite the unexpected impairment of monocyte/macrophage responses in G-CSF$^{-/-}$ mice during *Listeria* infections *(40,44,45)*, *Mycobacterium avium* infections were not exacerbated in G-CSF$^{-/-}$ mice, and high levels of interferon (IFN)-γ production accompanied infection with this pathogen *(46)*. *Candida* infection of G-CSF$^{-/-}$ mice was accompanied by a vigorous neutrophilia, exceeding the magnitude of that in wild-type mice, and early control of the pathogen load. However, after 1 wk of infection, deep tissue infection with high *Candida* pathogen loads persisted in G-CSF$^{-/-}$ mice at a time the infection was resolving in wild-type mice *(43)*.

The hematologic profile of G-CSFR$^{-/-}$ mice largely resembled that of the ligand-deficient mice, with chronic neutropenia, reduced marrow granulopoiesis, and a propensity of Gr-1+ marrow cells to undergo apoptotic death in vitro *(41)*. The G-CSFR$^{-/-}$ mice have enabled distinctions to be drawn between G-CSF-dependent and G-CSF-independent neutrophil functions. Neutrophil primary granule myeloperoxidase activity was normal, and neutrophil migration induced by chemical peritonitis was preserved. However, progenitor cell and neutrophil mobilization into the peripheral blood by cyclophosphamide and IL-8 was impaired *(47)*. Neutrophils from G-CSFR$^{-/-}$ mice had defective chemotactic responses to IL-8 and other chemoattractants in vitro, despite intact metabolic responses to several agents *(48)*. The intrinsic defect in G-CSFR$^{-/-}$ cells has enabled experiments to be designed to distinguish between cell-autonomous and -nonautonomous functions. For example, radiation chimeras were established with either wild-type or G-CSFR$^{-/-}$ hematopoietic cell populations in wild-type or G-CSFR$^{-/-}$ stromal backgrounds to study the phenomenon of G-CSF-stimulated progenitor cell mobilization. Expression of the G-CSFR on the hematopoietic cells (and then only a subpopulation of them) and not the stromal cells was necessary for G-CSF-stimulated mobilization to occur *(49)*, although interpretation of this experiment assumes that little reconstitution of the marrow stroma by the transplanted marrow cells occurred.

To define signals mediated specifically by the G-CSFR, gene-targeted mice have been generated in which the G-CSFR was replaced by a chimeric receptor comprising the extracellular and transmembrane portions of the G-CSFR (capable of binding G-CSF) connected to the intracellular portion of the EPOR *(50)*. Hematologically, these mice resemble G-CSFR$^{-/-}$ mice with peripheral blood neutropenia and a modest marrow granulopoietic defect. Although this chimeric receptor supported granulocytic lineage commitment and differentiation, some specific defects were demonstrable: there was impaired G-CSF-stimulated progenitor cell mobilization and reduced IL-8-induced chemotaxis *(50,51)*.

2.4. Granulocyte-Macrophage Colony-Stimulating Factor

Neutralizing polyclonal antibodies to MuGM-CSF have been characterized *(52)*, and well-characterized monoclonal anti-MuGM-CSF Abs *(53,54)* are now commercially available. Such Abs form the basis of enzyme-linked immunosorbent assays (ELISAs) for determination of immunoreactive MuGM-CSF levels and have been used to show specificity in MuGM-CSF bioassays. Although no studies attempting to neutralize basal levels of endogenously produced MuGM-CSF by passive immunization in vivo have been reported, Abs have been used to neutralize GM-CSF activity in disease models. The effect of GM-CSF pretreatment to aggravate lipopolysaccharide (LPS)-induced mortality and hepatic toxicity could be ameliorated by the administration of GM-CSF Abs *(55)*. Administration of an anti-GM-CSF Ab attenuated the severity of arthritis in two murine arthritis models, one in which erosive arthritis is induced by bovine serum albumin (BSA) and IL-1 administration *(56)*, and in one model of collagen-induced arthritis *(57)*.

A competitive antagonist of HuGM-CSF has been developed named E21R, which is a ligand analog in which amino acid 21 is changed from glutamic acid to arginine *(58)*. Owing to the high species specificity of GM-CSF, preclinical in vivo studies with the moiety were performed in baboons, administering E21R for up to 21 d *(59)* (Table 4). E21R resulted in a transient eosinophilia and neutrophilia and granulocyte infiltrates in lymph nodes and duodenal submucosa. The transient eosinophilia was unexpected but was also seen in patients receiving E21R on a phase 1 study *(59)*, and so is an effect of this agent accurately predicted by the animal model.

Two mouse lines with absolute GM-CSF deficiency owing to targeted gene disruption have been independently generated *(60,61)*; both lines show identical phenotypes. Baseline hematopoiesis is unperturbed despite GM-CSF deficiency *(61)*, although reduced frequencies of marrow CFU-E sensitive to low EPO concentrations in vitro have recently been documented *(31)*. During *M. avium* infection, GM-CSF$^{-/-}$ mice fail

Table 4
Animal Models of Reduced GM-CSF Levels or Signaling

Animal	*Method of reduced GM-CSF signaling*	*Major phenotypic consequences*	*Reference*
Mouse	Passive immunization with anti-MuGM-CSF antibodies	↓ LPS-induced mortality ↓ LPS hepatic toxicity	*55*
Mouse	Targeted disruption of GM-CSF gene	Normal basal hematopoiesis Pulmonary alveolar proteinosis ↓ hematopoiesis during chronic *M. avium* infection ↓ zymocel-induced hepatic granulomatous inflammation	*60–62, 68*
Mouse	Targeted disruption of IL-3/GM-CSF/IL-5 receptor β_c subunit	Normal basal hematopoiesis except ↓ eosinophil production Pulmonary alveolar proteinosis Failure to develop eosinophila to parasitic infections	*68, 69*
Baboon	Competitive peptide antagonist (E21R)	Transient eosinophilia and neutrophilia	*59*

ABBREVIATIONS: GM-CSF, granulocyte-macrophage colony-stimulating factor; LPS, lipopolysaccharide; IL, interleukin; Mu, murine; ↑, increased; ↓, decreased.

to sustain hematopoietic cell production *(62)*, suggesting a role for GM-CSF under emergency if not basal conditions of hematopoiesis. GM-CSF$^{-/-}$ mice have been exploited to examine the role of this factor in several models of inflammation; different effects have been seen in different models. Acute peritoneal inflammation after casein injection was normal in GM-CSF$^{-/-}$ mice *(63)*. GM-CSF deficiency delayed zymocel-induced hepatic granuloma formation and impaired monocyte infiltration and proliferation, although macrophages within granulomata expressed markers suggesting normal activation *(64)*. Normal activation of peritoneal macrophages was observed during *L. monocytogenes* infection *(45)*. GM-CSF deficiency attenuated inflammation in a murine model of arthritis induced by BSA and IL-1 injection *(56)* and also in murine models of immune-mediated glomerulonephritis *(65)*. GM-CSF$^{-/-}$ mice have moderately impaired reproductive capacity and reduced long-term survival *(66)*.

GM-CSF$^{-/-}$ mice develop a striking pulmonary pathology with extensive peribronchial B-cell infiltrates and alveolar accumulation of surfactant phospholipid, protein, and intra-alveolar macrophages, a disorder resembling pulmonary alveolar proteinosis *(60,61)*. The pathophysiology relates to impaired surfactant clearance and catabolism *(216)* and can be reversed by local GM-CSF expression *(67)*, evidence collectively indicating a local defect in alveolar macrophages.

GM-CSF signaling is initiated by ligand binding to a heterodimeric receptor comprising a specific α-subunit (GM-CSFRα) and a β-subunit (IL-3/GM-CSF/IL-5Rβ_c) shared in common with the analogously heterodimeric IL-3 and IL-5 receptors. (In mice, but not in humans, there are two rather than one IL-3 receptor β-subunits.) GM-CSF deficiency has been mimicked by targeted disruption of the IL-3/GM-CSF/IL-5Rβ_c gene *(68,69)*, and these mice develop a similar, but less severe, pulmonary pathology *(70)*.

Additionally, they showed additional manifestations of defective IL-5 signaling such as low baseline eosinophil numbers *(68)* and impaired eosinophil response to *Nippostrongylus brasiliensis (68,69,71)*. In this cell-autonomous model of the pulmonary disease, bone marrow transplantation with wild-type hematopoietic cells reversed the pulmonary pathology *(72)*, albeit not completely *(73)*. IL-3/GM-CSF/IL-5Rβ_c-deficient mice displayed an attenuated cutaneous reaction to *Leishmania major (74)*.

2.5. Interleukin-11

Despite its potent action on hematopoietic progenitor cell development in vitro, mice with a targeted disruption of the IL-11 receptor-α (IL-11Rα) had normal baseline hematopoiesis, immune function, and erythroid reserves *(75)* but displayed a defect in postimplantation decidualization that impaired the fertility of female mice *(76)*. Mice deficient in gp130, the partner of IL-11-Rα in the heterodimeric IL-11 receptor, display additional defects that reflect defective signaling from other ligands that share gp130 as a component of their heterodimeric receptors: IL-6, leukemia inhibitory factor (LIF), ciliary neurotropic growth factor (CNTF), oncostatin M, and cardiotropin (CT). Absolute gp130 deficiency results in embryonic lethality from multiple defects including impaired fetal liver hematopoiesis *(71)*. When embryonic lethality was circumvented by a genetically based inducible *Cre*-lox gene targeting approach, adult gp130-deficient mice developed multisystem defects including thrombocytopenia, leukocytosis, and impaired hematopoietic recovery after 5-fluorouracil (5-FU) stem-cell ablation or after antiplatelet antiserum *(77)*.

IL-11 has been neutralized in mice by passive immunization using a sheep anti-MuIL-11 Ab in a study investigating the role of IL-11 in bone changes after oophorectomy *(78)*.

2.6. Other Hematopoietic Growth Factors

Over the last decade, murine models of HGF deficiency have been generated for most factors, and in many cases, for their receptors (Tables 5 and 6).

2.7. Combined Hematopoietic Growth Factor Signaling Deficiencies

By combining genetically based factor-deficiencies, the interacting roles of growth factors can be studied in vivo. Sometimes interactions have been achieved by combining ligand-deficiency for one factor and receptor deficiency for another, often for reasons of utility and availability. Occasionally, genetic constraints due to the proximity of loci influence the approach. Some combinations merely result in the simple addition of the phenotypic traits of the two individual factor deficiencies, suggesting independent roles for the two factors. Others result in the emergence of new phenotypic features, or the accentuation of component phenotype traits, suggesting that one factor can assume a compensatory role in the deficiency phenotype of another factor, although compensation requires that activation of a process over the usual normal amount be shown as well. The emergence of new phenotypic traits in combination with deficiency genotypes allows for the possibility that independent, separately regulated mechanisms may contribute to a particular process, and the integrity of the process requires one or the other mechanism to be intact, but only when both mechanisms are impaired does the process fail.

Table 5
Genetic Models of Deficiency of CSFs and Other Factors Affecting Hematopoiesis in Mice

Factor	*Genetic basis (allele)*	*Major phenotypic features*[a]	*Reference*
G-CSF	Targeted gene disruption	–/– Chronic neutropenia	*40*
		↓ Progenitor cells	
		Infection vulnerability	
GM-CSF	Targeted gene disruption	–/– Unperturbed hematopoiesis	*60, 61*
		Alveolar proteinosis	
		Lung infections	
M-CSF	Natural point mutation *(op)*	–/– Osteopetrosis	*13, 20*
		↓ Monocyte/macrophages	
		↓ Osteoclasts	
SCF	Natural mutation *(Sl)*[b]	–/– Lethal *in utero*	*3, 5*
		Impaired hematopoiesis	
		+/– Pale coat	*3*
		Mild macrocytic anemia	
		Small gonads	
LIF	Targeted gene disruption	–/– Maternal infertility	*172*
		↓ Splenic CFC and CFU-S	*173*
		Normal peripheral blood	
IL-1β	Targeted gene disruption	–/– Fever-resistant	*174*
		↓ Acute-phase response	
		Hematopoiesis not analyzed	
IL-2	Targeted gene disruption	–/– Perturbed B-cell function	*175*
		Ulcerative colitis	*176*
IL-3	Transgenesis (antisense RNA, partial IL-3 deficiency only)	+/– Lymphoproliferative disorder	*177*
		Neurologic dysfunction	
IL-3	Targeted gene disruption	–/– ↓ Delayed-type hypersensitivity	*81, 82*
		↓ Tissue mast cells in nematode infection	

IL-4	Targeted gene disruption	–/– ↓ Th2 responses	*178*
		↓ Reactive eosinophilia	*178*
		↓ IgG1 switching	*179*
		↓ Mucosal immunity	*180*
IL-5	Targeted gene disruption	–/– Normal Th-dependent B-cell responses	*181*
		Normal immunoglobulins	
		Normal eosinophils ↑ in parasitic infection; normal parasite killing	
IL-6	Targeted gene disruption	–/–↓ Acute-phase and anti-infective response	*182, 183*
		↓ Mucosal immunity	*184*
		↓ Pre-CFU-S, CFU-S and lineage-committed CFCs	*185*
		↑ Bone turnover	*186*
IL-7	Targeted gene disruption	–/– ↓ B lymphopoiesis	*187*
		↓ Thymic cellularity	
		↓ Splenic lymphocytes	
EPO	Targeted gene disruption	–/– Lethal at E 13	*29*
		Hepatic erythropoiesis fails	
TPO	Targeted gene disruption	–/– ↓ Platelets (>80%)	*188, 189*
		↓ Marrow megakaryocytes and megakaryocyte-CFCs	
		↓ Megakaryocyte ploidy	
		+/– ↓ Platelets (67%)	*188, 189*

ABBREVIATIONS: CFC, colony-forming cell; CFU, colony-forming unit; EPO, erythropoietin; G-CSF, granulocyte colony-stimulating factor; GM-CSF, granulocyte-macrophage colony-stimulating factor; IL, interleukin; LIF, leukemia inhibitory factor; M-CSF, macrophage colony-stimulating factor; TPO, thrombopoietin; ↑, increased; ↓, decreased.

[a] Factor-deficient genotype indicated as heterozygous (+/–) or homozygous (–/–).

[b] Numerous different alleles exist. *Sl* refers to that originally described *(2,3)*. Other alleles are indicated by superscripts, e.g., Sl^d (Steel-Dickie): Sl^d/Sl^d and Sl/Sl^d mice are viable but severely anemic and sterile with black eyes and white coats *(190)*.

Table 6
Genetic Models of Chronic Deficiency of Components of Receptors for Factors Affecting Hematopoiesis in Mice

Ligands	*Receptor component*	*Genetic basis (allele)*	*Major phenotypic features*[a]	*Comments and comparison With ligand absence or impairment*	*Reference*
SCF	c-*kit*	Spontaneous and mutagen-induced mutation *(W)*[b]	–/– Perinatal lethality Severity macrocytic anemia Sterility Absent coat pigmentation +/– Normal hematopoiesis Fertile White spotting	Similar	*5,10,12*
IL-3	β_{IL3} (AIC2A)	Targeted gene disruption	–/– Normal	IL-3 signaling via αIL_3 βc receptor complex still possible; Basal hematopoiesis normal in IL-$3^{-/-}$ mice *(82)*	*68*
IL-3, IL-5 GM-CSF	βc (AIC2B)	Targeted gene disruption	–/– Lung alveolar proteinosis Normal CFC levels (assayed with SCF/IL-6/EPO) ↓ eosinophils ↓ reactive eosinophila	Resembles GM-$CSF^{-/-}$ mice *(60,61)* IL-$5^{-/-}$ mice have normal basal eosinophil numbers but ↓ reactive eosinophila *(181)*	*68,69*
IL-3	α_{IL3}	Spontaneous mutation	–/– IL-3 hyporesponsivness	Still have low numbers of high-affinity receptors on marrow cells; *probably not a null allele*	*191–194*
TPO	c-*mpl*	Targeted gene disruption	–/– Thrombocytopenia	Resembles $TPO^{-/-}$ mice *(195)*	*196, 197*
IL-2, IL-4, IL-7, IL-9, IL-15	γ, (γ_c)	Targeted gene disruption (X-linked gene)	–/– Males lacking γ_c: Perturbed T lymphopoiesis Perturbed B lymphopoiesis	Reflects IL-$2^{-/-}$ mice *(176)* Reflects IL-7-$receptor^{-/-}$ mice *(198)*	*203*

			Absent dendritic epidermal T cells Typhlitis and colitis	Not ulcerative as in IL-$2^{-/-}$ mice *(176)* or T-cell receptor α–/–, β–/– and β–/–, δ–/– mice *(199–202)*	
IL-2	β	Targeted gene disruption	–/– ↓ survival, activated CD4+ cells B-cell activation with IgG1 & IgE Perturbed T- and B-cell responses Hemolytic anemia Myeloproliferative disorder ↑ Splenic granulopoiesis	No colitis as in IL-$2^{-/-}$ mice *(176)*	*204*
IL-8	mIL-8Rh	Targeted gene disruption	–/– Splenomegaly B-cell hyperplasia ↑ Neutrophils and granulopoeisis ↓ Neutrophil migration	IL-$8^{-/-}$ mice not yet described	*205–207*
EPO	EPO-R	Targeted gene disruption	–/– Lethal at embryonic d 13 Failure of liver erythropoiesis CFU-E, BFU-E develop, but fail to survive	Resembles $EPO^{-/-}$ mice *(29)*	*29*
CSF-1 (M-CSF)	c-*fms*	Targeted gene disruption	–/– Osteopetrosis ↓ monocytes and tissue macrophages reproductive defects ↑ serum CSF-1 20-fold	Resembles *op/op* mice *(14)*	*24*

ABBREVIATIONS: SCF, stem cell factor; IL, interleukin; GM-CSF, granulocyte-macrophage colony-stimulating factor; TPO, thrombopoietin; CFU-E, colony-forming unit-erythroid; BFU-E, erythroid burst-forming unit; EPO, erythropoietin; CSF, colony-stimulating factor; ↑, increased; ↓, decreased.

[a] Factor-deficient genotype indicated as heterozygous (+/–) or homozygous (–/–).

[b] At least 27 alleles exist. *W* refers to that originally described *(10)* and molecularly characterized by Nocka et al. *(12)*. Other alleles are indicated by superscripts, e.g., W^v, a qualitatively different allele that occurred in C57BL/J6 results in homozygous mice that are viable but severely anemic, sterile, black-eyed, and white coated.

2.7.1. Combined Deficiencies Involving Erythropoietin

EPO-R$^{-/-}$ mice were interbred with GM-CSF$^{-/-}$ and IL-3$^{-/-}$ mice *(31)*. A reduced frequency of marrow CFU-E was observed in EPO-R$^{+/-}$ haploinsufficient GM-CSF$^{-/-}$ or IL-3$^{-/-}$ mice, although CFU-E frequencies were reduced in mice with isolated GM-CSF or IL-3 deficiency. This finding was of functional significance in the mice with combined factor signaling deficiencies, since GM-CSF$^{-/-}$EPO-R$^{+/-}$ and IL-3$^{-/-}$EPO-R$^{+/-}$ mice were more anemic after exposure to phenylhydrazine than mice of the single-component genotypes.

2.7.2. Combined Deficiencies Involving Granulocyte Colony-Stimulating Factor

G-CSF-deficient mice were interbred with GM-CSF-deficient mice to create mice deficient in both factors *(66)*. G-CSF$^{-/-}$GM-CSF$^{-/-}$ mice were more neutropenic than G-CSF$^{-/-}$ mice in the early neonatal period, had higher neonatal mortality, and showed a propensity to the development of the amyloidosis evident in G-CSF$^{-/-}$ mice. Mice deficient in G-CSF and IL-6 signaling have been generated, both by creating mice deficient in both ligands *(43)* and by creating G-CSFR$^{-/-}$IL-6$^{-/-}$ mice *(79)*. G-CSFR$^{-/-}$IL-6$^{-/-}$ mice had an exacerbated neutropenia compared with G-CSFR$^{-/-}$ mice *(79)*. Although infection of G-CSF$^{-/-}$ mice with *C. albicans* resulted in a neutrophilia with increased amounts of serum IL-6, indicating that factors other than G-CSF can drive the emergency granulopoietic response, G-CSF$^{-/-}$IL-6$^{-/-}$ mice also showed this phenomenon, indicating that IL-6 was not the sole driver of this infection-related granulopoietic response *(43)*. Thrombopoietin (TPO)-deficient mice and G-CSFR$^{-/-}$ mice have been interbred, testing the role of either factor in modulating the other-factor deficiency-phenotype. G-CSF deficiency did not further exacerbate the thrombocytopenia of TPO$^{-/-}$ mice, but TPO deficiency augmented the granulopoietic defect of G-CSFR$^{-/-}$ mice, with a consequent increased early infective mortality *(80)*.

2.7.3. Combined Deficiencies Involving Granulocyte-Macrophage Colony-Stimulating Factor

Since mice have a second IL-3 receptor (βIL-3), IL-3/GM-CSF/IL-5Rβ_c-deficient mice are not absolutely deficient in IL-3 signaling. IL-3-deficient mice have been generated by gene targeting *(81,82)*, but the close chromosomal location of GM-CSF and IL-3 precluded bringing these mutations together efficiently by interbreeding. GM-CSF deficiency has been combined with IL-3 deficiency by a sequential gene targeting approach *(83)*; these mice have a basal eosinophila but had impaired contact hypersensitivity reactions. They have also been used to evaluate the role of these cytokines in vivo in murine models of leukemia and myeloproliferative disease based on BCR-ABL and several leukemogenic TEL-tyrosine kinase fusion oncoproteins *(84,85)*; in all models, combined deficiency of these two factors did not impact on the in vivo phenotype of the model leukemia. Mice completely lacking GM-CSF, IL-3, and IL-5 signaling were generated by creating IL-3$^{-/-}$IL-3/GM-CSF/IL-5R$\beta_c^{-/-}$ mice; these mice have surprisingly normal basal hematopoiesis and showed normal hematopoietic responses to *L. monocytogenes* infection and after 5-FU administration *(86)*. GM-CSF$^{-/-}$IL-3$^{-/-}$IL-3/GM-CSF/IL-5R$\beta_c^{-/-}$ mice have been created, which sum to the same growth factor signaling defect *(83)*.

GM-CSF deficiency has been combined with CSF-1 (M-CSF) deficiency by interbreeding CSF-1-deficient *op* mutant mice with GM-CSF$^{-/-}$ mice *(87,88)*. Concomitant

CSF-1 (M-CSF) deficiency accentuated the pulmonary disease of GM-CSF-deficient mice, but mice deficient in both factors still had residual macrophages, indicating that other factors are still able to affect macrophage development and differentiation in vivo *(87)*. Conversely, GM-CSF deficiency was shown not to be the mediator of age-related corrections in macrophage development observed in *op/op* mice *(88)*.

GM-CSF deficiency has also been combined with TPO signaling deficiency by generating GM-CSF$^{-/-}$c-*mpl*$^{-/-}$ mice. On an inbred background, no further effect of GM-CSF deficiency on the thrombocytopenia of c-*mpl*$^{-/-}$ was observed. This study demonstrated one of the pitfalls of this approach: on a noninbred background, a partial amelioration of the c-*mpl*$^{-/-}$ thrombocytopenia was seen, suggesting existence of other modifier genes of this phenotype.

2.7.4. Combined Deficiencies Involving Interleukin-11

To combine IL-11 and TPO deficiency, IL-11R$\alpha^{-/-}$ mice and mice deficient in the TPO receptor c-*mpl* were interbred *(89)*. Despite the ability of pharmacologic doses of IL-11 to stimulate megakaryocytopoiesis and thrombopoiesis, combined IL-11R$\alpha^{-/-}$c-*mpl*$^{-/-}$ mice did not have accentuation of the platelet and megakaryocyte production defects that characterize c-*mpl* deficiency.

3. ANIMAL MODELS OF HEMATOPOIETIC GROWTH FACTOR EXCESS

Administration of an HGF to a normal animal superimposes an acute excess of circulating factor on otherwise normal hematopoiesis, potentially mimicking factor-driven emergency hematopoiesis. Numerous preclinical evaluations of this type have been done, and only some are summarized in this chapter. A particular advantage of this approach is its flexibility for comprehensive testing of the in vivo effects of combinations of multiple different factors, including enabling a range of scheduling issues to be evaluated.

Genetic models of HGF overproduction have the advantage of durability and provide additional information about the effects of chronic long-term exposure to the factor (Table 7). When the model is based on germline transgenesis, the model is able to be propagated, and populations of uniformly affected animals can be generated for study. Genetic approaches are particularly useful for evaluating the effects of excess factor production in vivo when there are limited amounts of factor available for direct administration and for defining the toxicity of long-term factor exposure.

3.1. Erythropoietin

Numerous studies have reported the effects of EPO administration to a wide range of species. Recombinant EPO administration induces polycythemia in a dose-related manner; summaries of these early preclinical studies are found in several comprehensive reviews *(90,91)*. Mice have also been used for comparative evaluations of the in vivo activity of the EPO-related moiety darbepoietin alfa, an EPO derivative with a modified polypeptide and glycosylation structure (reviewed in ref. *92*), and to demonstrate the activity of small-molecule EPO mimetics *(93)*. rHuEPO has a wide cross-species activity that apparently extends from mammals to fish *(94)*. Collectively, these studies indicate that in many species, EPO is a potent and highly specific stimulant of erythropoiesis.

A transgene including 0.4 kb of endogenous 5′ untranslated sequences flanking the 5 exons of the human genomic *EPO* gene sequences resulted in high serum EPO

Table 7
Genetic Models of Chronic Elevation of Hematopoietic Growth Factor Amounts in Mice

Factor	*Genetic basis of model*	*Reference*
EPO	Transgenesis	*95* *96* *97*
EPO	Reconstitution with hematopoietic cells infected with EPO-expressing recombinant retrovirus	*98*
G-CSF	Reconstitution with hematopoietic cells infected with G-CSF-expressing recombinant retrovirus	*104*
GM-CSF	Transgenesis	*107*
GM-CSF	Reconstitution with hematopoietic cells infected with GM-CSF-expressing recombinant retrovirus	*111*
IL-11	Transgenesis	*117* *118*
IL-11	Reconstitution with hematopoietic cells infected with IL-11-expressing recombinant retrovirus	*115* *114*

ABBREVIATIONS: EPO, erythropoietin; G-CSF, granulocyte colony-stimulating factor; GM-CSF, granulocyte-macrophage colony-stimulating factor; IL, interleukin.

concentrations and sustained polycythemia in mice *(95)*. Subsequent transgenic studies exploited the transcriptional activity of this short EPO promoter fragment to identify more distant but contiguous regulatory elements that together regulate EPO expression in liver and kidney and in response to hypoxia *(96,97)*. Murine reconstitution experiments using marrow cells over-expressing monkey EPO resulted in a severe, progressive, and ultimately fatal polycythemia with marked expansion of erythropoiesis *(98)*.

3.2. Granulocyte Colony-Stimulating Factor

Several studies reporting the effect of HuG-CSF administration to mice for short periods up to 3 wk are listed (Table 8). In a study of neutrophil kinetics after HuG-CSF administration to mice (10 μg/kg/d for 4 d), the peripheral blood neutrophil count increased 14.5-fold, but neutrophil half-life remained normal, and the neutrophilia resulted from a calculated 3.8 extra maturation divisions in neutrophil formation *(99)*. Even after only 4 d of HuG-CSF administration, bone marrow showed increased granulopoiesis morphologically. Later, weakly labeled neutrophils were released that presumably reflected maturation and release of neutrophils that were the progeny of immature neutrophil progenitor cells labeled at the time of tritiated thymidine pulsing. Interestingly, the number of peripheral blood monocytes increased during HuG-CSF administration (primarily owing to amplified release of labeled cells 6–9 h after HuG-CSF administration), and HuG-CSF-treated mice had markedly increased numbers of several types of circulating nonerythroid progenitor cells *(100)*. Therefore, although the major acute effect of excess G-CSF was on the distribution of neutrophils and their immediate precursors, the effect of G-CSF was not completely lineage-specific, as G-CSF administration also affected the distribution of monocytes and progenitor cells of other lineages. Nonhematopoietic effects were reported in these studies of short courses of G-CSF

Table 8
Studies of Excess G-CSF Amounts in Mice

Study type (reference)	Major phenotypic consequences: Hematologic	Major phenotypic consequences: Tissues/survival
Recombinant factor administration (16 μg/mouse/d, 14 d) *(208)*	↑ Blood neutrophils (×10) ↑ Splenic CFCs	Not assessed
Recombinant factor administration (3 μg/kg/d, 14 d) *(209)*	↑ Blood neutrophils (×9) ↑ Blood monocytes (×3) ↑ Spleen cellularity (×3–4) ↑ Splenic GM-CFCs	Not assessed
Recombinant factor administration (10–2,500 μg/kg/d, 4 d) *(210,211)*	↑ Blood neutrophils ↑ Marrow granulopoiesis ↓ Marrow cellularity ↓ Marrow CFCs and CFU-S	Not assessed (effects accentuated by splenectomy)
Recombinant factor administration (5 μg/kg/d, 8 d) *(100)*	↑ Peripheral blood CFC (multiple types)	Not assessed
Recombinant factor administration (10 μg/kg/d, 4 d) *(99)*	↑ Blood neutrophils (×14) early monocyte release (×17)	Not assessed
Recombinant factor administration (2.5 μg/d, 21 d) *(101)*	↑ Blood neutrophils (×20) ↑ Marrow granulopoiesis Splenomegaly	↑ Endosteal osteoclasts ↑ Medullary cavity ↑ Periosteal bone
Recombinant factor administration (10 μg/d, 10 d) *(212)*	↑ Splenic dendritic cells (×2.3) Normal dendritic cell IFN production	Not assessed
Reconstitution with hematopoietic cells infected with G-CSF-expressing recombinant retrovirus *(104)*	↑ $[\text{G-CSF}]_{\text{serum}}$ ↑ Blood neutrophils ↑ Blood CFCs	↑ Neutrophils in lung and liver No tissue damage Normal 30-wk survival
Recombinant PEGylated factor administration (30–1000 μg/kg, 1 dose) *(102,103)*	↑ Blood neutrophils proportional to dose for up to 6 d ↑ Blood CFCs	Not assessed

Abbreviations: CFC, colony-forming cell; G-CSF, granulocyte colony-stimulating factor; GM-CFC, granulocyte-macrophage colony-forming cell, CFU-S, spleen colony-forming unit; IFN, interferon; ↑, increased; ↓, decreased.

administration to mice, but after 21 d, femoral bone morphology was altered, with increased numbers of endosteal osteoclasts, periosteal bone deposition, and increased size of the medullary cavity *(101)*. A recently developed polyethylene glycol-conjugated form of filgrastim (pegfilgrastim) has also been evaluated after administration to mice and shown to share many of the granulopoietic effects of filgrastim, but for a sustained duration and with less dosing-related fluctuation *(102,103)*.

Chimeric G-CSF transgenesis in adult mice was achieved by reconstituting mice with marrow infected with a retrovirus leading to G-CSF overproduction *(104)*. These mice developed very high serum G-CSF concentrations (equivalent to 20–260,000 ng/mL recombinant HuG-CSF) but had normal survival of up to 30 wk. No tissue damage was seen despite considerable tissue infiltration with neutrophils, suggesting that high circulating G-CSF amounts are well tolerated for long periods

Table 9
Studies of Excess GM-CSF Amounts in Mice

Study type (reference)	Major phenotypic consequences: Hematologic	Major phenotypic consequences: Tissues/survival
Recombinant factor administration (18–600 ng/d, 6 d) *(150)*	↑ blood neutrophils (×2) ↑ Peritoneal macrophages ↑ Splenic hematopoiesis	Lung and liver macrophages
Recombinant factor administration (10 μg/kg/d, 4 d) *(99)*	↑ Blood neutrophils (×1.5) Early monocyte release (×2)	Not assessed
Recombinant factor administration (450 ng/d, 21 d) *(101)*	↑ Peritoneal macrophages Peripheral blood normal Bone marrow normal	↑ Endosteal osteoclasts ↑ Medullary cavity
Recombinant factor administration (1–10 μg/kg/d ≤ 11 wk) *(106)*	↑ Splenic hematopoiesis ↑ Peritoneal macrophages Peripheral blood normal	No toxicity
Transgenesis *(107–110, 213, 214)*	↑ $[\text{GM-CSF}]_{serum}$ ↑ $[\text{IL-1}]_{serum}$ ↑ Peritoneal macrophages Peripheral blood normal	Eye damage Muscle lesions Wasting Premature death
Reconstitution with hematopoietic cells infected with GM-CSF-expressing recombinant retrovirus *(111)*	↑ $[\text{GM-CSF}]_{serum}$ ↑ Blood granulocytes ↑ Blood macrophages	Lesions in liver, lung Lesions in muscle, eye Early death
Recombinant pegylated factor administration (2–5 μg/d, 5 d) *(212, 215)*	↑ Splenic dendritic cells (×12) Impaired dendritic cell IL-12 production	Not assessed

ABBREVIATIONS: IL, interleukin; GM-CSF, granulocyte-macrophage colony-stimulating factor; ↑, increased; ↓, decreased.

and that the resultant neutrophils are not innately destructive. The changes in distribution of hematopoiesis and hematopoietic cell types were similar to those observed after short courses of G-CSF administration, indicating that these changes can be sustained for long periods. Dysregulated G-CSF expression in hematopoietic cells did not result in malignant transformation.

3.3. Granulocyte-Macrophage Colony-Stimulating Factor

Several studies report the effects of MuGM-CSF administration to mice for short periods (≤3 wk) *(99,105)*, and one study assessed the effects of MuGM-CSF administration for 11 wk *(106)* (Table 9). A short course of MuGM-CSF administered either intravenously *(99)* or intraperitoneally *(105)* increased peripheral blood neutrophils only 1.5–2-fold, and the effects on myeloid kinetics were modest *(99)*. GM-CSF had similar effects on bone morphology to those observed in G-CSF-treated mice, despite its less dramatic effects on marrow myelopoiesis *(101)*. During 11-wk MuGM-CSF courses (1–10 μg/kg/d, sc administration), the short-term effects of MuGM-CSF to increase the relative frequency of marrow and splenic progenitor cells subsided (this was not owing to the development of circulating GM-CSF inhibitors), although the early increase in number and enhanced function of macrophages was sustained. Compared with G-CSF, excess amounts of GM-CSF had only modest effects on myelopoiesis, and with long-term administration, these effects were transient.

Two genetically based models of mice ectopically overexpressing GM-CSF are of interest. Transgenic mice carrying an MuGM-CSF transgene were characterized by high serum GM-CSF concentrations, ocular opacity and retinal damage, striated muscle lesions, and reduced survival with death at 2–4 mo, but the mice had unperturbed hematopoiesis *(107)*. The tissue lesions appeared to be mediated by autostimulated macrophages *(107–109)* and macrophage-derived cytokines such as IL-1α, tumor necrosis factor-α (TNF-α), and basic fibroblast growth factor *(109,110)*. In the second model, mice transplanted with marrow cells infected with a retrovirus leading to MuGM-CSF production had 100-fold higher amounts of serum GM-CSF as well as extensive neutrophil and macrophage infiltration in many tissues, and they died within 1 mo of transplantation *(111)*. The mice also had perturbed hematopoiesis: peripheral blood neutrophils, monocytes, and eosinophils were increased by 15-, 7-, and 9-fold, respectively, with reduced numbers of marrow progenitor cells and variable changes in number of splenic progenitor cells. The differences between these two genetic models of GM-CSF overproduction may be owing to the different types of cells overexpressing GM-CSF, the effect of the transplantation itself, and the 100-fold difference in GM-CSF production. Both models suggest that although high concentrations of GM-CSF are capable of driving myelopoiesis, the body tolerates these extremely high supraphysiologic circulating GM-CSF amounts poorly.

3.4. Interleukin-11

The effects of IL-11 administration in preclinical models have been comprehensively reviewed *(112,113)*. Genetic overexpression of human IL-11 was achieved in mice transplanted with marrow cells transduced with a retrovirus leading to IL-11 production *(114,115)*; mice had high concentrations of serum IL-11, moderately increased platelet counts, increased splenic myeloid progenitor cell numbers, and evidence of system chronic IL-11 toxicity (loss of fat tissue, thymic atrophy, eyelid inflammation, and occasional hyperactivity). Several models of stable germline IL-11-expressing transgenes exist. An IL-11 transgene driven by the *Mx* promoter resulted in mice with constitutive expression on IL-11 in bone and bone marrow cells (this promoter was selected because its transcriptional activity can be upregulated by IFN); the major phenotype of these mice was increased bone formation *(116)*. Transgenic mice with IL-11 expression restricted to the airways have been generated *(117)*, including an inducible model using the reverse tetracycline transactivator system *(118)*; these models have elucidated the role of IL-11 in airway inflammation, lung fibrosis, and the response to acute lung injury *(119)*.

4. ANIMAL MODELS OF HEMATOPOIETIC GROWTH FACTOR ADMINISTRATION AFTER CHEMOTHERAPY OR RADIOTHERAPY

HGFs have found their most prominent role clinically in supporting hematopoietic recovery after anticancer chemotherapy and myeloablative regimens. The development of these approaches and the therapeutic principles underpinning them are based on appropriate animal models. Some examples selected from the large number of such studies follow.

4.1. Granulocyte Colony-Stimulating Factor

Many studies focus primarily on hematopoietic parameters after chemotherapy. For example, HuG-CSF accelerated granulopoietic recovery after cyclophosphamide in mice *(120)* and rats *(121)*, after etoposide in mice *(122)*, and after mitoxantrone and cyclophosphamide combination therapy in dogs *(123)*. Animal models can allow evaluation of novel approaches to scheduling and drug delivery. The effectiveness of rectal administration of G-CSF by suppositories has been shown in cyclophosphamide-treated rabbits *(124)*.

Scheduling issues can be more readily evaluated in animal models than in patients, particularly when theoretical risks exist. The risks and benefits of different schedules of exogenous G-CSF administration before and after a cyclophosphamide dose have been studied in mice *(125)*. Exogenous G-CSF administration immediately before chemotherapy and continued after chemotherapy accelerated neutrophil recovery, although neutrophil nadirs were lower than with other schedules. Exogenous G-CSF administration stopping several days before therapy and restarting after chemotherapy resulted in the greatest granulopoietic effect. The effect of exogenous G-CSF to minimize the interval between cyclophosphamide administrations has been studied *(126)*. Another scheduling evaluation showed that with exogenous G-CSF administration through 7 d of etoposide therapy, protection from neutropenia could still be achieved *(122)*. A comparison of the granulopoietic effects of pegfilgrastim and filgrastim after 5-FU effectively addressed a scheduling issue *(103)*.

More sophisticated studies have modeled the infective complications of chemotherapy. To model culture-positive febrile neutropenic complications of chemotherapy, cyclophosphamide-treated mice were treated with intraperitoneal exogenous G-CSF for 4 d and challenged with bacterial and fungal pathogens *(P. aeruginosa, Serratia marcescens, Staphylococcus aureus, C. albicans) (127)*. This short G-CSF treatment protected mice from otherwise lethal inoculums of these pathogens, and synergism with antibiotics was demonstrated for *P. aeruginosa* infections. Another study assessed the effects of exogenous G-CSF and antibiotics in vancomycin-resistant *Enterococcus faecalis*-infected mice *(128)*. Cyclophosphamide was administered to induce neutropenia, *E. faecalis* was inoculated, and then exogenous G-CSF was administered either alone or with antibiotics in various doses. The combination of exogenous G-CSF and antibiotics was more effective at enhancing survival than either antibiotic or exogenous G-CSF alone. Beneficial effects of G-CSF on the course of Gram-positive infections have been documented after cyclophosphamide administration in mice *(129)*; interestingly, this study did not find comparable effects after irradiation.

Animal models are useful for evaluating novel agents in combination with or compared with HGF. SCH 14988 is a small molecule that enhances endogenous G-CSF production; it accelerated neutrophil recovery after cyclophosphamide administration in association with increased G-CSF concentrations *(130)*. In combination with exogenous G-CSF, dipyridamole and adenosine monophosphate enhanced post-5-FU granulopoietic recovery *(131)*.

4.2. Granulocyte-Macrophage Colony-Stimulating Factor

Murine studies of GM-CSF are complicated by the lack of cross-species reactivity of HuGM-CSF, necessitating the use of MuGM-CSF.

A brief report demonstrated efficacy of exogenous GM-CSF in a murine model of melphalan-induced neutropenia *(132)*. The duration of post-melphalan neutropenia was shortened, and the mortality was reduced by approx 50%. Exogenous GM-CSF was shown to accelerate neutrophil and platelet recovery in monkeys after total body irradiation and autologous marrow transplantation *(133,134)*.

In non-neutropenic mice, administration of exogenous GM-CSF increased the number of peripheral blood neutrophils and monocytes and number of peritoneal macrophages but did not alter the course of *Listeria monocytogenes* infection. In mice rendered neutropenic by either cyclophosphamide administration or irradiation, exogenous GM-CSF had little effect; even these quantitative changes were not observed *(135)*.

Dose-for-dose comparison of exogenous G-CSF and exogenous GM-CSF has been undertaken in mice *(126)*. GM-CSF had 5% of the potency of G-CSF on neutrophil counts. Interestingly, during exogenous G-CSF administration, neutrophils egressed to an inflammatory site, but this did not occur during exogenous GM-CSF administration, consistent with other studies describing reduced neutrophil mobility with exogenous GM-CSF exposure.

4.3. Erythropoietin

Anemia, although a common accompaniment of cancer, is not usually viewed as an acute complication of myelotoxic chemotherapy, although it is well recognized that chemotherapeutic agents and regimens are associated with anemia, particularly with multiple dosings or repeated courses. Recombinant EPO preparations were effectively the first HGF to be evaluated for their ability to stimulate hematopoietic recovery in murine models, e.g., after irradiation *(136)* or 5-FU *(137)*. Relatively few animal studies have directly examined the effects of exogenous EPO administration along with chemotherapy, although the role of exogenous EPO in alleviating the anemia associated with cancer and its treatment is well established *(138)*.

One particularly interesting study in mice combined 7 d of etoposide (VP-16) therapy with simultaneous exogenous EPO administration. At lower VP-16 doses with exogenous EPO, higher reticulocytes and hematocrits were observed, but overall a negative interaction between VP-16 and exogenous EPO was evident: VP-16 had a larger antierythropoietic effect in EPO-treated compared with non-EPO-treated animals *(122)*. Although combining this relatively non-cell cycle-specific agent with a lineage-specific growth factor resulted in net advantageous outcome over part of the chemotherapeutic agent's dose range, in fact over all doses, growth factor stimulation of erythropoiesis was found to occur but was largely cancelled out by the abrogative effect of concomitant cytotoxic drug administration.

A number of recent animal studies have focused on the effect of EPO-stimulated anemia alleviation to improve the anticancer efficacy of chemotherapeutic agents including cyclophosphamide *(139)* and cisplatin *(140)*, of radiotherapy *(141,142)*, and of phototherapy *(143)*. These beneficial effects are thought to result from improved oxygen delivery to tumors resulting in sensitization to the cytotoxic modality. In one instance, a murine myeloma model, exogenous EPO itself was observed to stimulate immunologically mediated tumor regression *(143,144)*.

4.4. Interleukin-11

The preclinical studies of IL-11 effects in the context of myelotoxic or myeloablative therapies have been comprehensively reviewed *(112,113)*. Studies were conducted in syngeneic mouse transplant models and in mice given radiotherapy, or chemotherapy, or a combination of these. Some studies included assessment of impact on modeled infectious and bleeding complications *(145)*. Exogenous IL-11 promoted hematopoietic recovery, including accelerated platelet recovery, but another beneficial effect consistently observed has been an IL-11-related reduction in gastrointestinal mucosal toxicity. High-dose exogenous IL-11 protected rats rendered neutropenic with cyclophosphamide from *P. aeruginosa* infection *(146)*.

There has been an ongoing interest in IL-11 combinations with other growth factors, for example, to drive a more rapid multilineage hematopoietic recovery, or to combine the mucosal protective effects of IL-11 with the granulopoietic potency of other agents. In one study, 5-FU-related mortality was abrogated by exogenous IL-11 plus exogenous SCF *(147)*. In the rat neutropenia and *P. aeruginosa* infection model, G-CSF did not prove protective alone, but IL-11 combined with G-CSF was more protective than IL-11 alone *(148)*; additionally, there was significantly superior mucosal integrity in the combination group at histologic analysis at a fixed post-treatment timepoint.

5. ANIMAL MODELS EVALUATING HEMATOPOIETIC GROWTH FACTOR SIGNALING IN PATHOLOGIC PROCESSES

The phenotypic characterization and experimental validation of the animal models included descriptions of several pathologic states such as acute inflammation or experimental infection in which the role of a particular HGF has been assessed. To understand particular nuances regarding the role of HGF signaling in disease pathogenesis, particularly at the level of the receptor, several models have been generated by targeted gene modification rather than disruption. Particularly interesting questions about the contribution of HGF to disease pathogenesis can be addressed by interbreeding two murine models together, or by exploiting the range of genetic backgrounds available and the transplantability of the hematopoietic system to assess the role of paracrine and host factor production in disease pathogenesis.

5.1. G-CSF, G-CSFR, and Neutrophil Elastase in Severe Chronic Neutropenia

Although G-CSF-deficient mice have life-long neutropenia, congenital or acquired neutropenia in humans caused by G-CSF deficiency itself has not been described. Approximately 20% of patients with severe chronic neutropenia have associated carboxyl truncations of the G-CSF receptor (G-CSFR) *(149,150)*, although these appear to be acquired somatic mutations rather than germline mutations *(150)*. Representative examples of this mutation have been modeled in mice by targeted gene modification. In one model, based on a G-CSFR truncated at position 715, mice displayed baseline neutropenia, a milder haploinsufficiency phenotype, and a hyperproliferative response to exogenous G-CSF resulting in neutrophilia *(151,152)*. In the other model, both heterozygous and homozygous mice displayed a normal basal granulopoietic phenotype with only a modest reduction in circulating neutrophil numbers, despite the lesion resulting in a hyperproliferative response to exogenous G-CSF in vivo *(153)*. The reason for the difference between the two models is not clear, although the gene-targeting strategy used retained the selectable marker in one model *(153)* but not the other *(151)*.

Recently, the genetic lesion resulting in cyclical neutropenia was located to the neutrophil elastase gene *(154)*. A high prevalence of heterozygous neutrophil elastase mutations in severe congenital neutropenia implicates these lesions epidemiologically in the pathogenesis of the disease *(155)*. Normal granulopoiesis was observed in a murine model of one of these mutations *(156)*, suggesting that the pathogenesis of the neutropenia may be more complex than the effects of a single mutation.

5.2. Erythropoietin Receptor and Familial Erythrocytosis

In contrast to the situation with the G-CSF receptor, heterozygous carboxyl truncations of the human EPOR are associated not with anemia but with polycythemia and are often transmitted in the germline *(157,158)*. A multistep targeted gene modification approach has been used to replicate one mutated HuEPO receptor (C5964 $\rightarrow$ G) in a murine model *(159)*. These mice show a haploinsufficiency phenotype with polycythemia. Mice homozygous for this mutation (a situation not observed clinically) develop severe polycythemia, but are viable.

5.3. Granulocyte-Macrophage Colony-Stimulating Factor in Pulmonary Disease and Other Experimental Disease Models

The development of alveolar proteinosis in GM-CSFR and GM-CSF-Rβ_C-deficient mice has highlighted the role of GM-CSF signaling in pulmonary pathophysiology. The pathogenic and therapeutic insights contributed by this model have been reviewed *(160)*. GM-CSF-deficient mice have been exploited to evaluate the contribution of GM-CSF in other lung pathology. The acute lung injury associated with an experimental model of acute pancreatitis was ameliorated in GM-CSF$^{-/-}$ mice despite comparable degrees of pancreatic inflammation *(161)*. Similarly, other immunologically mediated inflammatory diseases have been shown to be ameliorated in GM-CSF$^{-/-}$ mice including collagen-induced arthritis *(162)* and experimental autoimmune encephalitis *(163)*.

5.4. Hematopoietic Growth Factors in Myeloid Leukemia

The role of HGF signaling in leukemogenesis and the notion of growth factor dependence as a potential Achilles' heel of leukemic cells that could be targeted therapeutically have been recognized for several decades *(164)*. Genetic models of murine myeloid leukemia have been generated based on transgenic expression of several common fusion oncogenes, both for the transformation of marrow cells, which are then used to reconstitute recipient animals, or by germline transgenesis. These leukemia models, when combined with animals with defective HGF signaling, provide a means to assess the role that HGF signals play in the leukemogenic process. Several examples of this approach have been reported.

Mice deficient in the neurofibromatosis 1 (NF1) gene die *in utero (165,166)*, but NF1-deficient fetal liver cells induce a myeloproliferative disorder in transplant recipients reminiscent of the juvenile myelomonocytic leukemia (JML) seen in humans with NF1 *(167,168)*. Like their human counterparts, murine NF1$^{-/-}$ fetal hematopoietic cells show hypersensitivity to GM-CSF in vitro *(167,169)*. NF$^{-/-}$ and GM-CSF$^{-/-}$ mice were interbred and used as a source of NF1$^{-/-}$GM-CSF$^{-/-}$ fetal liver hematopoietic cells for transplant studies to test directly whether the GM-CSF production ability of the fetal liver cells themselves, the host stroma, or both contributed to the murine myeloproliferative phenotype *(170)*. GM-CSF production by either the host or engrafting cells was sufficient to induce the myeloproliferative disease, but the myeloproliferative process was suppressed when neither the host nor graft could make GM-CSF. Frankly myeloproliferative marrows transplanted into GM-CSF-deficient recipients resulted in an attenuated phenotype compared with GM-CSF-replete recipients. Exogenous GM-CSF treatment of secondary recipients (i.e., mice with NF1$^{-/-}$GM-CSF$^{-/-}$ graft cells into GM-CSF$^{-/-}$ recipients) unmasked the myeloproliferative phenotype. Collectively, these data present an elegant use of these animal models to implicate endogenous GM-CSF production and signaling as necessary for the full manifestation of this myeloproliferative disease.

Hematopoietic cells carrying other leukemogenic fusion oncogenes have been tested for their dependence on HGF in similar models. Marrow cells transduced to overexpress *BCR/ABL* resulted in identical diseases in transplant recipients regardless of whether the graft donor, transplant recipient, or both lacked either GM-CSF, or IL-3, or both these factors *(84)*. Similarly, mice deficient in both GM-CSF and IL-3 were used to show that three TEL-protein tyrosine kinase fusion oncogenes induced similar myeloproliferative disorders despite absence of factor production by both the donor cells and recipient animal *(85)*.

We have reported preliminary observations from an experiment in which mice carrying a leukemogenic PLZF-RARα transgene were backcrossed onto G-CSF-deficient or GM-CSF-deficient backgrounds. Surprisingly, mice carrying the invariably lethal PLZF-RARα transgene on a G-CSF-deficient background failed to develop chronic myeloproliferation and lived a normal life span, whereas GM-CSF-deficient mice carrying the transgene died over 6–18 mo, like their transgenic wild-type background counterparts *(171)*. These observations suggest that this murine myeloproliferative disorder requires signals exclusively provided by G-CSF for its full manifestation.

6. CONCLUSIONS

Although much can be learned about the cellular effects of HGFs from their activities in vitro, animal models have been indispensable for understanding the basic physiology of the HGFs. Loss-of-function models and overexpression models have particularly contributed to this understanding of physiologic roles. Animal studies are a mandatory part of the preclinical development of new biologic therapeutics, and many specific models of particular therapeutic scenarios have delineated the potential beneficial activities of HGF in current clinical use, including studies exploring dosing and scheduling parameters that inform the clinical use of these agents in the hematologic support of anticancer treatments, such as those described in later chapters of this book. The animal models have provided sometimes unexpected insights into the pathogenesis of both nonmalignant and malignant disease, which suggest possibilities for exciting new therapeutic approaches.

ACKNOWLEDGMENTS

Parts of this review are updated versions of previously unpublished portions of a thesis entitled “Physiological Role of Hematopoietic Growth Factors in Mice Revealed by Targeted Gene Disruption” submitted by G.J.L. for the Doctor of Philosophy degree at the University of Melbourne. G.J.L. was the recipient of a Wellcome Senior Research Fellowship in Medical Sciences in Australia (1997–2002). Thanks to Simone Pakin for excellent secretarial assistance.

REFERENCES

1. Rubinson DA, Dillon CP, Kwiatkowski AV, et al. A lentivirus-based system to functionally silence genes in primary mammalian cells, stem cells and transgenic mice by RNA interference. *Nat Genet* 2003; 33:401–406.
2. Sarvella PA, Russell LB. *Steel,* a new dominant gene in the mouse. *J Hered* 1956; 47:123–128.
3. Bennett D. Developmental analysis of a mutation with pleiotropic effects in the mouse. *J Morphol* 1956; 98:199–234.
4. Peters J, Selley R, Cocking Y. Mouse gene list. *Mouse Genomics* 1995; 93:184–357.
5. Russell ES. Hereditary anemias of the mouse: a review for geneticists. *Adv Genet* 1979; 20:357–459.
6. Anderson DM, Lyman SD, Baird A, et al. Molecular cloning of mast cell growth factor, a hematopoietin that is active in both membrane bound and soluble forms. *Cell* 1990; 63:235–243.
7. Huang E, Nocka K, Beier DR, et al. The hematopoietic growth factor KL is encoded by the *Sl* locus and is the ligand of the *c-kit* receptor, the gene product of the *W* locus. *Cell* 1990; 63:225–233.
8. Zsebo KM, Williams DA, Geissler EN, et al. Stem cell factor is encoded at the *Sl* locus of the mouse and is the ligand for the *c-kit* tyrosine kinase receptor. *Cell* 1990; 63:213–224.
9. Metcalf D. Lineage commitment of hemopoietic progenitor cells in developing blast cell colonies: influence of colony-stimulating factors. *Proc Natl Acad Sci USA* 1991; 88:11310–11314.
10. de Aberle SB. A study of the hereditary anemia of mice. *Am J Anat* 1927; 40:219–247.
11. Little CC, Cloudman AM. The occurrence of a dominant spotting mutation in the house mouse. *Proc Natl Acad Sci USA* 1937; 23:535–537.
12. Nocka K, Tan JC, Chiu E, et al. Molecular bases of dominant negative and loss of function mutations at the murine *c-kit*/white spotting locus: W^{37}, W^{v}, W^{41} and *W. EMBO J* 1990; 9:1805–1813.
13. Marks SC, Lane PW. Osteopetrosis, a new recessive skeletal mutation on chromosome 12 of the mouse. *J Hered* 1976; 67:11–18.
14. Yoshida H, Hayashi S, Kunisada T, et al. The murine mutation osteopetrosis is in the coding region of the macrophage colony stimulating factor gene. *Nature* 1990; 345:442–444.
15. Marks SC Jr. Morphological evidence of reduced bone resorption in osteopetrotic *(op)* mice. *Am J Anat* 1982; 163:157–167.
16. Felix R, Cecchini MG, Fleisch H. Macrophage colony stimulating factor restores *in vivo* bone resorption in the *op/op* osteopetrotic mouse. *Endocrinology* 1990; 127:2592–2594.
17. Shibata Y, Zsengeller Z, Otake K, Palaniyar N, Trapnell BC. Alveolar macrophage deficiency in osteopetrotic mice deficient in macrophage colony-stimulating factor is spontaneously corrected with age and associated with matrix metalloproteinase expression and emphysema. *Blood* 2001; 98:2845–2852.
18. Takahashi K, Umeda S, Shultz LD, Hayashi S, Nishikawa S. Effects of macrophage colony-stimulating factor (M-CSF) on the development, differentiation, and maturation of marginal metallophilic macrophages and marginal zone macrophages in the spleen of osteopetrosis (op) mutant mice lacking functional M-CSF activity. *J Leukoc Biol* 1994; 55:581–588.
19. Usuda H, Naito M, Umeda S, Takahashi K, Shultz LD. Ultrastructure of macrophages and dendritic cells in osteopetrosis *(op)* mutant mice lacking macrophage colony-stimulating factor (M-CSF/CSF-1) activity. *J Submicrosc Cytol Pathol* 1994; 26:111–119.
20. Wiktor-Jedrzejczak WW, Ahmed A, Szczylik C, Skelly RR. Hematological characterization of congenital osteopetrosis in *op/op* mouse. Possible mechanism for abnormal macrophage differentiation. *J Exp Med* 1982; 156:1516–1527.
21. Wiktor-Jedrzejczak W, Ratajczak MZ, Ptasznik A, Sell KW, Ahmed-Ansari A, Ostertag W. CSF-1 deficiency in the *op/op* mouse has differential effects on macrophage populations and differentiation stages. *Exp Hematol* 1992; 20:1004–1010.
22. Pollard JW, Hunt JS, Wiktor-Jedrzejczak W, Stanley ER. A pregnancy defect in the osteopetrotic *(op/op)* mouse demonstrates the requirement for CSF-1 in female fertility. *Dev Biol* 1991; 148:273–283.
23. Pollard JW, Hennighausen L. Colony stimulating factor 1 is required for mammary gland development during pregnancy. *Proc Natl Acad Sci USA* 1994; 91:9312–9316.
24. Dai XM, Ryan GR, Hapel AJ, et al. Targeted disruption of the mouse colony-stimulating factor 1 receptor gene results in osteopetrosis, mononuclear phagocyte deficiency, increased primitive progenitor cell frequencies, and reproductive defects. *Blood* 2002; 99:111–120.
25. Schooley JC, Garcia JF. Immunochemical studies of human urinary erythropoietin. *Proc Soc Exp Biol Med* 1962; 109:325–328.

26. Schooley JC, Garcia JF. Some properties of serum obtained from rabbits immunized with human urinary erythropoietin. *Blood* 1965; 25:204–217.
27. Schooley JC, Garcia JF, Cantor LN, Havens VW. A summary of some studies on erythropoiesis using anti-erythropoietin immune serum. *Ann NY Acad Sci* 1968; 149:266–280.
28. Coscarella A, Liddi R, Di Loreto M, et al. The rhGM-CSF-EPO hybrid protein MEN 11300 induces anti-EPO antibodies and severe anaemia in rhesus monkeys. *Cytokine* 1998; 10:964–969.
29. Wu H, Liu X, Jaenisch R, Lodish HF. Generation of committed erythroid BFU-E and CFU-E progenitors does not require erythropoietin or the erythropoietin receptor. *Cell* 1995; 83:59–67.
30. Wu H, Lee SH, Gao J, Liu X, Iruela-Arispe ML. Inactivation of erythropoietin leads to defects in cardiac morphogenesis. *Development* 1999; 126:3597–3605.
31. Jegalian AG, Acurio A, Dranoff G, Wu H. Erythropoietin receptor haploinsufficiency and in vivo interplay with granulocyte-macrophage colony-stimulating factor and interleukin 3. *Blood* 2002; 99:2603–2605.
32. Burns S, Arcasoy MO, Li L, et al. Purification and characterization of the yeast- expressed erythropoietin mutant Epo (R103A), a specific inhibitor of human primary hematopoietic cell erythropoiesis. *Blood* 2002; 99:4400–4405.
33. Motojima H, Kobayashi T, Shimane M, Kamachi S, Fukushima M. Quantitative enzyme immunoassay for human granulocyte colony stimulating factor (G-CSF). *J Immunol Methods* 1989; 118:187–192.
34. Omori F, Okamura S, Hayashi S, Yamaga S, Hirota Y, Niho Y. Measurement of human granulocyte-macrophage colony-stimulating factor (GM-CSF) by enzyme-linked immunosorbent assay. *Biotherapy* 1989; 1:161–167.
35. Shirafuji N, Asano S, Matsuda S, Watari K, Takaku F, Nagata S. A new bioassay for human granulocyte colony-stimulating factor (hG-CSF) using murine myeloblastic NFS-60 cells as targets and estimation of its levels in sera from normal healthy persons and patients with infectious and hematological disorders. *Exp Hematol* 1989; 17:116–119.
36. Lee MY, Fevold KL, Dorshkind K, Fukunaga R, Nagata S, Rosse C. In vivo and in vitro suppression of primary B lymphocytopoiesis by tumor-derived and recombinant granulocyte colony-stimulating factor. *Blood* 1993; 82:2062–2068.
37. Nelson S. Role of granulocyte colony-stimulating factor in the immune response to acute bacterial infection in the nonneutropenic host: an overview. *Clin Infect Dis* 1994; 18:S197–S204.
38. Hammond WP, Csiba E, Canin A, et al. Chronic neutropenia. A new canine model induced by human granulocyte colony-stimulating factor. *J Clin Invest* 1991; 87:704–710.
39. Coccia MA, Hartley C, Sutherland W, et al. Prolonged neutropenia in a novel mouse granulocyte colony-stimulating factor neutralizing auto-immunoglobulin G mouse model. *Exp Hematol* 2001; 29:59–67.
40. Lieschke GJ, Grail D, Hodgson G, et al. Mice lacking granulocyte colony-stimulating factor have chronic neutropenia, granulocyte and macrophage progenitor cell deficiency, and impaired neutrophil mobilization. *Blood* 1994; 84:1737–1746.
41. Liu F, Wu HY, Wesselschmidt R, Kornaga T, Link DC. Impaired production and increased apoptosis of neutrophils in granulocyte colony-stimulating factor receptor-deficient mice. *Immunity* 1996; 5:491–501.
42. Basu S, Hodgson G, Katz M, Dunn AR. Evaluation of role of G-CSF in the production, survival, and release of neutrophils from bone marrow into circulation. *Blood* 2002; 100:854–861.
43. Basu S, Hodgson G, Zhang HH, Katz M, Quilici C, Dunn AR. "Emergency" granulopoiesis in G-CSF-deficient mice in response to *Candida albicans* infection. *Blood* 2000; 95:3725–3733.
44. Zhan Y, Lieschke GJ, Grail D, Dunn AR, Cheers C. Essential roles for granulocyte-macrophage colony-stimulating factor (GM-CSF) and G-CSF in the sustained hematopoietic response of *Listeria monocytogenes*-infected mice. *Blood* 1998; 91:863–869.
45. Zhan Y, Basu S, Lieschke GJ, Grail D, Dunn AR, Cheers C. Functional deficiencies of peritoneal cells from gene-targeted mice lacking G-CSF or GM-CSF. *J Leukoc Biol* 1999; 65:256–264.
46. Mannering SI, Zhan Y, Gilbertson B, Lieschke GJ, Cheers C. T lymphocytes from granulocyte colony-stimulating factor–/– mice produce large quantities of interferon-gamma in a chronic infection model. *Immunology* 2000; 101:132–139.
47. Liu F, Poursine-Laurent J, Link DC. The granulocyte colony-stimulating factor receptor is required for the mobilization of murine hematopoietic progenitors into peripheral blood by cyclophosphamide or interleukin-8 but not flt-3 ligand. *Blood* 1997; 90:2522–2528.

48. Betsuyaku T, Liu F, Senior RM, et al. A functional granulocyte colony-stimulating factor receptor is required for normal chemoattractant-induced neutrophil activation. *J Clin Invest* 1999; 103:825–832.
49. Liu F, Poursine-Laurent J, Link DC. Expression of the G-CSF receptor on hematopoietic progenitor cells is not required for their mobilization by G-CSF. *Blood* 2000; 95:3025–3031.
50. Semerad CL, Poursine-Laurent J, Liu F, Link DC. A role for G-CSF receptor signaling in the regulation of hematopoietic cell function but not lineage commitment or differentiation. *Immunity* 1999; 11:153–161.
51. Semerad CL, Liu F, Gregory AD, Stumpf K, Link DC. G-CSF is an essential regulator of neutrophil trafficking from the bone marrow to the blood. *Immunity* 2002; 17:413–423.
52. DeLamarter JF, Mermod JJ, Liang CM, Eliason JF, Thatcher DR. Recombinant murine GM-CSF from *E. coli* has biological activity and is neutralized by a specific antiserum. *EMBO J* 1985; 4:2575–2581.
53. Abrams JS, Roncarolo MG, Yssel H, Andersson U, Gleich GJ, Silver JE. Strategies of anti-cytokine monoclonal antibody development: immunoassay of IL-10 and IL-5 in clinical samples. *Immunol Rev* 1992; 127:5–24.
54. Sander B, Hoiden I, Andersson U, Moller E, Abrams JS. Similar frequencies and kinetics of cytokine producing cells in murine peripheral blood and spleen. Cytokine detection by immunoassay and intracellular immunostaining. *J Immunol Methods* 1993; 166:201–214.
55. Tiegs G, Barsig J, Matiba B, Uhlig S, Wendel A. Potentiation by granulocyte macrophage colony-stimulating factor of lipopolysaccharide toxicity in mice. *J Clin Invest* 1994; 93:2616–2622.
56. Yang YH, Hamilton JA. Dependence of interleukin-1-induced arthritis on granulocyte-macrophage colony-stimulating factor. *Arthritis Rheum* 2001; 44:111–119.
57. Cook AD, Braine EL, Campbell IK, Rich MJ, Hamilton JA. Blockade of collagen-induced arthritis post-onset by antibody to granulocyte-macrophage colony-stimulating factor (GM-CSF): requirement for GM-CSF in the effector phase of disease. *Arthritis Res* 2001; 3:293–298.
58. Hercus TR, Bagley CJ, Cambareri B, et al. Specific human granulocyte-macrophage colony-stimulating factor antagonists. *Proc Natl Acad Sci USA* 1994; 91:5838–5842.
59. Olver IN, Hercus T, Lopez A, et al. A phase I study of the GM-CSF antagonist E21R. *Cancer Chemother Pharmacol* 2002; 50:171–178.
60. Dranoff G, Crawford AD, Sadelain M, et al. Involvement of granulocyte-macrophage colony-stimulating factor in pulmonary homeostasis. *Science* 1994; 264:713–716.
61. Stanley E, Lieschke GJ, Grail D, et al. Granulocyte/macrophage colony-stimulating factor-deficient mice show no major perturbation of hematopoiesis but develop a characteristic pulmonary pathology. *Proc Natl Acad Sci USA* 1994; 91:5592–5596.
62. Zhan Y, Cheers C. Haemopoiesis in mice genetically lacking granulocyte-macrophage colony stimulating factor during chronic infection with *Mycobacterium avium*. *Immunol Cell Biol* 2000; 78:118–123.
63. Metcalf D, Robb L, Dunn AR, Mifsud S, Di Rago L. Role of granulocyte-macrophage colony-stimulating factor and granulocyte colony-stimulating factor in the development of an acute neutrophil inflammatory response in mice. *Blood* 1996; 88:3755–3764.
64. Wynn AA, Miyakawa K, Miyata E, Dranoff G, Takeya M, Takahashi K. Role of granulocyte/macrophage colony-stimulating factor in zymocel-induced hepatic granuloma formation. *Am J Pathol* 2001; 158:131–145.
65. Kitching AR, Ru H, X, Turner AL, Tipping PG, Dunn AR, Holdsworth SR. The requirement for granulocyte-macrophage colony-stimulating factor and granulocyte colony-stimulating factor in leukocyte-mediated immune glomerular injury. *J Am Soc Nephrol* 2002; 13:350–358.
66. Seymour JF, Lieschke GJ, Grail D, Quilici C, Hodgson G, Dunn AR. Mice lacking both granulocyte colony-stimulating factor (CSF) and granulocyte-macrophage CSF have impaired reproductive capacity, perturbed neonatal granulopoiesis, lung disease, amyloidosis, and reduced long-term survival. *Blood* 1997; 90:3037–3049.
67. Huffman JA, Hull WM, Dranoff G, Mulligan RC, Whitsett JA. Pulmonary epithelial cell expression of GM-CSF corrects the alveolar proteinosis in GM-CSF-deficient mice. *J Clin Invest* 1996; 97:649–655.
68. Nishinakamura R, Nakayama N, Hirabayashi Y, et al. Mice deficient for the IL-3/GM-CSF/IL-5 beta c receptor exhibit lung pathology and impaired immune response, while beta IL3 receptor-deficient mice are normal. *Immunity* 1995; 2:211–222.

69. Robb L, Drinkwater CC, Metcalf D, et al. Hematopoietic and lung abnormalities in mice with a null mutation of the common beta subunit of the receptors for granulocyte-macrophage colony-stimulating factor and interleukins 3 and 5. *Proc Natl Acad Sci USA* 1995; 92:9565–9569.
70. Reed JA, Ikegami M, Robb L, Begley CG, Ross G, Whitsett JA. Distinct changes in pulmonary surfactant homeostasis in common beta-chain- and GM-CSF-deficient mice. *Am J Physiol Lung Cell Mol Physiol* 2000; 278:L1164–L1171.
71. Yoshida T, Ikuta K, Sugaya H, et al. Defective B-1 cell development and impaired immunity against *Angiostrongylus cantonensis* in IL-5R alpha-deficient mice. *Immunity* 1996; 4:483–494.
72. Nishinakamura R, Wiler R, Dirksen U, et al. The pulmonary alveolar proteinosis in granulocyte macrophage colony-stimulating factor/interleukins 3/5 beta c receptor-deficient mice is reversed by bone marrow transplantation. *J Exp Med* 1996; 183:2657–2662.
73. Cooke KR, Nishinakamura R, Martin TR, et al. Persistence of pulmonary pathology and abnormal lung function in IL-3/GM-CSF/IL-5 beta c receptor-deficient mice despite correction of alveolar proteinosis after BMT. *Bone Marrow Transplant* 1997; 20:657–662.
74. Scott CL, Roe L, Curtis J, et al. Mice unresponsive to GM-CSF are unexpectedly resistant to cutaneous *Leishmania major* infection. *Microbes Infect* 2000; 2:1131–1138.
75. Nandurkar HH, Robb L, Tarlinton D, Barnett L, Kontgen F, Begley CG. Adult mice with targeted mutation of the interleukin-11 receptor (IL11Ra) display normal hematopoiesis. *Blood* 1997; 90:2148–2159.
76. Robb L, Li R, Hartley L, Nandurkar HH, Koentgen F, Begley CG. Infertility in female mice lacking the receptor for interleukin 11 is due to a defective uterine response to implantation. *Nat Med* 1998; 4:303–308.
77. Betz UA, Bloch W, van den BM, et al. Postnatally induced inactivation of gp130 in mice results in neurological, cardiac, hematopoietic, immunological, hepatic, and pulmonary defects. *J Exp Med* 1998; 188:1955–1965.
78. Shaughnessy SG, Walton KJ, Deschamps P, Butcher M, Beaudin SM. Neutralization of interleukin-11 activity decreases osteoclast formation and increases cancellous bone volume in ovariectomized mice. *Cytokine* 2002; 20:78–85.
79. Liu F, Poursine-Laurent J, Wu HY, Link DC. Interleukin-6 and the granulocyte colony-stimulating factor receptor are major independent regulators of granulopoiesis in vivo but are not required for lineage commitment or terminal differentiation. *Blood* 1997; 90:2583–2590.
80. Kaushansky K, Fox N, Lin NL, Liles WC. Lineage-specific growth factors can compensate for stem and progenitor cell deficiencies at the postprogenitor cell level: an analysis of doubly TPO- and G-CSF receptor-deficient mice. *Blood* 2002; 99:3573–3578.
81. Lantz CS, Boesiger J, Song CH, et al. Role for interleukin-3 in mast-cell and basophil development and in immunity to parasites. *Nature* 1998; 392:90–93.
82. Mach N, Lantz CS, Galli SJ, et al. Involvement of interleukin-3 in delayed-type hypersensitivity. *Blood* 1998; 91:778–783.
83. Gillessen S, Mach N, Small C, Mihm M, Dranoff G. Overlapping roles for granulocyte-macrophage colony-stimulating factor and interleukin-3 in eosinophil homeostasis and contact hypersensitivity. *Blood* 2001; 97:922–928.
84. Li S, Gillessen S, Tomasson MH, Dranoff G, Gilliland DG, Van Etten RA. Interleukin 3 and granulocyte-macrophage colony-stimulating factor are not required for induction of chronic myeloid leukemia-like myeloproliferative disease in mice by BCR/ABL. *Blood* 2001; 97:1442–1450.
85. Tomasson MH, Williams IR, Li S, et al. Induction of myeloproliferative disease in mice by tyrosine kinase fusion oncogenes does not require granulocyte-macrophage colony-stimulating factor or interleukin-3. *Blood* 2001; 97:1435–1441.
86. Nishinakamura R, Miyajima A, Mee PJ, Tybulewicz VL, Murray R. Hematopoiesis in mice lacking the entire granulocyte-macrophage colony-stimulating factor/interleukin-3/interleukin-5 functions. *Blood* 1996; 88:2458–2464.
87. Lieschke GJ, Stanley E, Grail D, et al. Mice lacking both macrophage- and granulocyte-macrophage colony-stimulating factor have macrophages and coexistent osteopetrosis and severe lung disease. *Blood* 1994; 84:27–35.
88. Nilsson SK, Lieschke GJ, Garcia-Wijnen CC, et al. Granulocyte-macrophage colony-stimulating factor is not responsible for the correction of hematopoietic deficiencies in the maturing op/op mouse. *Blood* 1995; 86:66–72.
89. Gainsford T, Nandurkar H, Metcalf D, Robb L, Begley CG, Alexander WS. The residual megakaryocyte and platelet production in c-mpl-deficient mice is not dependent on the actions of interleukin-6, interleukin-11, or leukemia inhibitory factor. *Blood* 2000; 95:528–534.

90. Dunn CJ, Markham A. Epoetin beta. A review of its pharmacological properties and clinical use in the management of anaemia associated with chronic renal failure. *Drugs* 1996; 51:299–318.
91. Markham A, Bryson HM. Epoetin alfa. A review of its pharmacodynamic and pharmacokinetic properties and therapeutic use in nonrenal applications. *Drugs* 1995; 49:232–254.
92. Joy MS. Darbepoetin alfa: a novel erythropoiesis-stimulating protein. *Ann Pharmacother* 2002; 36:1183–1192.
93. Wrighton NC, Farrell FX, Chang R, et al. Small peptides as potent mimetics of the protein hormone erythropoietin. *Science* 1996; 273:458–464.
94. Taglialatela R, Della CF. Human and recombinant erythropoietin stimulate erythropoiesis in the goldfish *Carassius auratus. Eur J Histochem* 1997; 41:301–304.
95. Semenza GL, Traystman MD, Gearhart JD, Antonarakis SE. Polycythemia in transgenic mice expressing the human erythropoietin gene. *Proc Natl Acad Sci USA* 1989; 86:2301–2305.
96. Semenza GL, Dureza RC, Traystman MD, Gearhart JD, Antonarakis SE. Human erythropoietin gene expression in transgenic mice: multiple transcription initiation sites and cis-acting regulatory elements. *Mol Cell Biol* 1990; 10:930–938.
97. Semenza GL, Koury ST, Nejfelt MK, Gearhart JD, Antonarakis SE. Cell-type-specific and hypoxia-inducible expression of the human erythropoietin gene in transgenic mice. *Proc Natl Acad Sci USA* 1991; 88:8725–8729.
98. Villeval JL, Metcalf D, Johnson GR. Fatal polycythemia induced in mice by dysregulated erythropoietin production by hematopoietic cells. *Leukemia* 1992; 6:107–115.
99. Lord BI, Molineux G, Pojda Z, Souza LM, Mermod JJ, Dexter TM. Myeloid cell kinetics in mice treated with recombinant interleukin-3, granulocyte colony-stimulating factor (CSF), or granulocyte-macrophage CSF in vivo. *Blood* 1991; 77:2154–2159.
100. Roberts AW, Metcalf D. Granulocyte colony-stimulating factor induces selective elevations of progenitor cells in the peripheral blood of mice. *Exp Hematol* 1994; 22:1156–1163.
101. Lee MY, Fukunaga R, Lee TJ, Lottsfeldt JL, Nagata S. Bone modulation in sustained hematopoietic stimulation in mice. *Blood* 1991; 77:2135–2141.
102. Lord BI, Woolford LB, Molineux G. Kinetics of neutrophil production in normal and neutropenic animals during the response to filgrastim (r-metHu G-CSF) or filgrastim SD/01 (PEG-r-metHu G-CSF). *Clin Cancer Res* 2001; 7:2085–2090.
103. Molineux G, Kinstler O, Briddell B, Hartley C, McElroy P, Kerzic P, et al. A new form of filgrastim with sustained duration in vivo and enhanced ability to mobilize PBPC in both mice and humans. *Exp Hematol* 1999; 27:1724–1734.
104. Chang JM, Metcalf D, Gonda TJ, Johnson GR. Long-term exposure to retrovirally expressed granulocyte-colony-stimulating factor induces a nonneoplastic granulocytic and progenitor cell hyperplasia without tissue damage in mice. *J Clin Invest* 1989; 84:1488–1496.
105. Metcalf D, Begley CG, Williamson DJ, et al. Hemopoietic responses in mice injected with purified recombinant murine GM-CSF. *Exp Hematol* 1987; 15:1 9.
106. Pojda Z, Molineux G, Dexter TM. Effects of long-term in vivo treatment of mice with purified murine recombinant GM-CSF. *Exp Hematol* 1989; 17:1100–1104.
107. Lang RA, Metcalf D, Cuthbertson RA, et al. Transgenic mice expressing a hemopoietic growth factor gene (GM-CSF) develop accumulations of macrophages, blindness, and a fatal syndrome of tissue damage. *Cell* 1987; 51:675–686.
108. Cuthbertson RA, Lang RA. Developmental ocular disease in GM-CSF transgenic mice is mediated by autostimulated macrophages. *Dev Biol* 1989; 134:119–129.
109. Lang RA, Cuthbertson RA, Dunn AR. TNF alpha, IL-1 alpha and bFGF are implicated in the complex disease of GM-CSF transgenic mice. *Growth Factors* 1992; 6:131–138.
110. Cuthbertson RA, Lang RA, Coghlan JP. Macrophage products IL-1 alpha, TNF alpha and bFGF may mediate multiple cytopathic effects in the developing eyes of GM-CSF transgenic mice. *Exp Eye Res* 1990; 51:335–344.
111. Johnson GR, Gonda TJ, Metcalf D, Hariharan IK, Cory S. A lethal myeloproliferative syndrome in mice transplanted with bone marrow cells infected with a retrovirus expressing granulocyte-macrophage colony stimulating factor. *EMBO J* 1989; 8:441–448.
112. Du X, Williams DA. Interleukin-11: review of molecular, cell biology, and clinical use. *Blood* 1997; 89:3897–3908.
113. Turner KJ, Clark SC. Interleukin-11: Biological and clinical perspectives. In: Mertelsmann R, Herrmann F, eds., *Hematopoietic Growth Factors in Clinical Applications.* New York: Marcel Decker. 1995:315–336.

114. Hawley RG, Fong AZ, Ngan BY, de Lanux VM, Clark SC, Hawley TS. Progenitor cell hyperplasia with rare development of myeloid leukemia in interleukin 11 bone marrow chimeras. *J Exp Med* 1993; 178:1175–1188.
115. Paul SR, Hayes LL, Palmer R, et al. Interleukin-11 expression in donor bone marrow cells improves hematological con.itution in lethally irradiated recipient mice. *Exp Hematol* 1994; 22:295–301.
116. Takeuchi Y, Watanabe S, Ishii G, et al. Interleukin-11 as a stimulatory factor for bone formation prevents bone loss with advancing age in mice. *J Biol Chem* 2002; 277:49011–49018.
117. Tang W, Geba GP, Zheng T, et al. Targeted expression of IL-11 in the murine airway causes lymphocytic inflammation, bronchial remodeling, and airways obstruction. *J Clin Invest* 1996; 98:2845–2853.
118. Ray P, Tang W, Wang P, et al. Regulated overexpression of interleukin 11 in the lung. Use to dissociate development-dependent and -independent phenotypes. *J Clin Invest* 1997; 100:2501–2511.
119. Waxman AB, Einarsson O, Seres T, et al. Targeted lung expression of interleukin-11 enhances murine tolerance of 100% oxygen and diminishes hyperoxia-induced DNA fragmentation. *J Clin Invest* 1998; 101:1970–1982.
120. Barrios L, Poletti OH, Agustini MI. The influence of recombinant human granulocyte colony-stimulating factor on granulopoiesis in mice recovering from cyclophosphamide treatment. *Methods Find Exp Clin Pharmacol* 2000; 22:275–280.
121. Nohynek GJ, Plard JP, Wells MY, Zerial A, Roquet F. Comparison of the potency of glycosylated and nonglycosylated recombinant human granulocyte colony-stimulating factors in neutropenic and non-neutropenic CD rats. *Cancer Chemother Pharmacol* 1997; 39:259–266.
122. de Haan G, Engel C, Dontje B, Loeffler M, Nijhof W. Hemotoxicity by prolonged etoposide administration to mice can be prevented by simultaneous growth factor therapy. *Cancer Res* 1995; 55:324–329.
123. Henry CJ, Buss MS, Potter KA, Wardrop KJ. Mitoxantrone and cyclophosphamide combination chemotherapy for the treatment of various canine malignancies. *J Am Anim Hosp Assoc* 1999; 35:236–239.
124. Watanabe Y, Kiriyama M, Oe J, Kikuchi R, Mizufune Y, Matsumoto M. Pharmacodynamic activity (leukopoietic effect) of recombinant human granulocyte colony-stimulating factor (rhG-CSF) after rectal administration in rabbits with leukopenia induced by cyclophosphamide. *Biol Pharm Bull* 1996; 19:1064–1067.
125. Misaki M, Ueyama Y, Tsukamoto G, Matsumura T. Timing of recombinant human granulocyte colony-stimulating factor administration on neutropenia induced by cyclophosphamide in normal mice. *Br J Cancer* 1998; 77:884–889.
126. Hattori K, Orita T, Oheda M, Tamura M, Ono M. Comparative study of the effects of granulocyte colony-stimulating factor and granulocyte-macrophage colony-stimulating factor on generation and mobilization of neutrophils in cyclophosphamide-treated neutropenic mice. *In Vivo* 1996; 10:319–327.
127. Ono M, Matsumoto M, Matsubara S, Tomioka S, Asano S. Protective effect of human granulocyte colony-stimulating factor on bacterial and fungal infections in neutropenic mice. *Behring Inst Mitt* 1988; 216–221.
128. Onyeji CO, Nicolau DP, Nightingale CH, Bow L. Modulation of efficacies and pharmacokinetics of antibiotics by granulocyte colony-stimulating factor in neutropenic mice with multidrug-resistant *Enterococcus faecalis* infection. *J Antimicrob Chemother* 2000; 46:429–436.
129. Buisman AM, Langermans JA, van Furth R. Effect of granulocyte colony-stimulating factor on the course of infection with gram-positive bacteria in mice during granulocytopenia induced by sublethal irradiation or cyclophosphamide. *J Infect Dis* 1996; 174:417–421.
130. Fine JS, Cai XY, Justice L, et al. A specific stimulator of granulocyte colony-stimulating factor accelerates recovery from cyclophosphamide-induced neutropenia in the mouse. *Blood* 1997; 90:795–802.
131. Hofer M, Pospisil M, Weiterova L, et al. Combination of drugs elevating extracellular adenosine with granulocyte colony-stimulating factor promotes granulopoietic recovery in the murine bone marrow after 5-fluorouracil treatment. *Physiol Res* 2001; 50:521–524.
132. Douer D, Sagi O, Shaked N, Witz IP, Ramot B. Response to recombinant murine GM-CSF in melphalan treated mice. *Blood* 1987; 70:133a.
133. Monroy RL, Skelly RR, MacVittie TJ, et al. The effect of recombinant GM-CSF on the recovery of monkeys transplanted with autologous bone marrow. *Blood* 1987; 70:1696–1699.
134. Nienhuis AW, Donahue RE, Karlsson S, et al. Recombinant human granulocyte-macrophage colony-stimulating factor (GM-CSF) shortens the period of neutropenia after autologous bone marrow transplantation in a primate model. *J Clin Invest* 1987; 80:573–577.

135. Buisman AM, Langermans JA, van Furth R. Effect of granulocyte-macrophage colony-stimulating factor on the number of leucocytes and course of *Listeria monocytogenes* infection in naive and leucocytopenic mice. *Immunology* 1998; 93:73–79.
136. Naidu NV, Reddi OS. Effect of post-treatment with erythropoietin(s) on survival and erythropoietic recovery in irradiated mice. *Nature* 1967; 214:1223–1224.
137. Reissmann KR, Samorapoompichit S. Effect of erythropoietin on early recovery of erythropoiesis in mice after sublethal dose of 5-fluorouracil. *Proc Soc Exp Biol Med* 1968; 128:898–901.
138. Spivak JL. Recombinant human erythropoietin and the anemia of cancer. *Blood* 1994; 84:997–1004.
139. Thews O, Kelleher DK, Vaupel P. Erythropoietin restores the anemia-induced reduction in cyclophosphamide cytotoxicity in rat tumors. *Cancer Res* 2001; 61:1358–1361.
140. Silver DF, Piver MS. Effects of recombinant human erythropoietin on the antitumor effect of cisplatin in SCID mice bearing human ovarian cancer: a possible oxygen effect. *Gynecol Oncol* 1999; 73:280–284.
141. Stuben G, Thews O, Pottgen C, Knuhmann K, Vaupel P, Stuschke M. Recombinant human erythropoietin increases the radiosensitivity of xenografted human tumours in anaemic nude mice. *J Cancer Res Clin Oncol* 2001; 127:346–350.
142. Thews O, Koenig R, Kelleher DK, Kutzner J, Vaupel P. Enhanced radiosensitivity in experimental tumours following erythropoietin treatment of chemotherapy-induced anaemia. *Br J Cancer* 1998; 78:752–756.
143. Golab J, Olszewska D, Mroz P, et al. Erythropoietin restores the antitumor effectiveness of photodynamic therapy in mice with chemotherapy-induced anemia. *Clin Cancer Res* 2002; 8:1265–1270.
144. Mittelman M, Neumann D, Peled A, Kanter P, Haran-Ghera N. Erythropoietin induces tumor regression and antitumor immune responses in murine myeloma models. *Proc Natl Acad Sci USA* 2001; 98:5181–5186.
145. Du XX, Keller D, Goldman S, Williams DA. Functional effects of interleukin-11 treatment in vivo following bone marrow transplantation (BMT) and combined modality therapy in mice. *Exp Hematol* 1992; 20:768.
146. Opal SM, Jhung JW, Keith JC, et al. Recombinant human interleukin-11 in experimental *Pseudomonas aeruginosa* sepsis in immunocompromised animals. *J Infect Dis* 1998; 178:1205–1208.
147. de Haan G, Donte B, Engel C, Loeffler M, Nijhof W. Prophylactic pretreatment of mice with hematopoietic growth factors induces expansion of primitive cell compartments and results in protection against 5-fluorouracil-induced toxicity. *Blood* 1996; 87:4581–4588.
148. Opal SM, Jhung JW, Keith JC, Jr., Goldman SJ, Palardy JE, Parejo NA. Additive effects of human recombinant interleukin-11 and granulocyte colony-stimulating factor in experimental gram-negative sepsis. *Blood* 1999; 93:3467–3472.
149. Dong F, Brynes RK, Tidow N, Welte K, Lowenberg B, Touw IP. Mutations in the gene for the granulocyte colony-stimulating-factor receptor in patients with acute myeloid leukemia preceded by severe congenital neutropenia. *N Engl J Med* 1995; 333:487–493.
150. Tidow N, Pilz C, Teichmann B, et al. Clinical relevance of point mutations in the cytoplasmic domain of the granulocyte colony-stimulating factor receptor gene in patients with severe congenital neutropenia. *Blood* 1997; 89:2369–2375.
151. Hermans MH, Ward AC, Antonissen C, Karis A, Lowenberg B, Touw IP. Perturbed granulopoiesis in mice with a targeted mutation in the granulocyte colony-stimulating factor receptor gene associated with severe chronic neutropenia. *Blood* 1998; 92:32–39.
152. Hermans MH, Antonissen C, Ward AC, Mayen AE, Ploemacher RE, Touw IP. Sustained receptor activation and hyperproliferation in response to granulocyte colony-stimulating factor (G-CSF) in mice with a severe congenital neutropenia/acute myeloid leukemia-derived mutation in the G-CSF receptor gene. *J Exp Med* 1999; 189:683–692.
153. McLemore ML, Poursine-Laurent J, Link DC. Increased granulocyte colony-stimulating factor responsiveness but normal resting granulopoiesis in mice carrying a targeted granulocyte colony-stimulating factor receptor mutation derived from a patient with severe congenital neutropenia. *J Clin Invest* 1998; 102:483–492.
154. Horwitz M, Benson KF, Person RE, Aprikyan AG, Dale DC. Mutations in ELA2, encoding neutrophil elastase, define a 21-day biological clock in cyclic haematopoiesis. *Nat Genet* 1999; 23:433–436.

155. Dale DC, Person RE, Bolyard AA, et al. Mutations in the gene encoding neutrophil elastase in congenital and cyclic neutropenia. *Blood* 2000; 96:2317–2322.
156. Grenda DS, Johnson SE, Mayer JR, et al. Mice expressing a neutrophil elastase mutation derived from patients with severe congenital neutropenia have normal granulopoiesis. *Blood* 2002; 100:3221–3228.
157. de la Chapelle A, Traskelin AL, Juvonen E. Truncated erythropoietin receptor causes dominantly inherited benign human erythrocytosis. *Proc Natl Acad Sci USA* 1993; 90:4495–4499.
158. Prchal JT, Crist WM, Goldwasser E, Perrine G, Prchal JF. Autosomal dominant polycythemia. *Blood* 1985; 66:1208–1214.
159. Divoky V, Liu Z, Ryan TM, Prchal JF, Townes TM, Prchal JT. Mouse model of congenital polycythemia: homologous replacement of murine gene by mutant human erythropoietin receptor gene. *Proc Natl Acad Sci USA* 2001; 98:986–991.
160. Trapnell BC, Whitsett JA. GM-CSF regulates pulmonary surfactant homeostasis and alveolar macrophage-mediated innate host defense. *Annu Rev Physiol* 2002; 64:775–802.
161. Frossard JL, Saluja AK, Mach N, et al. In vivo evidence for the role of GM-CSF as a mediator in acute pancreatitis-associated lung injury. *Am J Physiol Lung Cell Mol Physiol* 2002; 283:L541–L548.
162. McQualter JL, Darwiche R, Ewing C, et al. Granulocyte macrophage colony-stimulating factor: a new putative therapeutic target in multiple sclerosis. *J Exp Med* 2001; 194:873–882.
163. Campbell IK, Rich MJ, Bischof RJ, Dunn AR, Grail D, Hamilton JA. Protection from collagen-induced arthritis in granulocyte-macrophage colony-stimulating factor-deficient mice. *J Immunol* 1998; 161:3639–3644.
164. Metcalf D. *Hemopoietic Colonies: In Vitro Cloning of Normal and Leukemic Cells.* Berlin, New York: Springer-Verlag. 1977.
165. Brannan CI, Perkins AS, Vogel KS, et al. Targeted disruption of the neurofibromatosis type-1 gene leads to developmental abnormalities in heart and various neural crest-derived tissues. *Genes Dev* 1994; 8:1019–1029.
166. Jacks T, Shih TS, Schmitt EM, Bronson RT, Bernards A, Weinberg RA. Tumour predisposition in mice heterozygous for a targeted mutation in Nf1. *Nat Genet* 1994; 7:353–361.
167. Largaespada DA, Brannan CI, Jenkins NA, Copeland NG. Nf1 deficiency causes Ras-mediated granulocyte/macrophage colony stimulating factor hypersensitivity and chronic myeloid leukaemia. *Nat Genet* 1996; 12:137–143.
168. Zhang YY, Vik TA, Ryder JW, et al. Nf1 regulates hematopoietic progenitor cell growth and ras signaling in response to multiple cytokines. *J Exp Med* 1998; 187:1893–1902.
169. Bollag G, Clapp DW, Shih S, et al. Loss of NF1 results in activation of the Ras signaling pathway and leads to aberrant growth in haematopoietic cells. *Nat Genet* 1996; 12:144–148.
170. Birnbaum RA, O'Marcaigh A, Wardak Z, et al. Nf1 and GM-CSF interact in myeloid leukemogenesis. *Mol Cell* 2000; 5:189–195.
171. Lieschke GJ, Pandolfi PP, Varma S. PLZF-RARα transgenic mice lacking G-CSF, but no those lacking GM-CSF, fail to develop lethal acute myeloid leukemia and live a normal lifespan. *Blood* 2002; 100:189a.
172. Stewart CL, Kaspar P, Brunet LJ, et al. Blastocyst implantation depends on maternal expression of leukaemia inhibitory factor. *Nature* 1992; 359:76–79.
173. Escary JL, Perreau J, Dumenil D, Ezine S, Brulet P. Leukaemia inhibitory factor is necessary for maintenance of haematopoietic stem cells and thymocyte stimulation. *Nature* 1993; 363:361–364.
174. Zheng H, Fletcher D, Kozak W, et al. Resistance to fever induction and impaired acute-phase response in interleukin-1 beta-deficient mice. *Immunity* 1995; 3:9–19.
175. Schorle H, Holtschke T, Hunig T, Schimpl A, Horak I. Development and function of T cells in mice rendered interleukin-2 deficient by gene targeting. *Nature* 1991; 352:621–624.
176. Sadlack B, Merz H, Schorle H, Schimpl A, Feller AC, Horak I. Ulcerative colitis-like disease in mice with a disrupted interleukin-2 gene. *Cell* 1993; 75:203–205.
177. Cockayne DA, Bodine DM, Cline A, Nienhuis AW, Dunbar CE. Transgenic mice expressing antisense interleukin-3 RNA develop a B-cell lymphoproliferative syndrome or neurologic dysfunction. *Blood* 1994; 84:2699–2710.
178. Kopf M, Le Gros G, Bachmann M, Lamers MC, Bluethmann H, Kohler G. Disruption of the murine IL-4 gene blocks Th2 cytokine responses. *Nature* 1993; 362:245–248.
179. von der Weid T, Kopf M, Kohler G, Langhorne J. The immune response to *Plasmodium chabaudi* malaria in interleukin-4-deficient mice. *Eur J Immunol* 1994; 24:2285–2293.

180. Vajdy M, Kosco-Vilbois MH, Kopf M, Kohler G, Lycke N. Impaired mucosal immune responses in interleukin 4-targeted mice. *J Exp Med* 1995; 181:41–53.

181. Kopf M, Brombacher F, Hodgkin PD, et al. IL-5-deficient mice have a developmental defect in CD5+ B-1 cells and lack eosinophilia but have normal antibody and cytotoxic T cell responses. *Immunity* 1996; 4:15–24.

182. Fattori E, Cappelletti M, Costa P, et al. Defective inflammatory response in interleukin 6-deficient mice. *J Exp Med* 1994; 180:1243–1250.

183. Kopf M, Baumann H, Freer G, et al. Impaired immune and acute-phase responses in interleukin-6-deficient mice. *Nature* 1994; 368:339–342.

184. Ramsay AJ, Husband AJ, Ramshaw IA, et al. The role of interleukin-6 in mucosal IgA antibody responses in vivo. *Science* 1994; 264:561–563.

185. Bernad A, Kopf M, Kulbacki R, Weich N, Koehler G, Gutierrez-Ramos JC. Interleukin-6 is required in vivo for the regulation of stem cells and committed progenitors of the hematopoietic system. *Immunity* 1994; 1:725–731.

186. Poli V, Balena R, Fattori E, et al. Interleukin-6 deficient mice are protected from bone loss caused by estrogen depletion. *EMBO J* 1994; 13:1189–1196.

187. von Freeden-Jeffry U, Vieira P, Lucian LA, McNeil T, Burdach SE, Murray R. Lymphopenia in interleukin (IL)-7 gene-deleted mice identifies IL-7 as a nonredundant cytokine. *J Exp Med* 1995; 181:1519–1526.

188. Bunting S, Widmer R, Lipari T, et al. Normal platelets and megakaryocytes are produced in vivo in the absence of thrombopoietin. *Blood* 1997; 90:3423–3429.

189. Carver-Moore K, Broxmeyer HE, Luoh SM, et al. Low levels of erythroid and myeloid progenitors in thrombopoietin-and c-mpl-deficient mice. *Blood* 1996; 88:803–808.

190. Bernstein SE. New mutants: 2. Steel Dickie. *Mouse News Lett* 1960; 23:33–34.

191. Hara T, Ichihara M, Takagi M, Miyajima A. Interleukin-3 (IL-3) poor-responsive inbred mouse strains carry the identical deletion of a branch point in the IL-3 receptor alpha subunit gene. *Blood* 1995; 85:2331–2336.

192. Ichihara M, Hara T, Takagi M, Cho LC, Gorman DM, Miyajima A. Impaired interleukin-3 (IL-3) response of the A/J mouse is caused by a branch point deletion in the IL-3 receptor alpha subunit gene. *EMBO J* 1995; 14:939–950.

193. Miyajima I, Levitt L, Hara T, et al. The murine interleukin-3 receptor alpha subunit gene: chromosomal localization, genomic structure, and promoter function. *Blood* 1995; 85:1246–1253.

194. Morris CF, Salisbury J, Kobayashi M, Townsend PV, Hapel AJ. Interleukin 3 alone does not support the proliferation of bone marrow cells from A/J mice: a novel system for studying the synergistic activities of IL-3. *Br J Haematol* 1990; 74:131–137.

195. de Sauvage FJ, Luoh S-M, Carver-Moore K, et al. Deficiencies in early and late stages of megakaryocytopiesis in TPO-KO mice. *Blood* 1995; 86:255a.

196. Gurney AL, Carver-Moore K, de Sauvage FJ, Moore MW. Thrombocytopenia in c-mpl-deficient mice. *Science* 1994; 265:1445–1447.

197. Kimura S, Roberts AW, Metcalf D, Alexander WS. Hematopoietic stem cell deficiencies in mice lacking c-Mpl, the receptor for thrombopoietin. *Proc Natl Acad Sci USA* 1998; 95:1195–1200.

198. Peschon JJ, Morrissey PJ, Grabstein KH, et al. Early lymphocyte expansion is severely impaired in interleukin 7 receptor-deficient mice. *J Exp Med* 1994; 180:1955–1960.

199. Itohara S, Mombaerts P, Lafaille J, et al. T cell receptor delta gene mutant mice: independent generation of alpha beta T cells and programmed rearrangements of gamma delta TCR genes. *Cell* 1993; 72:337–348.

200. Mombaerts P, Clarke AR, Hooper ML, Tonegawa S. Creation of a large genomic deletion at the T-cell antigen receptor beta-subunit locus in mouse embryonic stem cells by gene targeting. *Proc Natl Acad Sci USA* 1991; 88:3084–3087.

201. Mombaerts P, Clarke AR, Rudnicki MA, et al. Mutations in T-cell antigen receptor genes alpha and beta block thymocyte development at different stages. *Nature* 1992; 360:225–231.

202. Mombaerts P, Mizoguchi E, Grusby MJ, Glimcher LH, Bhan AK, Tonegawa S. Spontaneous development of inflammatory bowel disease in T cell receptor mutant mice. *Cell* 1993; 75:274–282.

203. Cao X, Shores EW, Hu-Li J, et al. Defective lymphoid development in mice lacking expression of the common cytokine receptor gamma chain. *Immunity* 1995; 2:223–238.

204. Suzuki H, Kundig TM, Furlonger C, et al. Deregulated T cell activation and autoimmunity in mice lacking interleukin-2 receptor beta. *Science* 1995; 268:1472–1476.

205. Cacalano G, Lee J, Kikly K, et al. Neutrophil and B cell expansion in mice that lack the murine IL-8 receptor homolog. *Science* 1994; 265:682–684.
206. Moore MW, Cacalano G, Wood WI. Neutrophilia in mice that lack the murine IL-8 receptor homolog. *Science* 1995; 269:591.
207. Shuster DE, Kehrli ME, Jr., Ackermann MR. Neutrophilia in mice that lack the murine IL-8 receptor homolog. *Science* 1995; 269:1590–1591.
208. Fujisawa M, Kobayashi Y, Okabe T, Takaku F, Komatsu Y, Itoh S. Recombinant human granulocyte colony-stimulating factor induces granulocytosis in vivo. *Jpn J Cancer Res* 1986; 77:866–869.
209. Moore MA, Warren DJ. Synergy of interleukin 1 and granulocyte colony-stimulating factor: in vivo stimulation of stem-cell recovery and hematopoietic regeneration following 5-fluorouracil treatment of mice. *Proc Natl Acad Sci USA* 1987; 84:7134–7138.
210. Molineux G, Pojda Z, Dexter TM. A comparison of hematopoiesis in normal and splenectomized mice treated with granulocyte colony-stimulating factor. *Blood* 1990; 75:563–569.
211. Pojda Z, Molineux G, Dexter TM. Hemopoietic effects of short-term in vivo treatment of mice with various doses of rhG-CSF. *Exp Hematol* 1990; 18:27–31.
212. O'Keeffe M, Hochrein H, Vremec D, et al. Effects of administration of progenipoietin 1, Flt-3 ligand, granulocyte colony-stimulating factor, and pegylated granulocyte-macrophage colony-stimulating factor on dendritic cell subsets in mice. *Blood* 2002; 99:2122–2130.
213. Gearing AJ, Metcalf D, Moore JG, Nicola NA. Elevated levels of GM-CSF and IL-1 in the serum, peritoneal and pleural cavities of GM-CSF transgenic mice. *Immunology* 1989; 67:216–220.
214. Metcalf D, Moore JG. Divergent disease patterns in granulocyte-macrophage colony-stimulating factor transgenic mice associated with different transgene insertion sites. *Proc Natl Acad Sci USA* 1988; 85:7767–7771.
215. Daro E, Pulendran B, Brasel K, et al. Polyethylene glycol-modified GM-CSF expands CD11b (high) CD11c (high) but not CD11b (low) CD11c (high) murine dendritic cells in vivo: a comparative analysis with Flt3 ligand. *J Immunol* 2000; 165:49–58.
216. Ikegami M, Ueda T, Hull W, et al. Surfactant metabolism in transgenic mice after granulocyte macrophage-colony stimulating factor ablation. *Am J Physiol* 1996; 270:L650–L658.

3 The Jak-Stat Pathway of Cytokine Signaling

Ben A. Croker, BSc *and Nicos A. Nicola*, PhD

CONTENTS

1. INTRODUCTION

Hematopoiesis is defined by progressive changes in cytokine receptor expression and a delicate balance of intracellular activators and negative regulators of cytokine signaling. Binding of cytokines to their cognate receptors activates downstream signaling pathways and induces biologic responses. The plethora of cytokines that exhibit common structural motifs and use common receptor subunits and signaling pathways supports the notion of a highly redundant system. Mutation or deletion of components of these cytokine-signaling pathways, however, have defined remarkably specific roles for some signaling elements in hematopoiesis and shown their importance in cell survival, proliferation, differentiation, and responses to infection, as well as their potential roles in tumorigenesis.

2. THE JAK-STAT SIGNALING PATHWAY

The proliferation and differentiation of peripheral blood progenitor cell (PBPC) populations to form myeloid, erythroid, and lymphoid populations is controlled by the actions of cytokines. Most cytokine receptors consist of a cytokine-specific binding subunit as well as a signal-transducing subunit, but, unlike many growth factor receptors, such as those for macrophage colony-stimulating factor (M-CSF) and epidermal growth factor (EGF), they generally lack intrinsic kinase activity, rather, cytokine binding to receptor subunits results in homo- or heterodimerization bringing signaling proteins associated with the cytoplasmic domains of the receptors in close contact with each other. The biologic actions of the hematopoietic family of

From: *Cancer Drug Discovery and Development*
Hematopoietic Growth Factors in Oncology: Basic Science and Clinical Therapeutics
Edited by: G. Morstyn, M. A. Foote, and G. J. Lieschke © Humana Press Inc., Totowa, NJ

cytokines are orchestrated by a number of signaling pathways, one of the most important being the Janus kinase-signal transducers and activators of transcription (Jak-Stat) signaling pathway.

The proximity of cytoplasmic tails of receptor subunits after cytokine binding allows the constitutively associated Jaks to cross-phosphorylate each other on tyrosine, further activating their kinase activity and resulting in additional tyrosine phosphorylation of the receptor and other signaling molecules. This action produces docking sites on the receptor for signaling molecules, such as Stat proteins that are subsequently also phosphorylated by Jak. Activated phosphorylated Stat proteins then dissociate from the receptor and homo- or heterodimerize in the cytoplasm before translocating to the nucleus by an ill-defined mechanism to activate transcription (Fig. 1). Other signaling pathways are activated in response to cytokine activation including Src and mitogen-activated protein (MAP) kinases that contribute to proliferation, differentiation, functional activation, and survival of cells. It is envisaged that the cell-specific actions of cytokines could be determined at multiple levels, including expression levels of the receptor and signaling components, presence of negative regulators, and crosstalk between cytokines.

Cytokine receptors are classified according to common structural motifs and can be broadly grouped into five categories: hematopoietin/interferon (IFN; class I/class II) family, receptor tyrosine or serine/threonine kinase family, tumor necrosis factor (TNF)/nerve growth factor (NGF) family, toll-like receptors, and seven-transmembrane receptor family.

This chapter focuses predominantly on the hematopoietin/IFN and tyrosine kinase receptor families. The hematopoietin/IFN receptors contain several conserved features including hematopoietin and IFN receptor domains, as well as fibronectin type III and immunoglobulin-like domains. The hematopoietin and IFN receptor domains contain conserved cysteine and tryptophan residues in their N-terminal region and, in the case of hematopoietin receptors, a conserved tryptophan-serine-X-tryptophan-serine (W-S-X-W-S) sequence in the C-terminus of the extracellular domain (where "X" refers to any amino acid residue). This motif is absent in class II receptors. In contrast, the receptor tyrosine kinase family, which includes receptors for M-CSF, platelet-derived growth factor (PDGF), and stem cell factor (SCF), contains immunoglobulin-like extracellular domains, and intracellular tyrosine kinase domains that distinguish them from other hematopoietic growth factor and IFN receptor family members.

Cytokine families that share similar biologic functions often share common receptor subunits and signaling pathways (Table 1). The gp130 signal-transducing, common receptor β-chain is shared by inflammatory cytokines such as interleukin (IL)-6 and IL-11, leukemia inhibitory factor (LIF), oncostatin M (OSM), ciliary neurotrophic factor (CNTF), and cardiotrophin-1 (CT-1). A unique ligand-binding α-chain provides specificity for each cytokine. The receptors for the hematopoietic family of cytokines, which include IL-3, IL-5, and granulocyte-macrophage colony-stimulating factor (GM-CSF), feature a unique ligand-binding α-chain but share a common β_c signal-transducing subunit. The IL-2 family of immunomodulatory cytokines features a common IL-2γ signal-transducing subunit (γC), shared by IL-2, IL-4, IL-7, IL-9, and IL-15. The β-subunit is an additional signal-transducing subunit for IL-2 and IL-15, and the α-subunit is a unique ligand-binding chain. The IFN family of cytokines signals through separate ligand-binding and signal-transducing chains. IFN-α signals through the IFN-α receptor (IFN-αR). The receptor for IFN-γ comprises both the

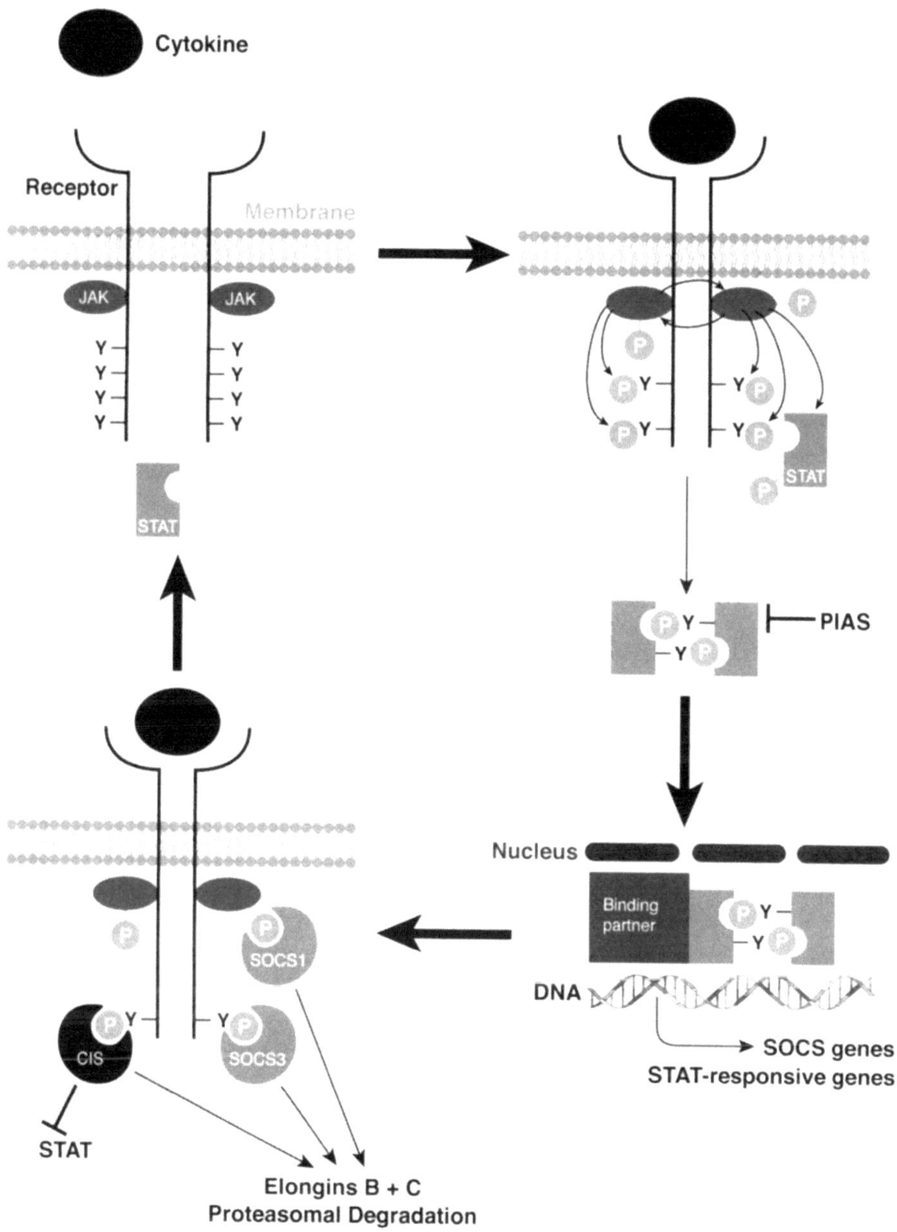

Fig. 1. The Jak-Stat signaling pathway is activated in response to cytokine stimulation. Binding of the ligand to the receptor induces dimerization of the receptor, allowing the constitutively associated Jaks to crossphosphorylate on tyrosine residues, thereby enhancing their kinase activity. Activated Jaks phosphorylate the receptor subunits on tyrosine residues, producing binding sites for Stat proteins, which are themselves phosphorylated by Jak. Phosphorylated Stat proteins dissociate from the receptor and homo- or heterodimerize before translocating to the nucleus, where they induce transcription of target genes. One family of Stat-inducible genes are the suppressors of cytokine signaling *(SOCS)* genes, which form part of a classical negative regulatory feedback mechanism to inhibit cytokine signaling by interfering with Jak kinase activity or by binding to the receptor and thereby preventing access of Stat molecules to phosphorylated tyrosine residues. In addition, SOCS proteins target binding partners for proteasomal degradation via the SOCS box domain. The protein inhibitor of activated Stat (PIAS) proteins can also interact with and inhibit the actions of activated Stat molecules.

Table 1
Hematopoietin (Class I) and Interferon (Class II) Family Receptors

Ligands	*Jak*	*STAT*
gp 130 family		
IL-6	Jak1, Jak2, Tyk2	Stat3, Stat1
IL-11	Jak1, Jak2, Tyk2	Stat3, Stat1
LIF (shares LIFR chain)	Jak1, Jak2, Tyk2	Stat3, Stat1
OSM (shares LIFR chain)	Jak1, Jak2, Tyk2	Stat3, Stat1
Leptin (gp130-related receptor)	Jak2	Stat4
CNTF (also shares LIFR chain)	Jak1, Jak2, Tyk2	Stat3, Stat1
CT-1 (also shares LIFR chain)	Jak1, Jak2, Tyk2	Stat3
IL-12 (gp130-related receptor)	Tyk2, Jak2	Stat4, Stat1, Stat3
IL-23		Stat4
NNT-1/BSF-3 (also shares LIF and CNTF chains)	Jak1, Jak2	Stat3, Stat1
IFN family		
IFN-α/β	Tyk2, Jak1	Stat1, Stat2, Stat3, Stat4, Stat5
IFN-γ	Jak1, Jak2	Stat1, Stat5
IL-10	Tyk2, Jak1	Stat3, Stat1, Stat5
IL-19		
IL-20		Stat3
IL-22	Jak1, Tyk2	Stat1, Stat3, Stat5
IL-3 (gp 140) family		
GM-CSF	Jak2	Stat5
IL-3	Jak2	Stat3, Stat5
IL-5	Jak2	Stat1, Stat3, Stat5
IL-2 (γC) family		
IL-2 (also shares common β-chain)	Jak1, Jak2, Jak3	Stat5, Stat3
IL-4	Jak1, Jak3	Stat6
IL-7	Jak1, Jak3	Stat5, Stat3, Stat1
IL-9	Jak1, Jak3	Stat5, Stat3
IL-15 (also shares common β-chain)	Jak1, Jak3	Stat5, Stat3
IL-21	Jak1, Jak3	Stat5, Stat3, Stat1
IL-13 (shares IL-4Rα chain but not γC)	Jak1, Jak2, Tyk2	Stat3, Stat6
IL-14 (shares α-chain)		
Single-chain family		
EPO	Jak2	Stat5
G-CSF	Jak1, Jak2, Tyk2	Stat1, Stat3, Stat5
GH	Jak2	Stat5
PRL	Jak1, Jak2, Jak3	Stat1, Stat3, Stat5
TPO	Jak2, Tyk2	Stat3, Stat5
Receptor tyrosine kinases		
M-CSF	Tyk2, Jak1	Stat1, Stat3, Stat5
EGF	Jak1, Jak2	Stat1, Stat3, Stat5
PDGF	Jak1, Jak2	Stat1, Stat3
HGF		Stat1, Stat3
SCF	Jak2	Stat1, Stat3, Stat5

(table continues)

Table 1
(continued)

Ligands	*Jak*	*STAT*
Unknown		
IL-17	Jak1, Jak2, Jak3	Stat1, Stat2, Stat3, Stat4
IL-18		Stat3
TSH	Jak1, Jak2	Stat3
Insulin		Stat1, Stat3, Stat5

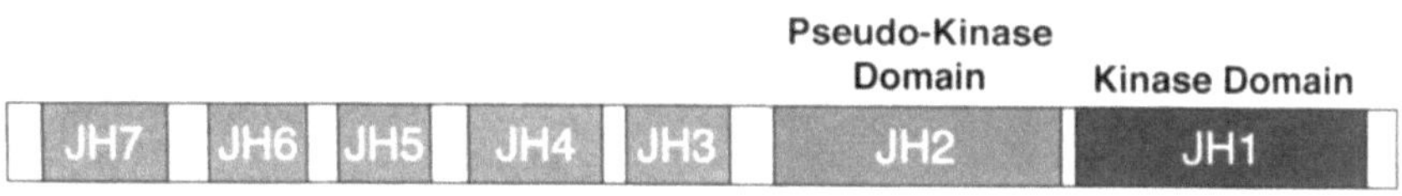

Fig. 2. Jaks are composed of multiple Jak homology (JH) domains. The JH1 domain has tyrosine kinase activity. The JH2 pseudokinase domain is thought to regulate kinase activity, whereas the JH6 and JH7 domains may interact with the receptor.

IFN-γR1 and IFN-γR2 subunits. Similarly, the receptor for IL-10 comprises both the IL-10R1 and IL-10R2 subunits.

The families of receptors for erythropoietin (EPO), growth hormone (GH), thrombopoietin (TPO), and prolactin (PRL) consist of homodimers of a single-receptor chain specific for each cytokine. Unlike the aforementioned cytokine receptors that lack intrinsic tyrosine kinase activity, the receptor tyrosine and serine/threonine kinases, such as receptors for EGF, M-CSF, and PDGF, can phosphorylate and activate signaling cascade components independently of Jak.

The receptor chains and receptor-associated Jaks are brought in close contact upon cytokine binding, allowing trans-phosphorylation on tyrosine. The Jaks contain four family members—Jak1, Jak2, Jak3, and Tyk2. They appear to be ubiquitously expressed, except for Jak3, in which expression is restricted to hematopoietic cells. Structurally, the Jaks are characterized by seven Jak homology (JH) domains (Fig. 2). The C-terminal tyrosine kinase JH1 and pseudokinase JH2 domains constitute a large portion of these 120–130-kDa proteins. The N-terminal JH3–JH7 domains are smaller, and their function is unclear. Studies suggest that the JH6–JH7 domains may be important for interaction with the receptor, whereas the JH2 pseudokinase domain (which lacks any detectable kinase activity) may be important for regulation of kinase activity.

2.1. Biologic Outcome of Jak/Stat Activation

Many of the biologic effects of cytokines are mediated by the Stat transcription factors. The Stat proteins are cytoplasmic proteins that are recruited to receptors and activated by tyrosine phosphorylation upon cytokine stimulation before translocating to the nucleus as dimers to initiate transcription of a wide range of genes (Fig. 3). This affects a plethora of cellular activities, as evidenced by the phenotype of mice deficient in Jaks and Stats. Despite the in vitro evidence suggesting a highly redundant system, deletion of individual Jaks and Stats resulted in highly specific effects on

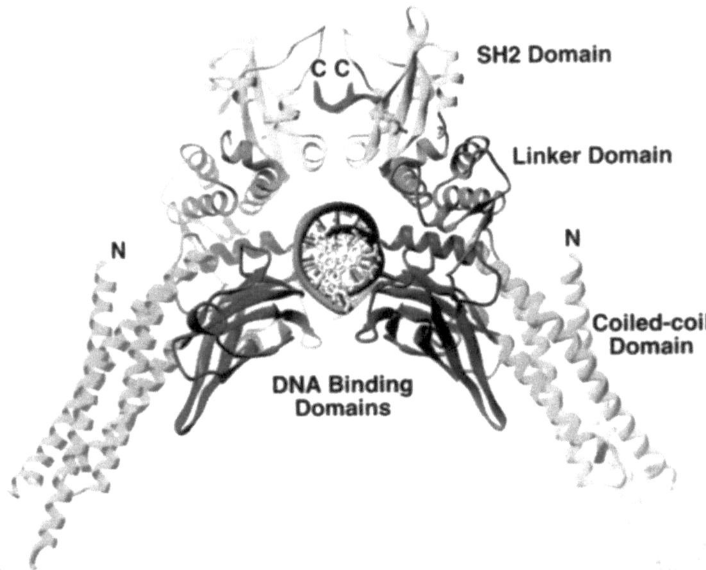

Fig. 3. Structure of Stat protein dimers. Stat proteins bind to the receptor through C-terminal SH2 domains and are phosphorylated on tyrosine (pY) and serine (pY) residues. Stat proteins homo- or heterodimerize by reciprocal SH2-pY interactions and translocate to the nucleus. Stats then bind DNA through the DNA-binding domain to initiate transcription. (Adapted from ref. *128*, with permission from J. Kuriyan.)

cytokine pathways, demonstrating nonredundant roles for these proteins. The results of these gene deletion studies are summarized below and in Table 2.

2.2. Jak1

Jak1-deficient mice are 40% smaller than littermates and die within 24 h of birth, probably as a result of failure of neurogenesis *(1)*. Signaling was ablated in response to IFN-γ, IFN-α, and IL-10, as well as cytokines that use the γC and gp130 chains. The absence of IL-7 signaling is thought to be largely responsible for a failure of lymphocyte development with an absence of T-lymphocyte development and a block in B-cell development at the transition from the pro-B to the pre-B cell. The response of Jak1-deficient macrophages, cardiomyocytes, and neurons to gp130 family members IL-6, CT-1, and LIF was severely perturbed.

2.3. Jak2

Jak2 can bind to receptors for TPO, GH, EPO, β-common chain-containing receptors (GM-CSF, IL-3, and IL-5), CT-1, PRL, G-CSF, and gp130-containing receptors (IL-6, CNTF, LIF, and OSM) *(2)*. Disruption of the ubiquitously expressed Jak2 results in embryonic lethality at E12.5 owing to the failure of definitive erythropoiesis *(3,4)*, a phenotype analogous to but more severe than that observed in mice deficient in the EPO receptor *(5)*. In the presence of EPO and IL-3, Jak2-deficient fetal liver cells failed to produce erythroid colony-forming units (CFU-E), erythroid blast-forming units (BFU-E), and mixed colony-forming units (CFU-Mix). Jak2-null cells failed to respond to TPO, GM-CSF, IL-3, and IFN-γ, and the number of progenitors was reduced in response to M-

Table 2
Phenotype of Mice Deficient for Jak, Stat, and SOCS Proteins

Gene	*Phenotype*
Jak1	Postnatal lethal owing to neurologic defect, defects in thymocyte and B-cell production
Jak2	E12.5 embryonic lethal—failure of definitive erythropoiesis
Jak3	Failure of lymphocyte development, increased apoptosis
Tyk2	Susceptible to bacteria and viral challenge
Stat1	Susceptible to bacteria and viral challenge and chemically induced tumors, defects in FGF-induced chondrocyte proliferation
Stat2	Susceptible to viral infection
Stat3	E7.5 embryonic lethal owing to defects in mesoderm; IL-6 activates Stat 1 signaling
Stat3 (conditional)	Increased granulocyte production, defects in hepatocyte acute-phase response, survival and proliferation of T cells, neuron survival, skin defects
Stat4	Loss of IL-12 responses; decreased NK cell activity, IFN-γ production and Th1 cell formation
Stat5a/b	Female infertility, same as for Stat5a and Stat5b, absent NK cells, reduced myeloid and lymphoid transformation by Tel-Jak2 but not v-Abl or BCR-Abl
Stat5a	Defects in mammary growth and lactation, T-cell proliferation, and GM-CSF-induced proliferation of macrophages
Stat5b	Defects in NK cell activity, growth, and male-specific gene expression in liver
Stat6	Defects in MHC class II expression, B- and T-cell proliferation, class switching to IgE, Th2 differentiation
CIS	Viable and fertile
SOCS1	Neonatal lethal owing to IFN-γ dependent inflammation
SOCS2	Gigantism
SOCS3	E 12.5 embryonic lethal owing to placental insufficiency
SOCS6	Modest growth retardation

ABBREVIATIONS: CIS, cytokine-inducible SH2 containing protein; DC, dendritic cell; FGF, fibroblast growth factor; GM-CSF, granulocyte-macrophage colony-stimulating factor; NK, natural killer; SOCS, suppressor of cytokine signaling; Stat, signal transducers and activators of transcription.

CSF and SCF. Development of lymphoid populations and responses to gp130-related cytokines and G-CSF were normal. Because of the embryonic lethality, it remains undefined what effect Jak2 deficiency has on PRL and growth hormone signaling.

2.4. Jak3

Jak3 binds to the γ common chain of the IL-2 family of cytokine receptors, whose signals are obligatory for lymphocyte development. Not unexpectedly, disruption of Jak3 in mice resulted in severe perturbations in lymphocyte development caused predominantly by defects in IL-7 signaling *(6–8)*, analogous to that observed in γ common chain-deficient mice *(9,10)*. In addition, a patient with mutations in both copies of the Jak3 allele displayed severe combined immunodeficiency *(11)*. B-cell development was blocked at the pre-B-cell stage, and T-lymphocyte development was severely affected, resulting in a reduction in thymic size and cellularity. Proliferation of Jak3-deficient T-cells was blunted in response to various mitogenic stimuli including IL-2, IL-4, IL-7, lipopolysaccharide (LPS), and activation of the T-cell receptor and T-cell co-receptor, CD28.

2.5. Tyk2

Tyk2 was originally isolated as a component involved in IFN-αR signaling. Deletion of Tyk2 in mice perturbed Stat3 activation in response to IFN-α/β and IL-12 and established a role for Tyk2 in innate and adaptive immunity *(12)*. Tyk2-deficient macrophages showed a decrease in Stat3 activation in response to IFN-α/β and IFN-γ and a decrease in IFN-γ and LPS-induced nitric oxide production. Mice deficient in Tyk2 had increased susceptibility to viral pathogens, such as vesicular stomatitis virus (VSV), lymphocytic choriomeningitis virus (LCMV), and vaccinia virus (VV), demonstrating defective antiviral IFN-dependent cytotoxic T-lymphocyte (CTL) activity. It is thought that Tyk2 serves to amplify and sustain specific cytokine responses through a Tyk2-Stat3 or Tyk2-Stat1 pathway rather than initiating signaling through IFN and gp130 receptors.

2.6. Stat1

In vitro studies suggested that Stat1 would be required for signaling downstream of a multitude of receptors including those for IFNs, gp130-related cytokines, PRL, and a variety of receptor tyrosine kinases. Disruption of the Stat1 gene in mice, however, interfered specifically with type 1 and type II IFN signaling pathways, demonstrating the remarkable specificity of Stat1, or perhaps suggesting that other Stat proteins are able to compensate for the loss of Stat1 in signaling pathways other than those for IFN. Stat1-deficient animals were born at the expected mendelian frequencies but were runted and generally died within 48 h of birth of opportunistic viral infections *(13)*.

Hematopoiesis was normal in adult Stat1-deficient animals bred under pathogen-free conditions; however, responses to IFN were absent. As a result, challenge with VSV, at a 10^6-fold lower dose than controls, was fatal for these mice *(14)*. Among other growth-inhibitory defects in Stat1-deficient mice was the lack of chondrocyte growth inhibition in response to fibroblast growth factor-1 (FGF-1) *(15)*.

2.7. Stat2

Type I IFN induces antiviral and antiproliferative effects in cells through the formation of Stat1/Stat2 heterodimers or Stat1 homodimers. Stat2-deficient primary mouse embryonic fibroblasts (PMEFs) responded poorly to IFN-α but normally to IFN-γ, whereas Stat2-deficient macrophages responded normally to IFN-α and IFN-γ, suggesting that IFN-α-induced gene upregulation in macrophages is Stat2-independent *(16)*. Stat2-deficient PMEFs were more sensitive to VSV in the presence or absence of IFN-α and IFN-γ. In these cells, the failure of an autocrine loop of induction of IFN-α by IFN-γ is believed to be responsible for the failure of IFN-γ to afford protection to the cells. Consistently, Stat2-null animals were more susceptible to VSV at doses up to 6 logs lower than for controls. Antagonism of T-cell proliferation by IFN-α after in vivo challenge with dexamethasone was absent in Stat2-deficient animals, resulting in enhanced recovery of thymic T-cell populations.

2.8. Stat3

Stat3 is activated in response to gp130-related cytokines as well as G-CSF, GM-CSF, leptin, and EGF. Unlike other members of the Stat family in which gene deletion affects specific signaling pathways, Stat3 gene ablation affects signaling downstream of a myriad of cytokine receptors *(17,18)*. Stat3 deficiency is embryonic lethal at E7 with a failure of mesoderm formation. Conditional gene deletion of Stat3 using a Cre-loxP strategy has overcome embryonic lethality and defined the roles of this protein in various adult mouse tissues. Conditional deletion of Stat3 impaired the acute-phase response in the liver, altered survival of neurons in the central nervous system, affected apoptosis in mammary epithelium as well as wound repair and keratinocyte migration in the skin, enhanced the inflammatory response, increased granulocyte production when targeted to macrophages and neutrophils, and perturbed survival and proliferation of T-lymphocytes *(19–21)*.

2.9. Stat4

This transcription factor is activated only in response to IL-12 *(22,23)*. Deletion of Stat4 in mice abrogated IL-12-induced IFN-γ production and skewed differentiation of CD4+ T-helper cells. Despite the normal development of Stat4-deficient mice, there was an increase in Th2 cells and a corresponding increase in IL-4, IL-5, and IL-10 production in vitro and when challenged with *Listeria monocytogenes (24)*.

2.10. Stat5

Stat5a and Stat5b are 95% identical in amino acid sequence and were assumed to be redundant for responses to GH, TPO, EPO, IL-2, GM-CSF, and PRL. Mice deficient in Stat5a and/or Stat5b have been generated, and they have both specific and redundant functions downstream of numerous cytokine receptors. Stat5a-deficient bone marrow-derived macrophages and T lymphocytes exhibited defects in proliferation in response to GM-CSF and IL-2, respectively *(25,26)*. Defects in T-cell proliferation and reductions in peripheral T-cell populations have been attributed at least in part to defects in IL-2-induced upregulation of the IL-2Rα chain. Disruption of Stat5a prevented mammary lobuloalveolar outgrowth during pregnancy and lactation after parturition, indicating a specific role for Stat5a in mammopoietic and lactogenic signaling *(27)*. Stat5b-deficient mice demonstrated impaired IL-2- and IL-15-induced proliferation of splenocytes, reductions in natural killer (NK) cell populations, and decreases in expression of IL-2Rβ chain and perforin *(28)*. Stat5b was required for the sexual dimorphism of body growth rates and gene expression in the liver, as well as for normal lactation, reproduction, fat deposition, and hair growth *(29)*. Deletion of both Stat5a and Stat5b abrogated responses to IL-2, IL-3, IL-5, IL-7, and GM-CSF, partially explaining reductions in B lymphocytes and peripheral T lymphocytes *(30,31)*. Using a competitive repopulation assay, it was shown that Stat5a/b is required for long-term repopulation of the hematopoietic compartment *(32)*. In addition, Stat5a/b mutant mice were significantly smaller than Stat5b-deficient animals, and the female infertility was caused by abnormal ovarian development and associated defects in progesterone secretion *(33)*.

2.11. Stat6

Stat6 is required for the actions of IL-4 on B and T lymphocytes. Stat6-deficient B lymphocytes have low proliferative capacity in response to IL-4 and submitogenic doses of anti-IgM antibody. Upregulation of the major histocompatibility complex (MHC) class II, as well as the low-affinity IgE receptor CD23, was abolished in response to IL-4 in the absence of Stat6. In T lymphocytes, Stat6 was essential for IL-4-induced proliferation and CD4+ T-cell differentiation and production of Th2 cytokines. When challenged with nematode, production of Th2-associated cytokines such as IL-4, IL-5, and IL-10, as well as Th2-type immunoglobulins such as IgG1 and IgE, was profoundly reduced *(34–36)*.

2.12. Regulation of the Jak-Stat Pathway

Numerous positive and negative regulatory mechanisms exist to modify the specificity, intensity, and duration of signals transduced from the cytokine receptor at the cell membrane to the promoter and enhancer elements of responsive genes in the nucleus. The action of Stat transcription factors is modulated by positive regulatory factors such as serine kinase pathways, chromatin remodeling proteins, and other transcription factors. Serine phosphorylation of Stat appears to modulate the transcriptional activity at defined Stat target promoters. Stat1 serine phosphorylation was shown to be important for the expression of IFN-γ target genes and for the recruitment of specific serine kinase pathways to individual Stat proteins to modulate activity at Stat-specific promoters *(37)*. Several reports have outlined the interaction of Stat proteins with other transcription factors and chromatin remodeling proteins. For example, Stat proteins have been shown to interact with CBP/p300, a chromatin remodeling protein, and numerous transcription factors such as NF-κB, PU.1, Sp1, c-Jun, and the glucocorticoid receptor *(38–45)*. It is perhaps oversimplified to view the action of dimerized Stat transcription factors in the nucleus independently of other interacting partners.

Given the diversity of actions of Stat proteins in cellular proliferation, differentiation, and survival, it is not surprising that multiple negative regulatory mechanisms also exist to control Stat activation.

First, prolonged engagement of the cytokine receptor by ligand and cell stimulation is limited by receptor endocytosis and degradation. For some cytokine/receptor systems, production of soluble receptors by receptor proteolysis or alternate mRNA splicing competes for the limiting amounts of ligand in the extracellular environment.

Second, degradation of signaling components by ubiquitin-mediated proteolysis also inhibits cytokine signaling. Proteasomal inhibitors prolong the activity of Jak and the activation of tyrosine-phosphorylated forms of Stat *(46–50)*. Candidates for coupling Jak and Stat to proteasomal degradation machinery include SOCS1 and SOCS3, which bind directly to Jak, receptors such as gp130, and elongins B and C *(51)*.

Third, Jaks are activated by tyrosine phosphorylation, and several phosphatases interact directly and deactivate Jak and Stat or bind to the receptor to inhibit signaling *(52–55)*. Mutation of SHP1 recruitment sites on the EPO receptor results in enhanced Jak activity and EPO signaling *(56)*. Similarly, prolonged Stat3 signaling was reported in gp130 mutant mice that failed to recruit the ubiquitously expressed SHP-2 phosphatase *(53)*. Expression of dominant negative Stat isoforms can interfere with signaling *(57–59)*.

Activated Stat proteins can be negatively regulated by interactions with protein inhibitor of activated Stat (PIAS) proteins, of which there are five family members. PIAS1 and PIAS3 bind to and inhibit Stat1 and Stat3, respectively *(60,61)*. The functions of the remaining three members of the PIAS family, PIASy, PIASxα and PIASxβ, remain unclear.

A fundamental negative regulatory mechanism of Jak-Stat cytokine signaling uses the suppressor of cytokine signaling (SOCS) proteins (reviewed in refs. *62* and *63*). The SOCS family has eight members—CIS (cytokine-induced SRC-homology 2 [SH2]protein) and SOCS1–7. This family is characterized by a central SH2 domain, a variable N-terminus, and a SOCS box motif at the C-terminus. Basal expression levels of SOCS family members are generally low but can be rapidly upregulated (often by the Stats themselves) in response to cytokine stimulation, thereby forming part of a classical negative feedback loop. The mechanism of Jak-Stat inhibition by SOCS proteins differs. For example, SOCS1 binds directly to tyrosine phosphorylated Jak through the SOCS SH2 domain and then inhibits kinase activity through the SOCS kinase inhibitory region (KIR), which is N-terminal of the SH2 domain and acts as a pseudosubstrate inhibitor. In contrast, SOCS3 has a higher binding affinity for the phosphorylated receptor than to Jak but nevertheless inhibits Jak activity by a similar mechanism to that of SOCS1. The SOCS box can bind to elongins B and C and through them to cullin 5 and RBX-1, to form an E3 ubiquitin ligase complex that targets SOCS-bound proteins for proteasome-mediated degradation *(51)*.

The critical role of SOCS proteins in the negative regulation of cytokine signaling is demonstrated by mice deficient in these proteins. SOCS1-deficient mice die within 3 wk of birth owing to IFN-γ-mediated fatty degeneration of the liver and infiltration of multiple organs including muscle, heart, lung, and pancreas with inflammatory cells *(64,65)*. SOCS2-deficient mice are characterized by gigantism caused by excessive signaling by the growth hormone/insulin-like growth factor-1 (IGF-1) axis *(66)*. SOCS3 deficiency is embryonic lethal owing to placental insufficiency *(67)*. A conditional deletion of SOCS3 using a Cre-loxP strategy will be required to elucidate the role of SOCS3 in specific adult mouse tissues. SOCS6-deficient animals have a mild growth retardation owing to abnormal responses to IGFs *(68)*. CIS-deficient mice appear to have no significant abnormalities.

3. ONCOGENIC CAPACITY OF THE JAK-STAT SIGNALING PATHWAY

Oncogenesis is a discontinuous, progressive transformation of cells into a malignant and metastatic cell population. Tumor development depends on alterations in the genome and aberrant proliferation owing to autonomous growth-promoting signals, unresponsiveness to extracellular and intracellular growth-inhibitory signals, and evasion of apoptosis. Subsequent progression of the cancer into a malignant and metastatic phenotype relies on unrestrained replicative potential, avoidance of immune surveillance, stimulation of angiogenesis, inappropriate tissue invasion, and metastasis. Coverage of all intracellular signaling pathways associated with oncogenesis is beyond the scope of this chapter, and we focus instead predominantly on the roles of the Jak-Stat pathway and selected members of the Src family protein tyrosine kinases as well as the SOCS proteins.

Although Stat transcription factors have not been implicated in DNA damage detection and repair systems, numerous reports outline their involvement in cell-cycle progression, apoptosis, and cytokine-induced survival, proliferation, and growth inhibition *(69–74)*. Indeed, numerous data show the presence of activated Stat proteins in a variety of cancers (reviewed in refs. *75* and *76*). Numerous studies indicate that activation of Jak-Stat pathways is required for transformation by the oncoprotein, v-src, which drives expression of c-myc, an important mediator of cell proliferation and differentiation *(77–82)*. It is important, however, to distinguish between a primary role for these proteins in disease progression and secondary consequences of tumorigenesis. To this end, it should be established both in cell lines and in animal models that activation or removal of a component of the signaling pathway, such as the Jak-Stat pathway, is essential or sufficient for cellular transformation or oncogenesis. The growth-suppressive functions of Stat1 indicate that it may be a potent tumor suppressor, evidenced by an increase in susceptibility to tumors in murine Stat1 knockout models. Numerous studies in cell lines and in vivo have shown the oncogenic potential of Jak1, Jak2, Jak3, Stat3, and Stat5. Circumstantial evidence in mouse models and methylation and expression patterns have indicated that SOCS proteins may also act as tumor-suppressor proteins.

Growth of tumors such as childhood acute lymphoblastic leukemia (ALL) is often dependent on cytokine stimulation, presumably through a paracrine or autocrine pathway, which induces phosphorylation and activation of receptors and associated signaling pathways, including the Jak-Stat pathway. Specific inhibition of Jak2 in ALL and acute myeloid leukemia (AML) by the tyrphostin AG490, a specific tyrosine kinase blocker, inhibited proliferation and induced apoptosis of leukemic cells without significant perturbations in hematopoiesis *(83,84)*. Another form of ALL is associated with a chromosomal translocation fusing the catalytic kinase domain of Jak2 with an ETS transcription factor family member TEL, also known as ETV6. TEL is characterized by a DNA-binding domain (conserved in ETS family members) and importantly, a helix-loop-helix oligomerization domain that allows TEL-Jak2 to dimerize and activate Jak2 kinase activity, thereby activating signaling pathways. Other common cytogenetic rearrangements resulting in neoplastic growth include TEL-ABL and TEL-AML fusions *(85–88)*. The TEL-Jak2 and TEL-ABL, but not BCR-ABL fusion proteins induced Stat3 and Stat5 activation and cytokine-independent growth of an IL-3-dependent BaF3 hematopoietic cell line *(84,89,90)*.

The growth-suppressive and proapoptotic activities of Stat1 in response to cytokines such as IFN-γ, TNF-α, and IL-6 are well documented. In the absence of Stat1, deficiencies occur in constitutive expression of caspases and IFN-γ-induced expression of caspase 1 and the cyclin-dependent kinase inhibitor $p21^{WAF1/CIP1}$ leading to an impairment of cell growth arrest and apoptosis *(91–94)*. An important step in tumor development is evasion of the immune system, in which IFN-γ plays an important role by upregulating expression of MHC proteins for antigen presentation. As described earlier, Stat1-

deficient mice are unresponsive to both type I and II IFN, and mice deficient in Stat1 or the IFN-γ receptor are more susceptible to spontaneous or chemical carcinogen-induced tumor development. The progression of tumor development is greater in mice deficient in both p53 and the IFN-γR than for p53-deficient mice, and the variety of tumors is more diverse *(95)*. Recent evidence indicates that IFN-γ can support effects on cell proliferation and induce an antiviral state independently of Stat1, suggesting that results obtained from mice deficient in IFN-γ may not necessarily be equivalent to those simply deficient in Stat1 *(96,97)*.

Extensive data describe activated Stat3 and Stat5 in tumors. Activating mutations of Stat3 and Stat5 and specific inhibition of Stat3 and Stat5 by gene deletion, antisense oligonucleotides, or dominant negative approaches have highlighted the importance of Stat3 and Stat5 in tumor formation. Mutations of Stat3 that allow spontaneous dimerization of the monomers in the absence of interactions between phosphorylated tyrosines and SH2 domains are sufficient to cause transformation and induce tumor formation in nude mice *(98)*. Inhibition of Stat3 signaling using antisense *Stat3* or by a Jak-selective tyrosine kinase inhibitor, AG490, restored the sensitivity of cells from patients with large granular lymphocyte (LGL) leukemia to Fas-mediated apoptosis *(99)*. Downregulation of Fas correlates with an increase in metastatic potential and resistance of tumors to chemically and physically induced apoptosis. This effect is mediated, at least in part, by an interaction between Stat3 and *c-jun*, which decreases expression of Fas *(100)*. Fas expression is increased in mice with a heterozygous disruption of *Stat3* or a homozygous deletion of *c-jun*. Furthermore, mutation of promoter binding sites for c-jun (AP-1) and Stat3 (GAS) increases Fas expression. Expression of dominant negative Stat3 increases Fas in a mouse melanoma model, decreases proliferation in a breast carcinoma model, and promotes apoptosis in a human myeloma cell line by inhibiting expression of the antiapoptotic protein Bcl-x_L *(100–102)*. Inhibition of Stat3 using antisense *Stat3* oligonucleotides inhibits proliferation and induces apoptosis in human prostate cancer cells and squamous cell carcinoma cell lines *(103,104)*. Inhibition of Stat3 in a murine head and neck xenograft tumor model using liposome-delivered plasmid antisense *STAT3* gene therapy inhibited proliferation and induced apoptosis in the tumor by downregulating expression of the antiapoptotic protein Bcl-x_L *(105)*. An activating mutation at Asp_{816} of c-kit, a receptor tyrosine kinase for SCF, is associated with numerous malignancies and is characterized by constitutive activation of Stat3. Overexpression of dominant negative Stat3 inhibited anchorage-independent growth of mutant c-kit cell lines and tumor formation in NOD/SCID mice *(106)*.

In these studies in which Stat3 function is inhibited by various approaches, it is assumed that the inhibition of proliferation and induction of apoptosis is directly linked to an absence of Stat3 function, and investigators have speculated on techniques of intervention in tumor formation by specific inhibition of Stat3. It was shown that Stat3-deficient, primary embryonic fibroblasts stimulated with IL-6 produce an IFN-γ-like response by activation of Stat1 and upregulation of IFN-γ-inducible genes, producing an antiviral response in the presence or absence of IFN-γ *(107)*. Stat3 conditional knockout mice display increased Stat1 activation in bone marrow *(21)*. It is unclear by what mechanism Stat3 provides specificity for IL-6 signaling and prevents activation of an IFN-γ-like Stat1-mediated response, but it has profound implications for the potential use of specific Stat3 inhibitors in the clinic.

Like Stat3, Stat5 also plays a fundamental role in regulation of proliferation, differentiation, and apoptosis of hematopoietic cells *(108)* by coordinating the expression of SOCS proteins as well as antiapoptotic genes such as *bcl-xL* and *pim-1* and growth-inhibitory genes such as $p21^{WAF1/Cip1}$. The TEL/Jak2 fusion protein, found in ALL and chronic myelogenous leukemia (CML), induced a myelo- and lymphoproliferative disease when TEL/Jak2 transformed bone marrow cells were transplanted into ablated recipients but had no effect on a *Stat*5a/b null background. *Stat*5a/b was not required for TEL/Jak2-induced growth factor-independent murine bone marrow-colony formation *(109)*. Importantly, expression of a constitutively active version of Stat5a in bone marrow recapitulated the phenotype of bone marrow transformed by TEL/Jak2. In acute promyelocytic leukemia (APL), a Stat5b-retinoic acid receptor α (RARα) fusion protein has been identified. RARα is a member of the nuclear hormone receptor family and serves to regulate differentiation and growth inhibition *(110)*. In this model, the Stat5b-RARα fusion protein altered transcription of target genes by binding retinoic acid response elements (RAREs) as a homodimer or as a heterodimer with the retinoid X receptor α (RXRα). In CML, BCR-ABL activates Stat5 through interactions with Jak *(111)*. Using a dominant negative approach, Stat5 activation was shown to be essential for proliferation, evasion of apoptosis, and tumor progression in a BCR-ABL-dependent model for leukemia in mice *(112)*. Overexpression of dominant negative Stat5a suppresses BCR-ABL-driven proliferation of Ba/F3 cells *(113)*. In the WAP-Tag transgenic mouse model for mammary cancer, 86% of the adenocarcinomas display activated Stat5a. Loss of one allele of Stat5a in transgenic mice reduced tumor incidence, reduced the size and time of first onset of tumors, and increased the apoptotic index of mammary cancer cells *(114)*. In mammary carcinoma cells, PRL induces proliferation by inducing cyclin D1 expression through a Jak2/Stat5 signaling pathway *(115)*.

Several studies indicate that insufficiency in negative regulation of Jak-Stat pathways by the SOCS proteins could contribute to oncogenesis *(116,117)*. SOCS1 inhibits transformation by TEL-Jak2, an activated c-KIT receptor, v-ABL and to a lesser degree BCR-ABL but not transformation induced by TEL-ABL, v-SRC, or RasV12 *(118–120)*. Mutation of the SH2 domain prevented SOCS1 inhibition of TEL-Jak2-induced cellular transformation, but not that of the mutant KIT receptor, indicating that more than one mechanism of tumor-suppressor activity exists for SOCS1. SOCS1 overexpression with TEL-Jak2 can prolong the latency period of murine bone marrow transplants compared with TEL-Jak2 alone. One mechanism for negative regulation of TEL-Jak2-mediated cellular proliferation is the SOCS-box dependent proteasomal degradation of TEL-Jak2 *(121)*. Importantly, SOCS1-deficient fibroblasts are more sensitive to transformation induced by TEL-Jak2 or activated KIT. Other studies have shown that the presence of SOCS1 does not necessarily inhibit the oncogenic activity of TEL-Jak2, which bypasses the actions of SOCS1 *(122)*. Similarly, constitutive expression of SOCS1 and SOCS3 in AML or cutaneous T-cell lymphoma may reflect the constitutive activation of cytokine-signaling pathways rather than reflecting inhibition of autocrine or paracrine cytokine-induced Stat3 activation *(123,124)*. In some human primary tumors, including human hepatocellular carcinoma and multiple myeloma, silencing of the *SOCS-1* gene by hypermethylation and loss of heterozygosity suggest a direct tumor suppressor role of SOCS-1 *(117,125–127)*.

4. CONCLUSIONS

An overwhelming body of literature describes aberrant Jak-Stat signaling in several human tumors. Specific inhibition of Jak and Stat in cell lines and animal models using chemical or peptide inhibitors, dominant negative proteins, and antisense oligonucleotides, as well as gene deletions have proved conclusively the importance of individual components of the Jak-Stat signaling pathway to oncogenesis. Inhibitors of the Jak-Stat pathway will be of significant value to current cancer treatment regimens. It would be envisaged that significant gains in treatment and patient outcomes will be achieved when these inhibitors are used in combination with improved diagnostic tools for understanding the unique biochemical profiles of tumors. Evidence indicates that inhibition of one signaling pathway can have unexpected effects on other signaling cascades, highlighting the importance of careful investigation of new therapeutics.

ACKNOWLEDGMENTS

The authors have been supported by the National Health and Medical Research Council, Canberra, Australia; the Cooperative Research Centres Program of the Australian Government; AMRAD Operations Pty. Ltd., Melbourne, Australia; and the National Institutes of Health, Grant CA22556

REFERENCES

1. Rodig SJ, Meraz MA, White JM, et al. Disruption of the Jak1 gene demonstrates obligatory and nonredundant roles of the Jaks in cytokine-induced biologic responses. *Cell* 1998; 93:373–383.
2. Kisseleva T, Bhattacharya S, Braunstein J, Schindler CW. Signaling through the JAK/STAT pathway, recent advances and future challenges. *Gene* 2002; 285:1–24.
3. Parganas E, Wang D, Stravopodis D, et al. Jak2 is essential for signaling through a variety of cytokine receptors. *Cell* 1998; 93:385–395.
4. Neubauer H, Cumano A, Muller M, et al. Jak2 deficiency defines an essential developmental checkpoint in definitive hematopoiesis. *Cell* 1998; 93:397–409.
5. Wu H, Liu X, Jaenisch R, Lodish HF. Generation of committed erythroid BFU-E and CFU-E progenitors does not require erythropoietin or the erythropoietin receptor. *Cell* 1995; 83:59–67.
6. Park SY, Saijo K, Takahashi T, et al. Developmental defects of lymphoid cells in Jak3 kinase-deficient mice. *Immunity* 1995; 3:771–782.
7. Thomis DC, Gurniak CB, Tivol E, Sharpe AH, Berg LJ. Defects in B lymphocyte maturation and T lymphocyte activation in mice lacking Jak3. *Science* 1995; 270:794–797.
8. Nosaka T, van Deursen JM, Tripp RA, et al. Defective lymphoid development in mice lacking Jak3. *Science* 1995; 270:800–802.
9. DiSanto JP, Muller W, Guy-Grand D, Fischer A, Rajewsky K. Lymphoid development in mice with a targeted deletion of the interleukin 2 receptor gamma chain. *Proc Natl Acad Sci USA* 1995; 92:377–381.
10. Cao X, Shores EW, Hu-Li J, et al. Defective lymphoid development in mice lacking expression of the common cytokine receptor gamma chain. *Immunity* 1995; 2:223–238.
11. Russell SM, Tayebi N, Nakajima H, et al. Mutation of Jak3 in a patient with SCID: essential role of Jak3 in lymphoid development. *Science* 1995; 270:797–800.
12. Karaghiosoff M, Neubauer H, Lassnig C, et al. Partial impairment of cytokine responses in Tyk2-deficient mice. *Immunity* 2000; 13:549–560.
13. Durbin JE, Hackenmiller R, Simon MC, Levy DE. Targeted disruption of the mouse Stat1 gene results in compromised innate immunity to viral disease. *Cell* 1996; 84:443–450.
14. Meraz MA, White JM, Sheehan KC, et al. Targeted disruption of the Stat1 gene in mice reveals unexpected physiologic specificity in the Jak-Stat signaling pathway. *Cell* 1996; 84:431–442.
15. Sahni M, Ambrosetti DC, Mansukhani A, et al. FGF signaling inhibits chondrocyte proliferation and regulates bone development through the STAT-1 pathway. *Genes Dev* 1999; 13:1361–1366.

16. Park C, Li S, Cha E, Schindler C. Immune response in Stat2 knockout mice. *Immunity* 2000 13:795–804.
17. Takeda K, Noguchi K, Shi W, et al. Targeted disruption of the mouse Stat3 gene leads to early embryonic lethality. *Proc Natl Acad Sci USA* 1997; 94:3801–3804.
18. Levy DE, Lee CK. What does Stat3 do? *J Clin Invest* 2002; 109:1143–1148.
19. Akaishi H, Takeda K, Kaisho T, et al. Defective IL-2-mediated IL-2 receptor alpha chain expression in Stat3- deficient T lymphocytes. *Int Immunol* 1998; 10:1747–1751.
20. Takeda K, Clausen BE, Kaisho T, et al. Enhanced Th1 activity and development of chronic enterocolitis in mice devoid of Stat3 in macrophages and neutrophils. *Immunity* 1999; 10:39–49.
21. Lee C, Raz R, Gimeno R, et al. STAT3 Is a negative regulator of granulopoiesis but is not required for G-CSF-dependent differentiation. *Immunity* 2002; 17:63–72.
22. Bacon CM, Petricoin EF 3rd, Ortaldo JR, et al. Interleukin 12 induces tyrosine phosphorylation and activation of STAT4 in human lymphocytes. *Proc Natl Acad Sci USA* 1995; 92:7307–7311.
23. Jacobson NG, Szabo SJ, Weber-Nordt RM, et al. Interleukin 12 signaling in T helper type 1 (Th1) cells involves tyrosine phosphorylation of signal transducer and activator of transcription (Stat)3 and Stat4. *J Exp Med* 1995; 181:1755–1762.
24. Kaplan MH, Sun YL, Hoey T, Grusby MJ. Impaired IL-12 responses and enhanced development of Th2 cells in Stat4-deficient mice. *Nature* 1996; 382:174–177.
25. Feldman GM, Rosenthal LA, Liu X, et al. STAT5A-deficient mice demonstrate a defect in granulocyte-macrophage colony-stimulating factor-induced proliferation and gene expression. *Blood* 1997; 90:1768–1776.
26. Nakajima H, Liu XW, Wynshaw-Boris A, et al. An indirect effect of Stat5a in IL-2-induced proliferation: a critical role for Stat5a in IL-2-mediated IL-2 receptor alpha chain induction. *Immunity* 1997; 7:691–701.
27. Liu X, Robinson GW, Wagner KU, et al. Stat5a is mandatory for adult mammary gland development and lactogenesis. *Genes Dev* 1997; 11:179–186.
28. Imada K, Bloom ET, Nakajima H, et al. Stat5b is essential for natural killer cell-mediated proliferation and cytolytic activity. *J Exp Med* 1998; 188:2067–2074.
29. Udy GB, Towers RP, Snell RG, et al. Requirement of STAT5b for sexual dimorphism of body growth rates and liver gene expression. *Proc Natl Acad Sci USA* 1997; 94:7239–7244.
30. Moriggl R, Topham DJ, Teglund S, et al. Stat5 is required for IL-2-induced cell cycle progression of peripheral T cells. *Immunity* 1999; 10:249–259.
31. Moriggl R, Sexl V, Piekorz R, Topham D, Ihle JN. Stat5 activation is uniquely associated with cytokine signaling in peripheral T cells. *Immunity* 1999; 11:225–230.
32. Bunting KD, Bradley HL, Hawley TS, et al. Reduced lymphomyeloid repopulating activity from adult bone marrow and fetal liver of mice lacking expression of STAT5. *Blood* 2002; 99:479–487.
33. Teglund S, McKay C, Schuetz E, et al. Stat5a and Stat5b proteins have essential and nonessential, or redundant, roles in cytokine responses. *Cell* 1998; 93:841–850.
34. Takeda K, Tanaka T, Shi W, et al. Essential role of Stat6 in IL-4 signalling. *Nature* 1996; 380:627–630.
35. Shimoda K, van Deursen J, Sangster MY, et al. Lack of IL-4-induced Th2 response and IgE class switching in mice with disrupted Stat6 gene. *Nature* 1996; 380:630–633.
36. Kaplan MH, Schindler U, Smiley ST, Grusby MJ. Stat6 is required for mediating responses to IL-4 and for development of Th2 cells. *Immunity* 1996; 4:313–319.
37. Kovarik P, Mangold M, Ramsauer K, et al. Specificity of signaling by STAT1 depends on SH2 and C-terminal domains that regulate Ser727 phosphorylation, differentially affecting specific target gene expression. *EMBO J* 2001; 20:91–100.
38. Bhattacharya S, Eckner R, Grossman S, et al. Cooperation of Stat2 and p300/CBP in signalling induced by interferon-alpha. *Nature* 1996; 383:344–347.
39. Look DC, Pelletier MR, Tidwell RM, Roswit WT, Holtzman MJ. Stat1 depends on transcriptional synergy with Sp1. *J Biol Chem* 1995; 270:30264–30267.
40. Aittomaki S, Pesu M, Groner B, et al. Cooperation among Stat1, glucocorticoid receptor, and PU.1 in transcriptional activation of the high-affinity Fc gamma receptor I in monocytes. *J Immunol* 2000; 164:5689–5697.
41. Martino A, Holmes JHt, Lord JD, Moon JJ, Nelson BH. Stat5 and Sp1 regulate transcription of the cyclin D2 gene in response to IL-2. *J Immunol* 2001; 166:1723–1729.
42. Ohmori Y, Schreiber RD, Hamilton TA. Synergy between interferon-gamma and tumor necrosis factor-alpha in transcriptional activation is mediated by cooperation between signal transducer and activator of transcription 1 and nuclear factor kappaB. *J Biol Chem* 1997; 272:14899–14907.

43. Zhang X, Wrzeszczynska MH, Horvath CM, Darnell JE Jr. Interacting regions in Stat3 and c-Jun that participate in cooperative transcriptional activation. *Mol Cell Biol* 1999; 19:7138–7146.
44. Stocklin E, Wissler M, Gouilleux F, Groner B. Functional interactions between Stat5 and the glucocorticoid receptor. *Nature* 1996; 383:726–728.
45. Wyszomierski SL, Rosen JM. Cooperative effects of STAT5 (signal transducer and activator of transcription 5) and C/EBPbeta (CCAAT/enhancer-binding protein-beta) on beta-casein gene transcription are mediated by the glucocorticoid receptor. *Mol Endocrinol* 2001; 15:228–240.
46. Kim TK, Maniatis T. Regulation of interferon-gamma-activated STAT1 by the ubiquitin-proteasome pathway. *Science* 1996; 273:1717–1719.
47. Wang D, Moriggl R, Stravopodis D, et al. A small amphipathic alpha-helical region is required for transcriptional activities and proteasome-dependent turnover of the tyrosine-phosphorylated Stat5. *EMBO J* 2000; 19:392–399.
48. Yu CL, Burakoff SJ. Involvement of proteasomes in regulating Jak-Stat pathways upon interleukin-2 stimulation. *J Biol Chem* 1997; 272:14017–14020.
49. Callus BA, Mathey-Prevot B. Hydrophobic residues Phe751 and Leu753 are essential for STAT5 transcriptional activity. *J Biol Chem* 2000; 275:16954–16962.
50. Haspel RL, Salditt-Georgieff M, Darnell JE Jr. The rapid inactivation of nuclear tyrosine phosphorylated Stat1 depends upon a protein tyrosine phosphatase. *EMBO J* 1996; 15:6262–6268.
51. Zhang JG, Farley A, Nicholson SE, et al. The conserved SOCS box motif in suppressors of cytokine signaling binds to elongins B and C and may couple bound proteins to proteasomal degradation. *Proc Natl Acad Sci USA* 1999; 96:2071–2076.
52. Irie-Sasaki J, Sasaki T, Matsumoto W, et al. CD45 is a JAK phosphatase and negatively regulates cytokine receptor signalling. *Nature* 2001; 409:349–354.
53. Ohtani T, Ishihara K, Atsumi T, et al. Dissection of signaling cascades through gp130 in vivo: reciprocal roles for STAT3- and SHP2-mediated signals in immune responses. *Immunity* 2000; 12:95–105.
54. Yi T, Mui AL, Krystal G, Ihle JN. Hematopoietic cell phosphatase associates with the interleukin-3 (IL-3) receptor beta chain and down-regulates IL-3-induced tyrosine phosphorylation and mitogenesis. *Mol Cell Biol* 1993; 13:7577–7586.
55. Yu CL, Jin YJ, Burakoff SJ. Cytosolic tyrosine dephosphorylation of STAT5. Potential role of SHP-2 in STAT5 regulation. *J Biol Chem* 2000; 275:599–604.
56. Klingmuller U, Lorenz U, Cantley LC, Neel BG, Lodish HF. Specific recruitment of SH-PTP1 to the erythropoietin receptor causes inactivation of JAK2 and termination of proliferative signals. *Cell* 1995; 80:729–738.
57. Caldenhoven E, van Dijk TB, Solari R, et al. STAT3beta, a splice variant of transcription factor STAT3, is a dominant negative regulator of transcription. *J Biol Chem* 1996; 271:13221–13227.
58. Kieslinger M, Woldman I, Moriggl R, et al. Antiapoptotic activity of Stat5 required during terminal stages of myeloid differentiation. *Genes Dev* 2000; 14:232–244.
59. Piazza F, Valens J, Lagasse E, Schindler C. Myeloid differentiation of FdCP1 cells is dependent on Stat5 processing. *Blood* 2000; 96:1358–1365.
60. Liao J, Fu Y, Shuai K. Distinct roles of the NH2- and COOH-terminal domains of the protein inhibitor of activated signal transducer and activator of transcription (STAT) 1 (PIAS1) in cytokine-induced PIAS1-Stat1 interaction. *Proc Natl Acad Sci USA* 2000; 97:5267–5272.
61. Chung CD, Liao J, Liu B, et al. Specific inhibition of Stat3 signal transduction by PIAS3. *Science* 1997; 278:1803–1805.
62. Alexander WS. Suppressors of cytokine signalling (SOCS) in the immune system. *Nat Rev Immunol* 2002; 2:410–416.
63. Nicola NA, Greenhalgh CJ. The suppressors of cytokine signaling (SOCS) proteins: important feedback inhibitors of cytokine action. *Exp Hematol* 2000; 28:1105–1112.
64. Alexander WS, Starr R, Fenner JE, et al. SOCS1 is a critical inhibitor of interferon gamma signaling and prevents the potentially fatal neonatal actions of this cytokine. *Cell* 1999; 98:597–608.
65. Starr R, Metcalf D, Elefanty AG, et al. Liver degeneration and lymphoid deficiencies in mice lacking suppressor of cytokine signaling-1. *Proc Natl Acad Sci USA* 1998; 95:14395–14399.
66. Metcalf D, Greenhalgh CJ, Viney E, et al. Gigantism in mice lacking suppressor of cytokine signalling-2. *Nature* 2000; 405:1069–1073.
67. Roberts AW, Robb L, Rakar S, et al. Placental defects and embryonic lethality in mice lacking suppressor of cytokine signaling 3. *Proc Natl Acad Sci USA* 2001; 98:9324–9329.

68. Krebs DL, Uren RT, Metcalf D, et al. SOCS-6 binds to insulin receptor substrate 4, and mice lacking the SOCS- 6 gene exhibit mild growth retardation. *Mol Cell Biol* 2002; 22:4567–4578.
69. de Veer MJ, Holko M, Frevel M, et al. Functional classification of interferon-stimulated genes identified using microarrays. *J Leukoc Biol* 2001; 69:912–920.
70. Bromberg JF. Activation of STAT proteins and growth control. *Bioessays* 2001; 23:161–169.
71. Takeshita T, Arita T, Higuchi M, et al. STAM, signal transducing adaptor molecule, is associated with Janus kinases and involved in signaling for cell growth and c-myc induction. *Immunity* 1997; 6:449–457.
72. Chapman RS, Lourenco PC, Tonner E, et al. Suppression of epithelial apoptosis and delayed mammary gland involution in mice with a conditional knockout of Stat3. *Genes Dev* 1999; 13:2604–2616.
73. Fukada T, Ohtani T, Yoshida Y, et al. STAT3 orchestrates contradictory signals in cytokine-induced G1 to S cell-cycle transition. *EMBO J* 1998; 17:6670–6677.
74. Epling-Burnette PK, Zhong B, Bai F, et al. Cooperative regulation of Mcl-1 by Janus kinase/Stat and phosphatidylinositol 3-kinase contribute to granulocyte-macrophage colony-stimulating factor-delayed apoptosis in human neutrophils. *J Immunol* 2001; 166:7486–7495.
75. Turkson J, Jove R. STAT proteins: novel molecular targets for cancer drug discovery. *Oncogene* 2000; 19:6613–6626.
76. Bromberg J. Stat proteins and oncogenesis. *J Clin Invest* 2002; 109:1139–1142.
77. Kiuchi N, Nakajima K, Ichiba M, et al. STAT3 is required for the gp130-mediated full activation of the c-myc gene. *J Exp Med* 1999; 189:63–73.
78. Turkson J, Bowman T, Garcia R, et al. Stat3 activation by Src induces specific gene regulation and is required for cell transformation. *Mol Cell Biol* 1998; 18:2545–2552.
79. Bromberg JF, Horvath CM, Besser D, Lathem WW, Darnell JE, Jr. Stat3 activation is required for cellular transformation by v-src. *Mol Cell Biol* 1998; 18:2553–2558.
80. Yu CL, Meyer DJ, Campbell GS, et al. Enhanced DNA-binding activity of a Stat3-related protein in cells transformed by the Src oncoprotein. *Science* 1995; 269:81–83.
81. Turkson J, Ryan D, Kim JS, et al. Phosphotyrosyl peptides block Stat3-mediated DNA binding activity, gene regulation, and cell transformation. *J Biol Chem* 2001; 276:45443–45455.
82. Bowman T, Broome MA, Sinibaldi D, et al. Stat3-mediated Myc expression is required for Src transformation and PDGF-induced mitogenesis. *Proc Natl Acad Sci USA* 2001; 98:7319–7324.
83. Meydan N, Grunberger T, Dadi H, et al. Inhibition of acute lymphoblastic leukemia by a Jak-2 inhibitor. *Nature* 1996; 379:645–648.
84. Spiekermann K, Biethahn S, Wilde S, Hiddemann W, Alves F. Constitutive activation of STAT transcription factors in acute myelogenous leukemia. *Eur J Haematol* 2001; 67:63–71.
85. Papadopoulos P, Ridge SA, Boucher CA, Stocking C, Wiedemann LM. The novel activation of ABL by fusion to an ets-related gene, TEL. *Cancer Res* 1995; 55:34–38.
86. Romana SP, Mauchauffe M, Le Coniat M, et al. The t(12; 21) of acute lymphoblastic leukemia results in a tel-AML1 gene fusion. *Blood* 1995; 85:3662–3670.
87. Golub TR, Barker GF, Bohlander SK, et al. Fusion of the TEL gene on 12p13 to the AML1 gene on 21q22 in acute lymphoblastic leukemia. *Proc Natl Acad Sci USA* 1995; 92:4917–4921.
88. Romana SP, Poirel H, Leconiat M, et al. High frequency of t(12;21) in childhood B-lineage acute lymphoblastic leukemia. *Blood* 1995; 86:4263–4269.
89. Lacronique V, Boureux A, Valle VD, et al. A TEL-JAK2 fusion protein with constitutive kinase activity in human leukemia. *Science* 1997; 278:1309–1312.
90. Peeters P, Raynaud SD, Cools J, et al. Fusion of TEL, the ETS-variant gene 6 (ETV6), to the receptor-associated kinase JAK2 as a result of t(9; 12) in a lymphoid and t(9; 15; 12) in a myeloid leukemia. *Blood* 1997; 90:2535–2540.
91. Kumar A, Commane M, Flickinger TW, Horvath CM, Stark GR. Defective TNF-alpha-induced apoptosis in STAT1-null cells due to low constitutive levels of caspases. *Science* 1997; 278:1630–1632.
92. Chin YE, Kitagawa M, Su WC, et al. Cell growth arrest and induction of cyclin-dependent kinase inhibitor p21 WAF1/CIP1 mediated by STAT1. *Science* 1996; 272:719–722.
93. Chin YE, Kitagawa M, Kuida K, Flavell RA, Fu XY. Activation of the STAT signaling pathway can cause expression of caspase 1 and apoptosis. *Mol Cell Biol* 1997; 17:5328–5337.
94. Bromberg JF, Horvath CM, Wen Z, Schreiber RD, Darnell JE Jr. Transcriptionally active Stat1 is required for the antiproliferative effects of both interferon alpha and interferon gamma. *Proc Natl Acad Sci USA* 1996; 93:7673–7678.
95. Kaplan DH, Shankaran V, Dighe AS, et al. Demonstration of an interferon gamma-dependent tumor surveillance system in immunocompetent mice. *Proc Natl Acad Sci USA* 1998; 95:7556–7561.

96. Gil MP, Bohn E, O'Guin AK, et al. Biologic consequences of Stat1-independent IFN signaling. *Proc Natl Acad Sci USA* 2001; 98:6680–6685.
97. Ramana CV, Gil MP, Han Y, et al. Stat1-independent regulation of gene expression in response to IFN-gamma. *Proc Natl Acad Sci USA* 2001; 98:6674–6679.
98. Bromberg JF, Wrzeszczynska MH, Devgan G, et al. Stat3 as an oncogene. *Cell* 1999; 98:295–303.
99. Epling-Burnette PK, Liu JH, Catlett-Falcone R, et al. Inhibition of STAT3 signaling leads to apoptosis of leukemic large granular lymphocytes and decreased Mcl-1 expression. *J Clin Invest* 2001; 107:351–362.
100. Ivanov VN, Bhoumik A, Krasilnikov M, et al. Cooperation between STAT3 and c-jun suppresses Fas transcription. *Mol Cell* 2001; 7:517–528.
101. Catlett-Falcone R, Landowski TH, Oshiro MM, et al. Constitutive activation of Stat3 signaling confers resistance to apoptosis in human U266 myeloma cells. *Immunity* 1999; 10:105–115.
102. Li L, Shaw PE. Autocrine-mediated activation of STAT3 correlates with cell proliferation in breast carcinoma lines. *J Biol Chem* 2002; 277:17397–17405.
103. Gao B, Shen X, Kunos G, et al. Constitutive activation of Jak-Stat3 signaling by BRCA1 in human prostate cancer cells. *FEBS Lett* 2001; 488:179–184.
104. Grandis JR, Drenning SD, Chakraborty A, et al. Requirement of Stat3 but not Stat1 activation for epidermal growth factor receptor-mediated cell growth In vitro. *J Clin Invest* 1998; 102:1385–1392.
105. Grandis JR, Drenning SD, Zeng Q, et al. Constitutive activation of Stat3 signaling abrogates apoptosis in squamous cell carcinogenesis in vivo. *Proc Natl Acad Sci USA* 2000; 97:4227–4232.
106. Ning ZQ, Li J, McGuinness M, Arceci RJ. STAT3 activation is required for Asp(816) mutant c-Kit induced tumorigenicity. *Oncogene* 2001; 20:4528–4536.
107. Costa-Pereira AP, Tininini S, Strobl B, et al. Mutational switch of an IL-6 response to an interferon-gamma-like response. *Proc Natl Acad Sci USA* 2002; 99:8043–8047.
108. Nosaka T, Kawashima T, Misawa K, et al. STAT5 as a molecular regulator of proliferation, differentiation and apoptosis in hematopoietic cells. *EMBO J* 1999; 18:4754–4765.
109. Schwaller J, Parganas E, Wang D, et al. Stat5 is essential for the myelo- and lymphoproliferative disease induced by TEL/JAK2. *Mol Cell* 2000; 6:693–704.
110. Dong S, Tweardy DJ. Interactions of STAT5b-RARalpha, a novel acute promyelocytic leukemia fusion protein, with retinoic acid receptor and STAT3 signaling pathways. *Blood* 2002; 99:2637–2646.
111. Shuai K, Halpern J, ten Hoeve J, Rao X, Sawyers CL. Constitutive activation of STAT5 by the BCR-ABL oncogene in chronic myelogenous leukemia. *Oncogene* 1996; 13:247–254.
112. Nieborowska-Skorska M, Wasik MA, Slupianek A, et al. Signal transducer and activator of transcription (STAT)5 activation by BCR/ABL is dependent on intact Src homology (SH)3 and SH2 domains of BCR/ABL and is required for leukemogenesis. *J Exp Med* 1999; 189:1229–1242.
113. Nosaka T, Kitamura T. Pim-1 expression is sufficient to induce cytokine independence in murine hematopoietic cells, but is dispensable for BCR-ABL mediated transformation. *Exp Hematol* 2002; 30:697–702.
114. Ren S, Cai HR, Li M, Furth PA. Loss of Stat5a delays mammary cancer progression in a mouse model. *Oncogene* 2002; 21:4335–4339.
115. Brockman JL, Schroeder MD, Schuler LA. PRL activates the cyclin D1 promoter via the Jak2/Stat pathway. *Mol Endocrinol* 2002; 16:774–784.
116. Nagai H, Kim YS, Lee KT, et al. Inactivation of SSI-1, a JAK/STAT inhibitor, in human hepatocellular carcinomas, as revealed by two-dimensional electrophoresis. *J Hepatol* 2001; 34:416–421.
117. Yoshikawa H, Matsubara K, Qian GS, et al. SOCS-1, a negative regulator of the JAK/STAT pathway, is silenced by methylation in human hepatocellular carcinoma and shows growth-suppression activity. *Nat Genet* 2001; 28:29–35.
118. Iwamoto T, Senga T, Naito Y, et al. The JAK-inhibitor, JAB/SOCS-1 selectively inhibits cytokine-induced, but not v-Src induced Jak-Stat activation. *Oncogene* 2000; 19:4795–4801.
119. Rottapel R, Ilangumaran S, Neale C, et al. The tumor suppressor activity of SOCS-1. *Oncogene* 2002; 21:4351–4362.
120. Frantsve J, Schwaller J, Sternberg DW, Kutok J, Gilliland DG. Socs-1 inhibits TEL-JAK2-mediated transformation of hematopoietic cells through inhibition of JAK2 kinase activity and induction of proteasome- mediated degradation. *Mol Cell Biol* 2001; 21:3547–3557.
121. Kamizono S, Hanada T, Yasukawa H, et al. The SOCS box of SOCS-1 accelerates ubiquitin-dependent proteolysis of TEL-JAK2. *J Biol Chem* 2001; 276:12530–12538.
122. Monni R, Santos SC, Mauchauffe M, et al. The TEL-Jak2 oncoprotein induces Socs1 expression and altered cytokine response in Ba/F3 cells. *Oncogene* 2001; 20:849–858.

123. Schuringa JJ, Wierenga AT, Kruijer W, Vellenga E. Constitutive Stat3, Tyr705, and Ser727 phosphorylation in acute myeloid leukemia cells caused by the autocrine secretion of interleukin-6. *Blood* 2000; 95:3765–3770.
124. Brender C, Nielsen M, Kaltoft K, et al. STAT3-mediated constitutive expression of SOCS-3 in cutaneous T-cell lymphoma. *Blood* 2001; 97:1056–1062.
125. Zardo G, Tiirikainen MI, Hong C, et al. Integrated genomic and epigenomic analyses pinpoint biallelic gene inactivation in tumors. *Nat Genet* 2002; 32:453–458.
126. Galm O, Yoshikawa H, Esteller M, Osieka R, Herman JG. SOCS-1, a negative regulator of cytokine signaling, is frequently silenced by methylation in multiple myeloma. *Blood* 2002; 27:27.
127. Nagai H, Kim Y, Konishi N, et al. Combined hypermethylation and chromosome loss associated with inactivation of SSI-1/SOCS-1/JAB gene in human hepatocellular carcinomas. *Cancer Lett* 2002; 186:59.
128. Chen X, Vinkemeier U, Zhao Y, et al. Crystal structure of a tyrosine phosphorylated STAT-1 dimer bound to DNA. *Cell* 1998; 93:827–839.

4 Small-Molecule and Peptide Agonists

A Literature Review

Ellen G. Laber, PhD and
C. Glenn Begley, MBBS, PhD, FRACP, FRCPath, FRCPA

CONTENTS

1. INTRODUCTION

Hematopoietic growth factors (HGFs) have proved to be clinically successful therapeutics; however, their size (15–70 kDa), conformational instability, susceptibility to proteolytic degradation, poor membrane penetration, antigenicity, high cost of production, and unfavorable pharmacokinetics can make them less than ideal drug candidates. Furthermore, the poor bioavailability of the native proteins requires that they be administered parenterally. It would be advantageous, therefore, to develop small-molecule agonists (and antagonists) of HGF receptors that are equipotent to their polypeptide counterparts but that lack some of the inherent drawbacks of large proteins. The identification and examination of smaller peptides that bind to and activate cytokine receptors may provide a better understanding of ligand-receptor interactions, which could be used to design orally available small-molecule cytokine mimetics rationally. Recent advances in both small-molecule and small-peptide agonists are reviewed here.

Activation of transmembrane receptors by growth factors and cytokines occurs when a ligand binds to a specific domain on the receptor, thereby inducing a conformational change *(1)* and triggering dimerization or oligomerization of receptor chains. Upon ligand binding, several members of the class I cytokine receptors form homodimers, including the erythropoietin receptor (EPOR), thrombopoietin receptor

From: *Cancer Drug Discovery and Development*
Hematopoietic Growth Factors in Oncology: Basic Science and Clinical Therapeutics
Edited by: G. Morstyn, M. A. Foote, and G. J. Lieschke © Humana Press Inc., Totowa, NJ

(TPOR), granulocyte colony-stimulating factor receptor (G-CSFR), growth hormone receptor (GHR), and prolactin receptor (PrR) *(2)*. Several studies have been reported that are directed toward discovering the precise details of the dimerization interfaces and the degree to which the unliganded receptors exist as dimers *(3–5)*. The results of these studies have shown structural and functional similarities between the class I cytokine receptors. Studies also have shown that receptor dimerization alone, although necessary for intracellular signaling, is not sufficient to produce signal transduction *(6)*. Until recently, mediation of this complex series of events seemed impossible by a small molecule or peptide; however, recent reports have shown that both small molecules and peptides can bind to and activate homodimeric cytokine receptors by acting as agonists and mimicking the effects of the natural proteins.

2. CONSTRUCTION AND SCREENING OF SMALL-MOLECULE AND PEPTIDE LIBRARIES

Cloning of hematopoietic receptors has provided targets to screen small molecules and peptides for hematopoietic agonist *(7)* and antagonist *(8)* activity. By constructing compound libraries and using high-throughput automation, hundreds of thousands of small molecules and peptides have been screened against these targets to identify, and subsequently optimize, lead molecules. Although the techniques for constructing small-molecule and peptide libraries are very different, the same types of high-throughput screening (HTS) assays (competitive binding and functional assays) are used to screen both classes of compounds.

2.1. Assays for Receptor Binding

Molecules must bind to the cytokine receptor before dimerization can occur. To screen for molecules that display receptor binding and to determine receptor-binding affinity, small-molecule and peptide libraries are screened against the immobilized extracellular domain (ECD) of a receptor or cells engineered to express the receptor. Molecules that demonstrate binding may be receptor antagonists. These molecules are devoid of intrinsic activity, but they block the response to the cytokine by interacting with the receptor. Once identified, receptor antagonists can be dimerized or oligomerized by way of various linking strategies to generate potential receptor agonists *(1)*.

2.2. Assays for Functional Activity

In functional assays, compounds are screened against a cell line that has, for example, been engineered to respond to a cytokine-induced signaling event using a light-generating luciferase reporter *(9)*. The cell line expresses the functional cytokine receptor of interest, and compounds that activate this receptor cause cells to emit light. Competitive binding assays identify compounds that bind to the receptor, whereas functional assays reveal compounds that initiate receptor activation, thereby identifying agonists directly.

2.3. Principles of Small-Molecule Library Construction

Small-molecule libraries usually comprise approx 10^6 organic compounds (molecular weights < 600 amu) that have been prepared by combinatorial and/or traditional medicinal chemistry techniques (classic synthesis). Because both traditional chemistry and combinatorial chemistry offer distinct advantages, they frequently are combined. Libraries also may contain natural product extracts that are isolated from native environmental sources.

Using traditional medicinal chemistry, one molecule at a time is synthesized through a series of solution-phase organic reactions. The advantages of this method include easy isolation and identification of individual molecules, creativity of molecule design, and ability to synthesize complex molecules that may be unavailable from other sources. The major disadvantage of using this method to construct small-molecule libraries is the extensive amount of time required.

In combinatorial chemistry, large numbers of structurally diverse molecules are produced by synthesizing all possible combinations from a set of smaller chemical entities *(10)*. Combinatorial chemical reactions are usually performed on solid phase, in which part of the target molecule is covalently attached to an insoluble support or resin. Then, split synthesis (see below) is used to generate the small-molecule library. Solid-supported chemistry was first optimized in peptide and oligonucleotide synthesis and subsequently applied to small-molecule synthesis. One advantage of generating combinatorial arrays in solid phase is that compounds are easily isolated by washing away reagents from the solid supports. Furthermore, reactions can be driven to completion using excess reagents. Another advantage of solid-phase combinatorial chemistry is that nucleotide, chemical, or radio-encoded tags can be attached to the solid support, which simplifies compound identification *(11)*.

Combinatorial chemistry can also be performed in solution using parallel array synthesis *(12)*. Dynamic combinatorial chemistry, in which the "building blocks" are assembled through reversible chemical reactions in the presence of the target ligand or receptor, is a recent method of preparing small-molecule libraries and offers a new dimension for combinatorial chemistry *(10,13)*.

2.3.1. Split Synthesis

The split synthesis strategy generates libraries of equimolar mixtures of compounds by using repetitive "split and mix" operations *(14)*. A quantity of polymer resin is first split into equal portions and placed into separate reaction vessels. Different chemical entities are attached to each portion of resin, the individual portions are recombined, and a second set of chemical entities is added. After mixing thoroughly, the polymer resin is reapportioned into the requisite number of reaction vessels *(11)*. This procedure allows all the possible combinations of the two sets of chemical entities to be incorporated. The split, react, and mix operations are repeated for each new set of chemical entities added. The total number of compounds generated by this method is obtained by multiplying together the number of chemical entities that are used in each synthesis step.

By incorporating automated systems into the split synthesis process, the time involved in executing the repetitive split and mix operations is greatly reduced *(15–17)*. The disadvantage of split synthesis is that pools (mixtures of compounds) are created; thus, deconvolution (i.e., identifying individual compounds from the mixtures) of the synthesized library is necessary. Fortunately, many solutions to the deconvolution problem have been developed, such as the positional scanning approach *(18)*, the orthogonal library method *(19)*, structural determination by automated analytical methods *(20,21)*, and various encoding strategies *(22–24)*.

2.3.2. Parallel Synthesis

In contrast to the mixtures of compounds that are produced by the split and mix procedure, individual compounds are generated through parallel synthesis *(25)*. In this technique, many compounds are synthesized in parallel in spatially separate reaction vessels. The advantage of this method is that the identity of each compound in a particular location is known and can be confirmed directly. Furthermore, when the library is assayed, individual compounds that demonstrate the desired activity are easily isolated.

Many automated systems for performing parallel synthesis have been reported *(26)*. The first system was introduced by Geyson and coworkers for the mapping of peptide epitopes *(27)* and later applied to the synthesis of small molecules. Subsequently, many other systems designed exclusively for small molecules were developed *(28,29)*.

2.4. Approaches to Peptide Library Construction

In the last 10 years, numerous strategies have been developed to identify peptides that mimic the biologic effects of HGFs *(30–32)*. These methods generate large recombinant-peptide libraries that are screened against immobilized receptor protein. The most common strategy for evaluating peptide libraries uses expression of peptides on bacteriophage (phage display). Other methods include lac repressor display, headpiece dimer display, and polysome display. These approaches have been reviewed *(33)*.

2.4.1. Phage Display

In phage display, mixtures of randomly assembled oligonucleotides are spliced into the genes that encode the filamentous bacteriophage coat proteins and transformed into bacteria *(31)*. Recombinant DNA techniques are used to produce large numbers of bacteriophage that carry random surface peptide sequences. This method generates libraries of up to 10^9 bacteriophage that are easily screened in competitive binding assays by incubating the altered phage with an immobilized cytokine receptor protein. The bacteriophage that demonstrate binding to the receptor are captured and eluted from the immobilized receptor, and the inserted peptide genes are sequenced *(9)*. This process typically identifies a consensus of the residues critical for binding. The consensus sequence can be used, with a new group of amino acids, to generate a second library of peptide genes that have a higher binding affinity for the receptor. After performing this procedure several times, individual peptides can be tested for cell-based receptor binding and biologic activity in functional assays. Typically, these high-affinity peptides are dimerized to generate potential receptor agonists.

2.4.2. Peptides-on-Plasmids

In the peptides-on-plasmids method (also referred to as lac repressor display) the nucleic acid sequences that will encode the library of random peptides are fused to the C-terminus of the *Escherichia coli* lac repressor *(34)*. This method is a clever strategy that allows for rapid selection of desired peptides. The DNA-binding activity of the repressor protein acts to link the peptides physically to the plasmid that encodes them by binding to the lac operator sequences on the plasmid. This linkage promotes the enrichment of specific polypeptides in the library by selecting the peptide-repressor-plasmid complexes using affinity purification with the desired receptor.

2.4.3. Headpiece Dimer and Polysome Display

The headpiece dimer method and polysome display are modifications of lac repressor display that allow for the recovery of higher affinity-peptides. DNA binding by the lac repressor occurs by a residue domain containing approx 60 amino acids: the "headpiece" domain. By creating dimers of this headpiece region, libraries of peptides can be constructed and displayed on the C-terminus of the headpiece dimer that retain the ability to interact with the plasmid that encodes them. Libraries of plasmids can then be screened by affinity chromatography so that the peptide-headpiece dimer-plasmid complex is purified. Transformation of *E. coli* permits rapid amplification of the selected plasmids, which can be used for repeated rounds of purification and ultimately submitted to DNA sequence analysis *(35)*.

A similar strategy is used in polysome display: expression of the peptide library is achieved using an in vitro transcription/translation system of a library of DNA molecules. As with the aforementioned approaches, the peptides are displayed in a complex with the encoding nucleic acid. However, polysome display is an in vitro method, so it does not require cellular expression of peptides; thus, larger libraries are constructed *(33)*.

3. CURRENT STATUS OF SMALL-MOLECULE AGONISTS FOR CYTOKINE RECEPTORS

Until recently, it was believed that small molecules were incapable of mimicking the action of polypeptides and were not large enough to bring two receptor molecules together. Within the past 5 years, however, several small-molecule agonists of G-CSFR, EPOR, and TPOR have been reported. Furthermore, the first oral, small-molecule TPOR agonist was reported to have entered human development in the fourth quarter of 2002.

3.1. G-CSF: SB 247464

SB 247464 was identified in a high-throughput, cell-based screen that detects compounds that activate the G-CSFR *(36)*. A moderately sized library of organic compounds was screened against a cell line that expressed a functional murine G-CSFR using a signal transducer and activator of transcription (Stat)-luciferase protein reporter gene. SB 247464 was 30% as effective as G-CSF at a 1 μ*M* concentration in the luciferase assay and displayed a biphasic dose-response curve. In terms of its ability to stimulate the proliferation of normal murine hematopoietic cells, SB 247464 was 25–80% as effective as G-CSF in murine progenitor cell (G-CFC) assays.

Scientists also demonstrated that SB 247464 phosphorylated the G-CSFR as well as Jak1, Jak3, Stat3, and Stat5 *(36)*. Subcutaneous administration of 30 mg/kg of SB 247464 twice daily to normal mice resulted in a fourfold increase in blood neutrophil counts after 4 d. This effect was equivalent to 50 μg/kg of recombinant (r)G-CSF administered to normal mice in the same manner (Fig. 1). From a clinical perspective, SB 247464 was specific for the mouse G-CSFR and had no measurable activity in a number of human myeloid G-CSF-responsive cell lines. Thus, the ECD of the murine G-CSFR was required for SB 247464 activity. Although the precise mechanism of action of SB 247464 remains unclear, the data suggest that the compound binds to a region other than the G-CSF binding site and mediates dimerization of the G-CSFR.

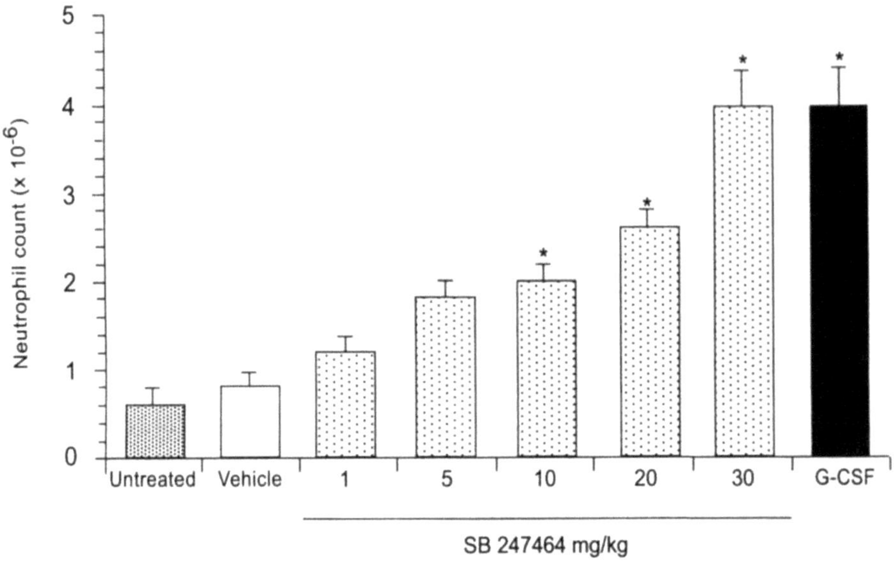

Fig. 1. Granulopoietic activity of SB 247464 in vivo. Female BDF-1 mice were given twice-daily subcutaneous injections of either granulocyte colony-stimulating factor (G-CSF) (50 µg/kg) in phosphate-buffered saline or SB 247464 dissolved in acidified H_2O (pH 4.0). Control animals received only acidified H_2O. After 4 d, blood was drawn, and the numbers of neutrophils were counted using a Technicon hematology analyzer. Each bar represents the average of five mice; error bars show standard error of mean (SEM). Asterisks indicate neutrophil counts that differ from those in untreated controls with a $p < 0.001$ by analysis of variance (ANOVA). (Reproduced with permission from ref. *36*. Copyright 1998 American Association for the Advancement of Science.)

3.2. EPO: Merck Compound

The recombinant EPO-binding protein (rEBP) is the ECD of the EPOR that has been produced in *E. coli,* refolded, and characterized for binding activity. It has been used extensively to screen peptide libraries in search of a peptide agonist of EPOR. Using HTS of a chemical library and rEBP, scientists at Merck Research Laboratories identified a small-molecule EPOR antagonist, a biphenyl indole, which they were able to oligomerize and convert into an EPOR agonist *(37)*. The antagonist inhibited binding of ^{125}I-EPO to rEBP with a median inhibitory concentration (IC_{50}) of 60 µ*M*. An EPOR agonist was synthesized by attaching eight copies of the small molecule antagonist to a polyamidoamino-octa-4-hydroxymethylbenzamide support using a chemical linker. This compound inhibited binding of ^{125}I-EPO to the rEBP with a IC_{50} of 4.4 µ*M* in the EPOR binding assay. Although both compounds were tested in an EPOR dimerization assay, only the small-molecule agonist induced dimerization of soluble EPOR.

The results from further experimentation showed that the biphenyl indole agonist could indeed function as a successful EPO mimetic *(37)*. Screening the compound against a cell line that expresses a functional human EPOR using a luciferase protein reporter gene driven by activated STAT transcription factors indicated that this agonist induced cellular transcription (Fig. 2) and proliferation in cells expressing EPOR. Furthermore, the Merck compound supported the proliferation of several tumor cell lines

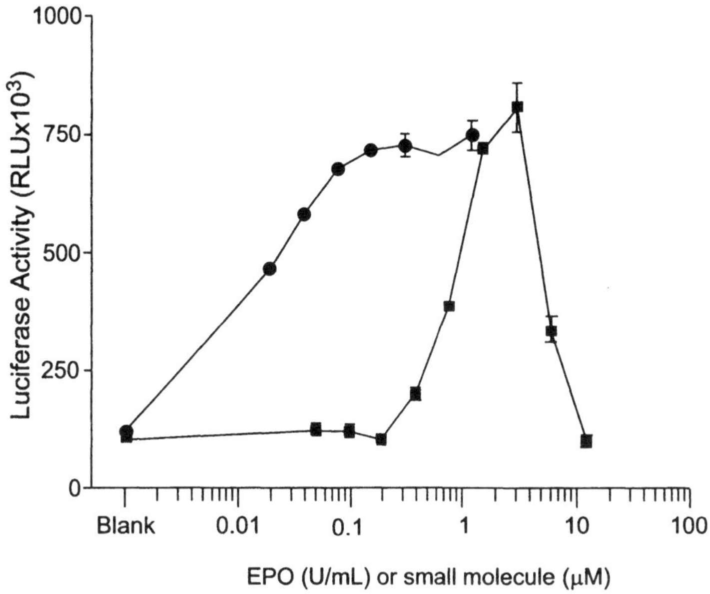

Fig. 2. Induction of luciferase activity in BAF3/LUC/EPOR cells expressing human EPOR. BAF3/LUC/EPOR cells containing a stably integrated luciferase gene under the control of a STAT-binding element were treated with varying amounts of erythropoietin (EPO) or small molecule for 16 h. The luciferase activity is expressed in relative light units (RLU). Data are the mean (± SEM) of two to three independent experiments performed in triplicate. The x-axis reflects the concentration of EPO (closed circles) or small molecule (closed squares) in unit/mL or μ*M*, respectively. Assays were performed in 1% dimethyl sulfoxide. (Adapted with permission from ref. *37*. Copyright 1999 National Academy of Sciences USA.)

that express human or mouse EPOR and induced differentiation of human progenitor cells into cells of erythrocytic lineage. Although recombinant human EPO (rHuEPO) was much more potent than the Merck agonist in all these experiments, an important proof of principle was obtained.

3.3. TPO: TM41

Kimura and coworkers *(38)* have reported that a small organic molecule, benzodiazepinone TM41, competes with TPO for binding to the receptor's extracellular region. A library of benzodiazepinones was synthesized and screened (using HTS automation) against the soluble form of human c-Mpl containing the ECD of c-Mpl and the human immunoglobulin Fc region (MPL-IgG). Several compounds were identified as dose-dependent inhibitors of TPO binding to MPL-IgG, but only TM41 was active in a cell-proliferation assay using UT-7/TPO cells (Fig. 3). TM41 also was shown to activate STAT5 in a human TPOR-dependent cell line and to be specific for c-Mpl, indicating that it does not activate other cytokine receptors.

3.4. TPO: SB 394725, SB 497115, and Related Compounds

Scientists at Ligand and GlaxoSmithKline (GSK) developed a high-throughput, cell-based screen that detects activation of STAT in response to TPO. A large library of

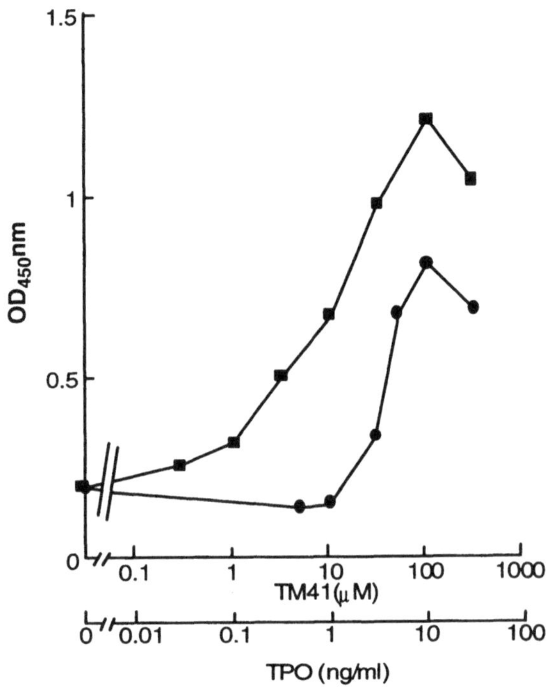

Fig. 3. Proliferative response of UT-7/TPO cells to TM41. UT/TPO cells were deprived of growth factor for 24 h and then plated at a density of 2×10^4 cells/well in Iscove's modified Dulbecco's medium (IMDM) containing 10% fetal calf serum (FCS) and incubated in the absence or presence of TM41 or thrombopoietin (TPO). After 3 d, the absorbance was measured. The values for TM41 (closed circles) and TPO (closed squares) shown are the means of triplicate determinations. (Adapted from ref. *38.*)

small molecules was screened against a TPO-responsive cell line (BAF-3B5/TPO) that was stably transfected with a luciferase reporter gene under the control of a STAT-responsive promoter. One of the molecules identified from this screen was optimized using traditional medicinal chemistry to generate SB 394725, a pyrazol-4-ylidenehydrazine that had an efficacy equivalent to that of TPO with a median effective concentration (EC_{50}) of 40 n*M* *(39)*.

Because the pyrazol-4-ylidenehydrazines had low-to-no oral absorption in both rodent and nonrodent species, another class of compounds from the initial HTS was examined. The salicylaldehyde thiosemicarbazones demonstrated weak TPOR agonist activity compared with the pyrazol-4-ylidenehydrazines; however, after medicinal chemistry optimization, the potency and efficacy of these compounds was significantly improved. For example, one biaryl derivative had an efficacy equivalent to that of TPO with an EC_{50} of 20 n*M* in a UT7/TPOR proliferation assay *(40)*.

Encouraged by the success of optimizing the salicylaldehyde thiosemicarbazones, scientists designed and examined a third series of TPO mimics, the naphtho[1,2-*d*]imidazoles *(41)*. Optimization of this series was achieved using parallel array synthesis, and as with the two previously described series of TPO mimics, the naphtho[1,2-*d*]imidazoles were completely selective for TPO-responsive cell lines vs other cytokine-responsive cell lines. SB 394725 and several of the salicylaldehyde thiosemicarbazones and naphtho[1,2-*d*]imidazoles were shown to stimulate the proliferation and differentiation of TPO-responsive cell lines and human bone marrow cultures with full TPO efficacy. One member of these three series of compounds, SB 497115, is currently in phase 1 clinical trials for hematologic diseases, including anemia and thrombocytopenia.

3.5. Evaluation of Small-Molecule Agonists

Evidence that small molecules can function as cytokine mimetics by inducing receptor dimerization is provided by the aforementioned examples; however, few reports indicate that small molecules are capable of disrupting protein-protein interactions *(8)*. Furthermore, none of the small molecules reported to date have shown the established safety and specificity of the recombinant counterparts to the native proteins. One reason that the discovery of small-molecule cytokine receptor agonists has proved so difficult is that the precise mechanism of receptor dimerization and the resulting complex series of intracellular events necessary for cytokine activity are not clearly understood. In addition, because only a few small molecules have been found to activate HGF receptors, preferred pharmacophores or structural arrays that could be used for rational drug design have not been identified. Nevertheless, considering the molecules together (Fig. 4), some similarities can be seen, and hypotheses relating molecule structure to function can be formulated.

All of the molecules contain multiple aromatic rings in fairly rigid conformations, perhaps indicating that some degree of rigidity in structure is necessary to prevent intramolecular hydrophobic collapse *(8)*. Several molecules are C2 symmetric (SB 247464, Fig. 4A; Merck EPOR agonist, not shown), suggesting that these molecules trigger receptor dimerization by bridging two receptor monomers. It is interesting to note that many of the molecules contain certain "privileged" pharmacophores *(42)* and protein turn mimetics *(43)*, such as benzodiazepinones (TM41, Fig. 4B), biphenyls (Merck EPOR antagonist, Fig. 4C; Ligand/GSK TPOR agonists, Fig. 4E and F), pyrazoles (SB 394725, Fig. 4D), and imidazoles (SB 247464, Fig. 4A; Ligand/GSK TPOR agonist, Fig. 4F). Finally, examination of the three Ligand/GSK TPOR agonists (Fig. 4D–F) reveals several structural features that seemingly are required for TPOR agonist activity: lipophilic functionality, acidic functionality on opposite ends of the molecule, and a heteroatom metal chelate in the central portion of the molecule *(41)*. As new small-molecule cytokine receptor agonists are discovered, additional structural trends may be identified. These trends may highlight some of the principles of small-molecule-protein interactions, which could be used to guide future rational drug design.

4. CURRENT STATUS OF PEPTIDE AGONISTS FOR CYTOKINE RECEPTORS

Many recombinant cytokines are successfully marketed as drugs, including recombinant forms of human growth hormone (hGH), EPO, G-CSF, interferon (IFN)-α, IFN-β, interleukin (IL)-2, and IL-11 *(44)*. Others are in late stages of clinical development. Scientists have been searching for smaller peptide cytokine agonists that mimic the activity of their larger counterparts to use as probes for understanding the detailed mechanisms of receptor activation. EPO mimetic peptide 1 (EMP1) was the first reported peptidomimetic *(45)*. Subsequently, small-peptide agonists of the EPO and TPO receptors, including the EMP1-related peptides AF13948 *(46)*, PK1 *(47)*, and GW395058 *(48)*, were reported.

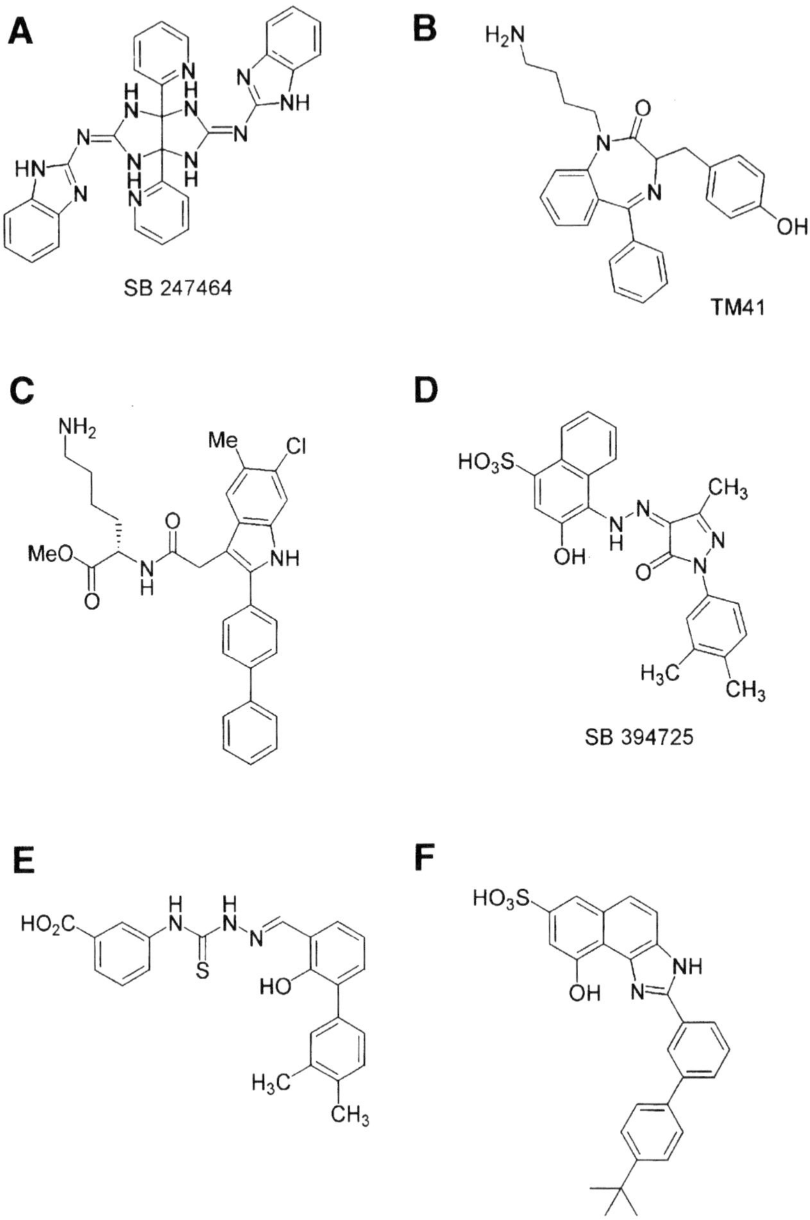

Fig. 4. Small-molecule hematopoietic growth factor agonists and antagonists. **(A)** G-CSFR agonist, SB 247464. **(B)** TPOR agonist, TM41. **(C)** EPOR antagonist, biphenyl indole. **(D)** TPOR agonist, SB 394725. **(E)** TPOR agonist, salicylaldehyde thiosemicarbazone. **(F)** TPOR agonist, naphtho[1,2-*d*]imidazole.

4.1. EPO: EMP1 and Related Peptides

Wrighton and coworkers *(45)* used phage display and EBP to identify peptides that would bind to the human EPOR. Phage-display mutagenesis of the lead molecule, an 8-amino-acid peptide sequence, produced a family of related peptides (20-mers) with approx

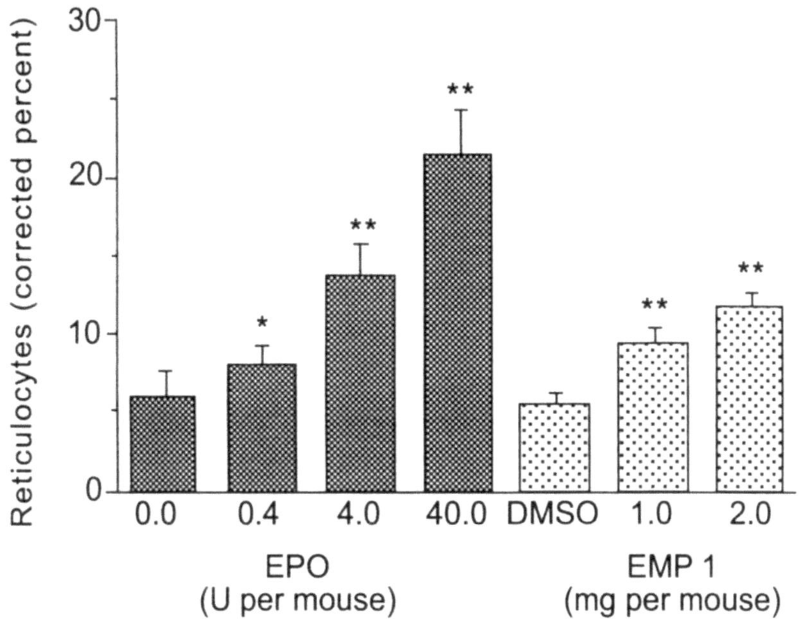

Fig. 5. Murine reticulocyte assay. Normal, untreated mice were treated with various amounts of either erythropoietin (EPO; solid bars, n = 10/dose group) or EPO mimetic peptide 1 (EMP1; dotted bars, n = 8/dose group), and the increase in reticulocytes was measured by flow cytometry. Peptide samples were solubilized in dimethyl sulfoxide (DMSO) and subsequently diluted with assay vehicle. Mean values are shown. *, $p < 0.01$; **, $p < 0.0001$ by ANOVA. (Reproduced with permission from ref. *45*. Copyright 1996 American Academy for the Advancement of Science.)

200 n*M* affinity for the human EPOR. The peptides were selective for the EPOR and demonstrated full EPOR agonist behavior in an EPO-dependent cell proliferation assay. None of the EPOR peptide ligands had complete homology with the primary sequence of EPO.

A representative peptide, EMP1, stimulated TF-1 cells in a dose-dependent manner with an IC_{50} of 100 n*M*. EMP1 is a cyclic peptide and has conserved amino acids at the 4, 9, 10, 12, 13, and 17 positions. EMP1 was found to induce the same intracellular phosphorylation pattern as EPO, to stimulate erythroid colony formation from precursor cells, and to be active in two in vivo models of EPO activity (Fig. 5) *(45)*. N- and C-terminal deletions of EMP1 produced a minimally active peptide, EMP20. Alanine-scanning substitutions *(49)* demonstrated that specific conserved residues were required for activity. A cyclic peptide was also found to be necessary for EPOR agonist behavior.

The activity of EMP1 was increased by covalent dimerization of the peptide in two ways *(50)*. In one method, two EMP1 peptides were joined through their N-termini using a difunctional polyethylene glycol (PEG) molecule. The EMP1-PEG dimer demonstrated marked improvements in both TF-1 cell binding affinity (IC_{50} = 28 n*M*) and cell proliferation (median effective dose [ED_{50}] = 2 n*M*) compared with the monomeric peptide (IC_{50} = 100 n*M* and ED_{50} = 100 n*M*, respectively). Scientists produced a chemical dimer of EMP1 by attaching the two peptides through a C-termini lysine-β-alanine branch. The correct intrachain disulfide bonds were formed by controlled oxidation and sequential removal of cysteine-residue protecting groups *(33)*. This method was even more effective than the PEG dimerization, improving both the binding and in vitro activity (IC_{50} = 0.75 n*M*, ED_{50} = 1 n*M*). Unfortunately, neither method generated a compound with in vivo activity that was comparable to that of rHuEPO. The in vivo equivalents to 0.025 U of rHuEPO were 3.8, 0.28, and 0.035 nmol for EMP1, PEG dimer, and chemical dimer, respectively, compared with 0.0000058 nmol for rHuEPO.

4.2. TPO: AF13948

Cwirla and coworkers *(46)* used several peptide library construction methods and covalent dimerization to produce AF13948, a 28-amino-acid peptide that was equipotent to the natural growth factor TPO in cell-based assays. Peptides that bind to TPOR were identified using both phage display and lac repressor display of random peptide libraries. Libraries were screened against the immobilized ECD of TPOR, and the resulting clones were categorized into two families and two subfamilies based on amino acid sequence homology.

Scientists constructed and screened several mutagenesis libraries to optimize the higher affinity sequences further. These libraries were constructed in the headpiece dimer and polysome vectors to generate even higher affinity ligands than those that were obtained using phage or lac repressor display. A 19-residue peptide (AF12434) obtained from these screens was then used as a template for additional mutagenesis to generate another library of peptides. This library produced a high-affinity peptide (AF12505, IC_{50} = 2 n*M*) that was subsequently covalently dimerized using the same branched-lysine strategy (chemical dimer) applied to the EMP series to generate AF13948 *(33)*. Dimer AF13948 was 4000 times as potent as the monomer AF12505 and equipotent to rHuTPO in the cell proliferation assay (Fig. 6). The peptide dimer also stimulated in vitro proliferation and maturation of megakaryocytes from human bone marrow cells and increased platelets by 80% in vivo *(46)*.

4.3. TPO: PK1

A family of potent TPOR ligands similar in sequence to one of the subfamilies identified by Cwirla and coworkers *(46)* was discovered independently by another group using phage display *(47)*. A 15-amino-acid random-phage peptide library was constructed by inserting a degenerate oligonucleotide into the amino terminus of the bacteriophage gene III protein. The library was screened against the ECD of human TPOR, and six clones that demonstrated binding were isolated. The peptide from one of these clones, PK1, stimulated the proliferation of TPO-dependent cells. In addition, mouse bone marrow cells were differentiated to megakaryocytes by modified forms of the PK1 peptide. No homology between PK1 and the primary amino acid sequences of human and mouse TPO was observed. By constructing and screening a mutagenesis library based on PK1, scientists discovered a consensus sequence of GCXLXXWXXGXC.

4.4. TPO: GW395058/3DP-3534

Although AF13948 was equipotent to native TPO in cell-based assays, 250 μg/kg of the peptide was required to produce the same results as 1 μg/kg of TPO in vivo. Thus, scientists pursued various techniques to optimize the activity, synthesis, and bioavailability of AF13948 *(48)*. The tryptophan residues in AF13948 were replaced by napthylalanines for ease of synthesis, and an alanine and a β-alanine were each replaced with

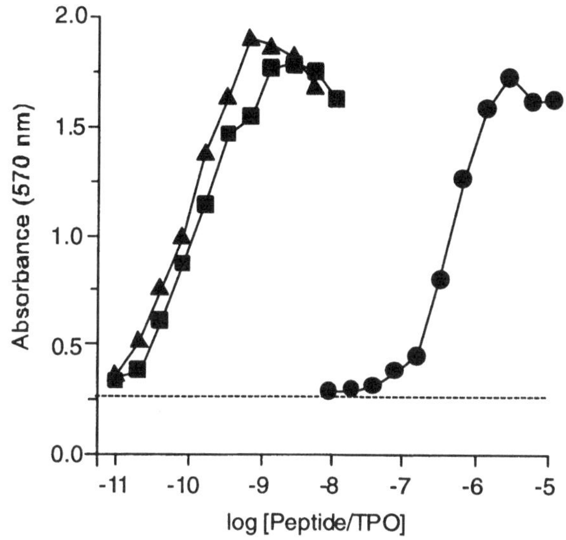

Fig. 6. Proliferative response of Ba/F3 HuTPOR cells to peptides AF12505 (closed circles), AF13948 (closed squares), and rHuTPO (closed triangles). Peptides were dissolved at 20 m*M* in dimethyl sulfoxide and serially diluted in a 96-well assay plate with an equal volume of medium (RPMI-1640 containing 10% fetal calf serum [FCS], 2 m*M* L-glutamine, 1 × antibiotics-antimycotics). Ba/F3 HuTPOR cells were added to each well at a density of 2×10^4 cells/well to attain the indicated concentration of peptide or thrombopoietin (TPO). After 48 h, proliferation was measured by a standard MTT assay (Promega). The dashed line indicates response in the absence of rHuTPO, AF12505, or AF13948. (Reproduced with permission from ref. *46*. Copyright 1997 American Academy for the Advancement of Science.)

sarcosine to remove the chiral centers from the molecule. The two amino termini were then conjugated to PEG (20,000 MW) to produce GW395058 (renamed 3DP-3534).

Aside from its potent in vitro activity, GW395058 was active in vivo, as demonstrated by its long plasma half-life (approx 50 h) and its ability to increase platelet counts and accelerate platelet recovery in mouse myelosuppression models (Fig. 7). *(48)*. The kinetics of GW395058 are similar to those of TPO, and although it shares no sequence homology, GW395058 does compete with the native protein for receptor binding. Compared with rHuTPO, GW395058 was not immunogenic in mice or rabbits. GW395058 also failed to produce antibodies to rHuTPO when administered to mice.

5. CONCLUSIONS

The interaction of a ligand with its cell surface receptor results in a complex series of engagement events that brings together multiple proteins in a specific three-dimensional arrangement. This interaction, and the resulting conformational change it triggers, generates a cascade of intracellular events that lead to the physiologic consequences unique to each growth factor. Given this complexity, it was perhaps surprising that both small molecules and peptides can mimic the effects of a growth factor. Recent studies, however, have clearly established this to be the case. Whether any of these molecules, or subsequent generations of them, will display the safety and specificity of the recombinant counterparts to the native proteins remains to be determined.

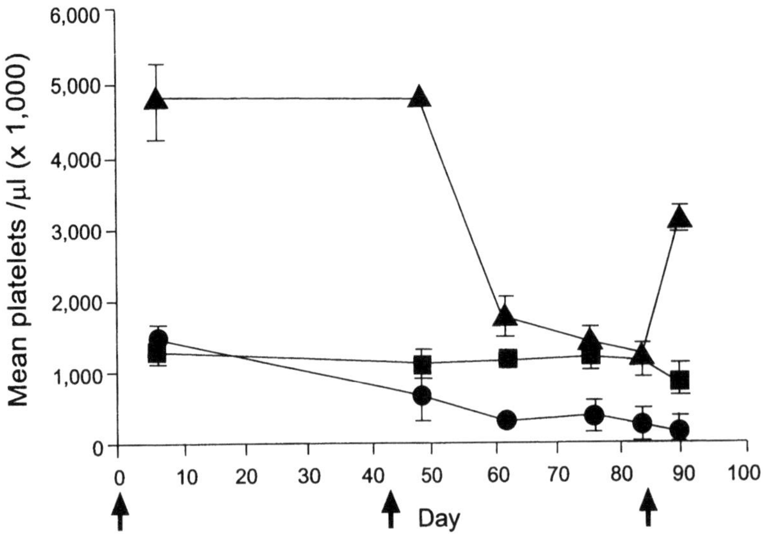

Fig. 7. Platelet responses in BALB/c mice to rHuTPO or GW395058. Average platelet counts in mouse blood samples are shown. Blood samples were obtained from BALB/c mice (*n* = 5/group; 3 dose cycles/group) that were receiving subcutaneous doses on d 1, 43, and 85 (arrows) of rHuTPO at 50 µg/kg, QD × 5/cycle (closed squares), GW395058 at 25 µg/kg, single dose/cycle (closed triangles), or vehicle (closed circles). (Reproduced with permission from ref. *48.* © AlphaMed Press 1066–5099.)

Safety and specificity are critical characteristics of candidate therapeutics, and the established profiles of protein therapeutics in these areas have set the bar very high.

It is also noteworthy that the area of protein therapeutics itself is evolving. The notion that a physiologic protein represents the ultimate in evolutionary development has been dispelled, at least from a therapeutic perspective. Site-directed mutagenesis of DNA encoding human EPO has resulted in a new protein, darbepoetin alfa, which not only has enhanced biologic properties but also retains the safety and specificity profiles of rHuEPO *(51).* Having demonstrated that proteins themselves can be improved, further advances are likely to occur that will make it more difficult for a small molecule to enter the therapeutic arena. However, the potential advantages offered in terms of oral delivery and cost of manufacture will ensure that small-molecule mimetics will continue to be an active area of on-going research.

REFERENCES

1. Boger DL, Goldberg J. Cytokine receptor dimerization and activation: prospects for small molecule agonists. *Bioorg Med Chem* 2001; 9:557–562.
2. Watowich SS, Wu H, Socolovsky M, Klingmuller U, Constantinescu SN, Lodish HF. Cytokine receptor signal transduction and the control of hematopoietic development. *Annu Rev Cell Dev Biol* 1996; 12:91–128.
3. Frank SJ. Minireview: receptor dimerization in GH and erythropoietin action. It takes two to tango, but how? *Endocrinology* 2002; 143:2–10.
4. Watowich SS. Activation of erythropoietin signaling by receptor dimerization. *Int J Biochem Cell Biol* 1999; 31:1075–1088.
5. Matthews DJ, Topping RS, Cass RT, Giebel LB. A sequential dimerization mechanism for erythropoietin receptor activation. *Proc Natl Acad Sci USA* 1996; 93:9471–9476.

6. Johnson DL, Farrell FX, Middleton SA, et al. Peptide mimetics of erythropoietin are powerful probes of receptor activation mechanisms. In: Fields GB, Tam JP, Barany G, eds., *Peptides for the New Millennium.* Boston: Kluwer Academic. 1999:536–538.
7. Kaushansky K. Hematopoietic growth factor mimetics. *Ann NY Acad Sci* 2001; 838:131–138.
8. Cochran AG. Antagonists of protein-protein interactions. *Chem Biol* 2000; 7:R85–R94.
9. Kaushansky K. Small molecule mimics of hematopoietic growth factors: improving on mother nature? *Leukemia* 2001; 15:673–674.
10. Ramstrom O, Lehn JM. Drug discovery by dynamic combinatorial libraries. *Nat Rev Drug Discovery* 2002; 1:26–36.
11. Thompson LA, Ellman JA. Synthesis and applications of small molecule libraries. *Chem Rev* 1996; 96:555–600.
12. Armstrong RW, Combs AP, Tempest PA, Brown SD, Keating TA. Multiple-component condensation strategies for combinatorial library synthesis. *Acc Chem Res* 1996; 29:123–131.
13. Otto S, Furlan R, Sanders J. Recent developments in dynamic combinatorial chemistry. *Curr Opin Chem Biol* 2002; 6:321–327.
14. Furka A, Sebestyen F, Asgedom M, Dibo G. General method for rapid synthesis of mulitcomponent peptide mixtures. *Int J Pept Protein Res* 1991; 37:487–493.
15. Lebl M, Krchnak V, Sepetov NF, et al. One-bead-one-structure combinatorial libraries. *Biopolymers* 1995; 37:177–198.
16. Zuckermann RN, Banville SC. Automated peptide-resin deprotection/cleavage by a robotic workstation. *Pept Res* 1992; 5:169–174.
17. Zuckermann RN, Kerr JM, Siani MA, Banville SC. Design, construction, and application of a fully automated equimolar peptide mixture synthesizer. *Int J Pept Protein Res* 1992; 40:497–506.
18. Dooley CT, Houghten RA. The use of positional scanning synthetic peptide combinatorial libraries for the rapid determination of opioid receptor ligands. *Life Sci* 1993; 52:1509–1517.
19. Deprez B, Williard X, Bourel L, Coste H, Hyafil F, Tartar A. Orthogonal combinatorial chemical libraries. *J Am Chem Soc* 1995; 117:5405–5406.
20. Vetter D, Tate EM, Gallop MA. Strategies for the synthesis and screening of glycoconjugates. 2. Covalent immobilization for flow cytometry. *Bioconjugate Chem* 1995; 6:319–322.
21. Needles MC, Jones DG, Tate EH, et al. Generation and screening of an oligonucleotide-encoded synthetic peptide library. *Proc Natl Acad Sci USA* 1993; 90:10700–10704.
22. Nikolaiev V, Stierandova A, Krchnak V, et al. Peptide-encoding for structure determination of nonsequenceable polymers within libraries synthesized and tested on solid-phase supports. *Pept Res* 1993; 6:161–170.
23. Nicolaou KC, Xiao XY, Parandoosh Z, Senyei A, Nova MP. Radiofrequency encoded combinatorial chemistry. *Angew Chem Int Ed Engl* 1995; 34:2289–2291.
24. Moran EJ, Sarshar S, Cargill JF, et al. Radiofrequency tag encoded combinatorial library method for the discovery of tripeptide-substituted cinnamic acid inhibitors of the protein tyrosine phosphatase PTP1B. *J Am Chem Soc* 1995; 117:10787–10788.
25. Houghten, RA. Parallel array and mixture-based synthetic combinatorial chemistry: tools for the next millennium. *Annu Rev Pharmacol Toxicol* 2000; 40:273–282.
26. Fodor SPA, Read JL, Pirrung MC, Stryer L, Lu AT, Solas D. Light-directed, spacially addressable parallel chemical synthesis. *Science* 1991; 251:767–773.
27. Geyson HM, Meloen RH, Barteling SJ. Use of peptide synthesis to probe viral antigens for epitopes to a resolution of a single amino acid. *Proc Natl Acad Sci USA* 1984; 81:3998–4002.
28. DeWitt SH, Kiely JS, Stankovic CJ, Schroeder MC, Cody DMR, Pavia MR. "Diversomers": an approach to nonpeptide, nonoligomeric chemical diversity. *Proc Natl Acad Sci USA* 1993; 90:6909–6913.
29. Meyers HV, Dilley GJ, Durgin TL, et al. Multiple simultaneous synthesis of phenolic libraries. *Mol Diversity* 1995; 1:13–20.
30. Georgiou G, Stathopoulos C, Daugherty PS, Nayak AR, Iverson BL, Curtiss R III. Display of heterogeneous proteins on the surface of microorganisms: from the screening of combinatorial libraries to live recombinant vaccines. *Nat Biotechnol* 1997; 15:29–34.
31. Lowman HB. Bacteriophage display and discovery of peptide leads for drug development. *Annu Rev Biophys Biomol Struct* 1997; 26:401–424.
32. Katz BA. Structural and mechanistic determinants of affinity and specificity of ligands discovered or engineered by phage display. *Annu Rev Biophys Biomol Struct* 1997; 26:27–45.

33. Dower WJ. Targeting growth factor and cytokine receptors with recombinant peptide libraries. *Curr Opin Chem Biol* 1998; 2:328–334.
34. Cull MG, Miller JF, Schatz PJ. Screening for receptor ligands using large libraries of peptides linked to the C terminus of the *lac* repressor. *Proc Natl Acad Sci USA* 1992; 89:1865–1869.
35. Gates CM, Stemmer WPC, Kaptein R, Schatz PJ. Affinity selective isolation of ligands from peptide libraries through display on a lac repressor "headpiece dimer". *J Mol Biol* 1996; 255:373–386.
36. Tian S-S, Lamb P, King A, et al. A small, nonpeptidyl mimic of granulocyte-colony-stimulating factor. *Science* 1998; 281:257–259.
37. Qureshi, SA, Kim RM, Konteatis Z, et al. Mimicry of erythropoietin by a nonpeptide molecule. *Proc Natl Acad Sci USA* 1999; 96:12156–12161.
38. Kimura T, Kaburaki H, Tsujino T, Ikeda Y, Kato H, Watanabe Y. A non-peptide compound which can mimic the effect of thrombopoietin via c-Mpl. *FEBS Lett* 1998; 428:250–254.
39. Duffy KJ, Darcy MG, Delorme E, et al. Hydrazinonaphthalene and azonaphthalene thrombopoietin mimics are nonpeptidyl promoters of megakaryocytopoiesis. *J Med Chem* 2001; 44:3730–3745.
40. Duffy KJ, Shaw AN, Delorme E, et al. Identification of a pharmacophore for thrombopoietic activity of small, non-peptidyl molecules. 1. Discovery and optimization of salicylaldehyde thiosemicarbazone thrombopoietin mimics. *J Med Chem* 2002; 45:3573–3575.
41. Duffy KJ, Price AT, Delorme E, et al. Identification of a pharmacophore for thrombopoietic activity of small, non-peptidyl molecules. 2. Rational design of naphthol[1,2-d]imidazole thrombopoietin mimics. *J Med Chem* 2002; 45:3576–3578.
42. Gordon EM, Barrett RW, Dower WJ, Fodor S, Gallop MA. Applications of combinatorial technologies to drug discovery. 2. Combinatorial organic synthesis, library screening strategies, and future directions. *J Med Chem* 1994; 37:1385–1401.
43. Fairlie DP, West ML, Wong AK. Towards protein surface mimetics. *Curr Med Chem* 1998; 5:29–62.
44. Whitty A, Borysenko CW. Small molecule cytokine mimetics. *Chem Biol* 1999; 6:R107–R118.
45. Wrighton NC, Farrell FX, Chang R, et al. Small peptides as potent mimetics of the protein hormone erythropoietin. *Science* 1996; 273:458–463.
46. Cwirla SE, Balasubramanian P, Duffin DJ, et al. Peptide agonist of the thrombopoietin receptor as potent as the natural cytokine. *Science* 1997; 276:1696–1699.
47. Kimura T, Kaburaki H, Miyamoto S, Katayama J, Watanabe Y. Discovery of a novel thrombopoietin mimic agonist peptide. *J Biochem* 1997; 122:1046–1051.
48. DeSerres M, Ellis B, Dillberger JE, et al. Immunogenicity of thrombopoietin mimetic peptide GW395058 in BALB/c mice and New Zealand white rabbits: evaluation of the potential for thrombopoietin neutralizing antibody production in man. *Stem Cells* 1999; 17:203–209.
49. Kallen K-J, Gr tzinger J, Rose-John S. New perspectives on the design of cytokines and growth factors. *Trends Biotechnol* 2000; 18:455–461.
50. Barbone FP, Johnson DL, Farrell FX, et al. New epoetin molecules and novel therapeutic approaches. *Nephrol Dial Transplant* 1999; 14(suppl 2):80–84.
51. Elliott S, Lorenzini T, Asher S, et al. Enhancement of therapeutic protein in vivo activities through glycoengineering. *Nat Biotechnol* 2003; 21:414–421.

II Hematopoietic Growth Factors

5 Granulocyte Colony-Stimulating Factor

Graham Molineux, PhD

CONTENTS

1. INTRODUCTION

Granulocyte colony-stimulating factor (G-CSF) is a major regulator of the development of antibacterial neutrophilic granulocytic leukocytes (neutrophils). In keeping with the functions of both G-CSF and neutrophils, the murine molecule was first purified from medium that had bathed the dissected lungs of animals previously treated with a bacterial cell-wall extract *(1)*. Several years later, the equivalent human molecule was reported in the supernatent from a carcinoma cell line that inadvertently expressed G-CSF in extraordinarily high concentrations *(2,3)*. The human material was found to be a glycoprotein of approx 19 kDa, which was variably acidic depending on the proportion of sialic acid in the carbohydrate component *(3)*. It was later found that the carbohydrate was optional for biologic activity and that the core protein comprised 174 amino acids *(4,5)* (Table 1).

Endogenous human G-CSF is the product of a single locus on chromosome 17q21-22 *(7)*, and its regulation is by both transcriptional and post-transcriptional processes *(8–10)* (Table 1).

The cloning and characterization of recombinant human G-CSF (rHuG-CSF) took place in the early 1980s and led to its expression in *Escherichia coli*, trials in humans, and approval of filgrastim (recombinant methionyl human [r-metHu]G-CSF) for administration to patients in the United States in 1991 *(1,6,11–15)*. A second, Chinese hamster ovary (CHO)-derived form (lacking the N-terminal methionine of the *E. coli*-derived version), was approved for human use in Europe in 1993 (lenograstim). The administration of rHuG-CSF to patients was initially for the treatment of cancer chemotherapy-induced neutropenia and the prevention of associated infections. Since those initial approvals, rHuG-CSF has been recommended for use in severe chronic neutropenia,

From: *Cancer Drug Discovery and Development*
Hematopoietic Growth Factors in Oncology: Basic Science and Clinical Therapeutics
Edited by: G. Morstyn, M. A. Foote, and G. J. Lieschke © Humana Press Inc., Totowa, NJ

Table 1
Summary of Characteristics of Human G-CSF

Characteristic	
Location of gene	Chromosome 17q11-22 (human)
Gene size	Approx 2500 nucleotides (approx 2.5 kb)
Number of exons	5
Protein produced	Proform
Glycosylation site	Thr 133
Disulfide bonds	Two (between 36 and 42, and 64 and 74)
Basic structure	Four helices arranged in antiparallel fashion; and sheet pleating
Receptor structure	Single 150-kDa chain-forming homodimer

Data from ref. *6*.

Table 2
Characteristics of the Forms of rHuG-CSF

Generic Name	*Amino acids; cell source*	*Expression system*	*Other information*
Filgrastim	175; bladder carcinoma cell line	*E. coli*	Nonglycosylated
Lenograstim	174; squamous carcinoma cell line	Chinese hamster ovary	Glycosylated
Nartograstim	174[a]	*E. coli*	Mutein form
Pegfilgrastim	175	*E. coli*	Nonglycosylated, pegylated
RO 25-8315	174	*E. coli*	Mutein form, pegylated

[a] Changes to amino acids 1, 3, 4, 5, and 17.

Data from ref. *6*.

aplastic anemia, support of hematopoiesis after bone marrow transplantation, support of induction and consolidation chemotherapy for acute myeloid leukemia, and prevention of infections in HIV-infected patients. It also has been used to mobilize transplantable stem cells to the blood of both patients with cancer and normal donors *(16)*.

2. BIOCHEMICAL IDENTITY OF VARIOUS FORMS OF rHuG-CSF

Various forms of rHuG-CSF have been developed and are available in different countries. Notably, filgrastim (Neupogen, Amgen), lenograstim (Granocyte, Chugai Pharmaceutical), and KW-2228 (Nartograstim, Kyowa-Hakko Kogyo) are variant G-CSFs described more fully in the following sections (Table 2).

2.1. Filgrastim (Neupogen)

r-metHuG-CSF (filgrastim) is a 175-amino acid protein produced in *E. coli*. Endogenous human G-CSF is a 204-amino acid glycoprotein including a 30-amino acid signal sequence that is removed from the secreted form. The bacterially synthesized version has an additional N-terminal methionine that aids stability in bacterial expression systems. Because of its origin, filgrastim is devoid of the *O*-linked carbohydrate on the threonine at position 133 of the endogenous protein *(17)* but retains all five cysteines typical of the human sequence (at positions 17, 36, 42, 64, and 74; the murine version lacks the Cys17). The latter four of these cysteines contribute to disulfide bonds that stabilize the structure as four antiparallel helices *(18)*.

r-metHuG-CSF was the first G-CSF to be approved for clinical use and has been used in more than 2 million patients worldwide *(16)*.

2.2. Lenograstim (Granocyte)

Lenograstim is another rHuG-CSF and is the result of expression in mammalian cells *(17)*. Although the gene is the same as that expressed in *E. coli* to produce filgrastim, this mammalian expression system does not require the extra methionine and hence possesses a 174-amino acid peptide core. In addition, the single *O*-linked carbohydrate chain typical of the endogenous molecule (at Thr133) is found in this form of G-CSF. The function of the carbohydrate is unclear, although several hypotheses have been proposed, including inhibition of proteolytic degradation and aggregation and increased serum half-life *(19–21)*, Cys17 being the apparent target in protein degeneration *(22)*. Although the activity of glycosylated rHuG-CSF has been shown to be greater than that of the nonglycosylated form in vitro *(23–26)*, the activity of the material in vivo is similar to the bacterially synthesized form in all respects *(5,27,28)* (with the exception of a single drug company-sponsored study *[29]*). So how, or indeed whether, the additional carbohydrate plays a role in vivo remains unclear.

2.3. KW-2228 (Nartograstim)

It is relatively commonplace to attach a radioactive tracer (often ^{125}I) to protein molecules to track their distribution in the body or to examine receptor interactions. G-CSF is a difficult molecule to radioiodinate because of its amino acid sequence. KW-2228 is a mutant version of G-CSF in which the amino acid sequence has been deliberately altered to allow the attachment of radioactive iodine *(30)*. The amino acid substitutions involved swapping the Thr1, Leu3, Gly4, Pro5, and Cys17 for alanine, threonine, tyrosine, arginine, and serine, respectively (recall that Cys17 is absent from murine G-CSF and does not affect disulfide bonding or activity, unlike the other four cysteines at positions 36, 42, 64, and 74). The mutein was found to be active and capable of detectable binding to G-CSF receptors *(30–32)*. Clinical studies have also shown the usefulness of this product in chemotherapy-induced neutropenia *(33)*. Preclinical studies in nonhuman primates have compared KW-2228 with both lenograstim and filgrastim and found all three preparations to have identical pharmacokinetic properties *(27)*.

2.4. Other Forms of Recombinant G-CSF

It has been reported that at least 18 forms of recombinant G-CSF are available in some countries in addition to the 3 forms described. Reference was found to only one specific form, Jilifen, however *(34)*. Details of the nature of the active ingredient are sparse, although it may be assumed that they are similar in nature to those listed in Subheadings 2.1. and 2.2.

2.5. Pegfilgrastim (Neulasta)

The attachment of polyethylene glycol (PEG) to proteins (pegylation) is a well-tested method of modifying their characteristics without substantially affecting their primary target *(34–40)*. The tactic has been used to extend serum residence time, reduce immunogenicity, protect from proteolytic degradation, and improve formulation characteristics *(41)*. Not surprisingly, pegylation of G-CSF has been reported several times *(42–46)*. The first, and to date only, pegylated G-CSF to be made available for clinical use is a derivative of filgrastim, pegfilgrastim, which was approved for human use in the United States, Canada, Australia, and Europe in 2002 *(47–51)*. The molecular nature of the derivation is a 20-kDa, linear PEG that is covalently attached to the N-terminus of filgrastim *(36)*. This material retains its ability to stimulate neutrophil production over a longer period because of its altered residence time in the circulation *(52)*. It also displays some unique pharmacokinetic properties that are more fully explained below (*see* Subheading 3.2.), but in effect presents a "self-regulating" form of rHuG-CSF ideal for use in chemotherapy-induced neutropenia.

2.6. Future Developments

Various methods of delivery have been investigated for rHuG-CSF including nebulization *(53)*, oral delivery for a pegylated derivative *(46)*, and rectal delivery *(54)*, though none of these forms are available for clinical use to date. Alternative molecular forms that interact with the G-CSF receptor have been suggested. A small-molecule drug that acts only on the murine receptor has been reported in addition to other molecular entities such as agonistic antibodies and mimetic peptides. It is not possible to predict which if any of the new approaches will come to fruition. All hold promise, but none have proven clinical usefulness.

3. MECHANISM OF G-CSF ACTION

3.1. The Cellular Targets of G-CSF

One of the properties that first allowed G-CSF to be purified was its ability to act as a so-called colony-stimulating factor (CSF). In this case, the colonies that were stimulated to grow consisted entirely of neutrophilic granulocytes, hence the name granulocyte colony-stimulating factor *(1)*.

This knowledge did little to assist in understanding the role that G-CSF plays in normal hematopoiesis; however, several approaches have illustrated what role G-CSF plays in both healthy and infected individuals.

G-CSF is normally difficult to detect in plasma since it is at concentrations of less than 10 pg/mL *(55)*. In other conditions, such as aplastic anemia, neutropenia, infection, and complicated pregnancy, concentrations may be substantially higher—up to 100,000 pg/mL *(56,57)*. Although these studies suggested that G-CSF may be detectable in complicated conditions like infection, especially when accompanying neutropenia, its role in normal hemostasis was not fully understood until the seminal work of Lieshke et al. *(58)*. These investigators produced a G-CSF knockout animal by targeted disruption of the gene in embryonal stem cells. This disruption produced an animal that was devoid of G-CSF for its entire existence and that had only 20–30% of a normal neutrophil count. This result may suggest that the remaining neutrophils were produced by a G-CSF-independent pathway, but the impaired ability of these animals to counter infection argued that not only was G-CSF involved in most baseline neutropoiesis but it also had an essential role in "emergency" neutropoiesis in response to bacterial infection. It may be argued that the absence of G-CSF, or indeed any other protein, from early in *in utero* life might not give a true representation of the function of the protein in normal adult life owing to the enforced use of redundant pathways. Later work in which G-CSF was deliberately neutralized in adult animals by causing G-CSF autoimmunity in mice, however, yielded a remarkably similar phenotype *(59)*.

At a cellular level, it has been shown that the absence of G-CSF effects (in this case owing to deletion of the G-CSF receptor *[60]*) increases the susceptibility of neutrophilic precursors to apoptosis, or programmed cell death. In examining the bone marrow of these G-CSFR$^{-/-}$ mice, it was found that cellularity was normal, progenitor numbers were only modestly reduced, and recognizable cells of the neutrophilic lineage were not significantly changed, with the exception of metamyelocytes and bands or segmented neutrophils. These cells are relatively mature compared with progenitor cells, but when bone marrow cells are exposed to G-CSF in vitro, it is the progenitor cells that proliferate and differentiate into recognizable neutrophils. This apparent incongruity is explained by considering the nature of the progenitor assays. When bone marrow cells are explanted in these semisolid cultures, a heterogeneous mixture of progenitor cells of widely varying potential is exposed to the cytokine environment provided. Those progenitors that will fulfill their potential and give rise to mature colonies of recognizable cells are obviously only those that survive, but also only those progenitors whose progeny also will survive to be seen in the mature colonies. In the presence of G-CSF, the G-CFC (granulocyte colony-forming cell) will survive and proliferate, but to observe the mature band and segmented neutrophils typically seen in the colonies, the intermediate myeloblasts and promyleocytes also must have survived, proliferated, and differentiated. So it is with these populations that G-CSF might be expected to have most of its effects.

This theory proved to be the case in in vivo studies in mice and humans. In studies reviewed by Lord *(61)*, it has been shown that the primary target of G-CSF is the promyleocyte/myeloblast population and that the accelerated neutrophil production under the influence of injected rHuG-CSF can be accounted for by the accelerated emigration of neutrophils from the bone marrow to the blood and by accompanying this acceleration with the insertion of a modest number of an extra amplification division. In addition, it was documented by both Lord and others *(60,62)* that moncytopoicsis is influenced profoundly by G-CSF, by mechanisms yet to be explained. Perhaps surprisingly, the longer lasting form of rHuG-CSF, pegfilgrastim, has exactly similar effects on neutrophil production kinetics to unmodified recombinant human G-CSF *(49)*, confirming that this pegylated derivative retains essentially the same biology as the parent molecule and differs significantly only in its pharmacokinetic properties.

3.2. Pharmacokinetics of G-CSF

rHuG-CSF has been administered to patients intravenously *(13,14)*, subcutaneously *(63)*, and intramuscularly *(64)*. In each case, the pharmacodynamic response, i.e., the neutrophil effect, is similar. Serum concentrations increase very quickly after intravenous infusion and peak within a matter of minutes at over 350 pg/mL *(13,14)*. Serum concentrations attained after subcutaneous administration also suggest a very rapid absorption *(15)*. The clearance of rG-CSF from the body has been examined in many species, and in all cases the serum half-life has been found to be between 1 and 2 h *(42,65,66)*. In humans, the half-life has been reported to be 4.7 h in the absence of neutrophils, but less than 2 h at higher absolute neutrophil counts (ANCs) *(67)*. The mode of clearance of the drug is of some interest not only because it is biologically appealing, but also because it has led to the development of derivatives with novel properties engineered to enhance the usefulness of the drug as a therapeutic.

Clearance of hematopoietic cytokines by blood cells has been reported for several important regulators, including thrombopoietin (TPO) *(68–71)*, erythropoietin (EPO) *(72)*, macrophage colony-stimulating factor (M-CSF) *(73,74)*, and G-CSF *(75)*. It has been suggested that homeostatic regulation may be an important process for the control of various blood cell types. In this model, the production of mature cell types in the blood would be promoted by a lineage-specific cytokine, and the mature cells would then negatively control their own number by being responsible for clearance of that very cytokine. To emphasize this point for G-CSF, the reciprocal relationship between G-CSF concentrations and neutrophil counts has been repeatedly reported *(76–79)*, as has the ability of neutrophils to destroy G-CSF in vitro *(80–82)*. Neutrophils have been shown, therefore, to be capable of removing a substantial amount of rHuG-CSF. In addition to this clearance mechanism, the role of the kidney in removal of rHuG-CSF from the body has been reported *(83–85)*. It is suggested by these observations that two mechanisms predominate in the clearance of rHuG-CSF from the body. One process, renal clearance, is of sufficient magnitude that to maintain effective serum concentrations, daily injections are required, even in conditions of absolute neutropenia. The other mechanism, mediated by neutrophils, is dependent on the number of neutrophils. It would be expected to be saturable and would lead to a progressive shortening of the rHuG-CSF half-life as neutrophils numbers increased; this is what was actually observed in early clinical studies *(75)*.

The implications of these combined mechanisms of clearance would be that stimulation of neutropoiesis would require frequent injections (since even in the total absence of neutrophils substantial amounts of rHuG-CSF would still be lost through the kidney) and as neutrophils numbers increase, rHuG-CSF would be more efficiently removed from the body. Understanding these factors led to the development of pegfilgrastim. This next-generation rHuG-CSF capitalizes on this dual mechanism of clearance in two ways: the chemical conjugation of G-CSF to a large PEG molecule renders it resistant to renal filtration owing to its disproportionate hydrodynamic size, yet its ability to interact with neutrophils in the same way as the parent molecule leaves neutrophil-mediated processes largely unchanged. These changes have several consequences for the therapeutic use of the drug. First, when injected in a neutropenic condition, it would be expected that circulating amounts would remain relatively constant until neutrophil recovery was significant. Second, when neutrophil numbers begin to accumulate owing to recovery from neutropenia, pegfilgrastim should be eliminated relatively quickly. Pegfilgrastim therefore represents a novel mechanism of action in that it capitalizes on the known pharmacokinetics of G-CSF to yield a molecule that is effectively self-regulating, remaining effective for periods of neutropenia of different duration. The limits of this flexibility must be fully explored, but preclinical and clinical data to date would appear to confirm the mechanism of action *(47,49,51,53,86,87)*. Table 3 compares the pharmacokinetics of pegfilgrastim and filgrastim.

3.3. Clinical Benefits of G-CSF

The dangers of neutropenia are manifold, whether that neutropenia is iatrogenic or congenital in nature since neutrophils play a critical role in protecting the body against

Table 3
Comparison of Filgrastim and Pegfilgrastim

Characteristic	*Filgrastim*	*Pegfilgrastim*
No. of amino acids	175	175
Cell source	*E. coli*	*E. coli*
Glycosylation	None	None
Pegylation	No	Yes
C_{max}	1.65–0.80 ng/mL for single 75-μg/kg dose	43.6–20 ng/mL for single 30-μg/kg dose
t_{max} (h)	5.5–1.8 for single 75-μg/kg dose	9.50–3.51 for single 30-μg/kg dose
Area under the curve	14.3–4.3 (0–24 h, ng·[h/L]) for single 75-μg/kg dose	887–336 (0–infinity, ng·[h/L]) for single 30-μg/kg dose

micro-organisms. The most intuitively obvious application of rHuG-CSF would be when endogenous amounts are low—it would not, for instance, be predicted that an autoimmune neutropenia involving destruction of neutrophils might respond to rHuG-CSF. Among iatrogenic neutropenias, chemotherapy-induced neutropenia in patients with cancer is widely discussed and is the best documented. It is in this setting that the first study of rHuG-CSF was performed. In 1987, Bronchud et al. *(12)* completed a small study in patients with lung cancer who received rHuG-CSF on alternating cycles of therapy. They noted a reduction in the severity of neutropenia in those cycles in which rHuG-CSF was administered. Since that time a large number of studies in a wide variety of chemotherapy regimes and other diseases have been published. These include lung cancer, lymphoma, breast cancer, bone marrow transplantation, testicular cancer, AIDS-related malignancies, myelodysplastic disorders, acute leukemia, congenital and cyclic neutropenias, and aplastic anemia, all of which are reviewed in Mortsyn et al. *(88)*.

Overall, the benefits of rHuG-CSF are that with its administration in chemotherapy- or radiotherapy-induced neutropenia, neutrophil recovery will begin sooner, proceed at a more rapid pace, and reduce the period when a patient might be in danger of developing febrile episodes. rHuG-CSF has few side effects, with bone pain being the only adverse effect of note, and it is normally managed with non-narcotic analgesics.

In addition to being used directly to increase neutrophil counts, rHuG-CSF can be used to mobilize precursor cells from the bone marrow to the blood, where they can be more easily collected. Although the mechanism of this effect remains largely unknown, by 1995 more than 80% of all transplants reported to the European Group for Blood and Marrow Transplantation (EBMT) were performed with cells harvested from the blood rather than the bone marrow *(89)*. These peripheral blood progenitor cells (PBPCs) have found use beyond the oncology setting, such as autoimmune disease *(90)*.

Currently, stem cells harvested from the peripheral blood after rHuG-CSF treatment represent one of several sources of stem cells (more strictly progenitor cells) that form the basis of so-called cell therapy. Alternative sources of such stem cells include umbilical cord blood, adult bone marrow, fetal tissues, and embryonal stem cells. The debate over the capacity of the cells from each of these sources is an active one, as are the ethical issues surrounding the use of each. Recent work, however, has indicated that early claims of stem cell plasticity (the ability to be "plastic," or flexible, with regard to contribution to other tissues) are becoming more widely appreciated and exploited *(91)*. Indeed, such is the level of excitement stemming from recent data indicating that PBPCs may be able to contribute to repair of the heart after myocardial infarction *(92)* that the entire August 2002 issue of the journal *Experimental Hematology* was dedicated to this question.

Additional uses for rHuG-CSF have been suggested, some supported by preliminary clinical data. Closure of fistulas in Crohn's disease has been reported *(93,94)*, as has quicker resolution of ulcers on the feet of patients with diabetes *(95)*.

In addition to these beneficial effects of rHuG-CSF, there have also been reports of side effects such as bone pain *(96,97)* and secondary leukemias. Leukemia evolving after rHuG-CSF in support of cancer therapy is a relatively rare event and may be associated with the exposure to mutagenic drugs such as topotecan. In other diseases, such as congenital neutropenias, it has been suggested that leukemia may be part of the normal evolution of the disease and that only the life-preserving effect of rHuG-CSF in early life allows the full expression later in life of the leukemic potential of some congenital neutropenias *(98,99)*. In the same population, the development of osteoporosis with extended rHuG-CSF treatment has been reported, although it remains unclear whether this is related to rHuG-CSF use or to a natural progression of the disease that is only expressed when rHuG-CSF allows the patients to survive long enough to develop symptoms *(100,101)*.

4. CONCLUSIONS

Various forms of rHuG-CSF have been available for clinical use for more than 10 years. rHuG-CSF increases neutrophil production and can reduce the possibility of bacterial or fungal infection. rHuG-CSF targets primarily cells within the bone marrow, reducing the time for them to mature and accelerating their release from the marrow to the circulation. It affects mature neutrophil function. Derivatives of G-CSF include a mutein and a PEG conjugate that have unique properties but retain the ability to influence the same biologic process as the parent molecule. Side effects of rHuG-CSF therapy are minor, usually involving only bone pain. In some circumstances, such as myelodysplastic syndromes and congenital neutropenias, the beneficial effects of rHuG-CSF may extend survival of patients long enough for the disease to evolve or progress.

REFERENCES

1. Nicola NA, Metcalf D, Matsumoto M, Johnson GR. Purification of a factor inducing differentiation in murine myelomonocytic leukemia cells. Identification as granulocyte colony-stimulating factor. *J Biol Chem* 1983; 258:9017–9023.
2. Welte K, Platzer E, Lu L, et al. Purification and biochemical characterization of human pluripotent hematopoietic colony-stimulating factor. *Proc Natl Acad Sci USA* 1985; 82:1526–1530.
3. Nomura H, Imazeki I, Oheda M, et al. Purification and characterization of human granulocyte colony-stimulating factor (G-CSF). *EMBO J* 1986; 5:871–876.
4. Nagata S, Tsuchiya M, Asano S, et al. Molecular cloning and expression of cDNA for human granulocyte colony-stimulating factor. *Nature* 1986; 319:415–418.
5. Souza LM, Boone TC, Gabrilove J, et al. Recombinant human granulocyte colony-stimulating factor: effects on normal and leukemic myeloid cells. *Science* 1986; 232:61–65.
6. Flynn J, Salvado AJ, Foote MA. Hematopoietic growth factors. In: Crommelin DJA, Sindelar RD, eds., *Pharmaceutical Biotechnology.* London: Harwood Academic. 193–215, 2002.

7. Kanda N, Fukushige S, Murotsu T, et al. Human gene coding for granulocyte-colony stimulating factor is assigned to the q21-q22 region of chromosome 17. *Somat Cell Mol Genet* 1987; 13:679–684.
8. Koeffler HP, Gasson J, Ranyard J, Souza L, Shepard M, Munker R. Recombinant human TNF alpha stimulates production of granulocyte colony-stimulating factor. *Blood* 1987; 70:55–59.
9. Ernst TJ, Ritchie AR, Demetri GD, Griffin JD. Regulation of granulocyte- and monocyte-colony stimulating factor mRNA levels in human blood monocytes is mediated primarily at a post-transcriptional level. *J Biol Chem* 1989; 264:5700–5703.
10. Nishizawa M, Nagata S. Regulatory elements responsible for inducible expression of the granulocyte colony-stimulating factor gene in macrophages. *Mol Cell Biol* 1990; 10:2002–2011.
11. Platzer E, Oez S, Welte K, et al. Human pluripotent hemopoietic colony stimulating factor: activities on human and murine cells. *Immunobiology* 1986; 172:185–193.
12. Bronchud MH, Scarffe JH, Thatcher N, et al. Phase I/II study of recombinant human granulocyte colony-stimulating factor in patients receiving intensive chemotherapy for small cell lung cancer. *Br J Cancer* 1987; 56:809–813.
13. Gabrilove JL, Jakubowski A, Scher H, et al. Effect of granulocyte colony-stimulating factor on neutropenia and associated morbidity due to chemotherapy for transitional-cell carcinoma of the urothelium. *N Engl J Med* 1988; 318:1414–1422.
14. Gabrilove JL, Jakubowski A, Fain K, et al. Phase I study of granulocyte colony-stimulating factor in patients with transitional cell carcinoma of the urothelium. *J Clin Invest* 1988; 82:1454–1461.
15. Morstyn G, Campbell L, Souza LM, et al. Effect of granulocyte colony stimulating factor on neutropenia induced by cytotoxic chemotherapy. *Lancet* 1988; 1:667–672.
16. Welte K, Gabrilove J, Bronchud MH, Platzer E, Morstyn G. Filgrastim (r-metHuG-CSF): the first 10 years. *Blood* 1996; 88:1907–1929.
17. Kubota N, Orita T, Hattori K, Oh-eda M, Ochi N, Yamazaki T. Structural characterization of natural and recombinant human granulocyte colony-stimulating factors. *J Biochem* 1990; 107:486–492.
18. Zink T, Ross A, Luers K, Cieslar C, Rudolph R, Holak TA. Structure and dynamics of the human granulocyte colony-stimulating factor determined by NMR spectroscopy: loop mobility in a four-helix-bundle protein. *Biochemistry* 1994; 33:8453–8463.
19. Oh-eda M, Hasegawa M, Hattori K, et al. O-linked sugar chain of human granulocyte colony-stimulating factor protects it against polymerization and denaturation allowing it to retain its biological activity. *J Biol Chem* 1990; 265:11432–11435.
20. Ono M. Physicochemical and biochemical characteristics of glycosylated recombinant human granulocyte colony stimulating factor (lenograstim). *Eur J Cancer* 1994; 30A(suppl 3):S7–11.
21. Wang C, Eufemi M, Turano C, Giartosio A. Influence of the carbohydrate moiety on the stability of glycoproteins. *Biochemistry* 1996; 35:7299–7307.
22. Arakawa T, Prestrelski SJ, Narhi LO, Boone TC, Kenney WC. Cysteine 17 of recombinant human granulocyte-colony stimulating factor is partially solvent-exposed. *J Protein Chem* 1993; 12:525–531.
23. Nissen C. Glycosylation of recombinant human granulocyte colony stimulating factor: implications for stability and potency. *Eur J Cancer* 1994; 30A(suppl 3):S12–14.
24. Pedrazzoli P, Gibelli N, Pavesi L, et al. Effects of glycosylated and non-glycosylated G-CSFs, alone and in combination with other cytokines, on the growth of human progenitor cells. *Anticancer Res* 1996; 16:1781–1785.
25. Mire-Sluis AR, Das RG, Thorpe R. The international standard for granulocyte colony stimulating factor (G-CSF). Evaluation in an international collaborative study. Participants of the Collaborative Study. *J Immunol Methods* 1995; 179:117–126.
26. Querol S, Cancelas JA, Amat L, Capmany G, Garcia J. Effect of glycosylation of recombinant human granulocytic colony-stimulating factor on expansion cultures of umbilical cord blood CD34+ cells. *Haematologica* 1999; 84:493–498.
27. Tanaka H, Tanaka Y, Shinagawa K, Yamagishi Y, Ohtaki K, Asano K. Three types of recombinant human granulocyte colony-stimulating factor have equivalent biological activities in monkeys. *Cytokine* 1997; 9:360–369.
28. Bonig H, Silbermann S, Weller S, et al. Glycosylated vs non-glycosylated granulocyte colony-stimulating factor (G-CSF)—results of a prospective randomised monocentre study. *Bone Marrow Transplant* 2001; 28:259–264.
29. Nohynek GJ, Plard JP, Wells MY, Zerial A, Roquet F. Comparison of the potency of glycosylated and nonglycosylated recombinant human granulocyte colony-stimulating factors in neutropenic and non-neutropenic CD rats. *Cancer Chemother Pharmacol* 1997; 39:259–266.

30. Uzumaki H, Okabe T, Sasaki N, et al. Identification and characterization of receptors for granulocyte colony-stimulating factor on human placenta and trophoblastic cells. *Proc Natl Acad Sci USA* 1989; 86:9323–9326.
31. Piao YF, Okabe T. Receptor binding of human granulocyte colony-stimulating factor to the blast cells of myeloid leukemia. *Cancer Res* 1990; 50:1671–1674.
32. Okabe M, Asano M, Kuga T, et al. In vitro and in vivo hematopoietic effect of mutant human granulocyte colony-stimulating factor. *Blood* 1990; 75:1788–1793.
33. Togawa A, Mizoguchi H, Toyama K, Urabe A, Ohasi Y, Takaku F. [Clinical evaluation of rhG-CSF in patients with neutropenia induced by chemotherapy for multiple myeloma]. *Rinsho Ketsueki J Clin Hematol* 2000; 41:115–122.
34. Hangzhou Jiuyuan Gene Engineering Co, Ltd. http://www.china-gene.com/f-cpjse.html; accessed 18 September 2002.
35. Roberts MJ, Bentley MD, Harris JM. Chemistry for peptide and protein PEGylation. *Adv Drug Deliv Rev* 2002; 54:459–476.
36. Kinstler O, Molineux G, Treuheit M, Ladd D, Gegg C. Mono-N-terminal poly(ethylene glycol)-protein conjugates. *Adv Drug Deliv Rev* 2002; 54:477–485.
37. Hinds KD, Kim SW. Effects of PEG conjugation on insulin properties. *Adv Drug Deliv Rev* 2002; 54:505–530.
38. Chapman AP. PEGylated antibodies and antibody fragments for improved therapy: a review. *Adv Drug Deliv Rev* 2002; 54:531–545.
39. Wang Y-S, Youngster S, Grace M, Bausch J, Bordens R, Wyss DF. Structural and biological characterization of pegylated recombinant interferon alpha-2b and its therapeutic implications. *Adv Drug Deliv Rev* 2002; 54:547–570.
40. Veronese FM, Caliceti P, Schiavon O, Sergi M. Polyethylene glycol-superoxide dismutase, a conjugate in search of exploitation. *Adv Drug Deliv Rev* 2002; 54:587–606.
41. Molineux G. Pegylation: engineering improved pharmaceuticals for enhanced therapy. *Cancer Treat Rev* 2002a; 28(Suppl A):13–16.
42. Eliason JF, Greway A, Tare N, et al. Extended activity in cynomolgus monkeys of a granulocyte colony-stimulating factor mutein conjugated with high molecular weight polyethylene glycol. *Stem Cells* 2000; 18:40–45.
43. Tanaka H, Satake-Ishikawa R, Ishidawa M, Matsuki S, Asano K. Pharmacokinetics of recombinant human granulocyte colony-stimulating factor conjugated to polyethylene glycol in rats. *Cancer Res* 1991; 51:3710–3714.
44. van Der Auwera P, Platzer E, Xu ZX, et al. Pharmacodynamics and pharmacokinetics of single doses of subcutaneous pegylated human G-CSF mutant (Ro 25–8315) in healthy volunteers: comparison with single and multiple daily doses of filgrastim. *Am J Hematol* 2001; 66:245–251.
45. van Spriel AB, van den Herik-Oudijk IE, van de Winkel JG. A single injection of polyethylene-glycol granulocyte colony-stimulating factor strongly prolongs survival of mice with systemic candidiasis. *Cytokine* 2000; 12:666–670.
46. Jensen-Pippo KE, Whitcomb KL, Deprince RB, Ralph L, Habberfield AD. Internal bioavailability of human granulocyte colony stimulating factor conjugated with poly(ethylene glycol). *Pharm Res* 1996; 13:102–107.
47. Molineux G, Kinstler O, Briddell B, et al. A new form of filgrastim with sustained duration in vivo and enhanced ability to mobilize PBPC in both mice and humans. *Exp Hematol* 1999; 27:1724–1734.
48. de Haan G, Ausema A, Wilkens M, Molineux G, Dontje B. Efficient mobilization of haematopoietic progenitors after a single injection of pegylated recombinant human granulocyte colony-stimulating factor in mouse strains with distinct marrow-cell pool sizes. *Br J Haematol* 2000; 110:638–646.
49. Lord BI, Woolford LB, Molineux G. Kinetics of neutrophil production in normal and neutropenic animals during the response to filgrastim (r-metHu G-CSF) or filgrastim SD/01 (PEG-r-metHu G-CSF). *Clin Cancer Res* 2001; 7:2085–2090.
50. Holmes FA, Jones SE, O'Shaughnessy J, et al. Comparable efficacy and safety profiles of once-per-cycle pegfilgrastim and daily injection filgrastim in chemotherapy-induced neutropenia: a multicenter dose-finding study in women with breast cancer. *Ann Oncol* 2002; 13:903–909.
51. Green M, Koelbl H, Baselga J, et al. A randomized, double-blind, phase III study of fixed-dose, single-administration pegfilgrastim vs daily filgrastim in patients receiving myelosuppressive chemotherapy. *Ann Oncol* 2003; 14:29–35.

52. Yowell SL, Crawford J, Holmes FA, Yang B, Liang BC. Sustained-duration, once-per-chemotherapy-cycle pegfilgrastim demonstrates highly efficient, self-regulating, neutrophil-dependent elimination. *Pharmacotherapy* 2001; 21:1281.
53. Niven RW, Prestrelski SJ, Treuheit MJ, Ip AY, Arakawa T. Protein nebulization II. Stabilization of G-CSF to air-jet nebulization and the role of protectants. *Int J Pharmaceutics (Amsterdam)* 1996; 127:191–201.
54. Watanabe Y, Kiriyama M, Oe J, Kikuchi R, Mizufune Y, Matsumoto M. Pharmacodynamic activity (leukopoietic effect) of recombinant human granulocyte colony-stimulating factor (rhG-CSF) after rectal administration in rabbits with leukopenia induced by cyclophosphamide. *Biol Pharm Bull* 1996; 19:1064–1067.
55. Kojima S, Matsuyama T, Kodera Y, et al. Measurement of endogenous plasma granulocyte colony-stimulating factor in patients with acquired aplastic anemia by a sensitive chemiluminescent immunoassay. *Blood* 1996; 87:1303–1308.
56. Cebon J, Layton JE, Maher D, Morstyn G. Endogenous haemopoietic growth factors in neutropenia and infection. *Br J Haematol* 1994; 86:265–274.
57. Umesaki N, Fukumasu H, Miyama M, Kawabata M, Ogita S. Plasma granulocyte colony stimulating factor concentrations in pregnant women. *Gynecol Obstet Invest* 1995; 40:5–7.
58. Lieschke GJ, Grail D, Hodgson G, et al. Mice lacking granulocyte colony-stimulating factor have chronic neutropenia, granulocyte and macrophage progenitor cell deficiency, and impaired neutrophil mobilization. *Blood* 1994; 84:1737–1746.
59. Coccia MA, Hartley C, Sutherland W, et al. Prolonged neutropenia in a novel mouse granulocyte colony-stimulating factor neutralizing auto-immunoglobulin G mouse model. *Exp Hematol* 2001; 29 59–67.
60. Liu F, Wu HY, Wesselschmidt R, Kornaga T, Link DC. Impaired production and increased apoptosis of neutrophils in granulocyte colony-stimulating factor receptor-deficient mice. *Immunity* 1996; 5:491–501.
61. Lord BI. Myeloid cell kinetics in response to haemopoietic growth factors. *Baillieres Clin Haematol* 1992; 5:533–550.
62. Lord BI, Molineux G, Pojda Z, Souza LM, Mermod JJ, Dexter TM. Myeloid cell kinetics in mice treated with recombinant interleukin-3, granulocyte colony-stimulating factor (CSF), or granulocyte-macrophage CSF in vivo. *Blood* 1991; 77:2154–2159.
63. Morstyn G, Campbell L, Lieschke G, et al. Treatment of chemotherapy-induced neutropenia by subcutaneously administered granulocyte colony-stimulating factor with optimization of dose and duration of therapy. *J Clin Oncol* 1989; 7:1554–1562.
64. Di Leo A, Bajetta E, Nole F, et al. The intramuscular administration of granulocyte colony-stimulating factor as an adjunct to chemotherapy in pretreated ovarian cancer patients: an Italian Trials in Medical Oncology (ITMO) Group pilot study. *Br J Cancer* 1994; 69:961–966.
65. Tanaka H, Tokiwa T. Pharmacokinetics of recombinant human granulocyte colony-stimulating factor studied in the rat by a sandwich enzyme-linked immunosorbent assay *J Pharmacol Exp Ther* 1990; 255:724–729.
66. Tanaka H, Kaneko T. Pharmacokinetic and pharmacodynamic comparisons between human granulocyte colony-stimulating factor purified from human bladder carcinoma cell line 5637 culture medium and recombinant human granulocyte colony-stimulating factor produced in *Escherichia coli*. *J Pharmacol Exp Ther* 1992; 262:439–444.
67. Kearns CM, Wang WC, Stute N, Ihle JN, Evans WE. Disposition of recombinant human granulocyte colony-stimulating factor in children with severe chronic neutropenia. *J Pediatr* 1993; 123:471–479.
68. Nichol JL, Hokom MM, Hornkohl A, et al. Megakaryocyte growth and development factor. Analyses of in vitro effects on human megakaryopoiesis and endogenous serum levels during chemotherapy-induced thrombocytopenia. *J Clin Invest* 1995; 95:2973–2978.
69. Marsh JC, Gibson FM, Prue RL, et al. Serum thrombopoietin levels in patients with aplastic anaemia. *Br J Haematol* 1996; 95:605–610.
70. Emmons RV, Reid DM, Cohen RL, et al. Human thrombopoietin levels are high when thrombocytopenia is due to megakaryocyte deficiency and low when due to increased platelet destruction. *Blood* 1996; 87:4068–4071.
71. Fielder PJ, Hass P, Nagel M, et al. Human platelets as a model for the binding and degradation of thrombopoietin. *Blood* 1997; 89:2782–2788.
72. Kato M, Kamiyama H, Okazaki A, Kumaki K, Kato Y, Sugiyama Y. Mechanism for the nonlinear pharmacokinetics of erythropoietin in rats. *J Pharmacol Exp Ther* 1997; 283:520–527.

73. Redman BG, Flaherty L, Chou TH, et al. Phase I trial of recombinant macrophage colony-stimulating factor by rapid intravenous infusion in patients with cancer. *J Immunother* 1992; 12:50–54.
74. Bauer RJ, Gibbons JA, Bell DP, Luo ZP, Young JD. Nonlinear pharmacokinetics of recombinant human macrophage colony-stimulating factor (M-CSF) in rats. *J Pharmacol Exp Ther* 1994; 268:152–158.
75. Layton JE, Hockman H, Sheridan WP, Morstyn G. Evidence for a novel in vivo control mechanism of granulopoiesis: mature cell-related control of a regulatory growth factor. *Blood* 1989; 74:1303–1307.
76. Stute N, Santana VM, Rodman JH, Schell MJ, Ihle JN, Evans WE. Pharmacokinetics of subcutaneous recombinant human granulocyte colony-stimulating factor in children. *Blood* 1992; 79:2849–2854.
77. Shimazaki C, Uchiyama H, Fujita N, et al. Serum levels of endogenous and exogenous granulocyte colony-stimulating factor after autologous blood stem cell transplantation. *Exp Hematol* 1995; 23:1497–1502.
78. Takatani H, Soda H, Fukuda M, et al. Levels of recombinant human granulocyte colony-stimulating factor in serum are inversely correlated with circulating neutrophil counts. *Antimicrob Agents Chemother* 1996; 40:988–991.
79. Sturgill MG, Huhn RD, Drachtman RA, Ettinger AG, Ettinger LJ. Pharmacokinetics of intravenous recombinant human granulocyte colony-stimulating factor (rhG-CSF) in children receiving myelosuppressive cancer chemotherapy: clearance increases in relation to absolute neutrophil count with repeated dosing. *Am J Hematol* 1997; 54:124–130.
80. Kuwabara T, Uchimura T, Kobayashi H, Kobayashi S, Sugiyama Y. Receptor-mediated clearance of G-CSF derivative nartograstim in bone marrow of rats. *Am J Physiol* 1995; 269:1–9.
81. Kuwabara T, Uchimura T, Takai K, Kobayashi H, Kobayashi S, Sugiyama Y. Saturable uptake of a recombinant human granulocyte colony-stimulating factor derivative, nartograstim, by the bone marrow and spleen of rats in vivo. *J Pharmaco Exp Ther* 1995; 273:1114–1122.
82. Kuwabara T, Kobayashi S, Sugiyama Y. Kinetic analysis of receptor-mediated endocytosis of G-CSF derivative, nartograstim, in rat bone marrow cells. *Am J Physiol* 1996; 271:1–84.
83. Tanaka H, Tokiwa T. Influence of renal and hepatic failure on the pharmacokinetics of recombinant human granulocyte colony-stimulating factor krn-8601 in the rat. *Cancer Res* 1990; 50:6615–6619.
84. Kuwabara T, Ishikawa Y, Kobayashi H, Kobayashi S, Sugiyama Y. Renal clearance of a recombinant granulocyte colony-stimulating factor, nartograstim, in rats. *Pharm Res* 1995; 12:1466–1469.
85. Fukuda M, Oka M, Ishida Y, et al. Effects of renal function on pharmacokinetics of recombinant human granulocyte colony-stimulating factor in lung cancer patients. *Antimicrob Agents Chemother* 2001; 45:1947–1951.
86. Schwab G, Roskos L, Molineux G, et al. A phase I study of sustained-duration filgrastim in normal volunteers. *Exp Hematol* 1998; 26:709.
87. Roskos LK, Yang B, Schwab G, et al. A cytokinetic model describes the granulopoietic effects of r-metHuG-CSF-SD/01 (SD/01) and the homeostatic regulation of SD/01 clearance in normal volunteers. *Clin Pharmacol Ther* 1999; 65:196.
88. Morstyn G, Dexter TM, Foote MA, eds. *Filgrastim (r-metHuG-CSF) in Clinical Practice,* 2nd ed. Totowa, NJ: Humana. 1998.
89. Gratwohl A, Hermans J, Baldomero H. Blood and marrow transplantation activity in Europe 1995. European Group for Blood and Marrow Transplantation (EBMT). *Bone Marrow Transplant* 1997; 19:407–419.
90. Tyndall A. Immunoablation and haemopoietic stem cell transplantation for severe autoimmune disease with special reference to systemic lupus erythematosus. *Lupus* 2001; 10:214–215.
91. Wulf GG, Jackson KA, Goodell MA. Somatic stem cell plasticity: current evidence and emerging concepts. *Exp Hematol* 2001; 29:1361–1370.
92. Orlic D, Kajstura J, Chimenti S, et al. Mobilized bone marrow cells repair the infarcted heart, improving function and survival. *Proc Natl Acad Sci USA* 2001; 98:10344–10349.
93. Korzenik JR, Dieckgraefe BK. Immunostimulation in Crohn's disease: results of a pilot study of G-CSF (R-methuG-CSF) in mucosal and fistulizing Crohn's disease. *Gastroenterology* 2000; 118:AGA A874–AGA A875.
94. Dejaco C, Gasche C, Poetzi R, Gangl A, Vogelsang H, Reinisch W. Safety and efficacy of granulocyte colony stimulating factor (G-CSF) for treatment of severe endoscopic postoperative recurrence in Crohn's disease (CD). *Gastroenterology* 2000; 118:AGA A566.

95. Edmonds M, Gough A, Solovera J, Standaert B. Filgrastim in the treatment of infected diabetic foot ulcers. Retrospective cost analysis of a phase II randomised clinical trial. *Clin Drug Invest* 1999; 17:275–286.
96. Froberg MK, Garg UC, Stroncek DF, Geis M, McCullough J, Brown DM. Changes in serum osteocalcin and bone-specific alkaline phosphatase are associated with bone pain in donors receiving granulocyte-colony-stimulating factor for peripheral blood stem and progenitor cell collection. *Transfusion* 1999; 39:410–414.
97. Kubista E, Glaspy J. Holmes FA, et al. Bone pain associated with once-per-cycle pegfilgrastim is similar to daily filgrastim in patients with breast cancer. *Clin Breast Cancer* 2003; 3:391–398.
98. Freedman MH, Bonilla MA, Fier C, et al. Myelodysplasia syndrome and acute myeloid leukemia in patients with congenital neutropenia receiving G-CSF therapy. *Blood* 2000; 96:429–436.
99. Tschan CA, Pilz C, Zeidler C, Welte K, Germeshausen M. Time course of increasing numbers of mutations in the granulocyte colony-stimulating factor receptor gene in a patient with congenital neutropenia who developed leukemia. *Blood* 2001; 97:82–1884.
100. Bishop NJ, Williams BM, Compston JC, Stirling DM, Prentice A. Osteoporosis in severe congenital neutropenia treated with granulocyte colony-stimulating factor. *Br J Haematol* 1995; 89:927–928.
101. Simon M, Lengfelder E, Reiter S, Hehlmann R. Osteoporosis in severe congenital neutropenia: Inherent to the disease or a sequela of G-CSF treatment? *Am J Hematol* 1996; 52:127.

6 Erythropoietic Factors

Clinical Pharmacology and Pharmacokinetics

Steven Elliott, PhD, *Anne C. Heatherington,* PhD, *and MaryAnn Foote,* PhD

CONTENTS

1. INTRODUCTION

In the 1950s, pioneering studies by Erslev and others conclusively demonstrated the presence of a humoral factor capable of stimulating erythropoiesis *(1,2)*. It was not until 1977, however, that Miyake et al. *(3)* isolated human erythropoietin (HuEPO) from the urine of severely anemic patients. Although preparation of the pure hormone allowed amino-acid sequencing of small EPO peptide fragments, it wasn't until 1983, with the use of unique probing strategies of a genomic library that the human *EPO* gene was cloned *(4)*. In this chapter, we review the clinical pharmacology of recombinant human erythropoietin (rHuEPO), including its chemistry, pharmacologic actions, pharmacokinetics, pharmacodynamics, and activity in various patient populations. In addition, newer erythropoietic proteins, such as darbepoetin alfa, as well as some ongoing research approaches to creating other new erythropoietic molecules, are discussed.

From: *Cancer Drug Discovery and Development*
Hematopoietic Growth Factors in Oncology: Basic Science and Clinical Therapeutics
Edited by: G. Morstyn, M. A. Foote, and G. J. Lieschke © Humana Press Inc., Totowa, NJ

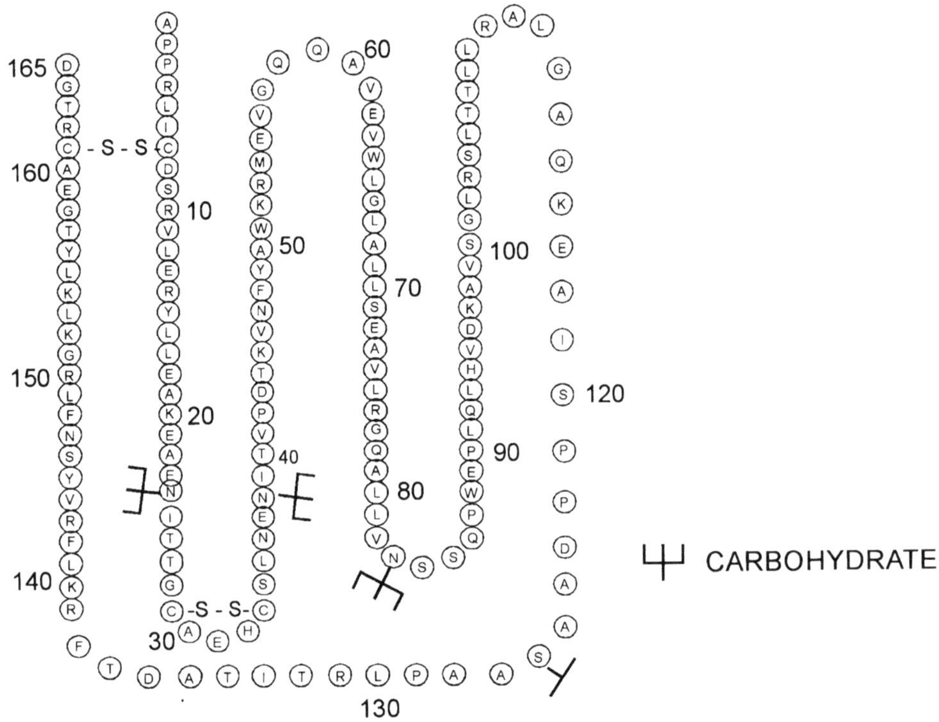

Fig. 1. EPO undergoes post-translational glycosylation at three specific asparagine residues (Asn24, Asn38, and Asn83) and one serine residue (Ser126).

2. CHEMISTRY

EPO, in both the endogenous and recombinant form, has a single polypeptide chain backbone composed of 165 amino acids *(5)*. rHuEPO forms a bundle of 4 α-helices that are folded into a compact globular structure *(6,7)*. Separate regions of the molecule contain the two EPO receptor-binding (EPOR) sites *(6,8)* of high (site 1: 1 n*M*) and low (site 2: 4 μ*M*) affinity *(9,10)*. Receptor activation occurs when one EPO molecule homodimerizes two EPOR molecules *(6,11)*.

EPO undergoes post-translational glycosylation at three specific asparagine residues (Asn24, Asn38, and Asn83) and one serine residue (Ser126) *(12,13)* (Fig. 1). In mammalian cells, the carbohydrate chains are typically of the complex type and contribute to approx 40% of the mass of the hormone *(14)*. The polypeptide backbone of the human EPO molecule has an invariant sequence and structure; however, the carbohydrate chains exhibit microheterogeneity in terms of composition and structure *(15–17)*. A negatively charged sialic acid molecule typically caps the end of each carbohydrate chain branch. As a consequence, the variable nature of the sialic acid content results in EPO isoforms with differences in charge.

The *N*-linked carbohydrates are important for retention of in vivo but not in vitro biologic activity *(16,18)*, and their sialic acid residues ensure, and promote, the molecule's survival in the circulation *(19)*.

Several rEPO molecules are used clinically, including epoetin alfa and epoetin beta. Epoetin alfa (marketed as Epogen®, Procrit®, Eprex®, and Erypo®) is available in most of the developed world, including the United States, Europe, Canada, Australia, and Asia. Epoetin beta (NeoRecormon®) is available in Europe and Japan. Both of these types of rHuEPO are produced in Chinese hamster ovary (CHO) cultures. No important differences in their clinical efficacy are apparent, and they are generally used interchangeably *(20)*. A novel glycosylation analog of EPO, darbepoetin alfa (Aranesp®) has the same safety profile and performs the same function as rHuEPO; however, it has a threefold increased serum half-life and increased in vivo potency, allowing for more flexible modes of administration, including extended dosing. Other rHuEPO moieties such as epoetin omega, are also marketed in Eastern Europe, Mexico, and South America.

3. SYNTHESIS OF ERYTHROPOIETIN

The primary site of EPO production in adults is the kidney, and peritubular cells are thought to be responsible for EPO synthesis *(20–22)*. The liver is a secondary site of EPO production, with synthesis occurring in both hepatocyes and fibroblastoid interstitial cells *(23)*. Recently, astrocytes and neurons within the central nervous system have been reported to express EPO *(24)*. No preformed stores of EPO exist, and plasma EPO concentrations are maintained at a constant concentration by basal production of the hormone *(25)*. Within a healthy individual, the plasma EPO concentration tends to be controlled tightly, but there is large interindividual variability (approximately normal range: 4–30 mU/mL). Plasma EPO concentrations have shown a small diurnal variation in some studies but not in others *(26,27)*.

Tissue hypoxia is a physiologic stimulus for EPO production, and numerous studies have shown an exponential increase in plasma EPO with increasing degrees of anemia *(1,20)*. Anemia (hematocrit $< 35\%$) and, as a consequence, tissue hypoxia regulate EPO expression at the gene level, and EPO concentrations can increase 100–1000-fold in response to anemia. The mechanism of hypoxic stimulation of EPO production is the focus of much investigation *(22,28)*. Under conditions of hypoxia, *EPO* gene transcription is activated when hypoxia-inducible factor-1 (HIF-1) binds to a hypoxia-responsive enhancer located in the 3′ flanking sequence of the *EPO* gene. HIF-1 is a heterodimer composed of an oxygen-sensitive HIF-1α and a constitutive HIF-1β *(29)*. This protein complex, in conjunction with other factors, signals *EPO* gene synthesis. The mechanism by which HIF-1α activity is regulated by oxygen is partially understood. HIF-1α contains proline residues within oxygen-dependent domains (ODDs) *(30)* that are hydroxylated by a family of prolyl hydroxylases (HIF-PH1, HIF-PH2, HIF-PH3, and HIF-PH4) *(31,32)*. HIF-PHs are iron-containing proteins that are positively regulated by oxygen. Under conditions of normoxia, HIF-PHs are active, which then hydroxylates HIF-1α. Hydroxylated HIF-1α is then targeted for destruction by the von Hippel Lindau tumor suppressor gene (pVHL), a component of protein ubiquitin ligase *(33)*. HIF-1α is also hydroxylated at an asparagine residue near its C-terminus by another oxygen-regulated hydroxylase, factor inhibiting HIF-1 (FIH) *(34,35)*. Hydroxylation of HIF-1α by FIH results in inhibition of HIF-1 association with a cofactor (p300) required for transcriptional activation of the *EPO* gene promoter. Under hypoxic conditions, HIF-PH and FIH are both inactive, allowing for increased levels of active HIF-1α/HIF-1β/p300 *EPO* gene transcription complexes and thereby resulting in increased *EPO* gene transcription.

4. ROLE OF ERYTHROPOIETIN IN ERYTHROPOIESIS

In healthy individuals, red blood cell (RBC) production matches RBC loss. This remarkable homeostasis is controlled primarily by changes in rates of RBC formation through alterations in EPO concentrations. EPO regulates erythropoiesis by promoting the survival, proliferation, and differentiation of erythroid progenitors *(28)*. Erythropoiesis encompasses the orderly differentiation of pluripotent, hematopoietic stem cells to mature erythrocytes. Erythropoiesis occurs primarily in the bone marrow and requires 10–14 d for the early progenitor cells, erythroid burst-forming units (BFU-E) to differentiate to erythrocytes. Later stage progenitors, erythroid colony-forming units (CFU-E), require approx 7 d; however, RBC counts increase within 1–2 d of EPO synthesis because cells even later in the differentiation process are present and responsive to EPO. The 1-d to 2-wk time period for RBC formation is relatively fast compared with the life span of an erythrocyte (60–120 d). The temporal mismatch indicates that changes in rates of RBC formation determine RBC counts.

A number of growth factors control the earliest steps of erythroid cell development, including stem cell factor (SCF), granulocyte-macrophage colony stimulating factor (GM-CSF), and several interleukins (ILs) *(22)*. The earliest cell committed to the erythroid lineage, the BFU-E, is weakly stimulated by EPO. Differentiation of BFU-E cells to the CFU-E stage does not absolutely require EPO, as shown in an elegant series of studies with knockout mice that lacked the *EPO* gene *(36)*. Steps subsequent to the CFU-E stage are EPO-dependent such that EPO is absolutely required for cell survival *(37)*. CFU-E differentiate into additional cell types, ultimately resulting in a reticulocyte. Enucleation of reticulocytes produces mature erythrocytes. The EPO requirement is lost at the last stages (orthochromic erythroblast) of erythropoiesis *(21)*.

EPO acts on erythroid precursor cells through its receptor (EPOR), a transmembrane protein that is a member of the type I cytokine receptor superfamily. Activation of EPOR occurs through homodimerization whereby one EPO molecule binds two EPORs on the surface of the CFU-E (approx 1000 EPORs/cell). EPOR homodimerization activates a number of signal transduction pathways, including Janus Kinase/Signal transducers and activators of transcription (JAK-STAT), phosphatidylinositol 3-kinase (PI3K), and RAS-mitogen-activated protein kinase (MAPK) *(21,22)*. Current research suggests that EPO exerts its control over erythropoiesis by preventing cell apoptosis (programmed cell death), thus allowing more red cell precursors to survive, proliferate, and induce erythroid-specific proteins *(37)*. Some of the apoptotic tendency of erythroid cells is attributed to proapoptotic molecules produced by hematopoietic cells, macrophages, inflammatory cytokines, and stromal cells. EPO prevents apoptosis by upregulation of antiapoptotic *Bcl* proteins (Bcl2, $BclX_L$,) and downregulation/inactivation of apoptotic proteins (BAD, a prodeath Bc12 family member, tumor necrosis factor-related apoptosis-inducing ligand (TRAIL) forkhead and caspases) *(38–43)*.

5. ENDOGENOUS EPO CONCENTRATIONS IN HEALTH AND DISEASE

Maintenance of normal plasma levels of endogenous EPO requires the synthesis of about 2–3 U/kg/d, or approx 1000–1500 U/wk for a 70-kg man *(44)*. No significant sex differences are found in endogenous EPO concentrations. In a study of athletes *(45)*, regular-to-moderate training did not appear to affect endogenous EPO concentrations.

The overexpression of EPO occurs in a number of adaptive and pathologic conditions. In response to acute hypoxic stress, such as severe blood loss or severe anemia, EPO production can increase 100- to 1000-fold, although the maximal bone marrow response to such stimulation is only a 4- to 6-fold increase in RBC production *(46)*. Overproduction of EPO with accompanying erythrocytosis may be an adaptive response to conditions that produce chronic tissue hypoxia, such as living at high altitude, chronic respiratory diseases, cyanotic heart disease, sleep apnea, smoking, localized renal hypoxia, or hemoglobinopathies with increased oxygen affinity *(21)*. Paraneoplastic production of EPO from tumors and cysts, including renal carcinomas, benign renal tumors, Wilms' tumors, hepatomas, liver carcinomas, cerebellar hemangioblastomas, adrenal gland tumors, and leiomyomas, can also result in high plasma concentrations of the hormone.

In chronic renal disease, up to 60% of patients are anemic (hemoglobin [Hb] concentration < 11 g/dL) before beginning dialysis *(47)*. Multiple mechanisms are involved *(22)*, but the most important are the inability of the diseased kidneys to produce an appropriate EPO response for the given degree of anemia or an inability to meet the increased red cell demands of uremic patients *(48,49)*. In addition, the uremic state itself appears to blunt the bone marrow response to EPO, perhaps through polyamines, inflammatory cytokines, and/or parathyroid hormone mediators *(22,50)*. It is of interest that chronically anemic dialysis patients who have acute hypoxic stress (from either acute bleeding or systemic hypoxemia) are able to increase their serum EPO concentrations at least partially, suggesting that kidney failure does not result in a complete inability to produce EPO *(51,52)*.

The anemia of cancer is also of multifactorial etiology. As with other anemias of chronic disease, including those associated with chronic infection and inflammatory disorders, there is decreased production of endogenous EPO *(53)*, cytokine-induced suppression of bone marrow function, disordered iron absorption and metabolism *(54)*, and decreased RBC survival. A number of other factors may also contribute to anemia in patients with cancer *(25)*; however, the amount of endogenous EPO increases transiently during the administration of some chemotherapeutic drugs *(55)*.

Finally, the anemias associated with infant prematurity, pregnancy, allogeneic bone marrow transplantation, and HIV infection are often characterized by inappropriately low EPO concentrations *(23)*.

6. ASSAYS FOR ERYTHROPOIETIN

The earliest EPO assays were bioassays that measured biologic effects of the test sample in intact animals or cultures of erythroid tissues *(1)*. Various endpoints were used, including ^{59}Fe uptake, production of BFU-E or CFU-E, or increase in Hb concentration or reticulocyte number. Bioassays are still used as reference assays for establishing the potency of rHuEPO in pharmaceutical development. In vitro assays are useful in determination of receptor interactions and response at the cellular level; however, in vitro activity is not necessarily predictive of in vivo activity *(56)*. A common in vivo assay, used to define the "erythropoietic unit," measures short-term erythropoietic activity (defined as the instantaneous rate of ^{59}Fe incorporation into heme 1–2 d after administration of the test agent *(57)*. This measure was appropriate when all erythropoietic molecules had similar serum half-lives; however, with the discovery of darbepoetin alfa, an erythropoietic molecule with a threefold longer serum half-life than that of rHuEPO *(58,59)* and increased in vivo activity *(56)*, it became apparent that this assay was ineffective at predicting biologic response, particularly at extended time periods. For example, darbepoetin alfa was three- to fourfold more potent than rHuEPO when the agents were administered three times per week *(59)*. The potency difference increased to approx 13-fold when the test agents were administered once per week. This observation indicated that erythropoietic molecules with pharmacokinetic properties different from that of the EPO reference standard will have a relative in vivo potency difference compared with rHuEPO that depends on the frequency of administration, route of administration, and other variables.

The purification of EPO allowed development of the immunoassay that is generally used today for both clinical and research purposes *(60)*. This assay has proved particularly useful clinically because there is only one circulating and biologically active form of EPO; there are no preformed stores of the hormone; and the molecule bears little homology to any other circulating hematopoietic growth factor (HGF) except for thrombopoietin (TPO), with which it shares approx 20% sequence identity *(61)*. Commercial EPO assays use immunoassays that detect the antibody/EPO complexes by hemagglutination inhibition, chemiluminescence of attached molecules, radioactivity counting (radioimmunoassay), or enzymatic production of a chromagen (enzyme immunoassays, including enzyme-linked immunosorbent assay [ELISA]) *(62)*. The limit of detection is generally in the range of 2–15 mU/mL, which covers normal endogenous EPO concentrations.

Because of the identity in amino acid sequence between rHuEPO and endogenous EPO, the assays used for most clinical, pharmacokinetic, and pharmacodynamic studies measured both endogenous and exogenous hormone. To correct for the inability of the assay to differentiate between the two entities, at least one, and up to three, blood samples were collected and assayed for their EPO content in these studies before the administration of rHuEPO. This baseline value was used for the concentration of endogenous EPO and was subtracted from each "on-drug" concentration measurement *(63,64)*. This correction is an approximation, however, since it assumes that endogenous EPO concentrations remain constant during the sampling period, although fluctuations in EPO concentrations are frequent *(26)*. The potential for error with this method is greater when low doses of rHuEPO are being evaluated, since the endogenous EPO contributes a larger percentage of the total *(65)*.

Very recently, an assay was developed to differentiate endogenous EPO from epoetin alfa and epoetin beta products in urine *(66)*. This assay detects immunoblotted EPO separated into different isoforms by isoelectric focusing. A key step was the development of double immunoblotting, which increased sensitivity sufficiently so that the small amounts of rHuEPO and endogenous EPO present in urine could be detected. The assay has been used to detect rHuEPO abuse by athletes. The same assay can detect immunoblotted darbepoetin alfa from urine samples *(67)*, and this assay was used to detect darbepoetin alfa abuse by athletes in the 2002 Winter Olympics.

7. PHARMACOKINETICS

7.1. Intravenous Administration in Healthy Volunteers

After intravenous administration, peak (15-min) plasma rHuEPO concentrations correlate linearly with dose; a dose of 50 U/kg produces peak concentrations of about 1000 mU/mL *(44)*. In single-dose studies, clearance decreases nonlinearly with increasing dose, resulting in a longer half-life of rHuEPO as the dose administered is increased *(65)*. In multiple-dose studies of intravenous rHuEPO in healthy subjects, however, clearance appears to increase over the initial period of multiple dosing *(70)*.

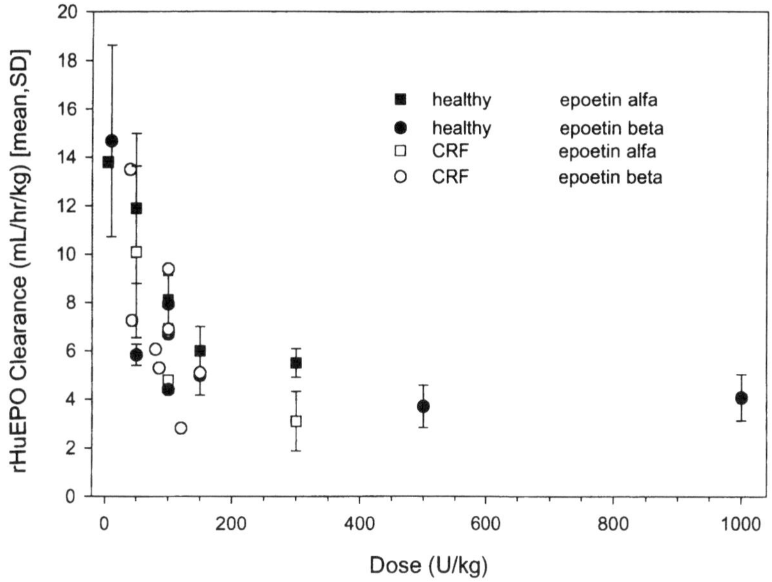

Fig. 2. Clearance of rHuEPO over a range of doses in healthy adults and patients with kidney disease, based on literature estimates. (From ref. *68*.)

Flaharty et al. *(65)* administered epoetin alfa in single iv doses of 10, 50,150, 500, and 1000 U/kg, and found a trend of decreasing clearance with increasing dose, with the most dramatic difference being between 10 and 50 U/kg (approx threefold decrease). The reduction in clearance resulted in longer half-lives as dose increased, i.e., from 4.4 h at 10 U/kg to 5.3 h at 50 U/kg and 8.5 h at 500 U/kg (range: 4.4–11.0 h). Over the dose range of 100–150 U/kg, clearance was approx 7 mL/h/kg, and terminal half-life was approx 5 h.

rHuEPO's dose-nonlinearity has not been well characterized. In one study, Veng-Pedersen et al. *(70)* administered single iv doses of epoetin alfa at three dose levels (10, 100, and 500 U/kg) in a three-way crossover study in 10 healthy volunteers. Again, clearance decreased as dose increased, which they ascribed primarily to a nonlinear, saturable mechanism obeying Michaelis-Menten kinetics.

Generally, one *(71)* or two *(72)* phases are evident in the serum concentration-time profiles. When only one phase was observed, it is likely that the early rapid phase was not captured (owing to sampling schedule and/or interindividual variation) and that the slower, later phase dominated. The volume of distribution was generally similar to that of plasma volume (40–60 mL/kg), indicating limited extravascular distribution *(65,69)*.

McMahon et al. *(69)* compared the single-dose and multiple-dose pharmacokinetics of epoetin alfa (150 and 300 U/kg iv) in a parallel design. At both dose levels, the mean clearance increased by 25% after five doses, resulting in a comparable reduction in terminal half-life. The largest change in clearance occurred between the first and second doses.

7.2. Subcutaneous Administration in Healthy Volunteers

Subcutaneously administered rHuEPO is absorbed slowly and incompletely, resulting in substantially lower serum concentration vs time profiles, an extended terminal half-life (24–79 h), and a bioavailability ranging from 20 to 40% compared to iv rHuEPO (*68*). The pharmacokinetic model that describes subcutaneous rHuEPO data is called "flip flop" because absorption, rather than elimination, is the rate-limiting step *(61,70)*. Peak serum levels are only about 5–10% of those achieved with an iv dose and are reached in most studies between 16 and 29 h *(74,75)*. Neither the rate nor the extent of absorption are dose dependent. Data from selected studies follow.

Cheung et al. *(74)* studied single-dose administration of epoetin alfa at eight dose levels ranging from 300 to 2400 U/kg with an extended sampling period post dose. A linear relationship existed between C_{max} and dose, and T_{max} generally occurred between 16 and 29 h post dose. The mean terminal half-life varied up to threefold (range: 24–79 h), with up to 100% interindividual variability, but there was no consistent effect of dose on half-life. For groups with lower variability (% coefficient of variation [CV] < 50%), the mean half-life was between 24 and 36 h. In another dose-ranging study, Sans et al. *(76)* determined the single-dose pharmacokinetics of epoetin beta at 30, 60, and 100 U/kg (n = 3/group). They noted a dose-proportional increase in area-under-the curve (AUC), a constant T_{max}, and no dose dependency for terminal half-life. In a third study, Hayashi et al. *(77)* used population pharmacokinetic analysis (nonlinear mixed effects modeling) to describe the data from a study of epoetin beta in 48 healthy volunteers (1500 and 3000 U). Using a one-compartment model with first-order absorption, they found no dose dependency in the parameter estimates.

Multiple dose studies of sc administered rHuEPO have provided disparate results. McMahon et al. *(69)* reported that C_{max} after five doses of 150 U/kg epoetin alfa was much increased relative to a single dose; however, after five doses of 300 U/kg, C_{max} was similar to its single-dose value. Sans et al. *(76)* found a significant decrease in AUC (between 57 and 90% of single-dose values) and C_{max} (between 47 and 76% of single-dose values) after three doses of epoetin beta at 30, 60, or 100 U/kg (n = 3/group). For each group, there was a concomitant increase in terminal half-life (by one- to twofold) and mean residence time (MRT), and a 5–9-h prolongation in mean T_{max}. In the study by Cheung et al. *(74)*, the pharmacokinetic properties of epoetin alfa did not change substantially between the first and the fourth weekly doses of 600 U/kg (n = 5).

Most assessments of the bioavailability of sc administered rHuEPO have not taken into account the nonlinearity of rHuEPO pharmacokinetics. To gain an accurate determination of bioavailability for a drug cleared in a nonlinear manner, it is necessary to determine the underlying intravenous kinetics and then quantify the subcutaneous bioavailability by modeling; however, published bioavailability estimates have been obtained by administration of the same dose intravenously and subcutaneously with comparison of AUC; this method tends to underestimate bioavailability, especially at lower doses of rHuEPO, at which the nonlinearity in clearance is most evident. With this caveat in mind, bioavailability estimates for subcutaneously administered rHuEPO range from about 20 to 40% when determined in crossover studies *(71,78,79)*.

7.3. Pharmacokinetics in Nephrology Patients: Intravenous Administration

Most pharmacokinetic studies in this population have evaluated anemic patients receiving dialysis who were rHuEPO-naive. Few studies have been published in patients who retain some degree of kidney function. Since rHuEPO is a therapy for these patients, the studies are limited in their ability to investigate dose ranges or fixed dose regimens.

In general, after intravenous administration, the pharmacokinetic properties of rHuEPO are nonlinear with respect to dose, with clearance being faster at lower doses. Additionally, clearance appears to increase over the initial period of multiple dosing. As with healthy volunteers, two phases are generally evident in the serum concentration-time profiles of nephrology patients *(64,80–82),* although three phases (triexponential) have been reported *(80).* The volume of distribution is similar to that of plasma volume (40–60 mL/kg) *(63,81,82,84).*

Single-dose intravenous pharmacokinetic studies have generally included few patients, and the data are difficult to interpret *(68).* For example, Egrie et al. *(85)* and Lim et al. *(86)* each investigated a range of doses; however, only summary pharmacokinetic parameters across all dose groups were provided. Yamazaki et al. *(87),* using doses of 3000 U (60 U/kg) and 6000 U (120 U/kg), stated that they observed dose-dependent increases in AUC and C_{max}; however, mean clearance at the low dose was slightly higher than at the high dose (3000 U: 7.26 mL/h/kg; 6000 U: 5.84 mL/h/kg).

Most studies comparing single-dose and multiple-dose pharmacokinetics in nephrology patients have found that clearance increases and/or terminal half-life decreases after multiple dosing *(63,82,85,86).* Additionally, some investigators have reported that after the initial change (i.e., after 2–3 wk), no subsequent changes occurred (*85*). Conversely, other investigators reported no substantiative change in pharmacokinetic properties from single-dose values, either after reaching a new steady-state Hb value *(88)* or after 56 d *(87).* Jensen et al. *(72)* found no differences in the pharmacokinetic properties of epoetin beta after long-term treatment except for a reduction in the volume of distribution. In several studies, single-dose pharmacokinetics were not assessed; however, the authors concluded that the multiple-dose kinetics had not changed by using literature comparisons *(89)* or by noting a lack of differences between short-term treatment and long-term treatment *(90).*

7.4. Pharmacokinetics in Nephrology Patients: Subcutaneous Administration

As with healthy volunteers, all studies that investigated both intravenous and subcutaneous dosing have shown that absorption is rate limiting *(78,80).* Bioavailability has ranged from 20 to 40%, and dose or time dependencies are not apparent.

Only a few studies have evaluated single-dose, sc administration in rHuEPO-naive nephrology patients *(68).* In the very few studies that have investigated a range of doses, no apparent dose dependency in pharmacokinetic properties was determined.

Similar to the literature in healthy volunteers, no studies took into consideration the nonlinearity in the disposition of rHuEPO. Average bioavailability estimates for subcutaneously administered rHuEPO in nephrology patients tend to lie between 30 and 50% when determined in crossover studies *(63,87).* Several investigators have reported lower estimates (14.1–23.0%) *(68).*

Only a few studies have investigated the multiple-dose pharmacokinetics of sc administered rHuEPO in nephrology patients. Kampf et al. *(91)* treated patients for 6 wk with 40 U/kg three times weekly and observed no change in the rate or extent of absorption. In a well-controlled, crossover study, Jensen et al. *(78)* observed no statistically significant changes in pharmacokinetic parameters (including absolute bioavailability) after a median treatment period of 7.8 mo. Schouten et al. *(92)* also found no significant differences in pharmacokinetic parameters determined after the first dose and after 1 yr of treatment.

7.5. Other Pharmacokinetic Issues Related to Nephrology Patients

7.5.1. Degree of Renal Dysfunction

Most pharmacokinetic studies in the nephrology population have been conducted in patients receiving dialysis. In a study aimed at investigating the impact of varying degrees of renal dysfunction (range of creatinine clearances: <3 to >80 mL/min per 1.73 m^2), Kindler et al. *(81)* administered epoetin beta at doses of 130–152 U/kg iv in 10 previously untreated patients. They found no relationship between the degree of renal dysfunction and either terminal half-life or clearance. Using a 48-h urine collection, they also determined (by radioimmunoassay) that renal clearance contributed only 1.86% to total rHuEPO clearance.

7.5.2. Mode of Dialysis

Loss of rHuEPO in the dialysate is minimal *(89,93–95))*. Additionally, although few direct comparisons are available, several authors have concluded that the mode of dialysis (i.e., hemodialysis or peritoneal dialysis) has no impact on the pharmacokinetics of rHuEPO administered either intravenously or subcutaneously *(78,94–96)*.

7.5.3. Intraperitoneal Administration for Peritoneal Dialysis Patients

Reported bioavailability estimates of rHuEPO after intraperitoneal administration are generally very low (3–7%) *(64,94)*, with a large proportion of the dose (80%) being lost in the effluent *(95)*. The feasibility of the intraperitoneal route increases if rHuEPO is injected into a dry peritoneum *(80)*; in fact, Bargman et al. *(97)* reported a ninefold increase in AUC after administration into a dry peritoneum compared with that injected with dialysate. Additionally, increasing the dwell time within the peritoneum enhances absorption *(80,98)*.

7.5.4. Comparison of Healthy Volunteers and Nephrology Patients

When the pharmacokinetic characteristics of rHuEPO in healthy volunteers and nephrology patients are compared across studies, they appear similar *(68)*; however, in the only within-study comparison found, Jensen et al. *(72)* compared the pharmacokinetics of 100 U/kg epoetin beta iv in healthy (n = 12) vs uremic/dialysis (n = 21) subjects. Compared with the healthy volunteers, uremic patients had a statistically significant slower clearance (4.3 vs 6.8 mL/h/kg) and longer terminal half-life (8.3 vs 4.9 h). Distribution parameters were similar. After subcutaneous dosing, peak rHuEPO concentrations were significantly reduced (113 vs 153 mU/mL) and bioavailability was significantly lower (23.7% vs 38.5%) in uremic patients. The rate of absorption, however, did not differ between the two groups. Pharmacokinetic differences were not attributable to dialytic loss.

7.5.5. Pediatric Nephrology Patients

Pharmacokinetics in pediatric nephrology patients appear to be broadly similar to those of adults, although no studies directly compare the two populations. With intravenous rHuEPO, the mean terminal half-life in children ranged from 5.6 to 10.9 h, and mean clearance ranged from 6.0 to 10.1 mL/h/kg *(99,100)*. After subcutaneous administration, absorption was rate-limiting; the mean terminal half-life ranged from 13.3 to 25.2 h *(101,102)*, and bioavailability estimates were 34–40% *(99–101)*.

In a study of 20 patients, Braun et al. *(100)* determined that the pharmacokinetic data of younger vs older children (aged 7–20 yr) were not significantly different. For intraperitoneal dosing, Kausz et al. *(103)*, using literature values for the comparison, concluded that (similar to adults) injection into a dry peritoneum increased bioavailability.

7.6. Pharmacokinetics in Other Populations

The pharmacokinetics of rHuEPO have been studied in several other populations. In a comparison between patients with liver cirrhosis and healthy volunteers, Jensen et al. *(104)* did not find any difference in the pharmacokinetic properties of intravenously administered epoetin beta (100 U/kg). Patients with chronic obstructive pulmonary disease had similar mean serum concentrations and no significant difference in terminal half-life (5.98 ± 0.67 h, $n = 7$) compared with healthy volunteers (5.87 ± 0.35 h, $n = 6$) *(105)*. The determination of the pharmacokinetic properties of rHuEPO in patients with myelodysplastic syndromes was complicated by the extremely high endogenous EPO concentrations of these patients (210–5984 mU/mL, $n = 10$) *(106)*. After an iv bolus of 150 U/kg, however, peak serum concentrations were approx 2- to 10-fold higher than predose values. The reported half-lives ranged from 3.9 to 20.0 h; the average value (11.3 h) was longer than that generally reported for healthy volunteers or nephrology patients. Clearance rate and baseline serum concentrations were significantly correlated; the authors speculated that there might be reduced clearance of EPO by the bone marrow of these patients.

7.7. Effect of Site of Injection

The site chosen for a subcutaneous injection of rHuEPO may affect its absorption. Macdougall et al. *(107)* demonstrated more extensive absorption when radiolabeled rHuEPO was injected into the thigh compared with the abdomen or arm. The $AUCs_{(0-\infty)}$ measured after injections into the arm and abdomen were 89 and 77%, respectively, of the $AUC_{(0-\infty)}$ measured after injection into the thigh. Jensen et al. *(108)*, however, concluded that the only notable difference in pharmacokinetics between epoetin beta (100 U/kg) injected into the thigh compared with the abdomen was a longer median MRT (32.7 vs 26.2 h, respectively), which they attributed to slightly slower absorption.

7.8. Mechanisms of Clearance

Despite 20 years of clinical usage of rHuEPO, the mechanism of its clearance and the site of degradation still are not definitive *(20)*. Based on clinical data showing that clearance is faster at lower doses, it is likely that there are at least two clearance mechanisms. Although Veng-Pedersen et al. *(70)* proposed that rHuEPO is cleared solely by nonlinear, saturable mechanism(s), Kato et al. *(109)* demonstrated both saturable and nonsaturable clearance components in rats.

Neither the liver nor the kidney is felt to play more than a minor role in EPO clearance *(20,68,110)*. At this time, an attractive hypothesis is that the intact EPO undergoes receptor-mediated endocytosis, after which it is degraded by intracellular lysosomes. Other receptor-bearing, nonerythrocytic tissues, such as endothelial cells, could also be involved in this metabolism *(20)*. Clearly, greater insight into the mechanisms governing the absorption and clearance of rHuEPO will be welcomed.

7.9. Summary

Combining the clearance values from both healthy volunteers and nephrology patients after single bolus doses of rHuEPO enables a broader picture regarding dose linearity to evolve. Despite interstudy differences, Fig. 2 clearly illustrates that the clearance of rHuEPO is dose dependent *(68)*. At doses > 200 U/kg, the clearance of rHuEPO is approximately constant, at 5 mL/h/kg. At doses < 200 U/kg, the clearance increases as dose decreases with a threefold increase in clearance observed at 10 U/kg. This relationship appears to be, independent of population (healthy subjects or patients with chronic renal failure) or type of rHuEPO (epoetin alfa vs epoetin beta). With subcutaneous administration, there are no clear patterns regarding dose and the rate or extent of absorption, and bioavailability (although perhaps erroneously estimated) consistently lies between 20 and 40%. Upon multiple dosing, most data suggest that after several weeks of treatment (at least with intravenous dosing), clearance of rHuEPO increases about 10–30%, with an accompanying decrease in terminal half-life *(68)*. Thereafter, despite continued dosing, no further changes occur. For the patient populations with available data, no significant interpopulation differences in the pharmacokinetic properties of rHuEPO are apparent.

8. PHARMACODYNAMICS OF rHuEPO

Erythropoietic responses to rHuEPO are generally measured by changes in reticulocyte count, Hb concentration, and hematocrit *(65)*. In an early study of healthy volunteers *(65)*, the mean peak reticulocyte response occurred 4–5 d after a single intravenous dose of rHuEPO. In another study assessing multiple iv doses, 25 patients on hemodialysis received rHuEPO three times weekly at doses of 15, 50,150, or 500 U/kg or placebo *(111)*. Hematocrit values increased in a striking, dose-dependent fashion, with increases apparent in most of the dose groups within the first week of administration.

A similar but more prolonged response was seen with subcutaneous dosing; administration of rHuEPO in ascending, single doses to healthy volunteers produced prompt increases in the number of circulating reticulocytes *(112)*. The magnitude of the response was proportional to the EPO AUC until the next to the highest dose was administered (a single dose of 1800 U/kg), whereupon saturation of the response was noted. In a multidose study, Cheung et al. *(112)* randomized 36 healthy volunteers to receive sc either 40,000 U of rHuEPO once weekly or 150 U/kg three times weekly for 4 wk. Increases in Hb concentration, number of RBCs, and percent reticulocytes were maintained throughout the dosing period.

The in vivo activity of rHuEPO also depends on another pharmacodynamic factor, the minimum effective concentration (MEC). The intravenous administration of rHuEPO requires approx 30% more drug than the subcutaneous administration *(113)* despite the markedly higher peak plasma levels and bioavailability of the intravenous dose. It appears that serum rHuEPO concentrations must be maintained above a critical threshold (i.e., the MEC) for effective erythropoiesis, and increased time above the critical threshold results in increased biologic response. Maintenance of this threshold concentration is best achieved through slower absorption and more prolonged elimination *(20,44,110)*. The increased in vivo activity of darbepoetin alfa *(56,59)* is caused by its ability to maintain the MEC over an extended period *(110)*.

9. DARBEPOETIN ALFA

9.1. Successful Glycoengineering

Although rHuEPO has revolutionized the treatment of serious anemias and has been proved both safe and effective, its use is complicated by its relatively short physiologic half-life and the need for frequent, parenteral administrations. By using glycoengineering to introduce additional *N*-linked carbohydrate attachment points into rHuEPO, a new molecule was created with a prolonged serum half-life and increased vivo activity. Darbepoetin alfa (Aranesp®) is now available in the United States, the European Union, Australia, and Canada.

The carbohydrate component of rHuEPO consists of three *N*-linked carbohydrates, attached to the amino nitrogen on asparagine at amino acid positions 24, 38, and 83, and an *O*-linked carbohydrate, attached to the oxygen on serine at amino acid position 126 *(5)*. A typical *N*-linked carbohydrate made by mammalian cells is a sugar polymer with two to four branches, each of which is capped by sialic acid. Variations in the amount of sialic acid in molecules create glycoforms with different biologic activity *(19)*. Studies on glycoforms of rHuEPO containing different sialic acid contents demonstrated a direct relationship between increased sialic acid content and increased in vivo activity, owing to prolongation of the molecule's half-life *(19)*.

Efforts to modify rHuEPO by adding additional sialic acid-containing *N*-linked carbohydrates were initiated. New *N*-linked glycosylation consensus sequences (Asn-Xxx-Thr/Ser, where "Xxx" is any amino acid except proline) were introduced into rHuEPO at various positions by site-directed mutagenesis. These changes had to be introduced in such a way that the resultant molecule was glycosylated efficiently and retained activity, conformation, and stability. To ensure that the molecule would activate EPOR, the amino acid changes were introduced into rHuEPO at a site distal to the receptor binding site *(56)*. This effort was aided by structure-function studies that defined the active sites of rHuEPO and the amino acids important for maintenance of structure *(8,114,116)*. With the selection of maximal carbohydrate and sialic acid content during purification, reduction in the potential for antibody formation may be achieved by increased shielding by carbohydrate of potential antibody epitopes and appropriate solubility and stability, thereby inhibiting formation of aggregates and other byproducts *(116,117)*.

As a result of five amino acid substitutions to the native molecule, two additional *N*-linked chains were attached to the new asparagine residues at positions 30 and 88. The new molecule (darbepoetin alfa) had near-normal in vitro activity, was glycosylated efficiently, and had a similar conformation and stability to rHuEPO. The carbohydrate content was increased from 40 to 51%, the approximate size from 30 to 37 kDa, and the maximum number of sialic acid residues from 14 to 22.

9.2. Actions of Darbepoetin Alfa on Erythropoiesis

Darbepoetin alfa stimulates erythropoiesis by the same mechanisms as those previously discussed for endogenous EPO. In vitro, the affinity of darbepoetin alfa for EPOR is less that that of rHuEPO; however, the increase in mean residence time of darbepoetin alfa results in a prolonged period of time above an erythropoietic threshold (Fig. 3) that more than compensates for the reduced receptor affinity, resulting in increased in vivo activity *(56,59)*.

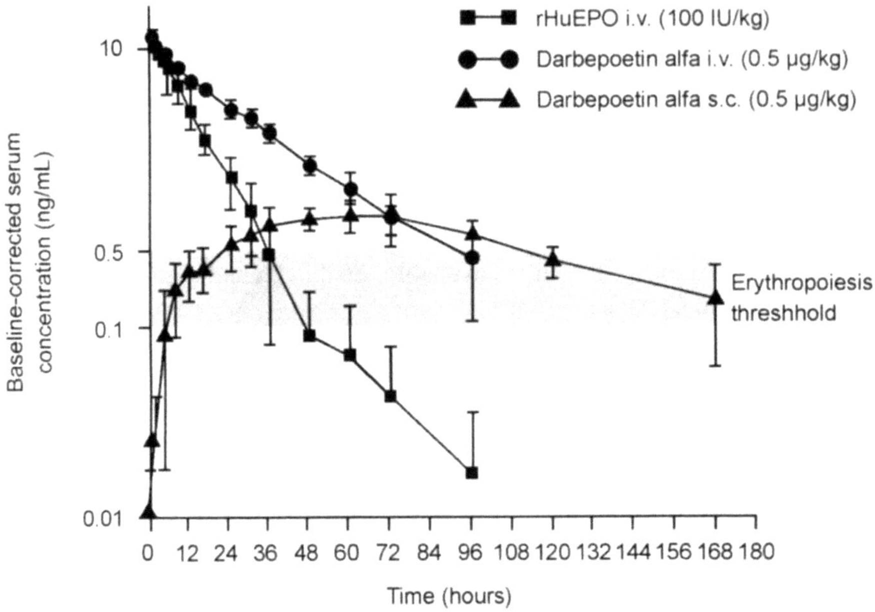

Fig. 3. Darbepoietin alfa has a longer serum half-life than rHuEPO (From ref. *119*.)

9.3. Pharmacokinetics and Pharmacodynamics of Darbepoetin Alfa

9.3.1. Animal Studies

Pharmacokinetic parameters of darbepoetin alfa were measured in rats and dogs *(59)*. The terminal half-life of darbepoetin alfa was increased relative to rHuEPO by almost three-fold in rats (6.9 vs 2.5 h), and the clearance decreased 3.7-fold (17.7 vs 48. mL/kg/h). The volumes of distribution of darbepoetin alfa and rHuEPO were the same and roughly equivalent to the volume of the serum compartment, approx 34 mL/kg, suggesting that distribution of the two proteins in the animal was similar. Similar results were observed in dogs, but the half-life of darbepoetin alfa was extended relative to that seen in rats (25 vs 6.9 h). In dogs, the terminal half-life of darbepoetin alfa was increased relative to rHuEPO by 3.5-fold, and the clearance was reduced 3.5-fold. Thus the glycoengineering successfully improved the pharmacokinetic parameters of darbepoetin alfa.

The effect of single injections of rHuEPO and darbepoetin alfa on Hgb concentration increase was explored in mice to determine relative in vivo activity *(56)*. An 18-fold higher amount of rHuEPO did not result in as great a response as the lower dose of darbepoetin alfa, indicating that darbepoetin alfa had a greater in vivo activity than that of rHuEPO. Mice were administered rHuEPO or darbepoetin alfa at various dosing intervals *(59)*. Threefold more rHuEPO than darbepoetin alfa was required to elicit a similar response when the drugs were administered three times per week. This difference increased to 13-fold when the molecules were administered at weekly intervals. Weekly dosing and every-other-week dosing intervals were also compared. Darbepoetin alfa was 6.4-fold more efficient when administered every other week compared with weekly dosing of rHuEPO. These results indicate that the relative potency difference of darbepoetin alfa compared with rHuEPO increased as the dosing interval increased. The differences were explained by the observed threefold greater serum half-life of darbepoetin alfa and thereby the prolonged period that darbepoetin alfa concentrations are above an erythropoietic threshold.

A rat model in which a chronic inflammatory state was generated resulted in anemia reminiscent of the anemia seen in patients with chronic inflammatory diseases (the anemia of chronic disease [ACD]) *(118)*. The anemic rats were treated with darbepoetin alfa, which corrected the anemia by increasing Hg concentration to baseline levels of approx. 16.0 g/dL (±0.17). This increase was achieved with administration of darbepoetin alfa on a once-every-2-wk schedule. The beneficial effect of darbepoetin alfa was even more evident when an up-front loading dose schedule was used.

9.3.2. Pharmacokinetics in Nephrology Patients

One of the first clinical trials in humans with darbepoetin alfa was performed in rHuEPO-naive patients receiving continuous ambulatory peritoneal dialysis *(119)*. The first phase compared the single-dose pharmacokinetics of an iv bolus dose of rHuEPO (100 U/kg) with an equivalent peptide mass of darbepoetin alfa. Darbepoetin alfa had an approx threefold longer mean terminal half-life than rHuEPO (25.3 vs 8.5 h, respectively, $p = 0.0008$), a more than twofold greater AUC (291± 8 vs 132 ± 8 ng/h/mL), and a fourfold lower clearance (1.6 ± 0.3 vs 4.0 ± 0.3 mL/h/kg), which was biphasic (Fig. 3). The volume of distribution was similar for the two molecules (52.4 ± 2.0 and 48.7 ± 2.1 mL/kg, respectively). Four days after the bolus, mean serum concentrations from darbepoetin alfa were substantially higher than those from rHuEPO (0.5 ng/mL vs 0.02 ng/mL, respectively). In the second phase of the study, six patients received sc darbepoetin alfa at the same dose they had received iv. The mean terminal half-life was approx 49 h (about twice that of iv darbepoetin alfa); C_{max} averaged about 10% of the iv value, T_{max} averaged 54 ± 5 h, and mean bioavailability was 37%.

In another study, hemodialysis patients were randomized to receive either darbepoetin alfa administered once weekly iv ($n = 17$), darbepoetin alfa administered three times weekly iv ($n = 15$), or rHuEPO iv administered three times weekly (n=15) *(58)*. Single-dose pharmacokinetics (obtained during the first day of dosing) were consistent with those from the prior study in patients on peritoneal dialysis *(119)*. Darbepoetin alfa (once/wk group) had an approx threefold longer mean terminal half-life than rHuEPO (17.8 vs 6.3 h, respectively), a fourfold greater AUC, and a fourfold slower clearance (2.0 vs 8.6 mL/h/kg). The volume of distribution was again similar for the two molecules (64.4 vs 60.4 mL/kg, respectively), suggesting little extravascular distribution. Darbepoetin alfa pharmacokinetic parameters showed essentially no changes in measurements taken at wk 1 and 12 and after attaining steady-state hemoglobin levels.

9.3.3. Pharmacokinetics of Darbepoetin Alfa in Other Populations

A pharmacokinetic study of darbepoetin alfa was done in 12 children (ages: 3–16 yr) with chronic renal disease, most of whom were on dialysis *(120)*. Patients were randomized to receive a 0.5-μg/kg single dose of darbepoetin alfa administered either iv or sc. Fourteen to 16 d later, the children received the identical dose by the alternate route. After iv administration, the drug's clearance was 2.3 mL/h/kg, and the terminal half-life was 22.1 h, similar to the 25.3 h reported in adults *(119)*. After sc administration, the terminal half-life was 43 h compared with 49 h in adults. On average, the children achieved maximum serum darbepoetin alfa concentrations after subcutaneous administration faster than did the adults (36 vs 54 h, respectively) *(119)*; the mean bioavailability for this population was 54%. The data suggest that the pharmacokinetic profile of darbepoetin alfa is similar in adults and children, except that absorption may be more rapid in children after subcutaneous administration. This same finding has been observed with rHuEPO *(99)*.

Heatherington et al. *(121)* reported on the use of darbepoetin alfa in anemic patients with nonmyeloid malignancies receiving multiple cycles of chemotherapy. Patients received darbepoetin alfa 2.25 μg/kg once weekly, starting on d 1 of chemotherapy and continuing for three chemotherapy cycles (given at 3-wk intervals). Blood samples were collected during chemotherapy cycles 1 and 3 for pharmacokinetic analysis. After a single dose during chemotherapy cycle 1, pharmacokinetic parameters for the first 12 patients included a clearance of 105 mL/h/kg, resulting in a terminal half-life of 39.7 ± 23.3 h and a mean residence time of 57.4 ± 29.0 h. These data support the dosing of intravenous darbepoetin alfa at intervals of once weekly or less in these patients.

In another report, Jumbe et al. *(122)* used clinical trial simulation techniques to evaluate fixed-dose vs weight-based dosing of darbepoetin alfa in patients with chemotherapy-induced anemia. A pharmacokinetic/pharmacodynamic model was developed using clinical data from 547 cancer patients who received darbepoetin alfa in various dosing regimens. Monte Carlo simulations were performed for weight-based (3 μg/kg every 2 wk) and fixed-dose (200 μg every 2 wk) regimens and were compared with the clinical data. For patients between 45 and 95 kg (over 90% of the population), the impact of a fixed dose on mean Hb change was negligible except at body weight extremes (<45 kg and >95 kg), suggesting that most chemotherapy patients would benefit equally from weight-based or fixed-dose darbepoetin alfa.

9.4. Pharmacodynamics of Darbepoetin Alfa in Patients

Clinical studies with darbepoetin alfa have been conducted in the United States, European Union, Australia, Canada, and Mexico. Several studies in the nephrology setting showed that darbepoetin alfa was effective at correcting anemia at a reduced dosing frequency. Randomized dose escalation studies compared once-weekly darbepoetin alfa (0.45 μg/kg) with twice-weekly rHuEPO (50 U/kg) in rHuEPO-naive predialysis patients *(123)*. Drug dosages were adjusted, as necessary, to maintain Hb concentrations in the study target range (11–13 g/dL). In both treatment groups there was a significant Hb response (mean Hb increase of 1.38 g/dL for darbepoetin alfa and 1.4 g/dL for rHuEPO. Similar proportions of the patients achieved an Hb response of 1 g/dL or greater from baseline by 24 wk, 93% of the 129 patients treated with darbepoetin alfa and 92% of the 37 patients treated with rHuEPO.

Conversion of dialysis patients from established rHuEPO therapy to darbepoetin alfa was addressed in two large clinical trials. In both studies the safety profiles of the rHuEPO and darbepoetin alfa groups was similar. The first trial, in North America, enrolled 507 hemodialysis patients into a randomized double-blind study, comparing patients who continued on three-times-weekly rHuEPO with those converting to darbepoetin alfa (once weekly plus twice-weekly placebo) *(124)*. After the 20-wk dose-titration phase, Hb concentration remained stable during the 8-wk follow-up phase and was comparable between the two groups. The second clinical trial, a European/Australian multicenter study, included hemodialysis and peritoneal dialysis patients who were randomized to darbepoetin alfa administered at either weekly intervals (if prior rHuEPO was given two or three times weekly) or at every-other-week dosing intervals (if prior rHuEPO dosing was weekly). The results suggested that that 97% of patients receiving weekly darbepoetin alfa and 95% of those on an alternate-week schedule could be successfully treated.

The ability of darbepoetin alfa to maintain Hb concentrations at reduced dosing intervals was evaluated in several clinical studies. Seventy-six rHuEPO-naive patients with chronic kidney disease (61 completed the treatment phase) were administered darbepoetin alfa at an every-two-weeks (q2w) dosing interval, and 97% reached the target Hb concentration Therefore darbepoetin administration could be used to treat anemia at every-other-week dosing intervals. Similarly, darbepoetin alfa administered to dialysis patients at q2w dosing intervals successfully maintained Hb concentrations in patients converted from rHuEPO. Hemoglobin was also successfully maintained in dialysis patients with darbepoetin alfa at even less frequent dosing intervals, q3w and q4w. Therefore it appears that darbepoetin alfa can be administered at less frequent intervals than rHuEPO.

Patients with cancer often have anemia caused by the inhibitory effects of the tumor, (inflammatory cytokines, destruction of bone marrow, bleeding) or anticancer treatment (chemotherapy or radiotherapy). The anemia can have profound negative effects on well-being and survival *(125)*. The efficacy of darbepoetin alfa antianemia treatment was demonstrated in cancer patients not receiving chemotherapy *(125)*. Patients, 102 primarily with lymphoid, breast, and prostate malignancies, were administered from 1.0 to 4.5 μg/kg/wk and studied for 12 wk. A 2-g/dL increase in Hb was observed in 66% or more of the patients. The 4.5-μg/kg/wk group had an even higher (92%) response rate.

Darbepoetin alfa has also been shown to treat anemia in a safe and effective manner in cancer patients receiving chemotherapy. In a multicenter, placebo-controlled study, patients with lung cancer receiving multicycle chemotherapy were randomized to darbepoetin alfa or placebo, and patients who completed the 28-wk study were assessed *(126)*. Patients treated with darbepoetin alfa required fewer transfusions (and had greater Hb responses) than patients receiving placebo. Other studies have suggested that darbepoetin alfa is safe and effective when administered at reduced dosing frequency (once every 1, 2, or 3 wk) *(125,127–129)*. Thus, darbepoetin alfa could be used to treat anemia in patients with reduced-dosing frequency.

10. ERYTHROPOIETIC FACTORS: RESEARCH DIRECTIONS

10.1. Introduction

Although rHuEPO is safe and effective, improvements in the properties of the molecule or its method of delivery are desirable. Endogenous EPO is naturally optimized for maintenance of an exquisite homeostasis; however, properties that are optimal for endogenous production and use may be suboptimal in a therapeutic agent. For example, rHuEPO must be administered frequently by injection, and the discomfort of injections and the inconvenience to the patient and health care provider burden both groups.

Several approaches are being pursued to prolong the activity of rHuEPO, including the exploration of sustained-release formulations and new delivery systems (such as infusion pumps) to maintain therapeutic drug concentrations for extended periods. Alternatively, chemical attachment of polymers to the protein may confer a longer half-life, as may modification of the protein itself by in vitro mutagenesis or through fusions between EPO and other peptides or proteins. The inherent limitations of rHuEPO because of its peptidic composition or mechanism of action may be bypassed entirely with new molecular entities such as small molecules or antibodies (EPO mimetics). Another approach involves the development of molecules that stimulate erythropoiesis by mechanisms such as those steps that occur before or after the receptor-activation step.

One new drug that has successfully met the above criteria has been the glycoengineering of rHuEPO to create darbepoetin alfa, an EPO glycosylation analog with a unique amino acid sequence and increased content of sialic acid-containing carbohydrate *(56)*. The extra carbohydrate attachments slow the clearance of the molecule and increase its in vivo biologic activity *(56,59,119)*. Darbepoetin alfa is as safe and effective as rHuEPO, but its less frequent dosing schedule adds both convenience and flexibility to patients and their health care providers.

Regardless of the avenue of development, any new drugs or new formulations should demonstrate efficacy, safety, and tolerability equal or superior to the current product. Because rHuEPO is highly effective at stimulating erythropoiesis with minimal side effects, it has created a high standard for these next generation products. Of particular importance for any new product is the avoidance of anti-EPO antibodies *(130)*. Antibody formation associated with new proteins, new drug entities, or new formulations is important not only because they could cause the new product to lose activity, but also because such antibodies might crossreact with endogenous EPO to produce pure red cell aplasia. Potential causes for antibody formation include not only the structure of the molecule itself, but also the breakdown products or aggregates generated during manufacture or storage. Accordingly, new drugs must be designed and manufacturing procedures put in place to minimize this risk.

With any new erythropoietic-stimulating protein, the clearance rate should match the desired use and effect. For example, in vivo erythropoiesis requires continuous stimulation of multiple receptors through multiple binding events *(113–133)*. Removal of sialic acid from carbohydrates or removal of *N*-linked carbohydrates entirely demonstrates increased receptor affinity and increased in vitro activity *(18)*. These molecules, however, have reduced in vivo activity because their more rapid clearance translates into fewer receptor binding events *(18,134)*. Increased concentrations can partially compensate for the increased clearance; however, these compounds must be administered more frequently to be fully efficacious. Extension in the serum half-life can increase efficacy, as demonstrated by the increased in vivo activity of darbepoetin alfa.

10.2. Erythropoietic Molecules With Changes in Stability or Receptor Binding Activity

Endogenous EPO activates the EPORs on precursor red cells through homodimerization, whereby two receptor binding sites on a single EPO molecule crosslink two receptors *(135)*. The two binding sites on rHuEPO have different affinities, high (approx. 1 n*M*) and low (approx 10 μ*M*) *(10)*. Initial binding is to the high-affinity binding site, followed by homodimerization of the receptor by binding to the low-affinity binding site *(9)*. Compounds that bind through the high-affinity site but do not dimerize because of reduced binding at the low-affinity site can function as antagonists *(8)*. Such molecules may have clinical utility for treatment of rHuEPO-induced, secondary polycythemias, and several such molecules have been described *(8,9)*.

10.3. Chemical Modification by Pegylation

Pegylation of proteins has been used successfully to increase the serum half-life of proteins *(136)*. Pegylation involves chemical attachment of the polymer polyethylene glycol (Peg), to reactive regions of proteins or carbohydrates. Pegylated molecules have an increased hydrodynamic size because they create a water shell around the molecule. The increased hydrodynamic size can result in reduced clearance and thus allow the vivo activity of the protein to be conferred for a longer period of time.

One potential problem with drugs made by solution or solid-phase chemistry can be poor specificity of conjugation in the chemical reaction or generation of undesirable byproducts. Many pegylation chemistries have been tried to reduce such undesirable outcomes *(137)*. The current chemistries typically target the reactive amino groups on lysine or the amino terminal amine. rHuEPO has eight lysines, some of which are part of the binding site *(6,8)*. Therefore, some pegylated EPO molecules may have low activity because PEG interferes with receptor binding and activation or results in structural alterations that interfere with receptor interaction.

Analogs of EPO might be able to increase specificity of PEG conjugation. Cysteine substitutions at targeted regions can allow addition of the conjugate to the sulfhydryl group with high specificity *(138,139)*. Another strategy is to make pegylated EPO synthetically: during synthesis, a PEG-conjugated amino acid could be introduced instead of the unconjugated amino acid. This approach allows specific targeting of particular amino- acid positions for PEG attachment, such as the glycosylation sites, and reduces heterogeneity and the potential for loss of activity. However, it is not clear whether these molecules will retain the same stability, activity, and lack of immunogenicity as their glycosylated counterparts.

10.4. Fusion Proteins

Several EPO fusion proteins have been reported, including EPO/IL-3 *(140)* and EPO/GM-CSF *(141)*. The theory behind the creation of such molecules is that the single fusion protein can provide the biologic activity of both molecules and ensure that both entities are present simultaneously. For example, enhanced erythropoiesis might well result from the co-administration of rHuIL-3, which acts on the earliest erythroid precursor cells, with rHuEPO, which acts on the more mature precursors. The larger size of the fusion protein also may impart increased activity for both partners because of reduced clearance. EPO dimer is another fusion protein that has been generated as a potential therapeutic *(142)*. Its increased size can reduce clearance, and the molecule may have increased activity owing to altered avidity to the receptor *(143)*.

Simultaneous administration by fusing two drugs can simplify dosing, especially when the two proteins have different pharmacokinetic parameters; however, the ability to adjust dosing independently of the fusion partners is lost. Other challenges in creating therapeutic fusion proteins are their potential immunogenicity *(141)* and possible loss of efficacy *(140)*, in that full activity of both proteins in fusion proteins may not occur.

10.5. EPO Mimetics

EPO mimetics are compounds that mimic the activity of EPO but bear no structural homology. EPO mimetics can have different biologic or biophysical properties from EPO that might allow a nonparenteral route of delivery.

Significant challenges are associated with the identification and development of a useful EPO mimetic. First, the molecule must be small enough to be delivered orally (preferably <600 Daltons) but large enough to retain full affinity for EPOR and to have an acceptable clearance. Also, the safety profiles of the compound and its breakdown products must be acceptable.

Several strategies are been used to identify EPO mimetics. One approach is to screen peptide and small-molecule libraries for compounds that can stimulate erythropoiesis using in vitro bioassays as screens. Another strategy is to identify molecules that directly bind to and agonize EPOR in a manner similar to that of rHuEPO. This latter strategy has been performed in two steps: the first step identifies compounds that bind EPOR, and the second step covalently links the compounds into bivalent dimers that can agonize the receptor by EPOR homodimerization.

Another approach to mimetic discovery is to modulate steps downstream from receptor activation, such as by inhibiting hematopoietic cell phosphatase (HCP) *(144)*. HCP is an enzyme that dephosphorylates and inactivates JAK2, a kinase that is part of the EPO signal transduction cascade *(11)*. Truncated EPORs lack the HCP binding site, and thus HCP cannot dephosphorylate JAK2, resulting in hypersensitivity of the receptor to EPO. Naturally occurring truncations have been described in humans; the affected individuals have increased Hgb concentrations but very low EPO concentrations *(135,145)*. Thus, small-molecule antagonists of HCP might result in increased EPOR activity that increases erythropoiesis in the absence of added EPO. Because HCP is a negative regulator for several other cytokine receptors, increases in the number of other hematopoietic cells may limit the usefulness of HCP inhibitors.

10.6. Gene Therapy

Controlled delivery of *EPO* genes to humans is another approach for EPO therapy. Early work in this field depended on direct injection of plasmid DNA containing constitutively active *EPO* genes into the muscles of mice *(146)*, resulting in a measurable increase in hematocrit. Several concerns became apparent from these studies, including inefficient and variable delivery of the *EPO* gene, with subsequent variations in EPO concentration. Although improvements in expression systems and better gene delivery methods have been reported *(147)*, current *EPO* gene therapy protocols still require repeated administration of *EPO* genes. In addition, there is concern that the therapy could be irreversible or cause altered gene expression and tumorigenicity.

Efforts to address the efficiency and irreversibility concerns have taken the form of developing implantable capsules containing *EPO*-expressing cells *(148)*. The capsules can be removed, halting EPO delivery. A further refinement has been to construct vectors whereby *EPO* expression is controlled by a small molecule such as tetracycline, enabling increased *EPO* expression in response to oral administration of the gene activator *(149)*. Other vectors have been developed whereby *EPO* expression is controlled by oxygen tension *(150)*, or methods are used that target the kidney for gene transfer *(151)*. Despite these advances, however, safe and controlled EPO delivery using gene therapy remains in the future.

10.7. Extended Release Formulations and Devices

New delivery systems, including devices that provided extended, controlled release of rHuEPO, could allow for smooth, sustained stimulation of erythropoiesis. Such devices necessitate that the molecule remain stable for a prolonged period. Another approach could be to introduce rHuEPO into a slow-release, biodegradable matrix that would erode at a predictable rate and release the protein in a controlled manner *(152,153)*.

To date, no slow-release process has been successful. The requirement for protein stability both during manufacturing and when implanted in the body has been a challenge, particularly when considering biodegradable matrices. Small amounts of contaminating rHuEPO aggregates, misfolded rHuEPO, or breakdown products would probably compromise not only efficacy but also safety (immunogenicity). Another concern is that too rapid breakdown of the matrix might result in an overdose of rHuEPO.

11. SUMMARY

Further progress is anticipated as new devices are developed. The future will be exciting as small-molecule EPO mimetics are discovered that will permit oral administration. Permanent correction of anemia may occur through gene therapy, allowing additional treatment opportunities. These developments will require extensive research and testing; however, many believe that this is not a question of if, but when.

REFERENCES

1. Kendall RG. Erythropoietin. *Clin Lab Haematol* 2001; 23:71–80.
2. Erslev A. Humoral regulation of red cell production. *Blood* 1952; 8:349–357.
3. Miyake T, Kung CK, Goldwasser E. Purification of human erythropoietin. *J Biol Chem* 1977; 252:5558–5564.
4. Lin FK, Suggs S, Lin CH, et al. Cloning and expression of the human erythropoietin gene. *Proc Natl Acad Sci USA* 1985; 82:7580–7584.
5. Lai PH, Everett R, Wang FF, Arakawa T, Goldwasser E. Structural characterization of human erythropoietin. *J Biol Chem* 1986; 261:3116–3121.
6. Syed RS, Reid SW, Li C, et al. Efficiency of signalling through cytokine receptors depends critically on receptor orientation. *Nature* 1998; 395:511–516.
7. Cheetham JC, Smith DM, Aoki KH, et al. NMR structure of human erythropoietin and a comparison with its receptor bound conformation. *Nature Struct Biol* 1998; 5:861–866.
8. Elliott S, Lorenzini T, Chang D, Barzilay J, Delorme E. Mapping of the active site of recombinant human erythropoietin *Blood* 1997; 89:493–502.
9. Matthews DJ, Topping RS, Cass RT, Giebel LB. A sequential dimerization mechanism for erythropoietin receptor activation. *Proceed Natl Acad Sci USA* 1996; 93:9471–9476.
10. Philo JS, Aoki KH, Arakawa T, Narhi LO, Wen J. Dimerization of the extracellular domain of the erythropoietin (EPO) receptor by EPO: one high-affinity and one low-affinity interaction. *Biochemistry* 1996; 35:1681–1691.
11. Youssoufian H, Longmore G, Neumann D, Yoshimura A, Lodish HF. Structure, function, and activation of the erythropoietin receptor. *Blood* 1993; 81:2223–2236.
12. Egrie JC, Strickland TW, Lane J, et al. Characterization and biological effects of recombinant human erythropoietin. *Immunobiology* 1986; 172:213–224.
13. Browne JKI, Cohen AM, Ergie JC, et al. Erythropoietin: gene cloning, protein structure, and biological properties. *Cold Spring Harb Symp Quant Biol* 1986; 51:693–702.
14. Davis JM, Arakawa T, Strickland TW, Yphantis DA. Characterization of recombinant human erythropoietin produced in Chinese hamster ovary cells. *Biochemistry* 1987; 26:2633–2638.
15. Sasaki H, Bothner B, Dell A, Fukuda M. Carbohydrate structure of erythropoietin expressed in Chinese hamster ovary cells by a human erythropoietin cDNA. *J Biol Chem* 1987; 262:12059–12076.

16. Takeuchi M, Kobata A. Structures and functional roles of the sugar chains of human erythropoietins. *Glycobiology* 1991; 1:337–346.
17. Rush RS, Derby PL, Smith DM, et al. Microheterogeneity of erythropoietin carbohydrate structure. *Anal Chem* 1995; 67:1442–1452.
18. Delorme E, Lorenzini T, Giffin J, et al. Role of glycosylation on the secretion and biological activity of erythropoietin. *Biochemistry* 1992; 31:9871–9876.
19. Egrie JC, Browne JK. Development and characterization of novel erythropoiesis stimulating protein (NESP). *Br J Cancer* 2001; 84:3–10.
20. Jelkmann W. Use of recombinant human erythropoietin as an anti-anemic and performance enhancing drug. *Curr Pharmaceut Biotech* 2000; 1:11–31.
21. Jelkmann W. Erythropoietin: structure, control of production, and function. *Physiol Rev* 1992; 72:449–489.
22. Fisher JW. Erythropoietin: physiology and pharmacology update. *Exp Biol Med (Maywood)* 2003; 228:1–14.
23. Spivak JL. The biology and clinical applications of recombinant erythropoietin. *Semin Oncol* 1998; 25(3 suppl 7):7–11.
24. Buemi M, Cavallaro E, Floccari F, et al. The pleiotropic effect of erythropoietin in the central nervous system. *J Neuropathol Exp Neurol* 2003; 62:228–236.
25. Spivak JL. Changing paradigms in anemia management. *Adv Studies Med* 2002; 22:610–619.
26. Roberts D, Smith DJ. Erythropoietin does not demonstrate circadian rhthym in healthy men. *J Appl Physiol* 1996; 80:847–851.
27. Pasqualetti P, Collacciani A, Casale R. Circadian rhythm of serum erythropoietin in myelodysplastic syndromes. *Eur Rev Med Pharmacol Sci* 2000; 4:111–115.
28. Lacombe C, Mayeux P. The molecular biology of erythropoietin. *Nephrol Dial Transplant* 1999; 14:22–28.
29. Jiang BH, Rue E, Wang GL, Roe R, Semenza GL. Dimerization, DNA binding, and transactivation properties of hypoxia-inducible factor 1. *J Biol Chem* 1996; 271:17771–17778.
30. Masson N, Willam C, Maxwell PH, Pugh CW, Ratcliffe PJ. Independent function of two destruction domains in hypoxia-inducible factor-alpha chains activated by prolyl hydroxylation. *EMBO J* 2001; 20:5197–5206.
31. Epstein AC, Gleadle JM, McNeill LA, et al. *C. elegans* EGL-9 and mammalian homologs define a family of dioxygenases that regulate HIF by prolyl hydroxylation. *Cell* 2001; 107:43–54.
32. Bruick RK, McKnight SL. A conserved family of prolyl-4-hydroxylases that modify HIF. *Science* 2001; 294:1337–1340.
33. Ivan M, Kondo K, Yang H, et al. HIFalpha targeted for VHL-mediated destruction by proline hydroxylation: implications for O_2 sensing. *Science* 2001; 292:464–468.
34. Hewitson KS, McNeill LA, Riordan MV, et al. Hypoxia-inducible factor (HIF) asparagine hydroxylase is identical to factor inhibiting HIF (FIH) and is related to the cupin structural family. *J Biol Chem* 2002; 277:26351–26355.
35. McNeill LA, Hewitson KS, Claridge TD, Seibel JF, Horsfall LE, Schofield CJ. Hypoxia-inducible factor asparaginyl hydroxylase (FIH-1) catalyses hydroxylation at the beta-carbon of asparagine-803. *Biochem J* 2002; 367:3–5.
36. Wu H, Liu X, Jaenisch R, Lodish HF. Generation of committed erythroid BFU-E and CFU-E progenitors does not require erythropoietin or the erythropoietin receptor. *Cell* 1995; 83:59–67.
37. Koury MJ, Bondurant MC. Maintenance by erythropoietin of viability and maturation of murine erythroid precursor cells. *J Cell Physiol* 1988; 137:65–74.
38. Gregoli PA, Bondurant MC. The roles of Bcl-X_L and apopain in the control of erythropoiesis by erythropoietin. *Blood* 1997; 89:630–640.
39. Chong ZZ, Kang JQ, Maiese K. Hematopoietic factor erythropoietin fosters neuroprotection through novel signal transduction cascades. *J Cereb Blood Flow Metab* 2002; 22:503–514.
40. Sawyer T, Jacobs-Helber SM. Unraveling distinct intracellular signals that promote survival and proliferation: study of erythroproietin, stem cell factor, and constitutive signaling in leukemic cells. *J Hematherapy Stem Cell Res* 2000; 9:21–29.
41. Kashii Y, Uchida M, Kirito K, et al. A member of Forkhead family transcription factors FKHRL, is one of the downstream molecules of phosphatidylinositol 3-kinase-AKT activation pathway in erythropoietin signal transduction. *Blood* 2000: 96:941–949.
42. Ghaffari S, Jagani Z, Kitidis C, Lodish HF, and Khosravi-Far R. Cytokines and BCR-ABL mediate suppression of TRAIL-induced apoptosis through inhibition of forkhead FOXO3a transcription factor. *Proc Natl Acad Sci* USA 2003; 100:6523–6528.

43. Zamai L, Secchiero P, Pierpaoli S. et al. TNF-related apoptosis-inducing ligand (TRAIL) as a negative regulator of normal human erythropoiesis. *Blood* 2000; 95:3716–3724.
44. Besarab A. Physiological and pharmacodynamic considerations for route of EPO administration. *Semin Nephrol* 2000; 20:364–374.
45. Soulliard A, Audran M, Bressolle F, Gareau R, Duvallet A, Chanal JL. Pharmacokinetics and pharmacodynamics of recombinant human erythropoietin in athletes. Blood sampling and doping control. *Br J Clin Pharmacol* 1996; 42:355–364.
46. Erslev AJ. Erythropoietin. *N Engl J Med* 1991; 324:1339–1344.
47. Jungers PY, Robino C, Choukroun G, Nguyen-Khoa T, Massy ZA, Jungers P. Incidence of anaemia, and use of epoetin therapy in pre-dialysis patients: a prospective study in 403 patients. *Nephrol Dial Transplant* 2002; 17:1621–1627.
48. Nissenson AR, Nimer SD, Wolcott DL. Recombinant human erythropoietin and renal anemia: molecular biology, clinical efficacy, and nervous system effects. *Ann Intern Med* 1991; 114:402–416.
49. Adamson JW, Eschbach JW. Treatment of the anemia of chronic renal failure with recombinant human erythropoietin. *Annnu Rev Med* 1990; 41:349–360.
50. Macdougall IC. Meeting the challenges of a new millennium: optimizing the use of recombinant human erythropoietin. *Nephrol Dial Transplant* 1998; 13 Suppl 2:23–27.
51. Kato A, Hishida A, Kumagai H, Furuya R, Nakajima T, Honda N. Erythropoietin production in patients with chronic renal failure. *Ren Fail* 1994; 16:645–651.
52. Ross RP, McCrea JB, Besarab A. Erythropoiein response to blood loss in hemodialysis patients is blunted but preserved. *ASAIO J* 1994; 40:M880–885.
53. Miller CB, Jones RJ, Piantadosi S, Abeloff MD, Spivak JL. Decreased erythropoietin response in patients with the anemia of cancer. *N Engl J Med* 1990; 322:1689–1692.
54. Bron D, Meuleman N, Mascaux C. Biological basis of anemia. *Semin Oncol* 2001; 28:1–6.
55. Pedain C, Herrero J, Kunzel W. Serum erythropoietin levels in ovarian cancer patients receiving chemotherapy. *Eur J Obstet Gynecol Reprod Biol* 2001; 98:224–230.
56. Elliott S, Lorenzini T, Asher S, et al. Enhancement of therapeutic protein in vivo activities through glycoengineering. *Nature Biotechnol* 2003; 21:414–421.
57. Cotes PM, Bangham DR. Bio-assay of erythropoietin in mice made polycythemic by exposure to air at reduced pressure. *Nature* 1961; 191:1065–1067.
58. Allon M, Kleinman K, Walczyk M, Kaupke C, et al. Pharmacokinetics and pharmacodynamics of darbepoetin alfa and epoetin in patients undergoing dialysis. *Clin Pharmacol Ther* 2002; 72:546–555.
59. Egrie JC, Dwyer E, Browne JK, Hitz A, Lykos MA. Darbepoetin alfa has a longer circulating half-life and greater in vivo potency than recombinant human erythropoietin. *Exp Hematol* 2003; 31:290–299.
60. Egrie JC, Cotes PM, Lane J, Gaines Das RE, Tam RC. Development of radioimmunoassays for human erythropoietin using recombinant erythropoietin as tracer and immunogen. *J Immunol Methods* 1987; 99:235–241.
61. Bartley TD, Bogenberger J, Hunt P, et al. Identification and cloning of a megakaryocyte growth and development factor that is a ligand for the cytokine receptor Mpl. *Cell* 1994; 77:1117–1124.
62 US Department of Health and Human Services, Food and Drug Administration, Center for Devices and Radiological Health. Guidance for industry: document for special controls for erythropoietin assay premarket notifications [510(k)s]: issued April 28, 1999. http://www.fda.gov/cdrh/ode/2241.html
63. Brockmoller J, Kochling J, Weber W, Looby M, Roots I, Neumayer HH. The pharmacokinetics and pharmacodynamics of recombinant human erythropoietin in haemodialysis patients. *Br J Clin Pharmac* 1992; 34:499–508.
64. Kampf D, Eckardt KU, Fischer HC, Schmalisch C, Ehmer B, Schostak M. Pharmacokinetics of recombinant human erythropoietin in dialysis patients after single and multiple subcutaneous administrations. *Nephron* 1992; 61:393–398.
65. Flaharty KK, Caro J, Erslev A, et al. Pharmacokinetics and erythropoietic response to human recombinant erythropoietin in healthy men. *Clin Pharmacol Ther* 1990; 47:557–564.
66. Lasne F, deCeaurriz J. Recombinant erythropoietin in urine. *Nature* 2000; 405:635.
67. Catlin DH, Breidbach A, Elliott S, Glaspy J. Comparison of the isoelectric focusing patterns of darbepoetin alfa, recombinant human erythropoietin, and endogenous erythropoietin from human urine. *Clin Chem* 2002; 48:2057–2059
68. Heatherington AC. Clinical pharmacokinetic properties of rHuEPO: a review. In: Molineux G, Foote MA, Elliot S, eds., *Erythropoietins and Erythropoiesis: Molecular, Cellular, Preclinical, and Clinical Biology*. Basel, Switzerland: Birkhauser. 2003; pp. 87–112.

69. McMahon FG, Vargas R, Ryan M, et al. Pharmacokinetics and effects of recombinant human erythropoietin after intravenous and subcutaneous injections in healthy volunteers. *Blood* 1990; 76:1718–1722.
70. Veng-Pedersen P, Widness JA, Pereira LM, Peters C, Schmidt RL, Lowe LS. Kinetic evaluation of nonlinear drug elimination by a disposition decomposition analysis. Application to the analysis of the nonlinear elimination kinetics of erythropoietin in adult humans. *J Pharm Sci* 1995; 84:760–767.
71. Salmonson T, Danielson BG, Wikstrom B. The pharmacokinetics of recombinant human erythropoietin after intravenous and subcutaneous administration to healthy subjects. *Br J Clin Pharmacol* 1990a; 29:709–713.
72. Jensen JD, Madsen JK, Jensen LW, Pedersen EB. Reduced production, absorption, and elimination of erythropoietin in uremia compared with healthy volunteers. *J Am Soc Nephrol* 1994; 5:177–185.
73. Boxenbaum H. Pharmacokinetic tricks and traps: flip-flop models. *J Pharm Pharmaceut Sci* 1998; 1:90–91.
74. Cheung WK, Goon BL, Guilfoyle MC, Wacholtz MC. Pharmacokinetics and pharmacodynamics of recombinant human erythropoietin after single and multiple subcutaneous doses to healthy subjects. *Clin Pharmacol Ther* 1998; 64:412–423.
75. Markham A, Bryson HM. Epoetin alfa. A review of its pharmacodynamic and pharmacokinetic properties and therapeutic use in nonrenal applications. *Drug Eval* 1995; 49:232–254
76. Sans T, Joven J, Vilella E, Masdeu G, Farre M. Pharmacokinetics of several subcutaneous doses of erythropoietin: potential implications for blood transfusions. *Clin Exp Pharmacol Physiol* 2000; 27:179–184.
77. Hayashi T, Kinoshita H, Yukawa E, Higuchi S. Pharmacokinetic anaylysis of subcutaneous erythropoietin administration with nonlinear mixed effect model including endogenous production. *Br J Clin Pharmacol* 1998; 46:11–19.
78. Jensen JD, Madsen JK, Jensen LW, Pedersen EB. Pharmacokinetics of epoetin in dialysis patients before and after correction of anaemia. *Drug Invest* 1994; 8:278–287.
79. Halstenson CE, Macres M, Katz SA, et al. Comparative pharmacokinetics and pharmacodynamics of epoetin alfa and epoetin beta. *Clin Pharmacol Ther* 1991; 50:702–712.
80. Ateshkadi A, Johnson CA, Oxton LL, Hammond TG, Bohenek WS, Zimmerman SW. Pharmacokinetics of intraperitoneal, intravenous, and subcutaneous recombinant human erythropoietin in patients on continuous ambulatory peritoneal dialysis. *Am J Kidney Dis* 1993; 21:635–642.
81. Kindler J, Eckardt KU, Ehmer B, et al. Single-dose pharmacokinetics of recombinant human erythropoietin in patients with various degrees of renal failure. *Nephrol Dial Transplant* 1989; 4:345–349.
82. Neumayer HH, Bröckmoller J, Fritschka E, Roots I, Scigalla P, Wattenberg M. Pharmacokinetics of recombinant human erythropoietin after SC administration and in long-term IV treatment in patients on maintenance hemodialysis. *Contrib Nephrol* 1989; 76:131–141.
83. Hughes RT, Cotes PM, Oliver DO, et al. Correction of the anaemia of chronic renal failure with erythropoietin: Pharmacokinetics studies in patients on haemodialysis and CAPD. *Contrib Nephrol* 1989; 76:122–130.
84. Nielsen OJ. Pharmacokinetics of recombinant human erythropoietin in chronic haemodialysis patients. *Pharmacol Toxicol* 1990; 66:83–86.
85. Egrie JC, Eschbach JW, McGuire T, Adamson JW. Pharmacokinetics of recombinant human erythropoietin (rHuEpo) administered to hemodialysis (HD) patients. *Kidney Int* 1988; 33:abstract p. 262.
86. Lim V, DeGowin R, Zavala D, et al. Recombinant human erythropoietin treatment in predialysis patients: a double-blind placebo-controlled trial. *Ann Intern Med* 1989; 110:108–114.
87. Yamazaki C, Watanabe Y, Sakamoto N. Pharmacokinetic study of recombinant human erythropoietin treatment in pre-dialysis end stage renal disease patients. *Nippon Jinzo Gakkai Shi* 1993; 35:1233–1242.
88. Cotes JM, Pippard MJ, Reid CD, Winearls CG, Oliver DP, Royston JP. Characterization of the anaemia of chronic renal failure and the mode of its correction by a preparation of human erythropoietin (r-HuEPO). An investigation of the pharmacokinetics of intravenous erythropoietin and its effects on erythrokinetics. *Q J Med* 1989; 70:113–137.
89. Gladziwa U, Klotz U, Baumer K, Zollinger R, Mann H, Sieberth HG. Pharmacokinetics of epoetin (recombinant human erythropoietin) after long term therapy in patients undergoing haemodialysis and haemofiltration. *Clin Pharmacokinet* 1993; 25:145–153.
90. Hughes RT, Cotes PM, Oliver DO, et al. Correction of the anaemia of chronic renal failure with erythropoietin: Pharmacokinetic studies in patients on haemodialysis and CAPD. *Contrib Nephrol* 1989; 76:122–130.

91. Kampf D, Kahl A, Passlick J, et al. Single-dose kinetics of recombinant human erythropoietin after intravenous, subcutaneous and intraperitoneal administration. Preliminary results. *Contrib Nephrol* 1989; 76:106–110.
92. Schouten JP, Voorhorst G, Helbing AR, Janssen JW, Diderich PP, Op de Hoek CT. Pharmacokinetics of epoetin in haemodialysis patients after subcutaneous administration: influence of chronic treatment. *Pharm World Sci* 1993; 15:252–256.
93. Petersen J, Kang MS, Hays MT. Erythropoietin can be administered during dialysis: a kinetic analysis. *ASAIO J* 1996; 42:27–33.
94. Macdougall IC, Roberts DE, Neubert P, Dharmasena AD, Coles GA, Williams JD. Pharmacokinetics of recombinant human erythropoietin in patients on continuous ambulatory peritoneal dialysis. *Lancet* 1989; 1:425–427.
95. Boelaert JR, Schurgers ML, Matthys EG, et al. Comparative pharmacokinetics of recombinant erythropoietin administered by the intravenous, subcutaneous, and intraperitoneal routes in continuous amulatory peritoneal dialysis (CAPD) patients. *Perit Dial Int* 1989; 9:95–98.
96. Stockenhuber F, Loibl U, Gottsauner-Wolf M, et al. Pharmacokinetics and dose response after intravenous and subcutaneous administration of recombinant erythropoietin in patients on regular haemodialysis treatment or continuous ambulatory peritoneal dialysis. *Nephron* 1991; 59:399–402.
97. Bargman JM, Jones JE, Petro JM. The pharmacokinetics of intraperitoneal erythropoietin administered undiluted or diluted in dialysate. *Perit Dial Int* 1992; 12:369–372.
98. Taylor CA, Kosorok MR, Zimmerman SW, Johnson CA. Pharmacokinetics of intraperitoneal epoetin alfa in patients on peritoneal dialysis using an 8-hour "dry dwell" dosing technique. *Am J Kidney Dis* 1999; 34:657–662.
99. Evans JH, Brockleank JT, Bowmer CJ, Ng PC. Pharmacokinetics of recombinant human erythropoietin in children with renal failure. *Nephrol Dial Transplant* 1991; 6:709–714.
100. Braun A, Ding R, Seidel C, Fies T, Kurtz A, Scharer K. Pharmacokinetics of recombinant human erythorpoietin applied subcutaneously to children with chronic renal failure. *Pediatr Nephrol* 1993; 7:61–64.
101. Cakar N. Ekim M, Tumer N, Yalcinkaya F, Akar N, Onaran HO. Pharmacokinetics of recombinant human erythropoietin in children with chronic renal failure. *Int Urol Nephrol* 1997; 29:377–383.
102. Montini G, Zacchello G, Perfumo F. Pharmacokinetics and pharmacodynamics of subcutaneous administration of r-HuEPO on CPD. A multicenter study from the Italian Registry of Pediatric CPD. *J Am Soc Nephrol* 1991; 2:283.
103. Kausz AT, Watkins SL, Hansen C, Godwin DA, Palmer RB, Brandt JR. Intraperitoneal erythropoietin in children on peritoneal dialysis: a study of pharmacokinetics and efficacy. *Am J Kidney Dis* 1999; 34:651–656.
104. Jensen JD, Jensen LW, Madsen JK, Poulsen L. The metabolism of erythropoietin in liver cirrhosis patients compared with healthy volunteers. *Eur J Haematol* 1995; 54:111–116.
105. Franek E, Wiecek A, Kozielski J, et al. Half-time of erythropoietin in patients with chronic obstructive pulmonary diseases. *Przegl Lek* 1996; 53:592–594.
106. Bowen D, Ehmer B, Neubert P, Lewis T, Jacobs A. The clearance of a single iv bolus of recombinant human erythropoietin from the serum of patients with myelodysplastic syndromes and its effects on erythropoiesis. *Exp Hematol* 1991; 19:613–616.
107. Macdougall IC, Jones JM, Robinson MI, Miles JB, Coles GA, Williams JD. Subcutaneous erythropoietin therapy: comparison of three different sites of injection. *Contrib Nephrol* 1991; 88:152–156.
108. Jensen JD, Jensen LW, Madsen JK. The pharmacokinetics of recombinant human erythropoietin after subcutaneous injection at different sites. *Eur J Clin Pharmacol* 1994; 46:333–337.
109. Kato M, Kamiyama H, Okazaki A, Kumaki K, Kato Y, Sugiyama Y. Mechanism for the nonlinear phamacokinetics of erythropoietin in rats. *J Pharmacol Exp Ther* 1997; 283:520–527
110. Macdougall IC. Once-weekly erythropoietic therapy: is there a difference between the available products? *Nephrol Dial Transplant* 2002; 17:2047–2051.
111. Eschbach JW, Egrie JC, Downing MR, et al. Correction of the anemia of end-stage renal diease with recombinant human erythropoietin: result of a phase I and II clinical trial. *N Engl J Med* 1987; 316:73–78.
112. Cheung W, Minton N, Gunawardena K. Pharmacokinetics and pharmacodynamics of epoetin alfa once weekly and three times weekly. *Eur J Clin Pharmacol* 2001; 57:411–418.
113. Kaufman JS, Reda DJ, Fye CL, et al. Subcutaneous compared with intravenous epoetin in patients receiving hemodialysis. Department of Veterans Affairs Cooperative Study Group on Erythropoietin in Hemodialysis Patients. *N Engl J Med* 1998; 339:578–583.

114. Elliott S, Chang D, Delorme E, et al. Isolation and characterization of conformation sensitive antierythropoietin monoclonal antibodies: effect of disulfide bonds and carbohydrate on recombinant human erythropoietin structure. *Blood* 1996; 87:2714–2722.
115. Elliott S, Lorenzini T, Chang D, et al. Fine-structure epitope mapping of antierythropoietin monoclonal antibodies reveals a model of recombinant human erythropoietin structure. *Blood* 1996; 87:2702–2713.
116. Lis H, Sharon N. Protein glycosylation. Structural and functional aspects. *Eur J Biochem* 1993; 218:1–27.
117. Endo Y, Nagai H, Watanabe Y, Ochi K, Takagi T. Heat-induced aggregation of recombinant erythropoietin in the intact and deglycosylated states as monitored by gel permeation chromatography combined with a low-angle laser light scattering technique. *J Biochem* 1992; 112:700–706.
118. Coccia MA, Cooke K, Stoney G, et al. Novel erythropoiesis stimulating protein (darbepoetin alfa) alleviates anemia associated with chronic inflammatory disease in a rodent model. *Exp Hematol* 2001; 29:1201–1209.
119. Macdougall IC, Gray SJ, Elston O, et al. Pharmacokinetics of novel erythropoiesis stimulating protein compared with epoetin alfa in dialysis patients. *J Am Soc Nepthrol* 1999; 10:2392–2395.
120. Lerner G, Kale AS, Warady BA, et al. Pharmacokinetics of darbepoetin alfa in pediatric patients with chronic kidney disease. *Pediatr Nephrol* 2002; 17:933–937.
121. Heatherington A, Schuller J, Dittrich C, the darbepoetin alfa 990146 Study Group, Mercer AJ, Rossi G. Intravenous (IV) administration of darbepoetin alfa to patients with nonmyeloid malignancies receiving multicycle chemotherapy; pharmacokinetic profiles. *Proc ASCO* 2002; 21:256b. Abstract 2844
122. Jumbe N, Yao B, Rovetti R, Rossi G, Heatherington AC. Clinical trial simulation of a 200-µg fixed dose of darbepoetin alfa in chemotherapy-induced anemia. *Oncology (Huntingt)* 2002; 16:37–44.
123. Locatelli F, Olivares J, Walker R, et al. Novel erythropoiesis stimulating protein for treatment of anemia in chronic renal insufficiency. *Kidney Int* 2001; 60:741–747.
124. Nissenson AR, Swan SK. Lindberg JS, et al. Randomized, controlled trial of darbepoetin alfa for the treatment of anemia in hemodialysis patients. *Am J Kidney Dis* 2002; 40:110–118.
125. Smith R. Applications of darbepoietin-alpha, a novel erythropoiesis-stimulating protein, in oncology. *Curr Opin Hematol* 2002; 9:228–233.
126. Vansteenkiste J, Pirker R, Massuti B, et al. Double-blind, placebo-controlled, randomized phase III trial of darbepoetin alfa in lung cancer patients receiving chemotherapy. *J Natl Cancer Inst* 2002; 94:1211–1220.
127. Glaspy J, Jadeja JS, Justice G, et al. A dose-finding and safety study of novel erythropoiesis stimulating protein (NESP) for the treatment of anaemia in patients receiving multicycle chemotherapy. *Br J Cancer* 2001; 84:17–23.
128. Glaspy JA, Jadeja JS, Justice G, et al. Darbepoetin alfa given every 1 or 2 weeks alleviates anaemia associated with cancer chemotherapy. *Br J Cancer* 2002; 87:268–276.
129. Glaspy JA, Tchekmedyian NS. Darbepoetin alfa administered every 2 weeks alleviates anemia in cancer patients receiving chemotherapy. *Oncology (Huntington)* 2002; 16:suppl 9.
130. Casadevall N, Nataf J, Viron B, et al. Pure red-cell aplasia and antierythropoietin antibodies in patients treated with recombinant erythropoietin. *N Engl J Med* 2002; 346:469–475.
131. Sawada K, Krantz SB, Sawyer ST, Civin Ci. Quantitation of specific binding of eryathropoietin to human erythorid colony-forming cells. *J Cell Physiol* 1988; 137:337–345.
132. Sawyer ST, Hankins WD. The functional form of the erythropoietin receptor is a 78-kDa protein: correlation with cell surface expression, endocytosis, and phosphorylation. *Proc Natl Acad Sci USA* 1993; 90:6849–6853.
133. Sawyer ST. Introduction: the erythropoietin receptor and signal transduction. *Ann NY Acad Sci* 1994; 718:185–190.
134. Fukuda M, Sasaki H, Fukuda MN. Structure and role of carbohydrate in human erythropoietin. *Adv Exp Med Biol* 1989; 271:53–67.
135. Watowich SS, Xie X, Klingmuller U, et al. Erythropoietin receptor mutations associated with familial erythrocytosis cause hypersensitivity to erythropoietin in the heterozygous state. *Blood* 1999; 94:2530–2532.
136. Delgado C, Francis GE, Fisher D. The uses and properties of PEG-linked proteins. *Crit Rev Ther Drug Carrier Syst* 1992; 9:249–304.
137. Francis GE, Fisher D, Delgado C, Malik F, Gardiner A, Neale D. PEGylation of cytokines and other therapeutic proteins and peptides: the importance of biological optimisation of coupling techniques. *Int J Hematol* 1998; 68:1–18.

138. Goodson RJ, Katre NV. Site-directed pegylation of recombinant interleukin-2 at its glycosylation site. *Biotechnology* 1990; 8:343–346.
139. He XH, Shaw PC, Tam SC. Reducing the immunogenicity and improving the in vivo activity of trichosanthin by site-directed pegylation. *Life Sci* 1999; 65:355–368.
140. Weich NS, Tullai J, Guido E, et al. Interleukin-3/erythropoietin fusion proteins: in vitro effectrs on hematopoietic cells. *Exp Hematol* 1993; 21:647–655.
141. Coscarella Carloni C, Liddi R, et al. Production of recombinant human GM-CSF-EPO hybrid proteins: in vitro biological characterization. *Eur J Haematol* 1987; 59:238–246.
142. Sytkowski AJ, Lunn ED, Risinger MA, Davis KL. An erythropoietin fusion protein comprised of identical repeating domains exhibits enhanced biological properties. *J Biol Chem* 1999; 274:24773–24778.
143. Sytkowski AJ, Lunn ED, Davis KL, Feldman L, Siekman S. Human erythropoietin dimers with markedly enhanced in vivo activity. *Proc Natl Acad Sci USA* 1998; 95:1184–1188.
144. Yi T, Zhang J, Miura O, Ihle JN. Hematopoietic cell phosphatase associates with erythropoietin (Epo) receptor after Epo-induced receptor tyrosine phosphorylation: identification of potential binding sites. *Blood* 1995; 85:87–95.
145. de la Chapelle A, Traskelin AL, Juvonen E. Truncated erythorpoietin receptor causes dominantly inherited benign human erythrocytosis. *Proc Natl Acad Sci USA* 1993; 90:4495–4499.
146. Naffakh N, Henri A, Villeval JL, et al. Sustained delivery of erythropoietin in mice by genetically modified skin fibroblasts. *Proc Natl Acad Sci USA* 1995; 92:3194–3198.
147. Meyer F, Finer M. Gene therapy: progress and challenges. *Cell Mol Biol* 2001; 47:1277–1294.
148. Dalle B, Payen E, Regulier E, et al. Improvement of mouse beta-thalassemia upon erythropoietin delivery by encapsulated myoblasts. *Gene Ther* 1999; 6:157–161.
149. Bohl D, Heard JM. Delivering erythropoietin through genetically engineered cells. *J American Soc Nephrol* 2000; 11:Suppl-62.
150. Payen E, Bettan M, Henri A, et al. Oxygen tension and a pharmacological switch in the regulation of transgene expression for gene therapy. *J Gene Med* 2001; 3:498–504.
151. Maruyama H, Higuchi N, Nishikawa Y, et al. Kidney-targeted naked DNA transfer by retrograde renal vein injection in rats. *Hum Gene Ther* 2002; 13:455–468.
152. Morlock M, Kissel T, Li YX, Koll H, Winter G. Erythropoietin loaded microspheres prepared from biodegradable LPLG-PEO-LPLG triblock copolymers: protein stabilization and in-vitro release properties. *J Control Release* 1998; 56:105–115.
153. Pistel KF, Bittner B, Koll H, Winter G, Kissel T. Biodegradable recombinant human erythropoietin loaded microspheres prepared from linear and star-branched block copolymers: influence of encapsulation technique and polyer composition on particle characteristics. *J Control Release* 1999; 59:309–325.

7 Thrombopoietin Factors

David J. Kuter, MD, DPhil

CONTENTS

1. INTRODUCTION

Thrombopoietin (TPO) was the name proposed by Kelemen in 1958 for the hematopoietic growth factor (HGF) presumed to regulate platelet production like erythropoietin (EPO) regulates erythrocyte production *(1,2)*. Despite almost 40 years of research efforts, TPO was finally purified in 1994 by five separate groups using several approaches. Two of the research groups purified the molecule directly from the plasma of thrombocytopenic mice *(3)* or sheep *(4)* using bioassays to detect the stimulation of megakaryocyte growth. The others purified TPO from thrombocytopenic animal plasma by affinity purification methods that used the previously described, presumed TPO receptor, c-mpl *(5,6)*. Finally, one group subjected a BaF3 cell line containing the presumed TPO receptor, c-mpl, to mutagenesis and selected for clones exhibiting exogenous factor-independent autocrine growth *(7)*.

Although all the molecules initially discovered had the same amino acid sequence, some groups called the molecule TPO and others called it megakaryocyte growth and

From: *Cancer Drug Discovery and Development*
Hematopoietic Growth Factors in Oncology: Basic Science and Clinical Therapeutics
Edited by: G. Morstyn, M. A. Foote, and G. J. Lieschke © Humana Press Inc., Totowa, NJ

Table 1
The Thrombopoietins (c-mpl Ligands)

Endogenous thrombopoietin (TPO)
Recombinant human thrombopoietin (rHuTPO)
Pegylated human growth and development factor (PEG-rHuMGDF)
Promegapoietin (TPO/IL-3 fusion protein)
Thrombopoietin peptide mimetics
Thrombopoietin nonpeptide mimetics

development factor (MGDF) *(5)*, c-mpl ligand *(6)*, or megapoietin *(4)*. MGDF was the name given to the 25- and 31-kDa amino-terminal fragments of full-length TPO purified from thrombocytopenic canine plasma that stimulated an increase in the size and number of megakaryocyte colonies in vitro *(8)*. Megapoietin was the name given the 31-kDa amino-terminal TPO fragment purified from thrombocytopenic sheep plasma based on its ability to stimulate an increase in the number and ploidy of megakaryocytes in culture *(4,9)*.

The name c-mpl ligand comes from the fact that before its identification as the TPO receptor, v-mpl was found to be a truncated hematopoietic cytokine receptor encoded by a murine retroviral oncogene that caused a myeloproliferative leukemia (hence the name "mpl") in mice *(10)*. When the full-length cellular homolog c-mpl was cloned in 1992 *(11)*, it was found to be present in megakaryocytes and platelets, and this led to the presumption, now known to be correct, that it was the TPO receptor. This information led many to attempt to find the ligand ("c-mpl ligand") that bound to the c-mpl receptor. In retrospect, it is now known that the c-mpl ligand is TPO and that c-mpl is the TPO receptor. The term "c-mpl ligand" is often used interchangeably with TPO, but it more appropriately describes a family of ligands that bind to c-mpl, including endogenous TPO, recombinant human TPO (rHuTPO), pegylated MGDF (PEG-rHuMGDF), promegapoietin (a fusion protein of interleukin [IL]-3 and TPO), and TPO mimetics (Table 1).

2. STRUCTURE

TPO is synthesized in the liver as a 353-amino acid precursor protein with a molecular weight of 36 kDa *(5,6,12)*. After the removal of the 21-amino acid signal peptide, the remaining 332 amino acids undergo glycosylation to produce a glycoprotein with a molecular weight of 80–90 kDa on sodium dodecyl sulfate-polyacrylamide gel electrophoresis (SDS-PAGE) and 57,539 Daltons by mass spectrometry *(13)*. The glycoprotein is then released into the circulation with no apparent intracellular storage in the liver.

TPO is a member of the four-helix-bundle cytokine superfamily and has a number of unusual properties (Fig. 1). First, it is much larger than most other regulators of blood cell production such as granulocyte colony-stimulating factor (G-CSF) and EPO. Second, it has an unusual structure in that it has two domains, an EPO-like domain (residues 1–153) and a carbohydrate-rich domain (residues 154–332) separated by a dibasic site of potential proteolytic cleavage (Arg153–Arg154). It is unclear whether this cleavage site is biologically relevant *(14)*.

The first 153 amino acids of the mature protein are 23% identical with human EPO *(15,16)* and 50% similar if conservative amino acid substitutions are considered. This

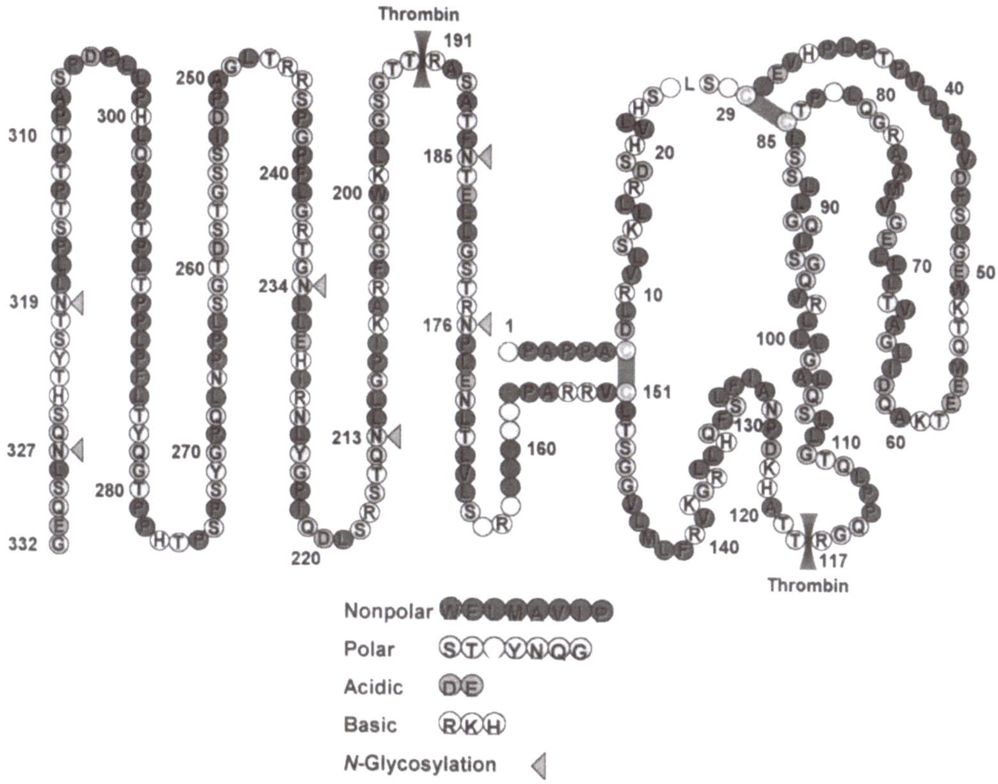

Fig. 1. The primary structure of human thrombopoietin. (Courtesy of Dr. T. Kato, Pharmaceutical Research Laboratory, Kirin Brewery, Takasaki, Gunma, Japan.)

region also contains four Cys residues, Cys7–Cys151 and Cys29–Cys85 *(17)*, comparable to those in EPO, which are highly conserved among different species. Replacement of Cys7 or Cys151 abrogates all activity, whereas disruption of Cys29 or Cys85 reduces activity *(18)*. This region also contains four α-helices as in EPO. All the TPO receptor binding activity is located in this region.

Amino acids 154–332 comprise a unique sequence that contains six *N*-linked glycosylation sites and is less well conserved among different species. It is rich in Ser, Thr, and Pro residues. Structure-function studies have shown that whereas the first 153 amino acids of the c-mpl ligand are all that are required for its thrombopoietic effect in vitro *(5,6)*, this truncated molecule has a markedly decreased circulatory half-life compared with the 20–40-h half-life of the native protein *(19)*. Paradoxically, the truncated molecule has a specific activity in vitro 20-fold greater than the full-length molecule *(20)*.

Glycosylation is an important post-translational modification of TPO. Other post-translational modifications, such as hydroxylation, methylation, or deamidation of TPO, are not evident. Presumably, the glycosylated second half of the molecule confers stability and prolongs the circulatory half-life. Similar carbohydrate sequences regulate the stability of EPO *(21)*. In addition, this part of the molecule assists in the secretion of the intact molecule from the hepatocytes by serving as a molecular chaperone or guide in protein folding; truncated muteins of this portion of the molecule have diminished secretion *(22)*. All six sites of *N*-glycosylation are found in residues 154–332. The *N*-glycans are of the complex type, with the core-fucosylated disialylated biantennary and trisialylated triantennary structures predominating. N_{185}FT and N_{234}GT appear to be 100% occupied, whereas N_{176}RT and N_{213}QT are partially occupied, and the status of N_{319}TS and N_{327}LS is uncertain *(13)*. In addition, there are 3 *O*-glycosylation sites (S1, T37, T110) in the EPO-like domain and at least 5 (T158, T159, S163, T192, T244) and possibly 16 others in the carbohydrate-rich domain. The *O*-glycans are of the mucin type with the monosialylated and disialylated GalGalNAc-S/T structures predominating. This formation has led to the proposal that the carbohydrate-rich domain of TPO can be further divided into two subdomains on the basis of sequence homology among the cloned sequences and glycosylation: an *N*-glycan domain (amino acids 154–246) and an *O*-glycan domain (amino acids 247–332) *(13)*.

Although the crystal-structure analysis of TPO has been completed, it has not been published. The areas of TPO that bind the TPO receptor are probably analogous to those of human growth hormone and EPO. Based on the similarity of these three cytokines, it has been proposed that Lys138 of helix D and Pro42 and Glu50 of loop AB may constitute one binding region, and Arg10 and Lys14 of helix A may constitute a second binding region that participates in the dimerization of TPO receptors *(23)*. This suggestion has been partly confirmed by monoclonal antibody (MAb) studies. Two MAbs that block TPO binding to its receptor have determinants in helix D *(24)*. These results again suggest that TPO has two receptor binding sites that help dimerize its receptor.

3. REGULATION OF THROMBOPOIETIN EXPRESSION

TPO mRNA is expressed in low amounts, primarily in liver parenchymal cells, and in even smaller amounts in the kidney *(25)*, skeletal muscle, heart, brain, testis, spleen *(26)*, and bone marrow *(27,28)*. To date physiologically relevant protein expression has been documented only in hepatocytes and possibly bone marrow cells *(27,29)*.

A single copy of the gene for TPO is on human chromosome 3q27–28 *(12,16,30)*. The gene spans approx 7 kb with seven exons, the first two of which are noncoding. The third exon contains part of the 5′-untranslated sequence and part of the signal peptide. The EPO-like region is coded for by exons 4–7, and the entire carbohydrate-rich domain is encoded by exon 7. Comparison with the *EPO* gene shows conservation of the boundaries of the coding exons except for the addition of the carbohydrate domain sequence in the final exon of the *TPO* gene.

Most studies have shown that expression of TPO does not appear to be regulated by any known stimuli at either a translational or transcriptional level. No endogenous or exogenous modulators have been uncovered that regulate TPO expression. TPO production appears to be constitutive, and the circulating concentrations are directly determined by the circulating platelet mass.

The 5′-flanking region of the *TPO* gene contains several possible regulatory regions including SP-1, AP-2, and NF-κB. Downstream of exon 1 are several GATA and Ets elements, but no TATA box or CAAT motif. The gene is located in a region of chromosome 3 in which there are many other genes containing iron-responsive elements, but no such elements have been detected in the TPO promoter.

In addition to the functional mRNA encoded (TPO-1), two other mRNA sequences are present owing to alternative splicing *(12,16,31,32)*. One variant has a deletion of

12 bp (amino acids 112–115 of the mature protein) at the junction of exons 6 and 7 but maintains the normal reading frame. In transfected cells, this protein is secreted 500-fold less than TPO-1, and the secreted protein is probably inactive *(16)*. The second variant is produced by a splice site within exon 7 that causes a frame shift and a protein predicted to contain 286 amino acids, the first 159 of which are identical to native TPO (including the signal peptide). This protein is synthesized in transfected cells, but it is unknown whether it is secreted or has any biologic effect *(31,32)*.

Further analysis of the expression of the human *TPO* gene has documented additional variant mRNA transcripts. Ten percent of all hepatic transcripts originate from a promoter in exon 1 (P1) and 90% from the dominant promoter site in exon 2 (P2). In addition, a splice variant in which exon 2 (containing much of the 5′ untranslated region) is skipped (P1ΔE2) is produced 2% of the time *(33)*. Although not abundant, the last transcript has much greater translational ability than does either of the other mRNAs.

A human mutation has demonstrated regulation of TPO at a translational level. Inherited thrombocythemia is an uncommon disorder that clinically affects a few families, similar to the more common, sporadic cases of essential thrombocythemia. Analysis of one of these families *(34)* has identified a single point mutation in the splice donor site of intron 3 of the *TPO* gene. This produces a new TPO mRNA with a normal protein coding region but with a shortened 5′ untranslated region that is more efficiently translated than normal TPO transcripts. This change results in more TPO protein synthesis, higher plasma TPO amounts, and chronically increased platelet counts. A similar mutation has been described in several other families *(35)*, but none of these mutations appears to be involved in the more common, sporadic cases of essential thrombocythemia *(36)*.

The nature of this translational regulation has been elucidated *(33)*. The TPO 5′ untranslated region is unusual in that it has eight AUG codons from which translation may be initiated. Only the eighth AUG results in a successful protein product, whereas the other AUG sites compete for ribosomal binding sites and markedly suppress effective TPO protein production. Elimination of some of the upstream AUG sites by mutation, deletion, or alternative splicing produces transcripts with fewer AUG sites, less competition for ribosome binding, and increased effective production of TPO protein. The families in which TPO is overproduced are characterized by the loss of some of these AUG sites *(34,35)*. Since TPO is such a highly potent HGF, it has been suggested that the presence of these extra AUG sites serves to guarantee against overproduction of TPO.

4. THROMBOPOIETIN FUNCTION

4.1. In Vitro Effects

TPO acts only through the c-mpl (TPO) receptor. Despite sharing considerable sequence and structural homology with EPO, TPO does not bind the EPO receptor and EPO does not bind the TPO receptor. Binding of TPO to its receptor causes receptor dimerization that has major effects on megakaryocyte precursors (megakaryocyte colony-forming cells [Meg-CFCs]) and megakaryocytes, including preventing apoptosis *(37)*; increasing megakaryocyte number, size, and ploidy *(4)*; and increasing the rate of cellular maturation. Increased megakaryocyte ploidy is associated with a gene dosage effect on the expression of lineage-specific proteins *(38)*. All these events are mediated through signal transduction pathways involving Janus kinase (JAK) signal transducers and activators of transcription (STAT), mitogen-activated protein (MAP) kinase, and other intracellular mediators.

Addition of TPO to isolated human CD34$^+$ cells can cause most cells to become megakaryocytes that shed platelets *(39)*. This last step, the shedding of platelets from megakaryocytes, however, does not require, and actually may be inhibited by, the presence of TPO *(40)*.

Although TPO affects late cellular maturation events only in megakaryocytes, it can stimulate in vitro early precursors of all lineages as well as pluripotential stem cells *(41)*. Approximately 70% of CD34$^+$ cells express the TPO receptor c-mpl *(42)*. Indeed, in some infants born with amegakaryocytic thrombocytopenia and a defective c-mpl receptor, the initial thrombocytopenia at birth often evolves over a few years into anemia and leukopenia as the marrow precursor cells die off, presumably owing to lack of TPO effect on multilineage precursors *(43,44)*. In general, TPO affects the growth of early progenitors of all lineages, including the pluripotential stem cells, but only affects the late maturation of megakaryocytes. Hence, it stimulates only the production of mature platelets in vitro and in vivo.

Binding of TPO to its receptor leads to internalization of the ligand-receptor complex that is the major clearance mechanism of TPO from the circulation *(4,9,45)*. Platelets, and probably megakaryocytes, are the sites of this activity; once internalized, TPO is degraded *(46–48)* with no recycling of the TPO receptor *(49)*.

4.2. In Vivo Effects in Animals

When administered to normal animals, TPO increases bone marrow and peripheral blood Meg-CFC, increases bone marrow megakaryocyte number size and ploidy, and increases platelet count. Interestingly, both erythroid and multipotential precursor cells are also increased in the bone marrow and peripheral blood, but not the erythrocytes or neutrophils.

After daily administration of a recombinant form of TPO (PEG-rHuMGDF) to normal baboons (Fig. 2), a predictable response occurs *(4,50,51)*. During the first 4 d of administration, bone marrow megakaryocyte ploidy increases to a maximum without change in platelet count. On d 5, the platelet count begins to increase and does so at a dose-dependent rate. With continued administration of TPO, a dose-dependent plateau platelet count is reached on d 8–12. A log-linear relationship exists between TPO dose and the plateau platelet count, with a maximum sixfold increase in the rate of platelet production (Fig. 2, inset). Upon stopping the growth factor, the platelet count returns to its baseline value over 10 d without a rebound thrombocytopenia. White and red blood cell counts are not affected.

Although TPO does not directly cause platelet activation, at pharmacologically high doses it does have a modest effect on mature platelets by increasing their reactivity to some aggregation stimuli; TPO-treated platelets require half as much adenosine diphosphate (ADP) for a response *(50,52)*. Other HGFs also reduce the threshold for platelet activation, but the clinical relevance is uncertain. This effect may be mediated by TPO-dependent activation of phosphatidylinositide 3-kinase (PI3K), which in turn phosphorylates Thr306 and Ser473 of platelet protein kinase Bα, an important anti-apoptotic protein *(53)*. However, TPO does not prevent apoptosis of platelets during ex vivo storage *(54,55)*.

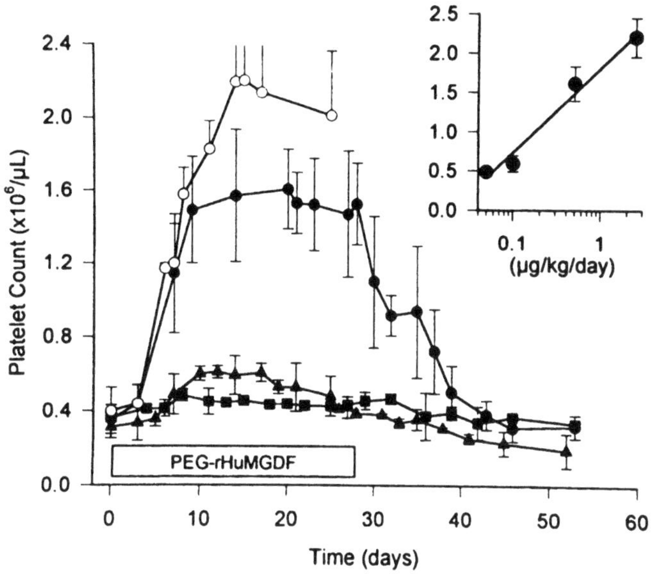

Fig. 2. The effect of recombinant thrombopoietin on the platelet count in vivo. Baboons were injected daily for 28 d with pegylated recombinant human megakaryocyte growth and development factor (PEG-rHuMGDF; horizontal bar) at doses of 0.05 (■; *n* = 3), 0.10 (▲; *n* = 3), 0.50 (●; *n* = 4), or 2.50 (○; *n* = 6) µg/kg/d. The inset shows the log-linear relationship between the administered dose and the fold-increase in platelet counts. White cell and red cell counts were not affected. (Reproduced with permission from ref. *51*.)

4.3. Normal Animal Physiology

Much has been learned about the normal physiology of TPO. First, TPO is the only physiologically relevant regulator of platelet production and acts to amplify the basal production rate of megakaryocytes and platelets. TPO is not necessary for megakaryocyte differentiation. When TPO or its receptor have been knocked out by homologous recombination in mice *(56–59)*, the megakaryocyte and platelet mass are reduced to approx 10% of normal, but the animals are healthy and do not spontaneously bleed (Fig. 3). The neutrophil and erythrocyte counts are normal. In animals in which only one of the *TPO* genes has been deleted, the platelet count is reduced to approx 65% of normal. If treated with other thrombopoietic growth factors such as IL-6, IL-11, and stem cell factor (SCF), such TPO-deficient mice modestly increase their platelet count *(60)*.

Second, TPO affects bone marrow precursor cells of all lineages. In the animals deficient in TPO or c-mpl, Meg-CFC are reduced to <5% of normal as expected, and the myeloid and erythroid precursor cells are also reduced to 20–30% of normal *(56,60)*, but with no change in the neutrophil or erythrocyte counts (Fig. 4). The normal counts in these animals are presumably maintained by the intact feedback mechanisms mediated by G-CSF and EPO. This finding supports the concept that TPO is an important stimulus for the growth of early progenitor cells of all lineages but only affects the late maturation of megakaryocytes and only stimulates platelet production.

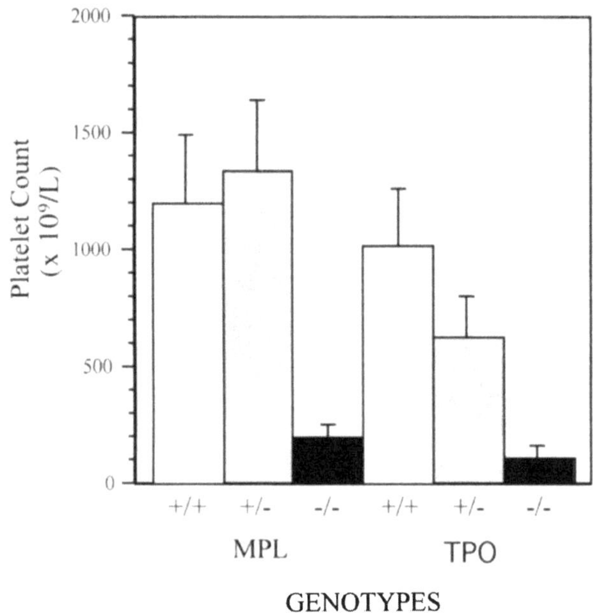

Fig. 3. Mice deficient in thrombopoietin (TPO) or its receptor (MPL) are thrombocytopenic. Platelet counts (+ SD) in normal (+/+) mice were compared with those in TPO or MPL homozygous (–/–) or heterozygous (+/–) deficient mice. (Adapted from refs. *59* and *58*.)

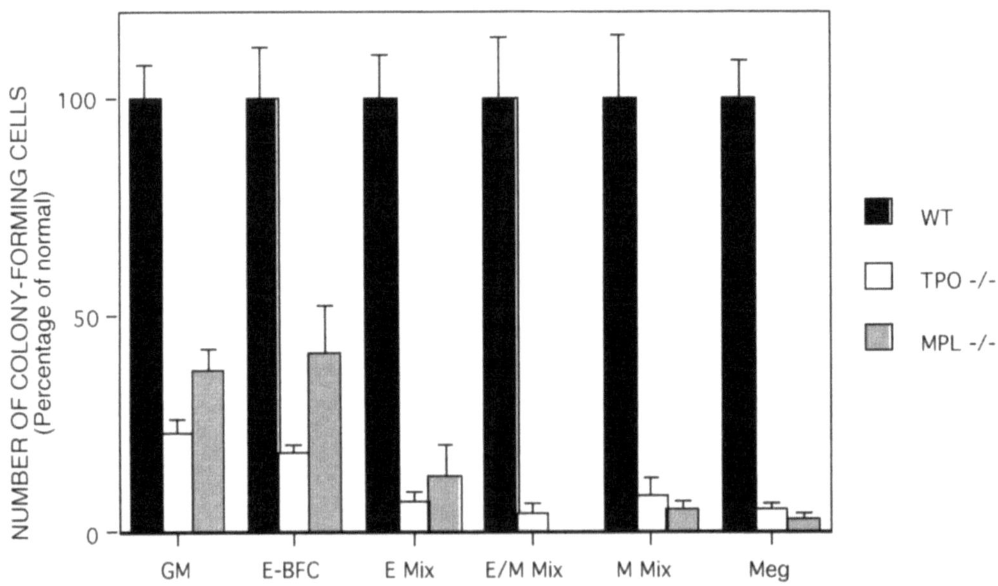

Fig. 4. Bone marrow progenitor cells of all lineages are decreased in mice deficient in thrombopoietin (TPO–/–) or its receptor (MPL–/–) compared with normal wild type (WT). Granulocyte-macrophage colony-forming cells (GM-CFC) (GM), erythroid burst-forming cells (E-BFC), and megakaryocyte-CFC (Meg), as well as mixed colonies (Mix-CFC) with erythroid component (E Mix), erythroid and megakaryocytic components (E/M Mix), or megakaryocytic with nonerythroid components (M-Mix) were enumerated (+ SD). (Adapted from ref. *60*.)

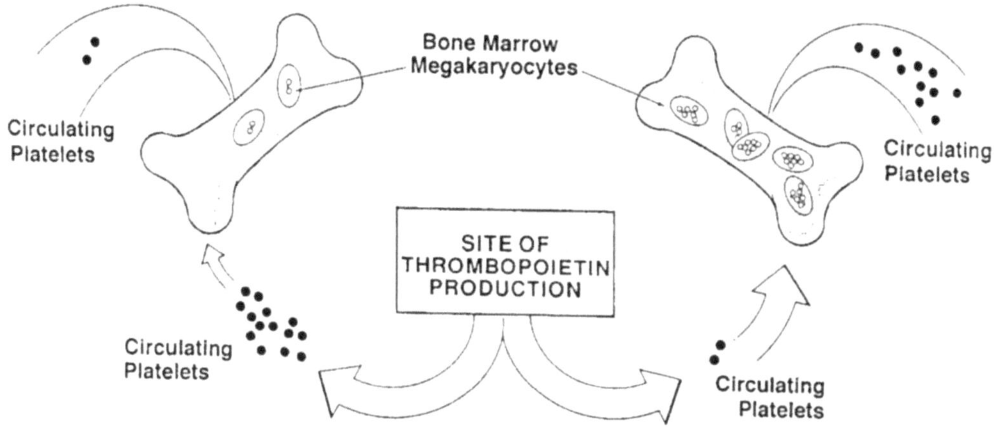

Fig. 5. The physiologic regulation of thrombopoietin levels. The constitutive hepatic production of thrombopoietin (center) is cleared by avid thrombopoietin receptors on platelets, resulting in normal levels when the platelet production is normal (left) and increased amounts when platelet production is reduced (right). The bone marrow megakaryocytes are stimulated as the circulating thrombopoietin concentration increases.

Third, TPO production is constitutive, and the circulating concentrations are directly determined by the circulating platelet mass (Fig. 5). Whereas the production of red blood cells is regulated by a cytochrome P-450 system that senses changes in the hematocrit and alters the rate of transcription of the *EPO* gene, there is no such sensor of the platelet mass *(4,9,45,61–64)*, rather, TPO mRNA is produced at the same rate in normal and thrombocytopenic individuals *(65)*. No drug or clinical condition has been shown to increase hepatic TPO production. Platelets and megakaryocytes contain high-affinity TPO (c-mpl) receptors that bind and clear TPO from the circulation and thereby directly determine the amount of circulating TPO. When platelet production is decreased, clearance of TPO is reduced and amounts increase.

This type of feedback system is not unusual in hematology. Indeed, both monocyte colony-stimulating factor (M-CSF) and G-CSF are normally regulated primarily by the amount of circulating monocytes and neutrophils, respectively. It appears that only for EPO is there a true sensor of the circulating blood cell mass that in turn alters production of this HGF. Transfusion of platelets into thrombocytopenic animals or humans decreases the amount of plasma TPO *(4,9,45,62,66)*, and similar results have been observed when normal platelets are transfused into c-mpl-deficient mice *(48)*. These findings indicate that TPO is constitutively synthesized in the liver and removed from circulation by binding to the c-mpl receptor on platelets and possibly bone marrow megakaryocytes.

Alternatively, some investigators have suggested that local production of TPO by bone marrow stromal cells may be increased during thrombocytopenia and may stimulate megakaryocyte growth *(29)*. Direct evidence to support the relative contribution of this mechanism to platelet production is lacking, and recent studies of hepatic TPO production make this mechanism unlikely *(67)*. These studies show that reduced hepatic production of TPO may play a major role in thrombocytopenia associated with liver disease. TPO is produced primarily in the liver, and thrombocytopenia in experimental animals seems to be proportional to the extent of liver resection *(68)*. In addition, after transplantation of healthy livers into TPO$^{-/-}$ mice, platelet counts returned toward normal, suggesting that most TPO is produced in the liver *(69)*. An association between low platelet counts (median: 84×10^9/L; range: $26–112 \times 10^9$/L) and low levels of TPO (median: <20 pg/mL; range: <20–182 pg/mL) has been reported in patients before orthotopic liver transplantation *(70,71)*. Within 4 d of orthotopic liver transplantation, amounts of TPO increased above normal and were accompanied by increased amounts of reticulated platelets. Fourteen days after transplantation, platelet counts were normal in 14/18 patients (median: 254×10^9/L; range: $70–398 \times 10^9$/L), and TPO concentrations returned to normal in 14/18 patients (median: 59 pg/mL; range: <20–639 pg/mL). No appreciable change in spleen size was observed. In multivariate analysis, the increase in TPO was the only variable that correlated with the increase in platelet count.

5. RECOMBINANT THROMBOPOIETINS AND THROMBOPOIETIN MIMETICS

A number of recombinant TPO and TPO mimetics have been generated and are under clinical development (Table 1). None has demonstrated clinical efficacy or been approved for marketing by regulatory agencies. Minimal pharmacologic data on these compounds are available.

5.1. rHuTPO

The amino acid sequence of rHuTPO (Genentech, South San Francisco, CA) is identical to that of endogenous TPO (Fig. 6 and Table 2). rHuTPO is produced in mammalian cells, is glycosylated, and has a circulatory half-life of 20–40 h. Nonetheless, its molecular weight is 90 kDa, less than the 95 kDa of the native molecule *(72)*.

5.2. PEG-rHuMGDF

PEG-rHuMGDF (Amgen, Thousand Oaks, CA), is a nonglycosylated, truncated molecule produced in *Escherichia coli* and composed of the first 163 amino acids of the native molecule that is then chemically coupled to a 20-kDa PEG moiety (Fig. 6 and Table 2) *(19)*. This half of the native molecule is 50% similar to EPO and contains the receptor binding domain but has a very short circulatory half-life and no biologic activity in vivo owing to the absence of the remaining, carbohydrate-rich portion of the native molecule. The addition of the PEG moiety serves to stabilize the molecule in circulation and replaces the carbohydrate domain. It has a half-life of 30–40 h *(73,74)*.

5.3. Promegapoietin

Promegapoietin *(75)*, is a molecular modification of TPO in which the receptor binding region is coupled to IL-3. This molecule can bind and activate both the TPO and IL-3 receptors. Administration of this molecule has been shown to increase platelet counts in animals, but it has been found to be immunogenic and is no longer under development *(75)*.

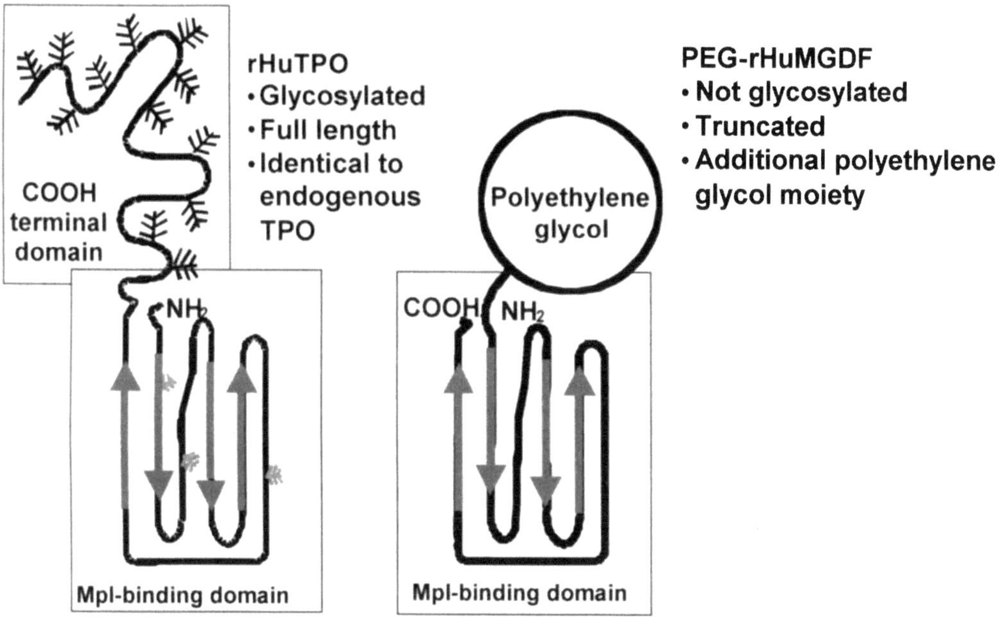

Fig. 6. Molecular structures of recombinant human thrombopoietin (rHuTPO) and pegylated recombinant human megakaryocyte growth and development factor (PEG-rHuMGDF) exhibit specific differences. rHuTPO is a glycosylated full-length thrombopoietin molecule, whereas PEG-rHuMGDF is a truncated molecule consisting of the receptor-binding portion of native thrombopoietin conjugated to a 20-kDa polyethylene glycol moiety. (Courtesy of Amgen, Thousand Oaks, CA.)

Table 2
Pharmacologic Characteristics of rHuTPO and PEG-rHuMGDF

Characteristic	*rHuTPO*	*PEG-rHuMGDF*
Terminal $t_{1/2}$ (h)	24–40	31
K_d for c-Mpl (pM)	150	150
Platelet clearance (mL/h/10^9)	1.28	1.28
Time to onset of effect in mice (d)	3	3
Time to peak effect in mice (d)	4–6	4–6
Truncation	No	Yes
Glycolsylation	Yes	No
Pegylation	No	Yes
Human route tested	Intravenous	Subcutaneous

ABBREVIATIONS: PEG-rHuMGDF, pegylated recombinant human megakaryocyte growth and development factor; rHuTPO, recombinant human thrombopoietin.

5.4. Thrombopoietin Peptide Mimetics

Great attention has been focused on the development of TPO peptide mimetics that activate the TPO receptor *(76,77)*. These mimetics are designed to bind to the TPO receptor but have no sequence homology with endogenous TPO. One is a dimer of two 14-amino acid peptides (AF13948) that has no sequence homology with TPO but

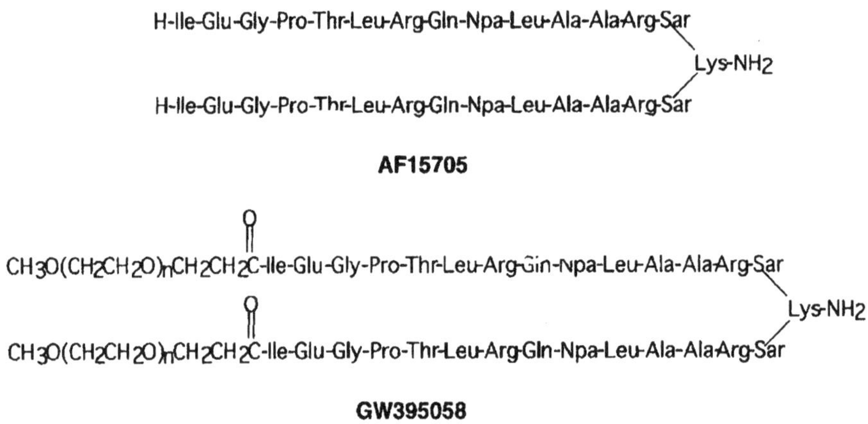

Fig. 7. The structure of some thrombopoietin peptide mimetics. AF15705 is a peptide dimer composed of two identical 14-amino acid chains linked by a lysine residue and modified to contain two sarcosine (sar) residues. GW395058 is formed by the conjugation of 20,000-Dalton polyethylene glycol to each of the paired peptides. Each of these peptide mimetics stimulates platelet production in mice and is nonimmunogenic. (Reproduced with permission from ref. *77*.)

avidly binds and activates the TPO receptor, c-mpl (Fig. 7) *(76)*. Although no longer in clinical development, AF13948 has been modified by amino acid substitution to yield AF15705, which was pegylated to produce GW395058 *(77)*. This peptide mimetic competes with TPO for binding to the TPO receptor but does not elicit neutralizing antibodies (Ab) in mice.

5.5. Thrombopoietin Nonpeptide Mimetics

Despite the reduced antigenicity of TPO peptide mimetics, with or without pegylation, recent efforts have focused on the development of nonpeptide, small-molecule mimetics *(78–81)*. These molecules elicit species-specific binding to the TPO receptor, are highly active, and allow for oral administration. Families of hydrazinonaphthalene (Fig. 8), azonaphthalene, semicarbazone, and naphtho[1,2-*d*]imidazole TPO mimetics have been described. They promote the proliferation of c-mpl-expressing cell lines, produce STAT5 phosphorylation, and stimulate human bone marrow CD34+ cells to mature into CD41+ megakaryocytes. They possess low molecular weights (MW < 500) and median effective concentration (EC_{50}) values of 1–20 n*M*. Preclinical studies have shown stimulation of platelet production identical with TPO; and human studies may begin soon.

5.6. Thrombopoietin-Potentiating Peptides

A peptide has been described that binds the EPO receptor at a site distant from the EPO binding site and prevents receptor-ligand internalization, thereby potentiating erythropoiesis *(82)*. An analogous TPO receptor-potentiating peptide has been developed that binds to c-mpl at a location distant from the TPO binding area and may prevent receptor internalization after TPO binding, thereby increasing TPO action. However, after showing no effect in a phase 1 trial, development of this molecule has been suspended.

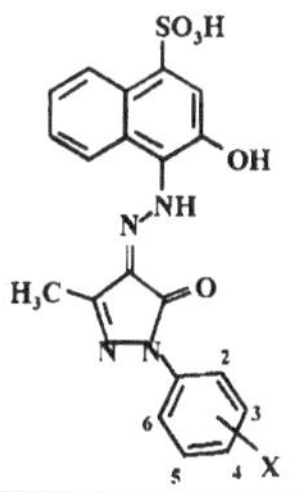	X	Luciferase		Proliferation		Differentiation	
		Efficacy (%TPO)	EC_{50} (μM)	Efficacy (%TPO)	EC_{50} (μM)	Efficacy (%TPO)	EC_{50} (μM)
25b	**3-Cl**	**34**	**2**	**45**	**0.5**	-	-
25c	**4-Cl**	**47**	**2**	**75**	**0.5**	-	-
25i	**4-CH_3**	**53**	**2**	**90**	**.05**	-	-
25j	**3-CF_3**	**62**	**0.04**	**120**	**0.07**	**95**	**0.1**
25k	**4-CF_3**	**39**	**0.1**	**100**	**0.05**	-	-
25m	**4-I**	**81**	**0.3**	**100**	**0.1**	**60**	**0.02**
25o	**3,4-diCl**	**67**	**0.2**	**70**	**0.05**	-	-
25p	**3,4-diCH_3**	**100**	**0.04**	**90**	**0.04**	**100**	**0.2**
25s	**4-$C(CH_3)_3$**	**86**	**0.02**	**100**	**0.001**	**100**	**0.03**

Fig. 8. Structure-function analysis of nonpeptide thrombopoietin mimetics. Various pyrazol-4-ylidenehydrazines were prepared as indicated (X) and tested for their efficacy vs recombinant thrombopoietin in several assays. The luciferase assay measures the extent of luciferase expression in a TPO-responsive cell line in which luciferase expression is driven by a STAT-responsive promoter. The proliferation assay measures the extent of growth of a TPO-dependent cell line (UT7/TPO). The differentiation assay measures the amount of CD41 cell expression when human bone marrow CD34+ cells are grown for 10 d. (Reproduced with permission from ref. *79.*)

6. EFFECT OF RECOMBINANT THROMBOPOIETIN IN DISEASE MODELS IN ANIMALS

The recombinant TPOs (rHuTPO and PEG-rHuMGDF) have undergone extensive testing in animal models of overexpression, chemotherapy, radiation therapy, radioprotection, bone marrow transplantation, stem cell expansion, HIV infection, and surgery. With only one exception, the results of these animal models have predicted the outcome of similar studies in humans. Only the enhanced white and red blood cell recovery seen in murine chemotherapy studies has never been seen in similar human chemotherapy trials.

6.1. Overexpression in Animal Models

Overexpression of TPO has been studied in three models. Mice in which TPO was overexpressed after transplantation of bone marrow cells transfected with MGDF had a more rapid platelet reconstitution than did control mice. Platelet counts increased four- to eightfold and remained increased. Mice had increased numbers of bone marrow and spleen megakaryocytes but ultimately developed marrow fibrosis, extramedullary hematopoiesis, hepatosplenomegaly, osteosclerosis, and anemia *(83,84).*

In a second model, murine bone marrow cells were transfected to a much higher degree with TPO cDNA and transplanted into mice. Whereas amounts of circulating

TPO barely remained detectable in the preceding experiment, amounts of TPO were persistently high in these mice during the entire course of the experiment. Early after transplantation, platelet and white blood cell counts increased, and hematocrits decreased. Megakaryocytes and granulocytes and their respective progenitor cells were markedly increased in the spleen, but erythroblasts and their precursor cells were decreased in the marrow. Later, the number of progenitor cells in the spleen decreased, extramedullary hematopoiesis was seen, the marrow and spleen developed marked fibrosis, and the bones developed osteosclerosis. The mice had reduced survival, and some developed leukemia *(85)*.

In a third model, normal mice and syngeneic mice with variable degrees of immune dysfunction (nude, SCID, NOD/SCID) were infected with adenovectors carrying human TPO cDNA. All mice had an increase in platelet count, but the increase was much higher in the SCID (T- and B-cell defect, minimal Ab response) and NOD/SCID (T- and B-cell defect, minimal Ab response, mononuclear phagocytes diminished in number and function) mice than in BALB/c (control) or nude mice (T-cell defect, impaired Ab production). The platelet count increase was proportional to the concentration of circulating TPO. The control mice subsequently developed Abs to human TPO that crossreacted with murine TPO, and the mice became thrombocytopenic. The SCID and NOD/SCID continued to express high concentration of TPO and did not develop Abs. They both developed hypercellular bone marrows; however, only the SCID mice developed osteosclerosis, myelofibrosis, and extramedullary hematopoiesis *(86)*.

These results suggest that chronic overexpression of low amounts of TPO in normal animals leads to thrombocytosis, marrow fibrosis, and osteosclerosis that mimics the human disorder of agnogenic myelofibrosis with myeloid metaplasia. With higher chronic expression, such changes may evolve into more significant fibrosis and possibly leukemic transformation. The fibrosis is not entirely mediated by TPO or the increased megakaryocyte mass but requires concomitant functional monocytes and/or macrophages.

6.2. Chemotherapy

When mice were treated with a combination of carboplatin and irradiation, they developed a life-threatening thrombocytopenia that resulted in the death of 95% of the animals. When the animals were treated instead with MGDF daily after the cytotoxic therapy, mortality was reduced to 15% and the animals experienced a reduction in the depth and duration of thrombocytopenia. In addition, the severity and duration of leukopenia and anemia were reduced *(19)*. In most similar animal models, the administration of recombinant TPO also reduced the depth and duration of thrombocytopenia and demonstrated multilineage recovery *(41,87,88)*, as suggested by in vitro data showing that TPO stimulates the growth of progenitor cells of most lineages.

6.3. Radiation Therapy

Nonhuman primates were treated with 700 cGy, ^{60}Co gamma, total body irradiation (TBI) and then daily with PEG-rHuMGDF, MGDF, rHuG-CSF, a combination of PEG-rHuMGDF and rHuG-CSF, or placebo. Treatment with MGDF, PEG-rHuMGDF, or PEG-rHuMGDF plus rHuG-CSF significantly decreased the duration of thrombocytopenia (platelet count $< 20 \times 10^9$/L for 0.25, 0, or 0.5 d, respectively) and the severity of the platelet nadir (28, 43, and 30 × 10^9/L, respectively) compared with the controls (12.2-d duration; nadir, 4 × 10^9/L) and elicited an earlier platelet recovery. Neutrophil regeneration was augmented in all cytokine protocols, and the combination of PEG-rMGDF and rHuG-CSF further decreased the duration of neutropenia compared with rHuG-CSF alone *(89)*.

6.4. Radioprotection

The potential for TPO to function as a radioprotectant is an area of special interest. In mice, administration of rHuTPO 2 h after exposure to sublethal TBI dramatically ameliorates the thrombocytopenia that is seen at d 10 in these mice *(90)*. Mice treated with rHuTPO before irradiation also have a higher platelet count nadir (739 × 10^9/L) than do mice that are untreated before irradiation (144 × 10^9/L); unirradiated control mice had a platelet count of 1123 × 10^9/L. This protective effect was enhanced when rHuTPO was administered close to TBI. Stem cells appeared to be highly sensitive to the effects of rHuTPO, possibly because it prevented apoptosis when given from 2 h before until 2 h after TBI. This very narrow window of protection underscores the importance of the timing of the administration of rHuTPO vis-à-vis irradiation. Furthermore, red and white blood cell counts appeared to be protected by the administration of rHuTPO close to the time of TBI *(90)*. These results suggest a major radioprotective effect of rHuTPO on progenitor cells in the bone marrow. This finding is in line with previous data suggesting that pluripotential stem cells are sensitive to the presence of TPO and that TPO can support their survival *(41,91)*. Similar results have been noted in subsequent studies that investigated the effect of rHuTPO in mice exposed to lethal doses of TBI *(92)*. Almost all the mice that received rHuTPO close to the time of irradiation survived, whereas all the mice that received placebo died within 30 d of receiving TBI. Furthermore, recovery of blood counts in all lineages improved in those mice that received rHuTPO within several hours of TBI.

Whether these results can be expanded to the chemotherapy setting has not been fully explored. Conceivably the antiapoptotic effects of TPO might reduce chemotherapy-induced apoptosis of pluripotential stem cells and ameliorate the pancytopenia of chemotherapy.

6.5. Bone Marrow Transplantation

In several animal models, recombinant TPO was administered after bone marrow infusion with no significant effect on the recovery of any lineage. These unexpected results led to further investigations in mice in which the donor animals were treated with recombinant TPO, and the TPO-stimulated marrow was transplanted into recipient animals (Fig. 9). This TPO-stimulated marrow transplantation reduced the duration of thrombocytopenia and allowed earlier recovery of erythrocytes *(93)*. It may be more important to use TPO to treat the stem cell donor than to treat the stem cell recipient, a conclusion also reached in human trials *(94)*.

6.6. Stem Cell Expansion Ex Vivo

Yagi and colleagues *(95)* showed that administration of TPO alone can sustain ex vivo expansion of hematopoietic stem cells in long-term bone marrow cultures (LTBMC) from mice. The continuous presence of TPO resulted in the generation of long- and short-term colony-forming cells and maintained the relative amount of high-proliferative-potential

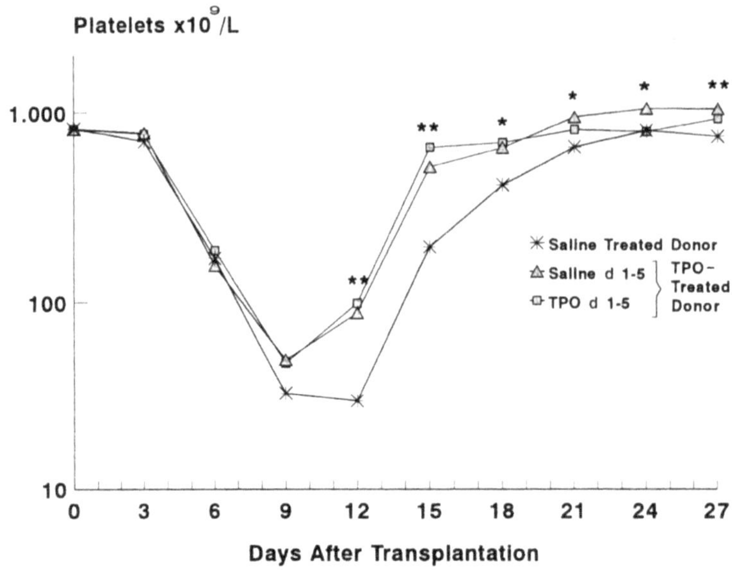

Fig. 9. Platelet recovery is improved when mice are transplanted with bone marrow from donor mice treated with thrombopoietin. Mice were transplanted with bone marrow cells from saline-treated or thrombopoietin (TPO)-treated donors. After infusion of marrow, mice were then treated with saline or TPO for 5 d. Marrow from TPO-treated mice produced earlier platelet engraftment than did marrow from untreated animals. The administration of thrombopoietin after marrow infusion was without effect. (Reproduced with permission from ref. *93*.)

colony-forming cells (HPP-CFCs). Most importantly, competitive repopulation studies found that the TPO-treated LTBMC cells were as effective as fresh marrow. Subsequent data suggest that the expanded population of stem cells, when transplanted into recipient mice, is adequate for the long-term repopulation.

6.7. HIV Infection

The thrombocytopenia of three HIV-infected nonhuman primates was rapidly reversed by infusion of PEG-rHuMGDF (Fig. 10) *(96)*. In these animals, the expanded megakaryocyte mass was presumably not producing adequate amounts of platelets owing to premature megakaryocyte apoptosis. Addition of TPO was felt to prevent premature megakaryocyte apoptosis and stimulate effective platelet production.

6.8. Surgical Thrombocytopenia

Approximately 40% of all platelet transfusions are used in surgical settings *(97)*. Preoperative and postoperative thrombocytopenia complicates surgical procedures and mandates platelet transfusions. Although no clinical studies have targeted this important area, one animal model is of interest. The administration of PEG-rHuMGDF to dogs 4 d before surgery decreased thrombocytopenia after cardiopulmonary bypass *(98)*. Despite its 5-d lag time before platelet increase, judicial administration of TPO before surgery may ameliorate preoperative and postoperative thrombocytopenia and reduce the need for platelet transfusions.

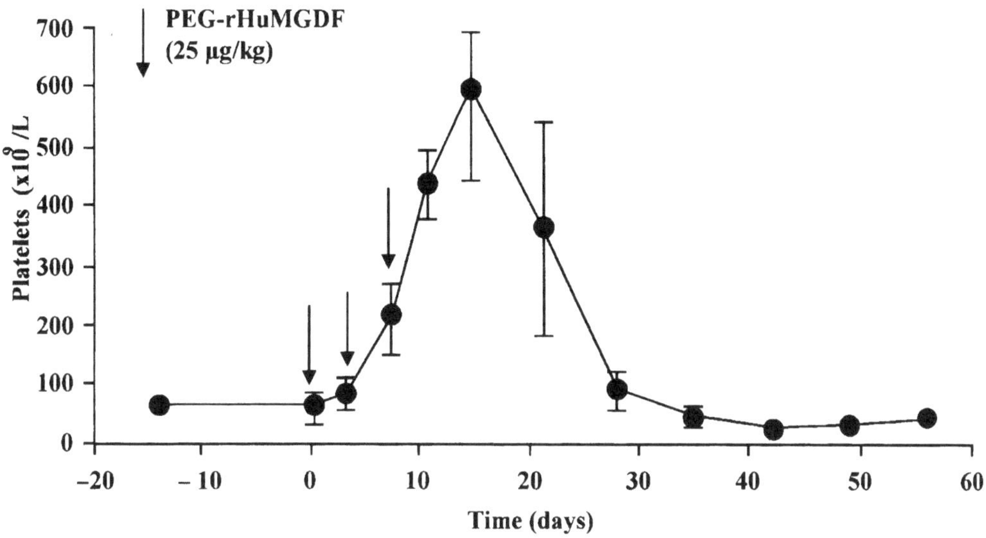

Fig. 10. Pegylated recombinant human megakaryocyte growth and development factor (PEG-rHuMGDF) increases the platelet count in HIV-infected baboons. Three thrombocytopenic, HIV-infected baboons were treated with three doses of PEG-rHuMGDF (arrows), and the platelet count was measured. (Reproduced with permission from ref. *96.*)

7. EFFECT OF RECOMBINANT THROMBOPOIETINS IN HEALTHY HUMANS AND CANCER PATIENTS BEFORE CHEMOTHERAPY

7.1. Thrombopoietin Increases Platelet Count in Healthy Humans

PEG-rHuMGDF has been given to healthy volunteers *(99)* and healthy apheresis donors *(100–102).* Treatment of apheresis donors with a single dose of PEG-rHuMGDF on d 1 produces a dose-dependent increase in the platelet count that begins on d 5 and peaks after 10–12 d (Fig. 11). A clear dose-response effect is seen. Compared with placebo-treated donors who had platelet counts of 225 × 10^9/L, donors treated with 1 or 3 µg/kg of PEG-rHuMGDF had median platelet counts of 336 × 10^9/L and 599 × 10^9/L, respectively. The donors experienced no adverse effects. The platelets produced had normal platelet aggregation responses in vitro and, when transfused into thrombocytopenic recipients, produced a dose-dependent increase in platelet count *(101).*

In addition to increasing the number of megakaryocytes and platelets, TPO affects the function of platelets. When TPO binds to its platelet receptor, it induces phosphorylation of the c-mpl receptor and a number of other molecules in several signal transduction pathways *(103–105)* but does not directly cause platelet activation. Such TPO treatment reduces by 50% the threshold for activation by other platelet agonists such ADP and collagen *(51).* It is unclear whether this is a clinically relevant effect.

7.2. Thrombopoietin Increases Platelet Count in Cancer Patients Before Chemotherapy

The stimulatory effects of PEG-rHuMGDF and rHuTPO on megakaryocyte and platelet production have been suggested in several clinical trials in patients before

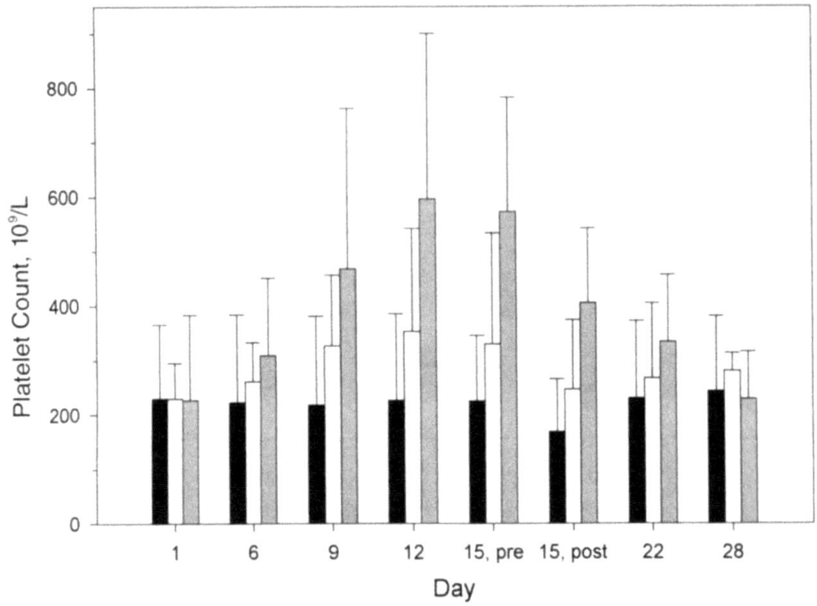

Fig. 11. PEG-rHuMGDF increases the platelet count in healthy humans. Healthy platelet apheresis donors were treated with a single dose of placebo (black bars), 1 μg/kg (white bars), or 3 μg/kg (gray bars) of PEG-rHuMGDF on d 1, and the platelet response was measured. There was no effect on the red or white cell count. (Reproduced with permission from ref. *100.*)

chemotherapy. When administered before chemotherapy as a daily subcutaneous injection, PEG-rHuMGDF produced a dose-dependent increase in peripheral blood platelet counts and a modest increase in megakaryocyte, erythroid, and myeloid progenitor cell counts in patients with advanced cancer *(106–110)*. No evidence of platelet activation or altered platelet function was observed with PEG-rHuMGDF administration *(111)*. rHuTPO has produced a dose-dependent increase in platelet counts in patients with sarcomas and gynecologic malignancies *(112–116)*. A phase 1–2 study examined the effect of rHuTPO on megakaryocyte and platelet production before chemotherapy with doxorubicin and ifosfamide in patients with sarcomas who were at high risk of developing chemotherapy-induced thrombocytopenia. When given intravenously before chemotherapy, a single dose of rHuTPO was associated with a dose-dependent increase in peripheral platelets that began on d 4 and peaked on d 12 in most patients *(113)*. This increase in platelet number was accompanied by a fourfold increase in bone marrow megakaryocytes and a marked expansion and mobilization of erythroid, myeloid, and megakaryocyte progenitor cells. A second trial investigated the clinical safety and activity of rHuTPO administered subcutaneously to previously treated patients with gynecologic malignancies before chemotherapy with carboplatin *(116)*. As observed in the previous study, administration of a single subcutaneous dose of rHuTPO before chemotherapy produced a modest dose-dependent increase in circulating platelet counts.

7.3. Thrombopoietin Promotes Mobilization of Peripheral Blood Progenitor Cells

Several pilot studies evaluated the activity of various doses and schedules of rHuTPO or PEG-rHuMGDF in combination with rHuG-CSF and chemotherapy as part of a mobilization regimen for stem cell transplantation *(94,107,117–120)*. In contrast to the peak progenitor cell numbers on d 5–7 usually obtained with rHuG-CSF alone, a peak on d 12–15 was produced by the combination of PEG-rHuMGDF and rHuGCSF. PEG-rHuMGDF produced a 250-fold increase in the number of circulating Meg-CFC, a 190-fold increase in GM-CFC, a 65-fold increase in erythroid blast-forming cells (E-BFC), and a 24-fold increase in CD34+ cells compared with patients receiving only chemotherapy and rHuG-CSF *(107)*. However, since a full pharmacodynamic response profile to PEG-rHuMGDF was not done in this study, the exact day of peak stem cell mobilization was not determined. In a separate study, the addition of rHuTPO to rHuG-CSF for chemotherapy mobilization regimens substantially increased $CD34^+$ yields. Treatment with rHuTPO in various doses and schedules reduced the number of aphereses needed to reach a target graft (i.e., $CD34^+ > 5 \times 10^6$/kg) and, compared with placebo treatment, increased the percentage of patients reaching a target graft (from 46% in the placebo group to 79% in the rHuTPO group), as well as the percentage of patients reaching the minimum target graft (i.e., $CD34^+ > 2 \times 10^6$/kg; from 75% in the placebo group to 94% in the rHuTPO group).

7.4. Thrombopoietin Helps Expand Primitive Stem Cells Ex Vivo

The role of TPO in the expansion and prolonged survival of primitive stem cells derived from bone marrow or umbilical cord blood has been the focus of several investigations. In one study, Piacibello and colleagues *(121)* showed that the use of HGF could expand human cord blood $CD34^+$ cells ex vivo by many million-fold in total number; the $CD34^+$ component and the lineage-specific progenitors increased proportionately. Although TPO alone and Flt-3 ligand alone were insufficient in stimulating sustained growth, a combination of the two growth factors accounted for this rapid increase in cell number during 24 wk in culture. However, whether the expanded cell population can be used clinically for transplantation has not been demonstrated.

8. ADVERSE EFFECTS OF RECOMBINANT THROMBOPOIETINS IN HUMAN TRIALS

8.1. Antibody Formation

Administration of multiple doses of PEG-rHuMGDF to some patients with cancer and healthy volunteers was associated with an abrogation of its pharmacologic effect as a result of the development of neutralizing Abs *(72,122–124)*. These Abs neutralized both the recombinant and endogenous TPO, causing thrombocytopenia. Thrombocytopenia occurred in 4/665 cancer/stem cell transplantation/leukemia patients given multiple doses and in 2/210 (1.2%) healthy volunteers who received two doses and in 11/124 (8.9%) healthy volunteers given three doses of PEG-rHuMGDF *(72,123)*. No subject developed neutralizing Abs or thrombocytopenia after a single injection. Evaluation of these thrombocytopenic subjects showed that the thrombocytopenia was caused by the formation of an IgG Ab to PEG-rHuMGDF that crossreacted with endogenous TPO and neutralized its biologic activity *(72,123,124)*. Because endogenous TPO is produced in a constitutive fashion by the liver, thrombocytopenia ensues. In two patients, thrombocytopenia was associated with anemia and neutropenia, suggesting an effect on a stem cell population *(72,124)*. PEG-rHuMGDF was withdrawn from clinical trials in the United States in September 1998 because of this adverse effect *(125)*.

A possible explanation for the immunogenicity of PEG-rHuMGDF administration may be that this molecule is truncated, nonglycosylated, and pegylated, in contrast to the full-length, glycosylated rHuTPO molecule (Table 2). In addition, PEG-rHuMGDF has usually been administered subcutaneously, whereas full-length native rHuTPO has been injected intravenously. Because TPO is a potent mobilizer of dendritic cells, injection of any form of TPO subcutaneously might enhance its immunogenicity. Support for this latter hypothesis comes from experiments in which PEG-ratMGDF was injected into rats once monthly for 3 mo by either a subcutaneous or intravenous route. Most animals treated subcutaneously developed neutralizing Abs and thrombocytopenia but not those treated intravenously *(126)*.

To date, the development of neutralizing Abs in patients treated with intravenous rHuTPO has not been reported, although one non-neutralizing Ab was found after subcutaneous injection of rHuTPO *(113,116)*.

8.2. Stimulation of Thrombocytosis and Thrombosis

In none of the closely followed animal or human studies with TPO has there been any evidence for increased thrombotic events, but three potentially prothrombotic attributes of TPO deserve attention. These molecules are extremely potent growth factors and can markedly increase the platelet count in a short period. The deposition of platelets in an extravascular shunt in baboons is directly related to the platelet count after PEG-rHuMGDF administration *(50,51)*. Since the extravascular shunt mimics an ulcerated atheroma in humans, these results show that except for its ability to increase the platelet count, PEG-rHuMGDF does not synergize with or exacerbate platelet deposition. Nonetheless, increasing the platelet count in individuals with active arterial thrombotic disease may exacerbate the cardiovascular disease.

When PEG-rHuMGDF or rHuTPO are added directly to platelets, they decrease by approximately 50% the threshold for activation by various agonists (ADP, collagen) in platelet aggregometry experiments *(50,51)*. This finding may not be clinically relevant since other HGFs do the same and have not been associated with thrombosis.

The production of young platelets is stimulated ("platelet tide"), and these peak in the circulation 4–5 d after administration of PEG-rHuMGDF to normal baboons or humans *(50,51)*. These younger platelets have a lower threshold for agonists and are more active in platelet aggregation experiments, but clinically these effects have not resulted in increased thrombosis in either animals or humans.

8.3. Stimulation of Tumor Growth

Since many hematopoietic malignancies express the TPO receptor c-mpl *(127)*, caution must be exercised in using TPO in this patient population. In acute leukemia studies, administration of PEG-rHuMGDF did not accelerate leukemia growth or increase the relapse rate *(128,129)*. The likelihood is small that TPO will stimulate nonhematopoietic tumor growth since c-mpl has not been detected on solid tumors *(130)*.

8.4. Bone Marrow Fibrosis

In several preclinical models, TPO was overexpressed in mice by retroviral or adenoviral vectors. Most of these mice developed extensive marrow fibrosis akin to that seen in agnogenic myelofibrosis with myeloid metaplasia *(84–86)*. This fibrosis is probably secondary to the high local bone marrow concentrations of TPO or other factors *(86)* in this murine model, as it has not been seen in nonhuman primates after prolonged administration or in humans receiving rHuTPO.

8.5. Interactions With Other Hematopoietic Growth Factors

In most of the studies with TPO in myeloablative and nonmyeloablative chemotherapy, patients also received myeloid growth factors. Although interactions of TPO with myeloid growth factors had been seen in one animal model *(131)*, none have been noted in any clinical study.

9. FUTURE DIRECTIONS

TPO studies have enormously expanded our understanding of platelet and megakaryocyte biology. The recombinant TPOs are highly potent stimulators of platelet production in both normal animals and humans. Preclinical studies have suggested that TPOs will reduce the thrombocytopenia associated with chemotherapy but not that from bone marrow transplantation. Benefits have also been seen in HIV-infected animals and in animals transplanted with stem cells expanded in vivo and ex vivo with TPO. Most of these preclinical animal findings have been confirmed in humans. However, no study has provided a clinically useful HGF, and no TPO has received marketing approval for human use, possibly for four major reasons. Foremost of these is the Ab formation observed with several full-length, recombinant TPOs that has stopped their development and cast a shadow on this entire class of HGFs. In addition, the platelet transfusion trigger has been continually reduced to 10×10^9/L in chemotherapy patients and made thrombocytopenia a less-pressing clinical issue *(132,133)*. Third, the pharmacology of TPO is not straightforward. Single doses on the first day after chemotherapy are as effective as daily doses for 7–10 d. Optimal regimens have not been elucidated and may differ with each indication. Finally, after the exhausting clinical development program of TPO, both industry and academia have lost enthusiasm for studies in this area.

With the first wave of TPO development completed, enthusiasm for a platelet growth factor is beginning to increase. This second wave of interest stems from exploring new TPO molecules and new indications. The TPO mimetics, especially the nonpeptide mimetics, are not antigenic but are potent stimulators of platelet production, and some may be administered orally. Although less common than in cancer chemotherapy patients, other disorders of thrombocytopenia may benefit from the administration of a TPO; these include idiopathic thrombocytopenia purpura, liver disease, myelodysplastic syndrome, surgery, and platelet apheresis donors *(67,126)*. Current studies with the second-generation TPOs may yield a clinically useful HGF.

ACKNOWLEDGMENTS

This work was supported in part by grants from the National Institutes of Health (HL54838, HL61272, and HL72299).

REFERENCES

1. Kelemen E. Thrombopoietin. *BMJ* 1970; 2:733–734.
2. Kelemen E, Cserhati I, Tanos B. Demonstration and some properties of human thrombopoietin in thrombocythaemic sera. *Acta Haematol* 1958; 20:350–355.
3. Kato T, Ogami K, Shimada Y, et al. Purification and characterization of thrombopoietin. *J Biochem* 1995; 118:229–236.
4. Kuter DJ, Beeler DL, Rosenberg RD. The purification of megapoietin: a physiological regulator of megakaryocyte growth and platelet production. *Proc Natl Acad Sci USA* 1994; 91:11104–11108.
5. Bartley TD, Bogenberger J, Hunt P, et al. Identification and cloning of a megakaryocyte growth and development factor that is a ligand for the cytokine receptor Mpl. *Cell* 1994; 77:1117–1124.
6. de Sauvage FJ, Hass PE, Spencer SD, et al. Stimulation of megakaryocytopoiesis and thrombopoiesis by the c-Mpl ligand. *Nature* 1994; 369:533–538.
7. Lok S, Kaushansky K, Holly RD, et al. Cloning and expression of murine thrombopoietin cDNA and stimulation of platelet production in vivo. *Nature* 1994; 369:565–568.
8. Hunt P, Li YS, Nichol JL, et al. Purification and biologic characterization of plasma-derived megakaryocyte growth and development factor. *Blood* 1995; 86:540–547.
9. Kuter DJ, Rosenberg RD. Appearance of a megakaryocyte growth-promoting activity, megapoietin, during acute thrombocytopenia in the rabbit. *Blood* 1994; 84:1464–1472.
10. Souyri M, Vigon I, Penciolelli JF, Heard JM, Tambourin P, Wendling F. A putative truncated cytokine receptor gene transduced by the myeloproliferative leukemia virus immortalizes hematopoietic progenitors. *Cell* 1990; 63:1137–1147.
11. Vigon I, Mornon JP, Cocault L, et al. Molecular cloning and characterization of MPL, the human homolog of the v-mpl oncogene: identification of a member of the hematopoietic growth factor receptor superfamily. *Proc Natl Acad Sci USA* 1992; 89:5640–5644.
12. Foster DC, Sprecher CA, Grant FJ, et al. Human thrombopoietin: gene structure, cDNA sequence, expression, and chromosomal localization. *Proc Natl Acad Sci USA* 1994; 91:13023–13027.
13. Hoffman RC, Andersen H, Walker K, et al. Peptide, disulfide, and glycosylation mapping of recombinant human thrombopoietin from Ser1 to Arg246. *Biochemistry* 1996; 35:14849–14861.
14. Kato T, Oda A, Inagaki Y, et al. Thrombin cleaves recombinant human thrombopoietin: one of the proteolytic events that generates truncated forms of thrombopoietin. *Proc Natl Acad Sci USA* 1997; 94:4669–4674.
15. Gurney AL, Wong SC, Henzel WJ, de Sauvage FJ. Distinct regions of c-Mpl cytoplasmic domain are coupled to the JAK-STAT signal transduction pathway and Shc phosphorylation. *Proc Natl Acad Sci USA* 1995; 92:5292–5296.
16. Gurney AL, Kuang WJ, Xie MH, Malloy BE, Eaton DL, de Sauvage FJ. Genomic structure, chromosomal localization, and conserved alternative splice forms of thrombopoietin. *Blood* 1995; 85:981–988.
17. Deane CM, Kroemer RT, Richards WG. A structural model of the human thrombopoietin receptor complex. *J Mol Graph Model* 1997; 15:170–1788, 185–188.
18. Wada T, Nagata Y, Nagahisa H, et al. Characterization of the truncated thrombopoietin variants. *Biochem Biophys Res Commun* 1995; 213:1091–1098.
19. Hokom MM, Lacey D, Kinstler OB, et al. Pegylated megakaryocyte growth and development factor abrogates the lethal thrombocytopenia associated with carboplatin and irradiation in mice. *Blood* 1995; 86:4486–4492.
20. Foster D, Hunt P. The biological significance of truncated and full-length forms of Mpl ligand. In: Kuter DJ, Hunt P, Sheridan W, Zucker-Franklin D, eds., *Thrombopoiesis and Thrombopoietins: Molecular, Cellular, Preclinical, and Clinical Biology.* Totowa, NJ: Humana. 1997:203–214.
21. Spivack JL, Hogans BB. The in vivo metabolism of recombinant human erythropoietin in the rat. *Blood* 1989; 73:90–99.
22. Foster D, Lok S. Biological roles for the second domain of thrombopoietin. *Stem Cells* 1996; 14:102–107.
23. Park H, Park SS, Jin EH, et al. Identification of functionally important residues of human thrombopoietin. *J Biol Chem* 1998; 273:256–261.
24. Pearce KH Jr, Potts BJ, Presta LG, Bald LN, Fendly BM, Wells JA. Mutational analysis of thrombopoietin for identification of receptor and neutralizing antibody sites. *J Biol Chem* 1997; 272:20595–20602.

25. Nomura S, Ogami K, Kawamura K, et al. Cellular localization of thrombopoietin mRNA in the liver by in situ hybridization. *Exp Hematol* 1997; 25:565–572.
26. Lok S, Foster DC. The structure, biology and potential therapeutic applications of recombinant thrombopoietin. *Stem Cells* 1994; 12:586–598.
27. Guerriero A, Worford L, Holland HK, Guo GR, Sheehan K, Waller EK. Thrombopoietin is synthesized by bone marrow stromal cells. *Blood* 1997; 90:3444–3455.
28. McCarty JM, Sprugel KH, Fox NE, Sabath DE, Kaushansky K. Murine thrombopoietin mRNA levels are modulated by platelet count. *Blood* 1995; 86:3668–3675.
29. Sungaran R, Markovic B, Chong BH. Localization and regulation of thrombopoietin mRNa expression in human kidney, liver, bone marrow, and spleen using in situ hybridization. *Blood* 1997; 89:101–107.
30. Schnittger S, de Sauvage FJ, Le Paslier D, Fonatsch C. Refined chromosomal localization of the human thrombopoietin gene to 3q27-q28 and exclusion as the responsible gene for thrombocytosis in patients with rearrangements of 3q21 and 3q26. *Leukemia* 1996; 10:1891–1906.
31. Chang MS, Hsu RY, McNinch J, Copeland NG, Jenkins NA. The gene for murine megakaryocyte growth and development factor (thrombopoietin, TPO) is located on mouse chromosome 16. *Genomics* 1995; 26:636–637.
32. Chang MS, McNinch J, Basu R, et al. Cloning and characterization of the human megakaryocyte growth and development factor (MGDF) gene. *J Biol Chem* 1995; 270:511–514.
33. Ghilardi N, Wiestner A, Skoda RC. Thrombopoietin production is inhibited by a translational mechanism. *Blood* 1998; 92:4023–4030.
34. Wiestner A, Schlemper RJ, van der Maas AP, Skoda RC. An activating splice donor mutation in the thrombopoietin gene causes hereditary thrombocythaemia. *Nat Genet* 1998; 18:49–52.
35. Kondo T, Okabe M, Sanada M, et al. Familial essential thrombocythemia associated with one-base deletion in the 5′-untranslated region of the thrombopoietin gene. *Blood* 1998; 92:1091–1096.
36. Li J, Xia Y, Kuter DJ. The platelet thrombopoietin receptor number and function are markedly decreased in patients with essential thrombocythaemia. *Br J Haematol* 2000; 111:943–953.
37. Zauli G, Vitale M, Falcieri E, et al. In vitro senescence and apoptotic cell death of human megakaryocytes. *Blood* 1997; 90:2234–2243.
38. Raslova H, Roy L, Vourc'h C, et al. Megakaryocyte polyploidization is associated with a functional gene amplification. *Blood* 2003; 101:541–544.
39. Choi ES, Hokom M, Bartley T, et al. Recombinant human megakaryocyte growth and development factor (rHuMGDF), a ligand for c-Mpl, produces functional human platelets in vitro. *Stem Cells* 1995; 13:317.
40. Choi ES, Hokom MM, Chen JL, et al. The role of megakaryocyte growth and development factor in terminal stages of thrombopoiesis. *Br J Haematol* 1996; 95:227–233.
41. Kaushansky K, Lin N, Grossmann A, Humes J, Sprugel KH, Broudy VC. Thrombopoietin expands erythroid, granulocyte-macrophage, and megakaryocytic progenitor cells in normal and myelosuppressed mice. *Exp Hematol* 1996; 24:265–269.
42. Solar GP, Kerr WG, Zeigler FC, et al. Role of c-mpl in early hematopoiesis. *Blood* 1998; 92:4–10.
43. Ihara K, Ishii E, Eguchi M, et al. Identification of mutations in the c-mpl gene in congenital amegakaryocytic thrombocytopenia. *Proc Natl Acad Sci USA* 1999; 96:3132–3136.
44. Van Den Oudenrijn S, Bruin M, Folman CC, et al. Mutations in the thrombopoietin receptor, mpl, in children with congenital amegakaryocytic thrombocytopenia. *Br J Haematol* 2000; 110:441–448.
45. Kuter DJ, Rosenberg RD. The reciprocal relationship of thrombopoietin (c-Mpl ligand) to changes in the platelet mass during busulfan-induced thrombocytopenia in the rabbit. *Blood* 1995; 85:2720–2730.
46. Li J, Xia Y, Kuter D. Interaction of thrombopoietin with the platelet c-mpl receptor in plasma: binding, internalization, stability and pharmacodynamics. *Br J Haematol* 1999; 106:345–356.
47. Fielder PJ, Hass P, Nagel M, et al. Human platelets as a model for the binding and degradation of thrombopoietin. *Blood* 1997; 89:2782–2788.
48. Fielder PJ, Gurney AL, Stefanich E, et al. Regulation of thrombopoietin levels by c-mpl-mediated binding to platelets. *Blood* 1996; 87:2154–2161.
49. Li J, Xia Y, Kuter DJ. Interaction of thrombopoietin with the platelet c-mpl receptor in plasma: binding, internalization, stability and pharmacokinetics. *Br J Haematol* 1999; 106:345–56.
50. Harker LA, Hunt P, Marzec UM, et al. Regulation of platelet production and function by megakaryocyte growth and development factor in nonhuman primates. *Blood* 1996; 87:1833–1844.

51. Harker LA, Marzec UM, Hunt P, et al. Dose-response effects of pegylated human megakaryocyte growth and development factor on platelet production and function in nonhuman primates. *Blood* 1996; 88:511–521.
52. Peng J, Friese P, Wolf RF, et al. Relative reactivity of platelets from thrombopoietin- and interleukin-6-treated dogs. *Blood* 1996; 87:4158–4163.
53. Kroner C, Eybrechts K, Akkerman JW. Dual regulation of platelet protein kinase B. *J Biol Chem* 2000; 275:27790–27798.
54. Snyder E, Perrotta P, Rinder H, Baril L, Nichol J, Gilligan D. Effect of recombinant human megakaryocyte growth and development factor coupled with polyethylene glycol on the platelet storage lesion. *Transfusion* 1999; 39:258–264.
55. Xia Y, Li J, Bertino A, Kuter DJ. Thrombopoietin and the TPO receptor during platelet storage. *Transfusion* 2000; 40:976–987.
56. Alexander WS, Roberts AW, Nicola NA, Li R, Metcalf D. Deficiencies in progenitor cells of multiple hematopoietic lineages and defective megakaryocytopoiesis in mice lacking the thrombopoietic receptor c-Mpl. *Blood* 1996; 87:2162–2170.
57. de Sauvage FJ, Villeval JL, Shivdasani RA. Regulation of megakaryocytopoiesis and platelet production: lessons from animal models. *J Lab Clin Med* 1998; 131:496–501.
58. de Sauvage FJ, Carver-Moore K, Luoh SM, et al. Physiological regulation of early and late stages of megakaryocytopoiesis by thrombopoietin. *J Exp Med* 1996; 183:651–656.
59. Gurney AL, Carver-Moore K, de Sauvage FJ, Moore MW. Thrombocytopenia in c-mpl-deficient mice. *Science* 1994; 265:1445–1447.
60. Carver-Moore K, Broxmeyer HE, Luoh SM, et al. Low levels of erythroid and myeloid progenitors in thrombopoietin- and c-mpl-deficient mice. *Blood* 1996; 88:803–808.
61. Kuter DJ. Thrombopoietin: biology, clinical applications, role in the donor setting. *J Clin Apheresis* 1996; 11:149–159.
62. Kuter DJ. The physiology of platelet production. *Stem Cells* 1996; 14:88–101.
63. Kuter DJ. Thrombopoietin: biology and clinical applications. *Oncologist* 1996; 1:98–106.
64. Kuter DJ. The regulation of platelet production. In: Kuter DJ, Hunt P, Sheridan W, Zucker-Franklin D, eds., *Thrombopoiesis and Thrombopoietins: Molecular, Cellular, Preclinical and Clinical Biology.* Totowa, NJ: Humana. 1997:377–395.
65. Stoffel R, Wiestner A, Skoda RC. Thrombopoietin in thrombocytopenic mice: evidence against regulation at the mRNA level and for a direct regulatory role of platelets. *Blood* 1996; 87:567–573.
66. Scheding S, Bergmann M, Shimosaka A, et al. Human plasma thrombopoietin levels are regulated by binding to platelet thrombopoietin receptors in vivo. *Transfusion* 2002; 42:321–327.
67. Kuter DJ. Whatever happened to thrombopoietin? *Transfusion* 2002; 42:279–283.
68. Siemensma NP, Bathal PS, Penington DG. The effect of massive liver resection on platelet kinetics in the rat. *J Lab Clin Med* 1975; 86:817–833.
69. Quin S, Fu F, Li W, Chen Q, de Sauvage FJ. Primary role of the liver in thrombopoietin production shown by tissue-specific knockout. *Blood* 1998; 92:2189–2191.
70. Peck-Radosavljevic M, Zacherl J, Meng YG, et al. Is inadequate thrombopoietin production a major cause of thrombocytopenia in cirrhosis of the liver? *J Hepatol* 1997; 27:127–131.
71. Peck-Radosavljevic M, Wichlas M, Zacherl J, et al. Thrombopoietin induces rapid resolution of thrombocytopenia after orthotopic liver transplantation through increased platelet production. *Blood* 2000; 95:795–801.
72. Li J, Yang C, Xia Y, et al. Thrombocytopenia caused by the development of antibodies to thrombopoietin. *Blood* 2001; 98:3241–3248.
73. Sheridan WP, Kuter DJ. Mechanism of action and clinical trials of Mpl ligand. *Curr Opin Hematol* 1997; 4:312–316.
74. Begley CG, Basser RL. Biologic and structural differences of thrombopoietic growth factors. *Semin Hematol* 2000; 37:19–27.
75. Giri JG, Smith WG, Kahn LE, et al. Promegapoietin, a chimeric growth factor for megakaryocyte and platelet restoration. *Blood* 1997; 90:580a.
76. Cwirla SE, Balasubramanian P, Duffin DJ, et al. Peptide agonist of the thrombopoietin receptor as potent as the natural cytokine. *Science* 1997; 276:1696–1699.
77. de Serres M, Ellis B, Dillberger JE, et al. Immunogenicity of thrombopoietin mimetic peptide GW395058 in BALB/c mice and New Zealand white rabbits: evaluation of the potential for thrombopoietin neutralizing antibody production in man. *Stem Cells* 1999; 17:203–209.

78. Erickson-Miller CL, Delorme E, Tian SS, et al. Discovery and characterization of a selective, non-peptidyl thrombopoietin receptor agonist. *Blood* 2000; 96:675a.
79. Duffy KJ, Darcy MG, Delorme E, et al. Hydrazinonaphthalene and azonaphthalene thrombopoietin mimics are nonpeptidyl promoters of megakaryocytopoiesis. *J Med Chem* 2001; 44:3730–3745.
80. Duffy KJ, Price AT, Delorme E, et al. Identification of a pharmacophore for thrombopoietic activity of small, non-peptidyl molecules. 2. Rational design of naphtho[1,2-d]imidazole thrombopoietin mimics. *J Med Chem* 2002; 45:3576–3578.
81. Duffy KJ, Shaw AN, Delorme E, et al. Identification of a pharmacophore for thrombopoietic activity of small, non-peptidyl molecules. 1. Discovery and optimization of salicylaldehyde thiosemicarbazone thrombopoietin mimics. *J Med Chem* 2002; 45:3573–3575.
82. Naranda T, Wong K, Kaufman RI, Goldstein A, Olsson L. Activation of erythropoietin receptor in the absence of hormone by a peptide that binds to a domain different from the hormone binding site. *Proc Natl Acad Sci USA* 1999; 96:7569–7574.
83. Yan XQ, Lacey D, Hill D, et al. A model of myelofibrosis and osteosclerosis in mice induced by overexpressing thrombopoietin (mpl ligand): reversal of disease by bone marrow transplantation. *Blood* 1996; 88:402–409.
84. Yan XQ, Lacey D, Fletcher F, et al. Chronic exposure to retroviral vector encoded MGDF (mpl-ligand) induces lineage-specific growth and differentiation of megakaryocytes in mice. *Blood* 1995; 86:4025–4033.
85. Villeval JL, Cohen-Solal K, Tulliez M, et al. High thrombopoietin production by hematopoietic cells induces a fatal myeloproliferative syndrome in mice. *Blood* 1997; 90:4369–4383.
86. Frey BM, Rafii S, Teterson M, Eaton D, Crystal RG, Moore MA. Adenovector-mediated expression of human thrombopoietin cDNA in immune-compromised mice: insights into the pathophysiology of osteomyelofibrosis. *J Immunol* 1998; 160:691–699.
87. Ulich TR, del Castillo J, Senaldi G, et al. Systemic hematologic effects of PEG-rHuMGDF-induced megakaryocyte hyperplasia in mice. *Blood* 1996; 87:5006–15.
88. Ulich TR, del Castillo J, Yin S, et al. Megakaryocyte growth and development factor ameliorates carboplatin-induced thrombocytopenia in mice. *Blood* 1995; 86:971–976.
89. Farese AM, Hunt P, Grab LB, MacVittie TJ. Combined administration of recombinant human megakaryocyte growth and development factor and granulocyte colony-stimulating factor enhances multilineage hematopoietic reconstitution in nonhuman primates after radiation-induced marrow aplasia. *J Clin Invest* 1996; 97:2145–2151.
90. Neelis KJ, Visser TP, Dimjati W, et al. A single dose of thrombopoietin shortly after myelosuppressive total body irradiation prevents pancytopenia in mice by promoting short-term multilineage spleen-repopulating cells at the transient expense of bone marrow-repopulating cells. *Blood* 1998; 92:1586–1597.
91. Kaushansky K. Thrombopoietin: more than a lineage-specific megakaryocyte growth factor. *Stem Cells* 1997; 15:97–103.
92. Mouthon MA, Van der Meeren A, Gaugler MH, et al. Thrombopoietin promotes hematopoietic recovery and survival after high-dose whole body irradiation. *Int J Radiat Oncol Biol Phys* 1999; 43:867–875.
93. Fibbe WE, Heemskerk DP, Laterveer L, et al. Accelerated reconstitution of platelets and erythrocytes after syngeneic transplantation of bone marrow cells derived from thrombopoietin pretreated donor mice. *Blood* 1995; 86:3308–3313.
94. Somlo G, Sniecinski I, ter Veer A, et al. Recombinant human thrombopoietin in combination with granulocyte colony-stimulating factor enhances mobilization of peripheral blood progenitor cells, increases peripheral blood platelet concentration, and accelerates hematopoietic recovery following high-dose chemotherapy. *Blood* 1999; 93:2798–2806.
95. Yagi M, Ritchie KA, Sitnicka E, Storey C, Roth GJ, Bartelmez S. Sustained ex vivo expansion of hematopoietic stem cells mediated by thrombopoietin. *Proc Natl Acad Sci USA* 1999; 96:8126–8131.
96. Harker LA, Marzec UM, Novembre F, et al. Treatment of thrombocytopenia in chimpanzees infected with human immunodeficiency virus by pegylated recombinant human megakaryocyte growth and development factor. *Blood* 1998; 91:4427–4433.
97. Kuter DJ. The use of PEG-rhuMGDF in platelet apheresis. *Stem Cells* 1998; 16:231–242.
98. Nakamura M, Toombs CF, Duarte IG, et al. Recombinant human megakaryocyte growth and development factor attenuates postbypass thrombocytopenia. *Ann Thorac Surg* 1998; 66:1216–1223.

99. Tomita D, Petrarca M, Paine T, Olson K, Roskos L, Cheung E. Effect of a single dose of pegylated human recombinant megakaryocyte growth and development factor (PEG-rHuMGDF) on platelet counts: implications for platelet apheresis. *Transfusion* 1997; 37:2S.
100. Kuter DJ, Goodnough LT, Romo J, et al. Thrombopoietin therapy increases platelet yields in healthy platelet donors. *Blood* 2001; 98:1339–1345.
101. Goodnough LT, Kuter DJ, McCullough J, et al. Prophylactic platelet transfusions from healthy apheresis platelet donors undergoing treatment with thrombopoietin. *Blood* 2001; 98:1346–1351.
102. Kuter D, McCullough J, Romo JD, et al. Treatment of platelet (PLT) donors with pegylated recombinant human megakaryocyte growth and development factor (PEG-rHuMGDF) increases circulating PLT counts (CTS) and PLT apheresis yields and increases platelet increments in recipients of PLT transfusions. *Blood* 1997; 90:579a.
103. Chen J, Herceg-Harjacek L, Groopman JE, Grabarek J. Regulation of platelet activation in vitro by the c-Mpl ligand, thrombopoietin. *Blood* 1995; 86:4054–4062.
104. Kubota Y, Arai T, Tanaka T, et al. Thrombopoietin modulates platelet activation in vitro through protein-tyrosine phosphorylation. *Stem Cells* 1996; 14:439–444.
105. Montrucchio G, Brizzi MF, Calosso G, Marengo S, Pegoraro L, Camussi G. Effects of recombinant human megakaryocyte growth and development factor on platelet activation. *Blood* 1996; 87:2762–2768.
106. Fanucchi M, Glaspy J, Crawford J, et al. Effects of polyethylene glycol-conjugated recombinant human megakaryocyte growth and development factor on platelet counts after chemotherapy for lung cancer. *N Engl J Med* 1997; 336:404–409.
107. Basser RL, Rasko JE, Clarke K, et al. Randomized, blinded, placebo-controlled phase I trial of pegylated recombinant human megakaryocyte growth and development factor with filgrastim after dose-intensive chemotherapy in patients with advanced cancer. *Blood* 1997; 89:3118–3128.
108. Basser RL, Rasko JE, Clarke K, et al. Thrombopoietic effects of pegylated recombinant human megakaryocyte growth and development factor (PEG-rHuMGDF) in patients with advanced cancer. *Lancet* 1996; 348:1279–1281.
109. Basser RL, Underhill C, Davis I, et al. Enhancement of platelet recovery after myelosuppressive chemotherapy by recombinant human megakaryocyte growth and development factor in patients with advanced cancer. *J Clin Oncol* 2000; 18:2852–2861.
110. Moskowitz C, Nimer S, Gabrilove J, et al. A randomized, double blind, placebo-controlled, dose finding, efficacy and safety study of PEG-rHuMGDF (M) in non-Hodgkin's lymphoma (NHL) patients (pts) treated with ICE (ifosfamide, carboplatin and etoposide). *J Clin Oncol* 1998; 17:76a.
111. O'Malley CJ, Rasko JE, Basser RL, et al. Administration of pegylated recombinant human megakaryocyte growth and development factor to humans stimulates the production of functional platelets that show no evidence of in vivo activation. *Blood* 1996; 88:3288–3298.
112. Vadhan-Raj S, Patel S, Broxmeyer HE, et al. Phase I–II investigation of recombinant human thrombopoietin (rhTPO) in patients with sarcoma receiving high dose chemotherapy (CT) with Adriamycin (A) and ifosfamide (I). *Blood* 1996; 88:448a.
113. Vadhan-Raj S, Murray LJ, Bueso-Ramos C, et al. Stimulation of megakaryocyte and platelet production by a single dose of recombinant human thrombopoietin in patients with cancer. *Ann Intern Med* 1997; 126:673–681.
114. Vadhan-Raj S, Verschraegen C, McGarry L, et al. Recombinant human thrombopoietin (rhTPO) attenuates high-dose carboplatin (C)-induced thrombocytopenia in patients with gynecological malignancy. *Blood* 1997; 90:580a.
115. Vadhan-Raj S, Patel S, Broxmeyer H, et al. Schedule-dependent reduction in thrombocytopenia by recombinant human thrombopoietin (rhTPO) in patients with sarcoma receiving high dose chemotherapy (CT) with Adriamycin (A) and ifosfamide (I). *J Clin Oncol* 1999; 18:52A.
116. Vadhan-Raj S, Verschraegen CF, Bueso-Ramos C, et al. Recombinant human thrombopoietin attenuates carboplatin-induced severe thrombocytopenia and the need for platelet transfusions in patients with gynecologic cancer. *Ann Intern Med* 2000; 132:364–368.
117. Gajewski J, Korbling M, Donato M, et al. Recombinant human thrombopoietin (rhTPO) for mobilization of peripheral blood progenitor cells (PBPC) for autologous transplantation in breast cancer: preliminary results of a phase I trial. *Blood* 1997; 90:97A.
118. Linker C, Anderlini P, Herzig R, et al. A randomized, placebo-controlled, phase II trial of recombinant human thrombopoietin (rhTPO) in subjects undergoing high dose chemotherapy (HDC) and PBPC transplant. *Blood* 1998; 92.

119. Rasko JE, Basser RL, Boyd J, et al. Multilineage mobilization of peripheral blood progenitor cells in humans following administration of PEG-rHuMGDF. *Br J Haematol* 1997; 97:871–880.
120. Murray LJ, Luens KM, Estrada MF, et al. Thrombopoietin mobilizes CD34+ cell subsets into peripheral blood and expands multilineage progenitors in bone marrow of cancer patients with normal hematopoiesis. *Exp Hematol* 1998; 26:207–216.
121. Piacibello W, Sanavio F, Garetto L, et al. Extensive amplification and self-renewal of human primitive hematopoietic stem cells from cord blood. *Blood* 1997; 89:2644–2653.
122. Crawford J, Glaspy J, Belani C, et al. A randomized, placebo-controlled, blinded, dose scheduling trial of pegylated recombinant human megakaryocyte growth and development factor (PEG-HUMGDF) with filgrastim support in non-small cell lung cancer (NSCLC) patients treated with paclitaxel and carboplatin during multiple cycles of chemotherapy. *Proc ASCO* 1998; 17:73a.
123. Yang C, Xia Y, Li J, Kuter DJ. The appearance of anti-thrombopoietin antibody and circulating thrombopoietin-IgG complexes in a patient developing thrombocytopenia after the injection of PEG-rHuMGDF. *Blood* 1999; 94:681a.
124. Basser RL, O'Flaherty E, Green M, et al. Development of pancytopenia with neutralizing antibodies to thrombopoietin after multicycle chemotherapy supported by megakaryocyte growth and development factor. *Blood* 2002; 99:2599–2602.
125. F-D-C-Reports. In brief: Amgen Megagen. *Pink Sheet* 1998; 60:27.
126. Kuter DJ, Begley CG. Recombinant human thrombopoietin: basic biology and evaluation of clinical studies. *Blood* 2002; 100:3457–3469.
127. Vigon I, Dreyfus F, Melle J, et al. Expression of the c-mpl proto-oncogene in human hematologic malignancies. *Blood* 1993; 82:877–883.
128. Schiffer CA, Miller K, Larson RA, et al. A double-blind, placebo-controlled trial of pegylated recombinant human megakaryocyte growth and development factor as an adjunct to induction and consolidation therapy for patients with acute myeloid leukemia. *Blood* 2000; 95:2530–2535.
129. Archimbaud E, Ottmann OG, Yin JA, et al. A randomized, double-blind, placebo-controlled study with pegylated recombinant human megakaryocyte growth and development factor (PEG-rHuMGDF) as an adjunct to chemotherapy for adults with de novo acute myeloid leukemia. *Blood* 1999; 94:3694–3701.
130. Columbyova L, Loda M, Scadden DT. Thrombopoietin receptor expression in human cancer cell lines and primary tissues. *Cancer Res* 1995; 55:3509–3512.
131. Molineux G, Hartley C, McElroy P, McCrea C, Kerzic P, McNiece I. An analysis of the effects of combined treatment with rmGM-CSF and PEG- rHuMGDF in murine bone marrow transplant recipients. *Stem Cells* 1997; 15:43–49.
132. Rebulla P, Finazzi G, Marangoni F, et al. The threshold for prophylactic platelet transfusions in adults with acute myeloid leukemia. *N Engl J Med* 1997; 337:1870–1875.
133. Rebulla P. Trigger for platelet transfusion. *Vox Sang* 2000; 78:179–182.

8 Stem Cell Factor and Its Receptor, c-Kit

Keith E. Langley, PhD

CONTENTS

1. INTRODUCTION

Inbred laboratory mice with a particular constellation of traits including defective hematopoiesis, melanogenesis (pigmentation), and gametogenesis (fertility) have been studied since the 1930s *(1–3)*. The molecular basis for these traits was uncovered with the findings in the late 1980s that the mutationally altered genetic loci in these mice, i.e., the *W* (dominant white spotting) locus or the *Sl* (steel) locus, correspond to the genes for the cell surface tyrosine kinase type receptor c-kit and its cognate ligand, stem cell factor (SCF), respectively. Subsequently, the functional roles of the SCF/c-kit ligand/receptor pair have been intensively studied in vitro and in vivo. The receptor is expressed by and required for normal functioning of various cell types in the affected tissue systems (embryonic and adult); appropriate receptor-mediated responses require SCF, generally expressed by stromal cells in the various tissue systems (e.g., bone marrow stromal cells for hematopoiesis, skin keratinocytes for melanocyte stimulation, gonadal Sertoli cells for male germ cells, or

From: *Cancer Drug Discovery and Development*
Hematopoietic Growth Factors in Oncology: Basic Science and Clinical Therapeutics
Edited by: G. Morstyn, M. A. Foote, and G. J. Lieschke

granulosa cells for female germ cells). The current state of knowledge of SCF/c-kit, particularly with respect to their role in the hematopoietic system, is reviewed in this chapter. In referencing the literature, primary citations are illustrative rather than exhaustive, and prior reviews (e.g., refs. *4–8*) are cited, especially for older work.

2. *W* AND *SL* PHENOTYPES

Numerous *W* mutations, mostly spontaneous in origin, and numerous *Sl* mutations, both spontaneous and generated by irradiation, have been described in mice *(1–4,6)*. The most severe of these mutations lead to extreme anemia and *in utero* or perinatal lethality. Mice with milder manifestations may be viable through adulthood and show varying degrees of the classic defects in hematopoiesis, melanogenesis, and gametogenesis. The range of *W* and *Sl* mutant phenotypes clearly indicates that c-kit and SCF play roles in cell migration, proliferation, differentiation, and function in these various tissue systems during embryonic development and/or in derivative adult tissues.

W and *Sl* mutant animals can be deficient in the migration of melanoblasts from the neural crest during embryogenesis and in homing of the presumptive melanocytes to the (epi)dermis and hair follicles. Differentiation of melanoblasts to mature melanocytes in the epidermis can be defective. The resulting phenotypes can include lack of pigmentation in various tissues, most notably the skin and coat hairs, leading to white spotting or coat-color dilution (and a resulting silver, roan, or steel appearance) either uniformly or ventrally. In addition, pigmentation in the iris of the eye can be impaired, but the retina is generally pigmented (i.e., black-eyed phenotype).

With respect to gametogenesis and fertility, *W* and *Sl* mutant animals can be deficient in the migration of primordial germ cells from the base of the allantois to the genital ridges during embryogenesis. Viable adults can have defects in oogenesis or spermatogenesis (particularly at the spermatogonia stages) and are typically sterile.

Normal embryonic hematopoiesis in the mouse occurs in the yolk sac blood islands during d 7–11 and then in the fetal liver until about d 17. Hematopoietic activity begins in the fetal spleen about d 15 and begins in fetal bone marrow near the end of gestation, continuing throughout life in both tissues. Mature hematopoietic status in the adult animal is reach by about 8–10 wk after birth. In *W* and *Sl* mutant animals, erythropoiesis and other aspects of hematopoiesis in the embryonic yolk sac and fetal liver can be impaired. Defects in hematopoiesis after birth are described in detail in Subheading 7.1.

In addition to the phenotypic characterizations, classical transplantation and embryo fusion studies established that, in all affected tissue types, the defects in *W* mutant animals were intrinsic to the affected cells and the defects in *Sl* mutant animals affected other cells in the microenvironment upon which the *W*-expressing cells were dependent *(1–4,6)*.

The elegant genetic and functional studies of the characteristics of *W* and *Sl* mutant animals provided a remarkably rich background for further studies after the products of the loci were identified as c-kit and SCF.

3. C-*KIT* GENE AND PROTEIN

The c-*kit* gene was originally cloned as a proto-oncogene (i.e., the cellular homolog of v-*kit*, an oncogene of the Hardy-Zuckerman 4 feline sarcoma virus) and localized to mouse chromosome 5 and to the syntenic human chromosomal region, the proximal long arm of human chromosome 4 *(4–7,9,10)*. The correspondence between *c-kit* and the *W* locus was established by studies showing that *W* mutant mice have mutational alterations in the c-*kit* gene *(4–7)*.

c-Kit is a member of the type III receptor tyrosine kinase family, which includes platelet-derived growth factor (PDGF) receptor, macrophage (M) colony-stimulating factor (CSF) receptor c-fms; and Flt3, the receptor for Flt3 ligand *(11,12)*. Like other members of the type III family, the c-*kit* gene contains 21 exons *(4–8)*. The open reading frame for the human c-*kit* gene encodes 976 amino acids, including an N-terminal hydrophobic signal sequence of 23 amino acids *(4–9)*. The extracellular portion of the receptor (amino acids 24–520) includes 5 immunoglobulin (Ig)-like domains; the hydrophobic transmembrane portion comprises 23 amino acids; and the intracellular portion of 433 amino acids includes a juxtamembrane domain, a characteristic "split kinase" catalytic domain, and a hydrophilic C-terminal domain. The split kinase domain has two kinase homology regions (amino acids 575–685 and 762–915) separated by a hydrophilic kinase insert region. Only the first of the kinase homology regions is catalytically active and binds ATP. The calculated molecular weight of the polypeptide representing amino acids 24–976 is approx 110 kDa. The extracellular portion has 10 sites of potential *N*-linked glycosylation, and the mature processed cell surface c-kit glycoprotein, carrying both *N*-linked and *O*-linked carbohydrate *(13,14)*, has a molecular weight of approx 145 kDa. The amino acid sequences of the extracellular portions of human c-kit and mouse c-kit are about 74% identical, the cytoplasmic portions are about 93% identical, and the overall identity is about 83% *(9,10)*.

Naturally occurring splice variation leads to an alternate form of c-kit, lacking amino acids 510–513 (human), that generally predominates over the longer form *(4,5,7)*. Any functional distinctions between these isoforms are not understood.

c-kit and the type III receptor tyrosine kinases are evolutionarily related to the type V family (vascular endothelial growth factor [VEGF] receptors), and (less so) to the type IV family (fibroblast growth factor [FGF] receptors) *(12)*. All have cytoplasmic portions with split kinase domains. Receptors in the type V family have seven Ig-like domains in their extracellular portion, and receptors in the type IV family have three.

4. *SCF* GENE AND PROTEIN: INTERACTIONS BETWEEN SCF AND C-KIT

In 1990 three research groups simultaneously reported the cloning of cDNAs for factors that proved to be the mouse *(15,16)*, rat *(17)*, and human *(17)* homologs of the ligand for c-kit *(4,6,7)*. Each of these groups also showed that the gene for the mouse factor, like the *Sl* gene, mapped to mouse chromosome 10; that mutant *Sl* genes corresponded to structural alterations in the cloned mouse gene; that the natural and recombinant factors could bind to cell surface c-kit; and that the natural and recombinant factors had biologic activities expected of a ligand for c-kit, e.g., stimulation of mast cell proliferation and stimulation of formation of hematopoietic colonies from bone marrow progenitor cells. The gene for the human factor maps to a region of chromosome 12 that is syntenic with the region of mouse chromosome 10 where the gene is located.

The factor encoded by the *Sl* gene is variously referred to in the literature as kit ligand (KL), mast cell growth factor (MGF), steel factor, and stem cell factor (SCF; term used in this chapter). The human gene includes eight exons representing an open reading frame for a membrane-associated protein of 273 amino acids *(4)*. Exon 1 includes a large 5′ untranslated region and part of the nucleotides encoding the hydrophobic signal sequence (amino acids –1 to –25); exons 2–6 include nucleotides encoding the rest of the signal sequence plus most of the extracellular portion (the extracellular portion is amino acids 1–189); exon 7 includes nucleotides encoding a small part of the extracellular portion plus the hydrophobic transmembrane portion (the transmembrane portion is amino acids 190–221); and exon 8 includes nucleotides encoding the cytoplasmic portion (amino acids 222–248) plus nucleotides that make up at least part of a very large 3′ untranslated region *(4,17)*. The mouse *SCF* gene also encodes 273 amino acids, and the amino acid sequence of mouse SCF is about 83% identical to that of human SCF *(4–7,15–17)*.

Both mouse SCF and human SCF are initially expressed as forms of 248 or 220 amino acids, depending on alternative mRNA splicing that includes or excludes exon 6 *(4–7)*. The extracellular region encoded by exon 6 (essentially amino acids 149–176) includes a proteolysis site such that a soluble form of SCF (amino acids 1–165) can be released from the 248-amino acid precursor. SCF220 lacks the exon 6-encoded amino acids and tends to remain membrane-associated. In the mouse, it has been shown that soluble forms can be released from SCF220 through cleavage at alternative sites of proteolysis, but the cleavage is probably less efficient than for SCF248 *(18)*.

Within the small cytoplasmic portion of the membrane-associated forms of SCF, it appears that amino acids 230–232 (GluGluAsp) and amino acid 238 (Leu) target SCF to the basolateral surfaces of polarized cells such as epithelial/keratinocytes in the skin and Sertoli cells in the testis *(19,20)*.

Soluble SCF exists in solution as a noncovalently associated dimer *(21)*, at least when the concentration is sufficiently high *(22)*. Each monomer has four Cys, which form intrachain disulfide bonds (Cys4–Cys89 and Cys43–Cys138) *(4,5)*. Soluble rat, mouse, and human SCF have three to four sites of potential *N*-linked glycosylation. Natural rat soluble SCF and recombinant human soluble SCF (isolated from the conditioned medium of Chinese hamster ovary [CHO] cells transfected with the full-length human cDNA) do in fact carry both *N*-linked and *O*-linked carbohydrate *(21)*, and the sites of complete or partial attachment of *N*-linked and *O*-linked carbohydrate have been assigned *(23)*. Glycosylation of SCF is not required for biologic activity either in vitro or in vivo. The *N*-linked glycosylation, especially that at Asn65 and Asn93 (human; these sites are glycosylated in some molecules but not in others) adversely affects in vitro binding to c-kit and biologic activity *(23)*. The membrane-associated forms of SCF appear to be dimeric as well *(24)* and are biologically active *(4,6,7)*.

Amino acids 1–141 represent a functional core of the soluble SCF monomer, sufficient for dimerization of SCF, receptor binding, and biologic activity *(25)*. The X-ray crystallographic structure of human SCF1–141 has been solved at 2.2 Å resolution *(26)*. Each monomer has an up-up-down-down 4-helix bundle structure, and monomers associate in a symmetric head-to-head fashion to form the dimer.

With respect to ligands for the related receptors in the type III receptor tyrosine kinase family, crystallographic structures of PDGF and M-CSF have been known for some time *(27)*, and that for Flt3 ligand *(28)* has been solved recently. SCF, M-CSF, Flt3 ligand, and

PDGF are all dimeric; the monomers are noncovalently associated in the cases of SCF and Flt3 ligand and disulfide-linked in the cases of M-CSF and PDGF. PDGF belongs to the Cys knot family, and its structure is quite different from those of SCF, M-CSF, and Flt3 ligand. The genes for the latter three have similar intron-exon structures; the mRNAs can undergo alternative splicing to include or exclude exon 6; all can analogously exist in soluble or membrane-associated forms; and intrachain disulfide bonds are generally homologous *(4,7,27)*. Based on these similarities, it had been anticipated that, although amino acid-sequence homology/identity is minimal, the ligands would have structural homology. The structures of the three ligands are in fact three-dimensionally very similar. All have the up-up-down-down 4-helix bundle structure, and the juxtaposition and orientation of the monomers within the dimer are similar.

Thus SCF, M-CSF, and Flt3 ligand are members of the large family of four-helix bundle proteins. The 4-helix bundle family has three subtypes: short chain, with relatively short α-helices; long chain, with relatively longer α-helices such that the overall 4-helix bundle structure is more elongated; and interferon (IFN)-like *(27)*. Many family members, growth hormone being a well studied example, are ligands for receptors of the hematopoietin receptor family *(27)*. These receptors do not have intrinsic kinase activity, but dimerization is necessary for the initiation of intracellular signaling. In the growth hormone/growth hormone receptor-binding paradigm, separate regions of monomeric ligand interact with similar regions of two receptor molecules to mediate receptor dimerization *(27,28)*.

SCF, M-CSF, and Flt3 ligand are members of the short-chain four-helix bundle subtype. Moreover, they in some sense represent a subtype within the short-chain subtype because they are all dimeric, and their receptors are type III receptor tyrosine kinases rather than hematopoietin receptors. The type III receptor tyrosine kinases initiate signal transduction by dimerization and autophosphorylation *(11)*. In their case, the receptor dimerization is mediated by ligand dimers, each ligand monomer interacting symmetrically with a receptor molecule. For example, SCF clearly forms a complex with the extracellular portion of c-kit in solution comprising two monomers of SCF and two molecules of the c-kit extracellular portion *(29,30)*.

SCF interacts with the outermost three of the five extracellular Ig-like domains of c-kit, particularly the second *(5,7)*. It is uncertain whether or not the fourth Ig-like domain is required for receptor dimerization *(5,7)*. The fifth Ig-like domain (i.e., the one closest to the membrane) appears to be required for proper presentation of cell surface c-kit for binding by SCF *(31)*, although a soluble form of c-kit (human) comprising Ig-like domains 1–4 readily binds SCF and dimerizes as a result *(5,7)*. Amino acids 553–563 in the cytoplasmic juxtamembrane portion of c-kit comprise a putative amphipathic α-helix that suppresses c-kit kinase activity and autophosphorylation in the absence of SCF *(32,33)*. Mutational and other structure/function studies have allowed proposals as to which regions of SCF interact with c-kit *(26)*, but atomic details await a solution of the structure of the SCF/c-kit complex.

VEGF is a dimeric Cys knot family member ligand with structural similarities to PDGF. VEGF receptors are members of the type V receptor tyrosine kinase family. Based in part on the crystallographic structure for interacting domains of VEGF and its receptor Flt-1 *(34)*, proposals for a generalized dimeric ligand/receptor tyrosine kinase dimerization mode have been put forth that would apply to SCF/c-kit, to additional ligand/receptor pairs for which the receptors are members of the type III and type V receptor tyrosine kinase families *(26,28,34)*, and to other much less related ligand/receptor tyrosine kinase pairs as well *(34)*.

Soluble human SCF binds to cell surface c-kit with high affinity (K_d approx 20–300 p*M*), and on some cells an additional lower affinity interaction (K_d approx 10–65 n*M*) has been discerned as well *(4,5,7,8)*. Rat and mouse SCFs bind to human c-kit reasonably well, but human SCF is essentially blind toward rat and mouse c-kit.

5. MOLECULAR BASIS OF *W* AND *SL* PHENOTYPES

Numerous different *W* and *Sl* mutant mice have been studied, and many of the underlying mutations have now been characterized at the molecular level *(6)*. *W*, the first "dominant white spotting" mutant described (in the early 1900s) *(2)*, is now known to represent a null mutation affecting c-kit mRNA splicing such that the c-kit polypeptide lacks a transmembrane domain, is not expressed at the cell surface, and lacks kinase activity *(4,6)*. Homozygous animals are severely affected with respect to hematopoiesis, melanogenesis, and gametogenesis and die within a week after birth *(1,2)*. Heterozygotes have some white spotting and coat color dilution but otherwise are relatively normal, and fertile. Therefore the *W* locus is semidominant. The W^v (*W*-viable) mutation represents a Thr660 → Met change in the first kinase homology region and confers reduced kinase activity *(4,6)*. Homozygous *(*W^v/W^v*)* animals are affected almost as severely as *W/W* animals, and most die within 3 wk after birth *(1,2)*. Heterozygotes *(*W^v*/+)* are affected somewhat more so than *W/+* heterozygotes with respect to all phenotypes, i.e., this mutation is dominant negative, probably as a result of an inhibitory effect of W^v monomers dimerizing with wild-type c-kit monomers. Mice of the compound heterozygous genotype W/W^v are the most studied and most used *W* mutants; they survive for a considerable period after birth and display all the characteristic phenotypes to a considerable extent (including sterility). W/W^v mice are generated by crosses of *W/+* mice and W^v/+ mice, both being viable and fertile. A fairly accurate generalization with respect to *W* mutations is that the extent of phenotypic defects correlates with the extent to which kinase activity is diminished *(6)*. Activating c-*kit* mutations have been described (*see also* Subheading 13).

Sl was the first "steel" mutant, named and described in 1956 *(3)*. It is now known to be a null mutation, with the entire locus deleted *(4,6)*. Homozygous animals are severely affected with respect to hematopoiesis, melanogenesis, and gametogenesis and die *in utero (1,3)*. Heterozygotes *(Sl/+)* have a moderate anemia plus some white spotting and coat color dilution but otherwise are relatively normal, and fertile. Therefore the *Sl* locus, like *W*, is semidominant.

The Sl^d (*Sl*-Dickie) mutation represents an intragenic deletion in the *Sl* gene such that a polypeptide of 183 amino acids (not counting the signal sequence) is made; the first 180 amino acids correspond to wild type, and the last 3 are novel *(4,6,7)*. This gene product lacks the transmembrane and cytoplasmic domains and consequently is secretable/soluble. The basolateral cell surface targeting sequences normally present in the cytoplasmic portion of SCF are of course missing. Homozygous *(*Sl^d/Sl^d*)* animals have a moderate macrocytic anemia, lack coat color, and are sterile but can be viable for up to 1 yr *(1,3)*. Heterozygotes *(*Sl^d*/+)* are similar to *Sl/+* animals with respect to all phenotypes. Mice of the compound heterozygous genotype Sl/Sl^d are probably the most studied of *Sl* mutants; they survive for up to 1 yr after birth, with severe macrocytic anemia, lack of coat color, and severe germ cell deficiency/sterility. *Sl/Sl^d^* mice are generated by crosses of *Sl*/+ mice and *Sl^d^*/+ mice, both of which are fertile. Amounts of SCF protein in *Sl/Sl^d^* mice appear to be reduced to a much greater extent than would be expected from the gene dosage effect alone *(35,36)*.

Analysis of Sl^{17H} mutant mice suggested some importance for the cytoplasmic portion of membrane-associated SCF. The Sl^{17H} allele is missing exon 8 (which encodes most of the 35-amino acid cytoplasmic portion) with a frameshift such that the resulting polypeptide has a 27-amino acid cytoplasmic portion of unique sequence *(4,6,7)*. Homozygotes (Sl^{17H}/Sl^{17H}) are affected (relatively mildly) in the hematopoiesis, melanocyte, and germ cell lineages. Based on in vitro studies of cells transfected with Sl^{17H}, expression of SCF protein at the cell surface is at most half of normal; dimerization of the cell surface SCF is decreased; and reasonably normal amounts of soluble SCF are released *(4,6,7,19,24,37)*. The basolateral-cell-surface-targeting sequences are altered, and an endocytosis-targeting sequence (in the unique cytoplasmic portion) may contribute to the decreased cell surface expression *(19,20)*.

Homozygous Sl^{17H}/Sl^{17H} mice, in which males are sterile whereas females are fertile, also represent an example of differential mutational effects in different affected tissues—a phenomenon that is quite common among the many *W* and *Sl* mutants *(4–7)*. In the case of Sl^{17H}/Sl^{17H}, it may be that basolateral localization of SCF (on Sertoli cells and on epithelial cells) is particularly important within the cellular and tissue architecture of the testis and skin (respectively), where SCF-dependent spermatocytes and melanocytes (respectively) are developing, and less important for hematopoiesis in bone marrow and spleen or for oogenesis in the ovary *(20)*. For other mutations, the phenomenon may reflect differences between the various tissues in the functional dependence on SCF/c-kit; or alterations (e.g., in upstream regulatory sequences) that affect expression in some tissues more so than in others *(6)*.

6. EXPRESSION OF SCF AND C-KIT MRNAS

Expression of SCF and c-kit mRNAs in tissues of the mouse during embryogenesis and after birth has been thoroughly studied by *in situ* hybridization *(38–41)*. A number of important results emerged from these studies:

1. During embryogenesis, expression of the mRNAs first becomes apparent with the start of organogenesis about d 8.5, and the patterns of expression become increasingly more specialized as organogenesis proceeds. For hematopoiesis, the localization of expression of the mRNAs matches the progression of hematopoiesis through yolk sac, liver, and bone marrow. For melanogenesis and gametogenesis, c-kit mRNA expression is apparent in the migrating cells, and SCF mRNA expression is apparent in a contiguous fashion in epithelial and stromal cells along the migratory routes and at the migratory destinations. The patterns are consistent with roles for SCF/c-kit in chemotaxis-directed migration; in proliferation; and in differentiation at the migratory destinations.
2. Expression of the mRNAs during embryogenesis is apparent in many tissues that were not known to be affected in *W* or *Sl* mutant mice. These tissues include various mesenteric tissues such as heart, lung, and gastrointestinal tract, as well as the developing central nervous system (CNS). The expression in the gastrointestinal tract and in the CNS are noteworthy. Subsequent work has clearly established that SCF and c-kit are required

for normal functioning of interstitial cells of Cajal, cells that govern the autonomic rhythmicity of the gastrointestinal tract, and that the rhythmicity can in fact be defective in *W* and *Sl* mutant mice *(42)*. On the other hand, despite consistent and strikingly contiguous patterns of expression of c-kit and SCF mRNA in CNS tissues, only slight CNS-related effects have been found in *W* and *Sl* mutant mice *(43–45)*. Contiguous expression of the RNAs also is observed during gestation in extraembryonic placental tissue *(41)*.

3. *In situ* c-kit and SCF mRNA analyses were done for embryos of two c-kit mutants (W^{37}/W^{37} and W^{v}/W^{v}) having defective c-kit mRNAs and for two *Sl* mutants, one (Sl^{d}/Sl^{d}) having defective SCF mRNA, and one *(Sl/Sl)* having no SCF mRNA *(41)*. In the *W* mutant embryos, cells expressing the defective mRNA were fewer or absent during embryogenesis in the tissues classically affected by the mutations (e.g., in the embryonic hematopoietic tissues), whereas cells expressing the (normal) SCF mRNA were present in the usual locations. In the *Sl* mutant embryos, cells expressing (normal) c-kit mRNA were similarly fewer or absent in the classically affected tissues; in the Sl^{d}/Sl^{d} mutant, cells expressing the defective SCF mRNA were present in the usual locations; in the *Sl/Sl* mutant, embryonic cells expressing SCF mRNA were of course not detected. Overall, the *in situ* hybridization analyses of the mutant embryos are consistent with a requirement for cells expressing functional SCF to direct the developmental migration and maturation of cells expressing functional c-kit. In tissues that express the mRNAs but are not known to be particularly affected by *W* and *Sl* mutations, e.g., the CNS, the patterns and localization of expression of defective or normal (depending on the mutant) c-kit and SCF mRNAs were not altered in the *W* and *Sl* mutant embryos.
4. For many of the tissues discussed, contiguous expression of SCF and c-kit mRNAs continued to be apparent by *in situ* hybridization after birth and into adulthood. Such tissues include hematopoietic tissues (bone marrow and spleen), the skin and hair follicles, the gonads, the gastrointestinal tract, and the CNS.

7. SCF/C-KIT IN HEMATOPOIESIS

Hallmarks of SCF/c-kit at the cellular level in hematopoiesis are early effects in lineage maturation (e.g., self-renewal, survival, proliferation) and (often very pronounced) synergies with the many other stimulatory and lineage-associated cytokines that also act during hematopoiesis. With respect to c-kit expression, the sequence during hematopoietic maturation appears to be as follows: very primitive c-kit^{-} stem cells → less primitive c-kit^{low} progenitors → lineage committed (but still largely lin^{-}) c-kit^{high} progenitors → lineage differentiated cells that lack c-kit expression (exceptions being mast cells, which express c-kit throughout their life span, dendritic cells, intraepithelial lymphocytes [IELs], and some natural killer [NK] cells; *see* relevant subheadings below). Responsiveness to SCF reflects the patterns of c-kit expression. Evidence supporting these general concepts will be discussed for the mouse and human species.

7.1. Hematopoietic Defects in W and Sl Mutant Mice

The extensive physiologic/genetic studies with *W* and *Sl* mutant mice show the erythroid and mast cell lineages to be the most dependent on SCF/c-kit (e.g., Sl/Sl^{d} and W/W^{v}, which retain enough SCF and c-kit functionality [respectively] to survive into adulthood, have macrocytic anemias; tissue mast cells are essentially absent), but the entire stem/progenitor compartment is also dependent *(1)*. Erythroid, myeloid, and megakaryocytic bone marrow cellularity and colony-forming unit (CFU)-S_{12} and CFU-C in the bone marrow are depleted *(1,4,6,46)*. Additional, more-subtle defects in hematopoietic lineages other than erythroid and mast cell are found *(1–4,6)*. Megakaryocytes are depleted and enlarged in the bone marrow, and neutrophils are depleted in the bone marrow, although manifestations with respect to circulating platelets and white blood cells are minimal. Thus multiple lineages are affected to various extents, consistent with a primary defect at the level of the multipotent stem/progenitor cell compartment and reduced output from that compartment.

Other important hematopoietic organs can be affected in *W* and *Sl* mutant mice, including the spleen *(1,47)* and thymus *(1–3,47)*. Sl^{wehi}/Sl^{wehi} mutant mice were found to have deficiencies in fetal thymic development suggestive of defects in the thymic microenvironment—the thymus was smaller than normal, with fewer lymphoid cells than normal; and immature thymocytes have been reported to be 2.5% as frequent in the *W/W* mutant mouse thymus compared with normal *(48)*. However, Sl/Sl^d and W/W^v mutant mice have normal numbers of circulating T cells and adequate T-cell function *(47,49)*.

As a consequence of the defective hematopoiesis, *W* and *Sl* mutant mice are characteristically radiosensitive and show extreme delays in onset of hematopoietic reconstitution after irradiation *(1,4)*. Mutant mice respond poorly to other hematopoietic stresses, including hypoxia (delayed erythropoietic responses), phenylhydrazine-induced red blood cell hemolysis, and 5-fluorouracil (5-FU)-induced or antiplatelet serum-induced thrombocytopenia *(1,4,5,50)*.

7.2. c-Kit Expression by Primitive Hematopoietic Cells and Progenitors (Mouse)

Given the early hematopoietic defects in *W* mutant mice, it is not surprising that c-kit plays an ongoing role in efforts to characterize hematopoietic progenitor cells including the most primitive self-renewing hematopoietic stem cell. In the normal adult mouse, approx 5–10% of bone marrow cells express c-kit at levels detectable by flow cytometry *(46,51–53)*. Approximately 50% of these c-kit$^+$ cells express myeloid lineage markers (e.g., Mac-1, Gr-1), and 50% are negative for lineage markers (lin$^-$) *(52)*. Cells with properties expected of early hematopoietic progenitors *(54,55)*, i.e., short-term (<30 d) radioprotection (STR) when transplanted to irradiated recipients, long-term (4–6 mo) multilineage reconstitution (LTR) when transplanted to irradiated recipients, and CFU-S_{12} activity, are greatly enriched in the c-kit$^+$lin$^-$ population and depleted in the c-kit$^+$lin$^+$ population, as are lineage-committed progenitors (CFU-C). In addition, of the various criteria that have been used to identify and select stem/progenitor populations *(55)*, e.g., cell surface markers such as Sca-1 (Ly-6A/E), Thy-1.1, CD34, H2-K, CD38, quiescence (poor vital dye [Rho123] uptake), lack of cycling, resistance to 5-FU (high proliferative potential colony-forming cells [HPP-CFC]) *(56)*, small size, and low density, cells meeting these criteria are enriched in the c-kit$^+$lin$^-$ population. Immature blast cells are c-kit$^+$ based on autoradiography showing direct binding of ^{125}I-SCF *(57)*.

Conversely, among the relatively rare Thy-1.1^{low}Sca-1$^+$Lin$^-$ population of primitive cells found in the bone marrow, 78% of cells are c-kit$^+$, and the Sca-1$^+$Lin$^-$c-kit$^+$ subpopulation (<0.1% of total bone marrow cells) is LTR$^+$ whereas the Sca-1$^+$Lin$^-$c-kit$^-$ subpopulation is LTR$^-$ *(58)*.

Most recently, several reports have focused on populations of rare cells that are small, low density, quiescent, and c-kit$^-$ *(54,55,59,60)*. Such cells may be very primitive (pre-CFU-S_{12}) and may give rise to pluripotent and multipotent c-kit$^+$ progenitor cells including CFU-S_{12}. They appear to have some or all of the following phenotypic properties in addition to c-kit$^-$: Sca-1$^+$CD34$^-$H2-K$^+$CD38$^+$Lin$^-$Rho123$^{low/int}$CFU-C$^-$CFU-$S_{12}$$^-$5-FU^{resistant}Cycling^{low}STR$^-$LTR$^-$. They may be highly dormant, with a delayed engraftment phenotype such that STR support is needed after transplantation to irradiated recipients, although extremely delayed engraftment (10–12 mo) has been shown in only one study *(54)*.

Other studies are consistent with the concept that hematopoiesis can proceed to a small degree without SCF/c-kit stimulus: genetically determined absence of SCF/c-kit depresses very early hematopoiesis, but does not completely prevent it, and severely curtails expansion of progenitors *(46,61)*. In the short term, in vivo administration of blocking antibody (Ab) against c-kit (e.g., Ab ACK2) ablates myeloid and erythroid hematopoiesis in the bone marrow, but not B lymphopoiesis *(52,53)*.

Thus these reports, plus others *(50,57)* that have examined c-kit expression and function at various stages of hematopoietic lineage maturation, suggest the sequence whereby very primitive c-kit$^-$ stem cells → less primitive c-kit^{low} progenitors → lineage committed (but still largely lin$^-$) c-kit^{high} progenitors → lineage differentiated cells that lack c-kit expression. c-Kit downregulation with lineage differentiation is discussed further in Subheading 12 *(62)*.

7.3. c-Kit Expression by Primitive Hematopoietic Cells and Progenitors (Human)

Since the mid-1980s, a major criterion for identification/selection of human hematopoietic stem and progenitor cells has been cell surface expression of the CD34 marker (although it has been proposed that a small CD34$^-$ population may be more primitive and may have LTR *[63]*). Approximately 1–4% of bone marrow cells are CD34$^+$, and 0.01% of (unmobilized) peripheral blood cells are CD34$^+$. As in the mouse, c-kit has proved to be an important marker also. Approximately 1–4% of bone marrow cells, 1–4% of fetal liver cells, and 0.1% of (unmobilized) nonadherent peripheral blood cells are c-kit$^+$ *(4,5,7,8)*. In the bone marrow, most CD34$^+$ cells (approx 75%) are also c-kit$^+$, and in the peripheral blood, about 50% of CD34$^+$ cells are also c-kit$^+$. Cells with immature blast-like morphology predominate in sorted CD34$^+$c-kit$^+$ populations. As a recent example of enrichment for primitive cells, CD34$^+$CD38$^-$CD33$^-$Rho123^{low}c-kit$^+$ cord blood cells were shown to be highly enriched in long-term culture-initiating cells (LTC-ICs) and myeloid-lymphoid initiating cells (ML-ICs) *(64)*. Committed hematopoietic progenitors are clearly c-kit$^+$; in vitro, blocking Ab against c-kit inhibits the formation of CFU-C (including erythroid burst-forming units (BFU-Es), granulocyte-macrophage colony-forming units (CFU-GMs), macrophage CFUs (CFU-Ms), and mixed CFUs (CFU-Mix). In semisolid cultures *(4,65)*. As in the mouse, it has been proposed that the most primitive stem cells may be c-kit^{low} or c-kit$^{<low}$/c-kit$^-$ *(60)*, and there is evidence that very primitive hematopoietic progenitors are not totally SCF/c-kit-dependent *(66)*.

7.4. Effects of SCF on Primitive Progenitor Cells In Vitro

In liquid cultures of bone marrow-derived primitive progenitors (of varying purity), SCF alone generally does little more than maintain survival of c-kit$^+$ cells identified as primitive progenitors by the criteria referred to in Subheadings 7.2. and 7.3. *(4,5,7)*.

However, along with various combinations of other relatively early-acting cytokines (such as interleukin [IL]-3, IL-6, or granulocyte-macrophage [GM] CSF), SCF can promote the expansion of such cells. Studies include assessments of bone marrow-derived or cord blood-derived LTR *(67–70)*, CFU-S_{12} *(67)*, pre-CFC *(71)*, HPP-CFC *(72)*, blast cells *(57)*, multipotent cells *(73,74)*, LTC-IC/extended(E)-LTC-IC *(70,74)*, and cells expressing relevant cell surface markers *(67)*.

7.5. Effects of SCF on Erythroid, Myeloid, and Megakaryocytic Lineages In Vitro

In erythroid and myeloid liquid and semisolid cultures (i.e., culture conditions include erythroid and myeloid lineage-associated cytokines) of committed progenitors of varying purity from bone marrow, cord blood, fetal liver, and peripheral blood, SCF can dramatically enhance the expansion and differentiation of CFUs *(4–7)*. The culture conditions often include one or more of the other relatively early-acting cytokines as well. The progeny obtained typically reflect the later acting lineage-associated cytokines that are present. In semisolid cultures, the effects of SCF are often seen as dramatic increases in the number and size of CFU-C, probably resulting from direct synergistic action of SCF on c-kit$^+$ lineage-committed progenitors. The synergy by SCF has been demonstrated repeatedly with erythropoietin (EPO) for BFU-E; with granulocyte (G)-CSF and GM-CSF for CFU-G and CFU-GM; with M-CSF for CFU-M; with thrombopoietin/megakaryocyte growth and development factor (TPO/MGDF) for CFU-megakaryocyte (CFU-Meg); and with cytokine combinations for CFU-Mix *(4–7,51,57,71,75–78)*. That the action of SCF is largely direct has been demonstrated by studies with purified cell populations, sequential additions of cytokines *(57,75,77,79)*, limiting dilution *(76)*, single-cell plating *(69,72,77,80)*, and autoradiography using ^{125}I-SCF *(50,57,65)*.

The expression of c-kit and action of SCF during human erythroid lineage maturation in culture have been dissected in some detail *(65,76,79,81)*. Blocking Ab against c-kit inhibits BFU-E formation but does not inhibit CFU-E formation in bone marrow cultures containing EPO and SCF. c-Kit expression, and the ability of SCF to enhance the generation of BFU-E, starts to decline after approximately d 6–9 of in vitro culture, i.e., at about the time of BFU-E to CFU-E transitioning. Expression of transferrin receptor is downregulated in parallel with downregulation of c-kit expression, whereas glycophorin expression is upregulated in parallel. Observations that SCF can stimulate production of fetal hemoglobin by human erythroid cells in culture suggest effects occurring after the onset on hemoglobinization *(4,5,7,80,81)*.

The etiologies of the (relatively rare) bone marrow failure syndromes such as Diamond-Blackfan anemia (DBA), Fanconi's anemia, aplastic anemia, and myelodysplastic syndromes (MDSs) are quite heterogeneous and poorly understood, but SCF/c-kit defects have not been implicated. DBA (a congenital pure red blood cell aplasia) was initially considered a candidate for SCF and/or c-kit defects because of the erythroid specificity, but Southern blotting analyses and sequencing of cDNA from patients have revealed no alterations in these genes *(82,83)*. The hematopoietic progenitors that are present, usually at much reduced levels, in the bone marrow of patients with these disorders generally appear to express c-kit normally and can be expanded and directed toward erythroid and myeloid differentiation at least somewhat in vitro in response to SCF along with other cytokines such as EPO, IL-3, GM-CSF, and G-CSF *(82,84–87)*.

The same is true for bone marrow from patients with human immunodeficiency virus (HIV)-associated myelosuppression *(88)*.

7.6. SCF/c-Kit and Lymphopoiesis

7.6.1. T Lymphopoiesis

During mouse embryogenesis, numbers of c-kit$^+$ cells in fetal liver and in fetal thymus reach a maximum at about d 15 and then decline; stromal/epithelial cells in the fetal thymus synthesize SCF mRNA *(89)*. Thymic defects have been noted in *Sl* and *W* mutant animals (Subheading 7.1.) In c-kit$^-$/γ_c^- mice, T-lymphoid hypocellularity in the thymus is extreme, and T-cell receptor (TCR)-β chain rearrangement repertoire formation is essentially absent; this severe phenotype probably reflects a normal requirement for cooperation between c-kit signaling and IL-7 receptor signaling *(48)*. In addition, wild-type fetal liver cells can reconstitute T lymphopoiesis when transferred to immunodeficient mice (RAG-2$^-$ or RAG-2$^-$/γ_c^-), but *W/W*-mutant fetal liver cells do so only partially *(90,91)*. Taken together, these observations suggest requirements for c-kit expression in progenitor cells and for SCF expression in the microenvironment during the very early stages of thymocyte maturation in the mouse thymus. The effects of blocking Ab against c-kit, administered in in vitro thymus organ cultures, support these conclusions and suggest a role for c-kit/SCF in the transition and commitment of T-cell progenitors from bone marrow to thymus *(92,93)*.

Progression in T-cell maturation from very primitive triple-negative (CD4$^-$CD8$^-$CD3$^-$) progenitors to pro-T cells, to pre-T cells, to subsequent terminal differentiation with expression of CD4 and/or CD8 has been delineated (*TCR* gene rearrangements occur at about the pro-T cell to pre-T-cell transition). c-Kit is expressed up until the terminal differentiation stages *(5,7,48,89,92,94,95)*. SCF is contiguously expressed by thymic stromal cells (human) *(94,96)*.

Several studies of the effects of SCF on immature thymocytes and on T cells in vitro have been reported. SCF in combination with cytokines such as IL-2, IL-3, and IL-7 or with thymic stromal cells supported the growth of adult very primitive thymocytes and pro-T thymocytes (mouse *[97]* and human *[94,98]*) but not more mature thymocytes or T cells (mouse; *[92,95]*).

In vivo administration of SCF to normal mice *(99)* or baboons *(100)* over periods of several weeks leads to observable but modest (two- to fourfold) increases in the numbers of circulating lymphocytes. The numbers tend to decrease toward baseline before the end of dosing.

7.6.2. Intraepithelial Lymphocytes

A particular class of adult mouse T cells, the CD8$^-$TCR-γδ IELs found in the intestine, seem to be dependent on SCF/c-kit in adult mice. These cells mature and undergo recombinational *TCR* gene rearrangements independently of the thymus; are juxtaposed with intestinal epithelial cells in vivo; and are thought to contribute to host first-line immune protection against bacterial and viral infection in the intestinal mucosa. TCR-γδ IEL populations become greatly depleted in *W/W*^{v} and *Sl/Sl*^{d} mice, both in the small intestine and in the large intestine, in an age-dependent fashion that starts approx 6 wk after birth *(47,101)*. In parallel, the TCR-αβ IEL population proliferates extensively and undergoes alterations with respect to CD4/CD8 subset ratios, in the small intestine of *W/W*^{v} mice *(47,101)*. Thus IEL homeostasis is disrupted, particularly in the small intestine. c-Kit mRNA and cell surface c-kit protein are expressed by TCR-γδ IELs from normal mice *(47,101,102)*, c-kit protein is expressed by potential IEL precursor cells in the intestinal epithelium *(103)* and is variably expressed by TCR-αβ IEL from normal mice *(47,102)*, and SCF mRNA can be expressed by intestinal epithelial cells *(101)*. In vitro, SCF selectively induces proliferation of TCR-γδ IELs but not TCR-αβ IELs and enhances the activation (IFN-γ production and cytolytic activity) of IELs by IL-2 and anti-TCR-γδ Ab *(102,104,105)*. In vivo administration of SCF in mice can expand the IEL populations *(102)*.

7.6.3. B Lymphopoiesis

SCF/c-kit appears to play stimulatory but not obligatory roles in B lymphopoiesis, more so in the mouse system than in the human. *W/W* mutant mice are not at all deficient with respect to B-cell maturation during embryogenesis *(90)*. Fetal liver progenitor populations from *W/W* mutant mice vs wild-type mice are equally proficient in reconstituting B lymphopoiesis when transplanted to immunodeficient recipients *(89–91)*. In vivo administration of blocking Ab against c-kit to adult mice abrogates all hematopoietic lineages except the B-cell lineage, which is actually enhanced and expanded, possibly because progenitors are blocked from progressing along other lineage maturation paths *(53)*. Thus, of the hematopoietic cell lineages, B lymphopoiesis is probably the least affected by SCF/c-kit; SCF/c-kit can be stimulatory but clearly are not obligatory.

In the mouse, c-kit is heterogeneously expressed in the earlier stages of B-cell maturation, i.e., pro-B (TdT^+, $B220^-$) and pre-B ($B220^+$, $c\mu^+$, sIg^-) *(89)*. Loss of c-kit expression seems to coincide with maturation (including Ig rearrangement in the pre-B stage) and lineage restriction *(53,106)*, and mature B cells are c-kit$^-$ *(89)*. In culture, SCF, supplied exogenously or produced by cocultured stromal cells, can enhance the recruitment of pro-B cells from a primitive $Sca\text{-}1^+c\text{-}kit^+Flt3^-Lin^{-/low}$ population when present along with IL-7 and Flt3 ligand *(107)* and can greatly expand the output of maturing B cells when present along with IL-7 *(107–109)*, but its absence does not limit the progression of B-cell maturation.

7.7. Natural Killer Cells

NK cells are a subset of large granular lymphocytes that are important for the innate immune responses to viral infection and malignant transformation. NK cells express inhibitory receptors that recognize self MHC class I and thereby prevent lysis of normal cells. Virally infected cells and tumor cells that evade the MHC-restricted T-cell response by downregulating the MHC class I expression become targets for NK-mediated Ab-independent cytolytic killing *(110,111)*. In humans, NK cells derive from $CD34^+$ progenitors in the bone marrow. Mature NK cells are characteristically $CD56^+CD3^-$, tend to traffic to and concentrate in the spleen, but also represent about 10–20% of circulating lymphocytes. Approximately 90% of circulating NK cells express FcRγIII (CD16), which enables Ab-dependent cell-mediated cytotoxicity (ADCC) as an additional mechanism of target cell killing. The remaining 10% express CD56 at high density ($CD56^{bright}$); are $CD16^{-/dim}c\text{-}kit^+$; constitutively express the high-affinity ($\alpha\beta\gamma_c$-chains) and intermediate-affinity (αβ-chains) IL-2 receptors, making them particularly responsive to IL-2 *(111)*; and represent one of the first lymphocyte subsets to repopulate recipients of autologous or allogeneic bone marrow transplantation. Physiologically, IL-15 appears to be a critical cytokine for NK cell development

(111). IL-15 is stromal cell-derived. The IL-15 receptor complex on target cells shares homology and subunits with the IL-2 receptor complex; its α-chain is homologous to that of the IL-2 receptor complex, and its β- and γ_c-chains are identical to those of the IL-2 receptor complex. Importantly, the immune role of NK cells includes secretion of immunoregulatory cytokines such as IFN-γ and tumor necrosis factor (TNF)-α.

In the human system, it has been shown in vitro that SCF synergistically and extensively promotes the IL-2-mediated or IL-15-mediated generation of $CD5^+CD3^-$ cytolytic NK cells from bone marrow-derived ($CD34^+$) *(111,112)* or fetal liver-derived ($CD34^+CD38^+$) *(113)* precursors; and that SCF and Flt3 ligand can each upregulate expression of the IL-15 receptor α-subunit and the IL-2/IL-15 receptor β-subunit in bone marrow-derived $CD34^+$ cells, thereby making the cells responsive to IL-15 *(111)*. In addition, SCF synergistically enhances the low-dose, IL-2-mediated proliferation of the $CD56^{bright}CD3^-CD16^-c\text{-}kit^+$ subset of NK cells obtained from the circulation *(111)*. SCF alone maintains survival of this $CD56^{bright}$ subset in vitro, by an antiapoptotic mechanism, i.e., Bcl-2 upregulation *(111)*.

With respect to NK cell development in mice, reduced amounts of natural killing have been noted in young W/W^v mice *(114)*. In a study involving transplantation of *W/W* fetal liver cells to alymphoid ($T^-B^-NK^-$) $RAG2/\gamma_c^{-/-}$ mice, NK cell reconstitution in the bone marrow and spleen was only partial (40–50%), and the reconstituted NK cells had cytolytic activity approx 50% of normal on a per cell basis, suggesting that c-kit signaling is not absolutely required for commitment to the NK lineage but is required for normal and complete NK cell proliferation and lineage maturation *(91)*.

The ontogeny of mouse NK cells seems to parallel that in humans. In vitro, IL-7, Flt3 ligand, and (to a lesser extent) SCF enable a maturation sequence whereby $c\text{-}kit^+Sca\text{-}2^+$ Lin^- bone marrow cells acquire IL-2/IL-15 receptor expression and progress to mature NK cells ($NK1.1^+CD3^-$ in the mouse) upon exposure to IL-2 or IL-15 plus bone marrow-derived stroma *(115)*. With mature splenic NK cells in vitro, SCF has been shown to decrease apoptosis and maintain viability *(91)*. In vivo administration of SCF to normal mice for 7 d led to a 1.5–2-fold expansion of NK cellularity in the spleen and bone marrow *(116)*, and administration of SCF with low-dose IL-2 for 8 wk led to synergistic expansion of functional NK cells in the bone marrow, spleen, and peripheral blood (three- to fourfold greater than that seen with low-dose IL-2 alone) *(111)*.

7.8. Dendritic Cells

Dendritic cells are among the cells that act as sentinels for the immune system *(117,118)*. They develop from bone marrow-derived progenitors that can be identified at low amounts in the peripheral blood; they are found (also in low numbers) in many nonlymphoid tissues including skin and mucosa; and they show heterogeneity with respect to maturation, phenotypes, and function. Relatively immature dendritic cells capture antigen (Ag) at tissue sites and undergo activation that involves migration to lymph nodes as well as processing (including proteolysis) and presentation of Ags as peptide complexes with MHC class I and class II molecules to T lymphocytes along with costimulatory signals (e.g., B7.1 = CD80, and B7.2 = CD86) necessary for activation of Th1 and Th2 lymphocytes.

Dendritic cells have received much attention for possible immunotherapy and cellular therapies against infectious diseases and cancers *(117,118)*. Experimental approaches have included expansion of dendritic cells in vivo, as well as expansion ex vivo, to be given back to the patient with or without other manipulations such as prior exposure to relevant tumor Ags or retroviral transfection to introduce tumor Ags or costimulatory molecules. Ex vivo therapeutic approaches require that large numbers of functional dendritic cells be generated, and culturing has been extensively studied in mouse and human systems *(117,118)*. For both species, it appears that GM-CSF with TNF-α can preferentially induce maturation of the dendritic cell lineage from progenitors present in various starting populations *(7,117,118)*. Early-acting hematopoietic factors, including SCF and Flt3 ligand, can enhance by orders of magnitude the yields of dendritic cells, probably by expanding the progenitor populations on which GM-CSF and TNF-α act *(7,117–120)*. The starting populations in many of the in vitro culture studies have been bone marrow, fetal liver, cord blood, or peripheral blood cells enriched (directly or indirectly) for c-kit$^+$ cells. Thus, in dendritic cell maturation, SCF can again synergize with other, later acting factors.

7.9. Mast Cells and Basophils

Mast cells represent the bone marrow-derived hematopoietic lineage probably most dependent on SCF/c-kit, for maturation, survival, proliferation, and function. Mast cells develop from bone marrow progenitors that are Thy-1^{low}c-kit$^+$ in the mouse and CD34$^+$c-kit$^+$ in the human *(121,122)*. In both species, c-kit is expressed throughout the progression from progenitors to mature cells, and the progression is dependent in part on SCF *(4,5)*. Progenitor cells migrate from the bone marrow to tissue sites where maturation occurs *(121)*. Mature mast cells can persist in tissues for months to years *(123)*.

Mast cells participate both in acquired (e.g., IgE-dependent) and innate immune responses and tend to be present in tissues that interface between the organism and its environment (e.g., skin, respiratory tract, gastrointestinal tract) *(121,122)*. The IgE-dependent roles of mast cells in allergic reactions, hay fever, and asthma are well established *(121–123)*. Allergens and Ags recognize and crosslink specific IgE bound to the cell surface high-affinity IgE receptor, FcεRI, to trigger acute hypersensitivity reactions, late-phase reactions, and chronic inflammatory reactions by release of preformed mediators present in the cytoplasmic granules (biogenic amines, proteoglycans, neutral proteases, TNF-α) and *de novo* synthesized mediators (leukotrienes, prostaglandins, cytokines).

Mast cells display considerable maturational, phenotypic, and functional diversity *(121,122,124)*. Connective tissue mast cells, found in dermal and submucosal tissue layers, tend to be constitutively present and are particularly dependent on SCF/c-kit. Intraepithelial, or mucosal, mast cells are dependent on SCF/c-kit, but are also dependent on and responsive to cytokines derived from the Th2 class of T-helper lymphocytes, e.g., IL-3, IL-4, IL-9, and IL-10. Phenotypic and functional differences are complex and not fully elucidated *(122,124)*. For example, mucosal mast cells appear to vary by tissue location with respect to their expression of preformed and *de novo* synthesized mediators *(124)*.

Sl and *W* mutant mice have detectable mast cell progenitors in the bone marrow *(5)*, but typically are completely deficient in tissue mast cells *(1–3)*. Conversely, administration of SCF in vivo increases the numbers of tissue mast cells in normal mice, rats, or nonhuman primates and restores numbers in *Sl* mutant mice, but not in *W* mutant mice *(4,5,121,122,125)*. In mutant mice that survive through adulthood (e.g., W/W^v), tissue mast cells can be reconstituted by administration of (genetically compatible) mast cells cultured, in vitro to generate mast cell knock-in mice that have proved useful in studying mast cell functions in vivo *(49,121,122)*. Based on studies using such approaches, it is clear that mast cells contribute to host defense against bacteria. The mechanism is IgE-independent and appears to be mediated at least in part by TNF-α released from mast cell granules upon binding of bacterial components to surface receptors on the mast cell or upon binding of complement-opsonized bacteria to complement receptors on mast cells *(121,123,126,127)*. Mast cells may contribute to protection against bacterial infections in humans also *(128)*. In vivo administration of SCF enhances the protection against bacterial infection in normal mice and in mast cell knock-in mice, but not in *W/W^v^* mast cell-deficient mice, indicating that the enhanced protection is at least partially owing to an effect of SCF on mast cells *(121,123)*. The enhanced protection may involve increases in the numbers of tissue mast cells and/or alterations in mast cell phenotype.

A beneficial role for mast cells is evident with respect to parasite infections (nematodes, worms, helminths) in the intestine *(122)*. Blocking Abs against c-kit and SCF have been used in vivo in mice to show that SCF/c-kit contribute to development of the intestinal mastocytosis and eosinophilia normally induced by *Trichinella spiralis* (intestinal nematode), and for nematode expulsion from the gut; Th2 lymphocyte-derived cytokines are also required *(122,124)*.

In other experiments with in vivo administration of SCF in mice, local intradermal administration has been shown to cause a local inflammatory response, with swelling and morphologic evidence of mast cell degranulation *(4,5)*. It is also of note that chronic systemic administration of SCF to mice, with corresponding increases in tissue mast cells, surprisingly did not result in increased severity of an IgE-mediated anaphylactic response *(4,5)*.

A large body of in vitro studies contributes to our understanding of the importance of SCF/c-kit with respect to mast cells and provides insight into the in vivo physiology. In mouse and human systems, SCF is capable of stimulating mast cells in vitro with respect to maturation, survival, proliferation, and function. Initiation of maturation from bone marrow-derived progenitors probably has an absolute requirement for SCF, with developmental fate tending toward the connective tissue type if other factors are not present, and toward the mucosal type if other factors such as IL-3 are present *(121,122,124)*. Following leads from studies of human mast cell maturation in vitro *(124,129,130)*, mouse bone marrow cultures containing SCF, IL-6, and IL-10 have been shown to mature partially, to a point at which addition of IL-3 is necessary for further maturation toward mucosal-type mast cells *(131)*. Similarly, other prior studies of mouse mast cells in vitro have demonstrated that SCF can influence and/or promote maturation (e.g., as monitored by granule contents), survival (e.g., antiapoptotic effects), proliferation, chemotaxis, integrin-mediated adhesion to fibronectin, and activation (e.g., release of granule contents including the cytokines IL-6 and TNF-α) *(4,5,132)*. It has been possible to culture mature connective tissue-type mast cells from embryonic stem cells under conditions that include SCF with leukemia inhibitory factor (LIF), IL-3, and IL-6; these cells survive and function when adoptively transferred in vivo to mast cell-deficient *W/W^v^* mice, such that this system provides the opportunity to study effects of various mutations, including mutations that are otherwise embryonic lethal *(133)*.

SCF stimulates the proliferation and maturation of human mast cells in vitro as well, from bone marrow, peripheral blood, cord blood, and fetal liver, with enhancement by

IL-3 in some cases *(4,5)*. An important advance has been the culturing of pure populations of mature mast cells (capable of IgE-mediated activation) from cord blood mononuclear cells in the presence of SCF, IL-6, and prostaglandin E_2 *(129)*. More recently, it has been found that cord blood mononuclear cells cultured with SCF, IL-6, and IL-10 give rise to partially mature mast cells, which can then mature further in response to various Th2 cytokines, including IL-2, IL-5, and IL-9 *(130)*. Otherwise, SCF has been shown to enhance IgE-mediated activation (e.g., release of histamine, leukotriene, and prostaglandin) and chemotaxis, in primary human lung or uterus mast cells in vitro *(4,5)*.

Basophils share many of the functional (phagocytic and activational) properties of mast cells with respect to innate and acquired immunity *(122)*; however, in contrast to mast cells, mature basophils circulate in the peripheral blood, are recruited to tissue sites, are short lived (i.e., a few days), and differ somewhat with respect to mediators released upon activation. Basophils appear to express c-kit, but much less intensely than do mast cells *(4,5)*, and generally are regulated more by IL-3 than by SCF *(121,122)*. As with human mast cells, SCF has been shown to enhance IgE-mediated activation of human basophils in vitro *(4,5)*.

7.10. Ex Vivo Manipulation of Mouse and Human Hematopoietic Progenitors

7.10.1. Ex Vivo Expansion

SCF has been an important component of conditions for ex vivo expansion of hematopoietic stem/progenitor cells in liquid culture for transplantation, in mouse and human systems *(5,7,134)*. From selected human ex vivo expansion studies, SCF (with other cytokines such as IL-3, IL-6, G-CSF, EPO, and MGDF) is seen to be a critical component for expansion in suspension culture of $CD34^+$ cells from bone marrow, cord blood, or mobilized peripheral blood *(5,7,77,78,134)*. Depending on the starting population, and on the cytokine combinations used, maintenance or expansion of primitive cells ($CD34^+$, LTC-IC/E-LTC-IC, LTR^+) *(70,74)* and extensive expansion of erythroid, myeloid, and megakaryocytic progenitors and more differentiated cells occurs over periods of 1–3 wk. Some evidence indicates that hematopoietic stem/progenitor cells may have better LTR if they are not cycling *(135,136)*, and if they express CXCR4, the receptor for the chemokine stromal cell-derived factor (SDF)-1, and other integrin-type adhesins that may facilitate homing. SCF may have a potential clinical benefit in both of these respects: by returning ex vivo expanded cells to relative quiescence before transplantation *(137)* and by upregulating expression of CXCR4 *(137)*. Several groups have shown that clinical transplantation of mobilized peripheral blood progenitor cells (PBPCs) expanded ex vivo with a cocktail of cytokines that included MGDF, G-CSF, and SCF is promising in terms of short-term recovery of neutrophils *(139–141)* and platelets *(140)* after myeloablative chemotherapy; in these studies, unmanipulated PBPCs were transplanted along with the ex vivo-expanded PBPCs.

7.10.2. Gene Therapy

Retroviral DNA is unable to pass the nuclear envelope, such that at least one round of mitosis is a requirement for infection/DNA integration. SCF, typically along with other cytokines such as IL-3, IL-6, Flt3 ligand, and TPO, has been a critical component for enhancing retrovirally mediated gene transfection into primitive hematopoietic cells in developing the ex vivo portions of gene therapy protocols *(5,7,142–144)*.

Transfection is highly efficient in murine systems, but less so for nonhuman primate and human. SCF probably contributes to initiation of target cell cycling *(145–147)* and may also upregulate binding sites for amphotrophic retroviral vectors on the target cells *(148)*. In the human system, various reports have described transfection of genes including neomycin resistance, murine adenosine deaminase, glucocerebrosidase (deficient in the lysosomal storage disorder Gaucher's disease), and multidrug resistance (MDR) into LTC-IC and committed hematopoietic progenitors from human bone marrow, cord blood, and peripheral blood *(5,7,142–144)*.

7.11. Hematopoiesis-Related Effects of SCF in Animals

Some in vivo studies with SCF have been mentioned above, in Subheadings 7.6.1., 7.6.2., 7.7., and 7.9.

In general, preclinical in vivo studies with SCF have been done in mice, rats, dogs, and nonhuman primates with the species-homologous form of recombinant soluble SCF *(4,5)*. Effects seen with respect to hematopoiesis have usually been reversible upon cessation of treatment.

In *Sl/Sl^d* mice, long-term administration of SCF brought about dose-related correction of the macrocytic anemia, significant increases in white blood cell and platelet counts, and marked increase in CFU-S in the bone marrow and spleen *(4,5,7,50,67)*. In normal mice and rats administered optimal doses of SCF for 7–21 d, peripheral blood leukocytosis (mostly neutrophilia) was observed; there were tendencies toward erythroid and lymphoid hypoplasia in the marrow; mast cell hyperplasia was apparent in the marrow, spleen, and other tissues (lung, gastrointestinal tract), but IgE-dependent Ag-induced anaphylactic reactions were surprisingly decreased in SCF-treated vs control animals (Subheading 7.9.) *(4,5,99,125,149,150)*. Observations with respect to stem and progenitor cells in the bone marrow, spleen, and peripheral blood compartments are of particular interest—several studies suggest that administration of SCF affects the proliferation, trafficking, and localization of very primitive hematopoietic cells (e.g., competitive LTR units) and hematopoietic progenitor cells (e.g., CFU-S). Early on, relatively quiescent primitive cells and progenitors appear to be mobilized to the peripheral blood and traffic to the spleen, such that numbers are increased in both of these compartments, and primitive cells and progenitors in the bone marrow are stimulated to cycling and proliferation *(116,149–154)*. Thus a redistribution, with substantial increase in overall numbers, occurs. Subsequently (e.g., by d 14), numbers in the bone marrow may be greatly expanded *(155)*. That proliferative and antiapoptotic effects on primitive cells and progenitors begin early is consistent with observations that SCF administered during the day before 5-FU administration sensitizes mice to hematopoietic suppression/ablation by the 5-FU *(156,157)*.

Rodent studies of the effects of SCF in combination with other cytokines (e.g., G-CSF, GM-CSF) have in some cases been consistent with the synergies seen in vitro. Observations with respect to the marrow, spleen, and peripheral blood upon multiday co-administration of SCF and G-CSF were similar to those with administration of SCF alone except for pronounced synergistic increase in peripheral-blood neutrophils; greater-than-additive increase in peripheral-blood progenitors; and pronounced splenic extramedullary granulopoiesis, erythropoiesis, and megakaryocytopoiesis *(4,5,99)*. SCF also synergistically enhanced IL-2-mediated expansion of functional NK cells in the spleen, bone marrow, and peripheral blood of mice (Subheading 7.7.) *(111)*. Some in vivo synergy with EPO, mostly at the level of erythroid progenitors (BFU-E and CFU-E), has been described *(158)*.

In baboons, optimal doses of SCF given for 28 d caused dose-related increases in bone marrow cellularity and bone marrow hematopoietic progenitors *(4,5,7,100)*. Multilineage increases in white blood cells were pronounced. Hematocrit increased slightly, whereas platelet counts were unchanged. Numbers of peripheral blood hematopoietic progenitors (CFC and $CD34^+$ cells) increased up to 300-fold. Mast cell hyperplasia was apparent in several tissues, including lung, liver, and spleen; was reversible after discontinuation of SCF; and was not associated with obvious histologic or clinical indications of mast cell activation *(4,5,121,122)*.

The synergy observed with SCF in combination with G-CSF in increasing numbers of progenitor cells in the peripheral blood of mice *(99)* led to systematic preclinical studies, in mice, dogs, and baboons, on the ability of the SCF/G-CSF combination (compared with G-CSF alone) to mobilize PBPCs that will repopulate marrow in transplantation settings *(5,7,159,160)*. The doses of SCF used in these studies were low and produced minimal effects if used alone. When the low-dose SCF was combined with optimal doses of G-CSF, the combinations were synergistic. PBPCs mobilized by SCF plus G-CSF rescued lethally irradiated animals, leading to multilineage, complete, and long-term hematopoietic reconstitution. These studies provided support for human clinical investigations that were done subsequently *(160)* (*see* Subheading 8).

The effects of SCF have been studied when it was administered directly in animal models of hematopoietic recovery or reconstitution. In a mouse irradiation model *(161)*, and in a severe combined immunodeficiency-human (SCID–Hu) model *(162)*, SCF was protective when given just before irradiation (i.e., during the preceding 24 h). The protective mechanism appeared to involve, at least in part, SCF-induced cycling and expansion of the hematopoietic progenitor population *(5,163)*. SCF given just before 5-FU was sensitizing to 5-FU rather than protective *(156,157)*; however, when given daily starting 7 d before 5-FU, SCF was protective, probably reflecting the greater expansion of progenitors over the longer period *(152,164)*.

In a mouse model of sublethal irradiation, SCF administered after the irradiation enhanced the recovery of progenitors in the bone marrow and spleen as well as circulating white blood cells and platelets *(165)*. SCF in combination with G-CSF synergistically promoted granulocyte recovery when administered after cyclophosphamide treatment *(166)*. In a mouse model of total body irradiation followed by bone marrow transplantation, SCF given after transplantation stimulated hematopoietic recovery, primarily erythroid *(167)*.

8. CLINICAL USE

Based on preclinical studies, clinical development of SCF has been directed toward using the combination of recombinant human SCF (rHuSCF; ancestim) and rHuG-CSF (filgrastim) to increase the mobilization of PBPCs vs that obtained with rHuG-CSF alone, for harvesting and autologous transplantation after myeloablative therapy in patients with cancer. Results of these studies have been reviewed in detail *(160)*. In several cancer patient populations, two- to threefold enhancement of mobilized and harvestable PBPCs was obtained. rHuSCF (ancestim) is approved in Canada, Australia, and New Zealand for use with rHuG-SCF (with or without PBPCs-mobilizing chemotherapy) to provide a sustained increase in the PBPCs capable of engraftment, to increase the proportion of patients reaching the PBPC target, and to reduce the number of leukaphereses required to collect a target number of PBPCs. Its use has not been approved in other regions, including the United States, Europe, and Japan.

Because of the potential for mast cell activation, the use of rHuSCF is contraindicated in patients with asthma, severe allergy, or other significant IgE-mediated hypersensitivity, and patients are given premedication with H1 and H2 antihistamines and a bronchodilator. Transient injection-site wheel-and-flare reactions with associated mast cell degranulation, and occasional (<10%) melanocyte-mediated injection-site hyperpigmentation, occur. In approx 500 patients who received rHuSCF (with premedication) in clinical studies, severe but manageable systemic allergic-like reactions with cutaneous and respiratory involvement occurred at a frequency of approx 3%.

9. SIGNAL TRANSDUCTION: SCF SYNERGY

Multiple pathways and effectors have been implicated in intracellular signaling downstream from c-kit activation and phosphorylation *(168)*. These pathways/effectors include phosphatidylinositol 3 kinase (PI3K)/Akt; Janus Kinase/signal transducers and activators of transcription (JAK/STAT); Ras/Raf/mitogen-activated protein kinase (MAPK); Src-family kinases; protein kinase C (PKC); and phospholipase c-γ (PLC-γ)/inositol phosphates/diacylglycerol. Considerable progress has been made in identifying Tyr and Ser/Thr residues in the cytoplasmic portion of c-kit whose phosphorylation/dephosphorylation dictate initial intracellular molecular interactions with c-kit; integration and crosstalk between pathways, including pathways initiated by other cytokines and regulators; functional consequences of signaling through different pathways; and differences in signaling pathways and signaling consequences as a function of cell lineage and stage of maturation.

Additive and complementary intracellular signal transduction that promotes cell cycling and proliferation and inhibits apoptosis is probably the major mechanism by which the synergies of SCF with other cytokines and effectors come about *(168)*. Various studies illustrate signaling routes potentially facilitated by SCF:

1. In the MO7e human megakaryocytic leukemia cell line, SCF synergy with GM-CSF may represent enhancement of Ras-Raf-MAPK signaling that promotes cell cycling and proliferation by induction of early response genes (c-Fos, JunB, c-Myc) and induction of the cyclin-dependent kinase (Cdk) inhibitor $p21^{cip-1}$ (such that Cdk2 activity and phosphorylation of retinoblastoma protein [Rb] is increased) *(168,169)*. Similarly, in purified human erythroid progenitor cells, markedly synergistic activation of MAPK by EPO and SCF has been shown *(170)*.
2. MO7e-G cells (MO7e cells transfected with the G-CSF receptor) proliferate additively/synergistically in response to SCF and G-CSF *(171)*. The combination of SCF and G-CSF, compared with each alone, leads to enhanced proliferation associated with c-fos induction, downregulation of $p27^{kip-1}$ (Cdk inhibitor), hyperphosphorylation of Rb, phosphorylation-based hyperactivation of STAT3, and shortening of G_0/G_1 time; STAT3 may serve as a point of integration for signaling through the Ras-Raf-MAPK and PI3K/Akt pathways in these cells *(171)*.
3. In the HB60-5 murine erythroblastic cell line, which proliferates in response to SCF plus EPO in combination and differentiates in response to EPO alone, SCF appears to keep the cells in a proliferating, cycling, undifferentiated state by downregulation of $p27^{kip-1}$

and p15 (Cdk inhibitors), upregulation of Cdc25A (phosphatase that activates Cdks), and associated upregulation of c-Myc *(172)*

4. In purified human erythroid progenitor cells, SCF can inhibit apoptosis by means of PI3K activation and Akt phosphorylation *(173);* and by means of uncoupling Fas ligation from caspase activation *(174,175)* in a way that is dependent on Src-family kinase(s) *(174)* and may occur through upregulation of an inhibitor of FLICE (caspase-activating enzyme) *(175).*
5. In some cell types, SCF appears to inhibit apoptosis by means of effects on Bcl family members, e.g., phosphorylation (and inactivation) of the proapoptotic protein Bad *(176)* and upregulation of the antiapoptotic protein Bcl-2 *(111).*

SCF synergy also may occur by crosstalk with other cytokine receptors. For example, SCF by itself stimulates Ser/Thr phosphorylation of the IL-3 receptor β-subunit in a murine bone marrow-derived cell line *(168).* In the murine erythroid progenitor cell line HCD57, SCF by itself stimulates not only Tyr phosphorylation of the EPOR *(177,178),* but also physical association between c-kit and the EPO receptor *(177,179);* however, the functional consequences of these receptor interactions are not completely clear *(178,180,181).* SCF-stimulated phosphorylation of the EPO receptor has been seen with purified human erythroid progenitor cells *(170).*

SCF can influence the adhesion properties of various cell types. In hematopoietic cells, SCF can increase the avidity of the integrins very late antigen (VLA)-4 and VLA-5 for partners such as vascular cell adhesion molecule-1 (VCAM-1) and fibronectin *(5).* These adhesion molecule interactions can in turn mediate intracellular proliferative signals.

10. VARIOUS FUNCTIONAL EFFECTS OF SCF

Like most cytokines, SCF initiates a broad range of functional effects on c-kit-expressing cells *(4–8).* A number of these effects—antiapoptosis/survival, cell cycling/proliferation, differentiation/maturation, adhesion, potentiation of secretion (mast cells), chemotaxis, and motility—have been referred to in preceding sections.

10.1. Soluble vs Membrane-Associated SCF

The possibility of soluble and membrane-associated forms of SCF (*see* Subheading 4.) raised questions as to their comparative functions. The fact that Sl^d/Sl^d and Sl/Sl^d mutant mice (*see* Subheading 5.) display the classical pleiotropic *Sl* mutant defects implied that absence of membrane-associated SCF is detrimental (but the overall level of expression of functional SCF is probably much reduced in these mice as well *[35,36]*).

Furthermore, cells expressing SCF248 maintain substantial steady-state amounts of membrane-associated SCF, and, conversely, cells expressing SCF220 have higher levels of membrane-associated SCF but do release detectable amounts of soluble SCF by cleavage at an alternate extracellular site (at or near amino acids 178–181) *(4–7,18,23).* Transgenic mice expressing SCF with the primary and alternate proteolytic cleavage sites both altered have been generated; the SCF, referred to as membrane-restricted, remains primarily membrane-associated and is biologically active *(4–7).*

Several studies have suggested functional differences between soluble and membrane-associated SCF forms *(4–7).* With respect to hematopoiesis, cultures of human $CD34^+$ hematopoietic progenitors with stromal cells expressing SCF248 were better at sustaining long-term in vitro hematopoiesis than cultures with stromal cells expressing

SCF220. Stromal cells expressing membrane-restricted SCF supported the growth of the murine erythroid cell line HCD57, whereas stromal cells expressing SCF248 did not *(179)*. In vivo, membrane-restricted SCF or SCF248 were transgenically introduced into *Sl/Sl*^{d} mice; the membrane-restricted SCF was more effective in restoring total bone marrow cellularity and correcting anemia, but less effective in restoring bone marrow myeloid cellularity *(179)*. Keratinocyte-targeted transgenic expression of SCF248 in vivo produced a dermal mastocytosis phenotype, whereas expression of membrane-restricted SCF did not *(182)*.

Mechanistically, it appears that membrane-associated SCF (compared with soluble SCF) may interact with c-kit on targets cells to prolong the lifetime of c-kit at the target-cell surface and to prolong intracellular signaling in the target cells *(183)*; in the cocultures of membrane-restricted SCF stromal cells with HCD57 cells, phosphorylation of the EPO receptor was prolonged, and physical association between c-kit and the EPO receptor (as previously reported by others *[177]*) could be shown *(179)*. In an in vitro study with the murine, SCF-dependent, erythroid progenitor cell line G1E-ER2, coculture with stromal cells expressing membrane-restricted SCF or SCF220 increased proliferation and cell cycle progression (possibly by way of increased Ras-Raf-MAPK signaling) and decreased apoptosis, more so than did coculture with stromal cells expressing SCF248 *(184)*. Because membrane-associated SCF and membrane-associated c-kit can mediate cell-cell binding, it is also likely that relative levels of soluble vs membrane-associated SCF regulate the extent of cosignaling initiated by other molecular associations between the cell surfaces (i.e., juxtamembrane signaling) and influence localization, migration, and trafficking of SCF-expressing and/or c-kit-expressing cells.

12. REGULATION OF C-KIT AND SCF

The promoters of the mouse and human c-*kit* genes lack any TATA boxes or CCAAT sequences, but there are numerous sites for binding of transcription factors, including Sp-1, AP-2, Ets, Myb, SCL (tal-1), GATA-1, and MITF *(4,6,8)*. The promoter of the *SCF* gene has not been extensively characterized, but multiple transcription factor binding sites (including a TATA box and sites for Sp-1 and AP-2) have been identified for both mouse *(185)* and human *(186)*.

The alternate splicing of exon 6 to generate SCF248 vs SCF220 presents possibilities for functional regulation. In normal mice, the ratio of expression of mRNAs for SCF248 and SCF220 differs between tissues (the ratio is approx 3:1 in bone marrow), and the ratio seems to be subject to modulation within a given cell type *(4–7)*.

Soluble c-kit, i.e., the extracellular portion, is found at very high concentration in normal human serum—approx 325 ng/mL, which represents a molar excess of approx 30-fold over the concentration of soluble SCF in serum (3 ng/mL, itself relatively high compared with that for most cytokines) *(4,5,7,14)*. Soluble c-kit can bind and thereby potentially sequester soluble or membrane-associated SCF and has been shown to block SCF action when supplied exogenously in vitro *(5,7,187)*. Whether or not it has a physiologically important role of this type is not known. Several cell types (hematopoietic cells, mast cells, endothelial cells) release soluble c-kit in vitro *(5–8)*, potentially subject to stimulation through PKC *(6,8)*. The cleavage site is within the fifth Ig domain *(31)*, probably very close to the transmembrane portion. In vivo, amounts of soluble c-kit appear to be increased in clinical disorders in which the prevalence of c-kit-expressing cells is a feature, e.g., acute myeloid leukemia (AML) *(8)* and mastocytosis *(188,189)*.

c-Kit is downregulated with maturation in most hematopoietic lineages, including the erythroid. Proteolytic release of soluble c-kit may represent one means of downregulating amounts of c-kit at the cell surface. Another means is internalization upon SCF binding. SCF c-kit complexes can be internalized rapidly (<30 min) by association with clathrin *(190)*, capping, and endocytosis of the coated pits *(5)*. Internalization requires that c-kit be activated with respect to its kinase activity; in DA-1 cells (murine lymphoma cell line) transfected with c-*kit*, SCF-induced association of c-kit with clathrin was dependent on PI3K *(190)*, and in MO7e cells, the steps after clathrin association were dependent on a Src family kinase(s) *(191)*. The internalized c-kit is degraded in lysosomes or ubiquitinated and targeted for degradation by proteasomes *(5,6)*.

At the level of gene transcription, various other cytokines can lead to downmodulation of c-kit, including transforming growth factor-β (TGF-β) and TNF-α, both of which tend to be inhibitory toward hematopoiesis *(6,8)*. In the erythroid lineage, it is possible that SCL (tal-1) drives c-kit transcription at early stages *(192)* but inhibits it later as part of a pentameric complex that also contains Rb (along with E2A, Lmo-2, and Ldb1) *(193)*. Under some circumstances, Sp-1 or GATA-1 may also be components of the transcription factor complexes regulating c-kit expression *(194)*.

13. TUMORS

c-*Kit* was initially characterized on the basis of an oncogenic variant, i.e., v-*kit (10)*. As with many cytokine/growth factor receptors, numerous reports of c-kit expression on different types of tumor cells have appeared (e.g., mastocytosis, gastrointestinal stromal tumor (GIST), AML, seminoma, small-cell lung cancer [SCLC], ovarian carcinoma, breast cancer, and melanoma [*195–197*]). It is apparent that many of these tumors derive from tissues that normally express c-kit. YB5.B8, the first monoclonal Ab against c-kit (unbeknownst at the time) was raised as an antitumor-Ag Ab using AML cells as immunogen *(8)*.

For two relatively rare tumor types, mastocytoma and GIST, c-kit is highly expressed in almost all cases and is usually mutationally altered such that the c-kit kinase is constitutively activated *(32,168,189,195)*. Most adult-onset mastocytomas have the D816V mutation, an activating mutation situated near the kinase active site. Most GISTs have mutations in the cytoplasmic juxtamembrane region, representing a putative amphipathic α-helix thought to regulate c-kit kinase activity negatively. c-Kit is expressed in most cases of AML (earlier stage blasts) and seminoma, and activating mutations occur, albeit infrequently *(195)*. For these and other tumors (e.g., SCLC) expressing c-kit that is not mutationally activated, functional activation of c-kit by SCF (autocrine or paracrine) has frequently been shown in vitro, but whether or not such activation contributes to in vivo tumorgenicity remains unclear.

The recent introduction of potent small-molecule kinase inhibitors (of varying mechanisms, potencies, and specificities) into clinical testing and practice has focused attention on c-kit-expressing tumors, particularly GIST. STI571 (imatinib), a potent inhibitor of the chronic myelogenous leukemia (CML) BCR-ABL fusion protein kinase, has achieved impressive clinical results in the CML setting *(195)*. STI571 potently inhibits PDGFR kinase activity and c-kit kinase activity, and early clinical testing in the GIST setting has been promising *(195,198,199)*. At the doses used, STI571 generally does not produce side effects reflecting action on other c-kit-dependent cell types. STI571 does not inhibit c-kit activated by the D816V mutation and therefore is unlikely to be clinically effective in the mastocytoma setting. Other inhibitors may prove effective as single agents in mastocytosis. Clinical studies with inhibitors that potentially target c-kit kinase activity have been initiated in the c-kit$^+$ AML setting *(195)*. It may be that for AML and other c-kit-expressing tumors in which c-kit kinase is not mutationally activated, the contributions of the SCF/c-kit axis to tumorgenesis are minimal or partial, but c-kit kinase inhibitors could find clinical use in combination with other anticancer agents.

c-Kit tends to be expressed in the early stages of melanomas and breast cancers but is downregulated with tumor progression *(196,197)*. The transcription factor AP-2 can activate c-kit expression, and in the case of melanomas, the downregulation of c-kit appears to be secondary to loss of AP-2. Ectopic expression of AP-2 or c-kit in advanced-stage melanoma cells can inhibit their growth and metastasis in models in vivo and can increase their susceptibility to SCF-induced apoptosis in vitro *(200,201)*.

14. CONCLUSIONS

The roles of SCF/c-kit in hematopoiesis during development and in the adult animal, and their analogous roles for other organismic processes including melanogenesis and gametogenesis, dictate that SCF/c-kit will continue to provide fertile ground for the study of mechanisms by which tissue development and homeostasis are regulated. c-Kit expression by hematopoietic stem/progenitor cells, and potentially by candidate stem cells of other adult tissues (e.g., oval cells in the liver as well as cardiac multipotential cells *[202]*), is also relevant to current efforts to understand the basis of adult tissue regeneration and apparent plasticity of stem cells found in various adult tissues such as bone marrow, brain, and skeletal muscle *(61,202–204)*.

ACKNOWLEDGMENTS

The author thanks C. Glenn Begley and Graham Molineux for reviewing the manuscript.

REFERENCES

1. Russell ES. Hereditary anemias of the mouse: a review for geneticists. *Adv Genet* 1979; 20:357–459.
2. Silvers WK. Dominant spotting, patch, and rump-white. In: *The Coat Colors of Mice: A Model for Mammalian Gene Action and Interaction.* New York: Springer-Verlag. 1979:206–223.
3. Silvers WK. Steel, flexed-tailed, splotch, and varitint-waddler. In: *The Coat Colors of Mice: A Model for Mammalian Gene Action and Interaction.* New York: Springer-Verlag. 1979:242–252.
4. Galli SJ, Zsebo KM, Geissler EN. The kit ligand, stem cell factor. *Adv Immunol* 1994; 55:1–96.
5. Broudy VC. Stem cell factor and hematopoiesis. *Blood* 1997; 90:1345–64.
6. Besmer P. Kit-ligand–stem cell factor. In: Garland JM, Quesenberry PJ, Hilton DJ, eds., *Colony-Stimulating Factors: Molecular and Cellular Biology.* New York: Marcel Dekker. 1997:369–404.
7. Lyman SD, Jacobsen SE. c-Kit ligand and Flt3 ligand: stem/progenitor cell factors with overlapping yet distinct activities. *Blood* 1998; 91:1101–1134.
8. Ashman LK. The biology of stem cell factor and its receptor c-kit. *Int J Biochem Cell Biol* 1999; 31:1037–1051.
9. Yarden Y, Kuang W-J, Yang-Feng T, et al. Human proto-oncogene c-*kit:* a new cell surface receptor tyrosine kinase for an unidentified ligand. *EMBO J* 1987; 6:3341–3351.

10. Qiu F, Ray P, Brown K, et al. Primary structure of c-*kit:* relationship with the CSF-1/PDGF receptor kinase family—oncogenic activation of v-*kit* involves deletion of extracellular domain and C terminus. *EMBO J* 1988; 7:1003–1011.
11. Heldin C-H. Dimerization of cell surface receptors in signal transduction. *Cell* 1995; 80:213–223.
12. Rousset D, Agnes F, Lachaume P, Andre C, Galibert F. Molecular evolution of the genes encoding receptor tyrosine kinase with immunoglobulin-like domains. *J Mol Evol* 1995; 41:421–429.
13. Majumder S, Brown K, Qiu F-H, Besmer P. c-kit protein, a transmembrane kinase: identification in tissues and characterization. *Mol Cell Biol* 1988; 8:4896–4903.
14. Wypych J, Bennett LG, Schwartz MG, et al. Soluble kit receptor in human serum. *Blood* 1995; 85:66–73.
15. Huang E, Nocka K, Beier DR, et al. The hematopoietic growth factor KL is encoded by the *Sl* locus and is the ligand of the c-kit receptor, the gene product of the *W* locus. *Cell* 1990; 63:225–233.
16. Anderson DM, Lyman SD, Baird A, et al. Molecular cloning of mast cell growth factor, a hematopoietin that is active in both membrane bound and soluble forms. *Cell* 1990; 63:235–243.
17. Martin FH, Suggs SV, Langley KE, et al. Primary structure and functional expression of rat and human stem cell factor DNAs. *Cell* 1990; 63:203–211.
18. Tajima Y, Moore MAS, Soares V, Ono M, Kissel H, Besmer P. Consequences of exclusive expression in vivo of kit-ligand lacking the major proteolytic cleavage site. *Proc Natl Acad Sci USA* 1998; 95:11903–11908.
19. Wehrle-Haller B, Weston JA. Altered cell-surface targeting of stem cell factor causes loss of melanocyte precursors in Steel^{17H} mutant mice. *Dev Biol* 1999; 210:71–86.
20. Wehrle-Haller B, Imhof BA. Stem cell factor presentation to c-kit. Identification of a basolateral targeting domain. *J Biol Chem* 2001; 276:12667–12674.
21. Arakawa T, Yphantis DA, Lary JW, et al. Glycosylated and unglycosylated recombinant-derived human stem cell factor are dimeric and have extensive regular secondary structure. *J Biol Chem* 1991; 266:18942–18948.
22. Hsu Y, Wu G, Mendiaz EA, et al. The majority of stem cell factor exists as monomer under physiological conditions. *J Biol Chem* 1997; 272:6406–6415.
23. Lu HS, Clogston SL, Wypych J, et al. Post-translational processing of membrane-associated recombinant human stem cell factor expressed in Chinese hamster ovary cells. *Arch Biochem Biophys* 1992; 298:150–158.
24. Tajima Y, Huang EJ, Vosseller K, Ono M, Moore MAS, Besmer P. Role of dimerization of the membrane-associated growth factor kit ligand in juxtacrine signaling: the Sl^{17H} mutation affects dimerization and stability phenotypes in hematopoiesis. *J Exp Med* 1998; 187:1451–1461.
25. Langley KE, Mendiaz EA, Liu N, et al. Properties of variant forms of human stem cell factor recombinantly expressed in *Escherichia coli*. *Arch Biochem Biophys* 1994; 311:55–61.
26. Jiang X, Gurel O, Mendiaz EA, et al. Structure of the active core of human stem cell factor and analysis of binding to its receptor Kit. *EMBO J* 2000; 19:3192–3203.
27. Sprang SR, Bazan JF. Cytokine structural taxonomy and mechanisms of receptor engagement. *Curr Opin Struct Biol* 1993; 3:815–827.
28. Savvas SN, Boone T, Karplus PA. Flt3 ligand structure and unexpected commonalities of helical bundles and cystine knots. *Nat Struct Biol* 2000; 7:486–491.
29. Philo JS, Wen J, Wypych J, Schwartz MG, Mendiaz EA, Langley KE. Human stem cell factor dimer forms a complex with two molecules of the extracellular domain of its receptor, Kit. *J Biol Chem* 1996; 271:6895–6902.
30. Lemmon MA, Pinchasi D, Zhou M, Lax I, Schlessinger J. Kit receptor dimerization is driven by bivalent binding of stem cell factor. *J Biol Chem* 1997; 272:6311–6317.
31. Broudy VC, Lin NL, Sabath DF. The fifth immunoglobulin-like domain of the Kit receptor is required for proteolytic cleavage from the cell surface. *Cytokine* 2001; 15:188–195.
32. Ma Y, Cunningham ME, Wang X, Ghosh I, Regan L, Longley BJ. Inhibition of spontaneous receptor phosphorylation by residues in a putative α-helix in the KIT intracellular juxtamembrane region. *J Biol Chem* 1999; 274:13399–13402.
33. Longley BJ, Reguera MJ, Ma Y. Classes of c-*KIT* activating mutations: proposed mechanisms of action and implications for disease classification and therapy. *Leuk Res* 2001; 25:571–576.
34. Wiesmann C, de Vos AM. Variations on ligand-receptor complexes. *Nat Struct Biol* 2000; 7:440–442.
35. Williams DE, Eisenman J, Baird A, et al. Identification of a ligand for the c-kit proto-oncogene. *Cell* 1990; 63:167–174.

36. Flanagan JG, Chan DC, Leder P. Transmembrane form of the kit ligand growth factor is determined by alternative splicing and is missing in the *Sl^d* mutant. *Cell* 1991; 64:1025–1035.
37. Kapur R, Cooper R, Xiao X, Weiss MJ, Donovan P, Williams DA. The presence of novel amino acids in the cytoplasmic domain of stem cell factor results in hematopoietic defects in Steel^{17H} mice. *Blood* 1999; 94:1915–1925.
38. Matsui Y, Zsebo KM, Hogan BLM. Embryonic expression of a haematopoietic growth factor encoded by the *Sl* locus and the ligand for c-*kit*. *Nature* 1990; 347:667–669.
39. Orr-Urtreger A, Avivi A, Zimmer Y, Givol D, Yarden Y Lonai P. Developmental expression of c-kit, a proto-oncogene encoded by the *W* locus. *Development* 1990; 109:911–923.
40. Keshet E, Lyman SD, Williams DE, et al. Embryonic RNA expression patterns of the c-kit receptor and its cognate ligand suggest multiple functional roles in mouse development. *EMBO J* 1991; 10:2425–2435.
41. Motro B, van der Kooy D, Rossant J, Reith A, Bernstein A. Contiguous patterns of c-kit and steel expression: analysis of mutations at the *W* and *Sl* loci. *Development* 1991; 113:1207–1221.
42. Sanders KM, Ördög T, Ward SM. Physiology and pathophysiology of the interstitial cells of Cajal: from bench to bedside. IV. Genetic and animal models of GI motility disorders caused by loss of interstitial cells of Cajal. *Am J Physiol Gastrointest Liver Physiol* 2002; 282:G747–G756.
43. Motro B, Wojtowicz JM, Bernstein A, van der Kooy D. Steel mutant mice are deficient in hippocampal learning but not long-term potentiation. *Proc Natl Acad Sci USA* 1996; 93:1808–1813.
44. Katafuchi T, Li AJ, Hirota S, Kitamura Y, Hori T. Impairment of spatial learning and hippocampal synaptic potentiation in c-kit mutant rats. *Learn Memory* 2000; 7:383–392.
45. Kondo T, Katafuchi T, Hori T. Stem cell factor modulates paired-pulse facilitation and long-term potentiation in the hippocampal mossy fiber-CA3 pathway in mice. *Brain Res* 2002; 946:179–190.
46. Ikuta K, Weissman IL. Evidence that hematopoietic stem cells express mouse c-kit but do not depend on steel factor for their generation. *Proc Natl Acad Sci USA* 1992; 89:1502–1606.
47. Puddington L, Olson S, Lefrancois L. Interactions between stem cell factor and c-*kit* are required for intestinal immune system homeostasis. *Immunity* 1994; 1:733–739.
48. Di Santo JP, Rodewald H-R. In vivo roles of receptor tyrosine kinases and cytokine receptors in early thymocyte development. *Curr Opin Immunol* 1998; 10:196–207.
49. Galli SJ, Kitamura Y. Animal models of human disease. Genetically mast-cell-deficient W/W^v and Sl/Sl^d mice. Their value for the analysis of the roles of mast cell in biologic responses in vivo. *Am J Pathol* 1987; 127:191–198.
50. Hunt P, Zsebo KM, Hokom MM, et al. Evidence that stem cell factor is involved in the rebound thrombocytosis that follows 5-fluorouracil treatment. *Blood* 1992; 80:904–911.
51. Okada S, Nakauchi H, Nagayoshi K, et al. Enrichment and characterization of murine hematopoietic stem cells that express c-*kit* molecule. *Blood* 1991; 78:1706–1712.
52. Ogawa M, Matsuzaki Y, Nishikawa S, et al. Expression and function of c-kit in hemopoietic progenitor cells. *J Exp Med* 1991; 174:63–71.
53. Rico-Vargas SA, Weiskopf B, Nishikawa S, Osmond DG. c-kit expression by B cell precursors in mouse bone marrow. Stimulation of B cell genesis by in vivo treatment with anti-c-kit antibody. *J Immunol* 1994; 152:2845–2852.
54. Ortiz M, Wine JW, Lohrey N, Ruscetti FW, Spence SE, Keller JR. Functional characterization of a novel hematopoietic stem cell and its place in the c-kit maturation pathway in bone marrow cell development. *Immunity* 1999; 10:173–182.
55. Randall TD, Weissman IL. Characterization of a population of cells in the bone marrow that phenotypically mimics hematopoietic stem cells: resting stem cells or mystery population? *Stem Cells* 1998; 16:38–48.
56. Bradley TR, Hodgson GS. Detection of primitive macrophage progenitor cells in mouse bone marrow. *Blood* 1979; 54:1446–1450.
57. Metcalf D, Nicola NA. Direct proliferative actions of stem cell factor on murine bone marrow cells *in vitro:* effects of combination with colony-stimulating factors. *Proc Natl Acad Sci USA* 1991; 88:6239–6243.
58. Okada S, Nakauchi H, Nagayoshi K, Nishikawa S-I, Miura Y, Suda T. In vivo and in vitro stem cell function of c-*kit*- and Sca-1-positive murine hematopoietic cells. *Blood* 1992; 80:3044–3050.
59. Jones RJ, Collector MI, Barber JP, et al. Characterization of mouse lymphohematopoietic stem cells lacking spleen colony-forming activity. *Blood* 1996; 88:487–491.

60. Ikehara S. Pluripotent hematopoietic stem cells in mice and humans. *Proc Soc Exp Biol Med* 2000; 233:149–155.
61. Miller CL, Rebel VI, Lemieux ME, Helgason CD, Lansdorp PM, Eaves CJ. Studies of *W* mutant mice provide evidence for alternate mechanisms capable of activating hematopoietic stem cells. *Exp Hematol* 1996; 24:185–194.
62. Weissman IL, Anderson DJ, Gage F. Stem and progenitor cells: origins, phenotypes, lineage commitments, and transdifferentiations. *Annu Rev Cell Dev Biol* 2001; 17:387–403.
63. Bonnet D. Haematopoietic stem cells. *J Pathol* 2002; 197:430–440.
64. Liu H, Verfaille CM. Myeloid-lymphoid initiating cells (ML-IC) are highly enriched in the rhodamine-c-kit$^+$CD33$^-$CD38$^-$ fraction of umbilical cord CD34$^+$ cells. *Exp Hematol* 2002; 30:582–589.
65. Broudy VC, Lin N, Zsebo KM, et al. Isolation and characterization of a monoclonal antibody that recognizes the human c-kit receptor. *Blood* 1992; 79:338–346.
66. Sutherland HJ, Hogge DE, Cook D, Eaves CJ. Alternative mechanisms with and without steel factor support primitive human hematopoiesis. *Blood* 1993; 81:1465–1470.
67. Bodine DM, Orlic D, Birkett NC, Seidel NE, Zsebo KM. Stem cell factor increases colony-forming unit-spleen number in vitro in synergy with interleukin-6, and in vivo in *Sl/Sl^d* mice as a single factor. *Blood* 1992; 79:913–919.
68. Li CL, Johnson GR. Murine hematopoietic stem and progenitor cells: I. Enrichment and biologic characterization. *Blood* 1995; 85:1472–1479.
69. Ema H, Takano H, Sudo K, Nakauchi H. In vitro self-renewal division of hematopoietic stem cells. *J Exp Med* 2000; 192:1281–1288.
70. Piacibello W, Sananip F, Severino A, et al. Engraftment in nonobese diabetic severe combined immunodeficient mice of human CD34$^+$ cord blood cells after ex vivo expansion: evidence for the amplification and self-renewal of repopulating stem cells. *Blood* 1999; 93:3736–3749.
71. Migliaccio G, Migliaccio AR, Valinsky J, et al. Stem cell factor induces proliferation and differentiation of highly enriched murine hematopoietic cells. *Proc Natl Acad Sci USA* 1991; 88:7420–7424.
72. Williams N, Bertoncello I, Kavnoudias H, Zsebo K, McNiece I. Recombinant rat stem cell factor stimulates the amplification and differentiation of fractionated mouse stem cell populations. *Blood* 1992; 79:58–64.
73. Miller JS, McCullar V, Punzel M, Lemischka IR, Moore KA. Single adult human CD34$^+$/Lin$^-$/CD38$^-$ progenitors give rise to natural killer cells, B-lineage cells, dendritic cells, and myeloid cells. *Blood* 1999; 93:96–106.
74. Kobari L, Pflumio F, Giarraana M-C, et al. In vitro and in vivo evidence for the long-term multilineage (myeloid, B, NK, and T) reconstitution capacity of ex vivo expanded human CD34$^+$ cord blood cells. *Exp Hematol* 2000; 28:1470–1480.
75. Heyworth CM, Whetton AD, Nicholls S, Zsebo KM, Dexter TM. Stem cell factor directly stimulates the development of enriched granulocyte-macrophage colony-forming cells and promotes the effects of other colony-stimulating factors. *Blood* 1992; 80:2230–2236.
76. Dai CH, Krantz SB, Zsebo KM. Human burst-forming units-erythroid need direct interaction with stem cell factor for further development. *Blood* 1991; 78:2493– 2497.
77. Bernstein ID, Andrews RG, Zsebo KM. Recombinant human stem cell factor enhances the formation of colonies by CD34$^+$ and CD34$^+$lin$^-$ cells, and the generation of colony-forming cell progeny from CD34$^+$lin$^-$ cells cultured with interleukin-3, granulocyte colony-stimulating factor, or granulocyte-macrophage colony-stimulating factor. *Blood* 1991; 77:2316–2321.
78. Migliaccio G, Migliaccio AR, Druzin M, Giardina PJV, Zsebo KM, Adamson JW. Effects of recombinant human stem cell factor (SCF) on the growth of human progenitor cells *in vitro*. *J Cell Physiol* 1991; 148:503–509.
79. Uoshima N, Ozawa M, Kimura S, et al. Changes in c-Kit expression and effects of SCF during differentiation of human erythroid progenitor cells. *Br J Haematol* 1995; 91:30–36.
80. Gabbianelli M, Testa U, Massa A, et al. Hemoglobin switching in unicellular erythroid culture of sibling erythroid burst-forming units: kit ligand induces a dose-dependent fetal hemoglobin reactivation potentiated by sodium butyrate. *Blood* 2000; 95:3555–3561.
81. Wojda U, Leigh KR, Njoroge JM, et al. Fetal hemoglobin modulation during human erythropoiesis: stem cell factor has late effects related to the expression pattern of CD117. *Blood* 2003; 101:492–497.
82. Olivieri NF, Grunberger T, Ben-David Y, et al. Diamond-Blackfan anemia: heterogenous response of hematopoietic progenitor cells in vitro to the protein product of the steel locus. *Blood* 1991; 78:2211–2215.

83. Spritz RA, Freedman MH. Lack of mutations of the MGF and KIT genes in Diamond-Blackfan anemia. *Blood* 1993; 81:3165.
84. Alter BP, Knobloch ME, He L, et al. Effect of stem cell factor on in vitro erythropoiesis in patients with bone marrow failure syndromes. *Blood* 1992; 80:3000–3008.
85. Bagnara GP, Strippoli P, Bonsi L, et al. Effect of stem cell factor on colony growth from acquired and constitutional (Fanconi) aplastic anemia. *Blood* 1992; 80:382–387.
86. Wodnar-Filipowicz A, Tichelli A, Zsebo KM, Speck B, Nissen C. Stem cell factor stimulates the in vitro growth of bone marrow cells from aplastic anemia patients. *Blood* 1992; 79:3196–3202.
87. Soligo DA, Campiglio S, Servida F, et al. Response of myelodysplastic syndrome marrow progenitor cells to stimulation with cytokine combinations in a stroma-free long-term culture system. *Br J Haematol* 1996; 92:548–558.
88. Miles SA, Lee K, Hutlin L, Zsebo KM, Mitsuyasu RT. Potential use of human stem cell factor as adjunctive therapy for human immunodeficiency virus-related cytopenias. *Blood* 1991; 78:3200–3208.
89. Palacios R, Nishikawa S-I. Developmentally regulated cell surface expression and function of c-kit receptor during lymphocyte ontogeny in the embryo and adult mice. *Development* 1992; 115:1133–1147.
90. Takeda S, Shimizu S, Rodewald HR. Interactions between c-kit and stem cell factor are not required by B-cell development in vivo. *Blood* 1997; 89:518–525.
91. Colucci F, Di Santo JP. The receptor tyrosine kinase c-kit provides a critical signal for survival, expansion, and maturation of mouse natural killer cells. *Blood* 2000; 95:984–991.
92. Godfrey DI, Zlotnik A, Suda T. Phenotypic and functional characterization of c-kit expression during intrathymic T cell development. *J Immunol* 1992; 149:2281–2285.
93. Matsuzaki Y, Gyotoku J, Ogawa M, et al. Characterization of c-kit positive intrathymic stem cells that are restricted to lymphoid differentiation. *J Exp Med* 1993; 178:1283–1292.
94. deCastro CM, Denning SM, Langdon S, et al. The c-kit proto-oncogene receptor is expressed on a subset of human $CD3^-CD4^-CD8^-$ (triple negative) thymocytes. *Exp Hematol* 1994; 22:1025–1033.
95. Godfrey DI, Kennedy J, Mombaerts P, Tonegawa S, Zlotnik A. Onset of TCR-beta gene rearrangement and role of TCR-beta expression during $CD3^-CD4^-CD8^-$ thymocyte differentiation. *J Immunol* 1994; 152:4783–4792.
96. Galy AHM, Malefyt RD, Barcena A, Peterson SM, Spits H. Untransfected and SV40-transfected fetal and postnatal human thymic stromal cells. *Thymus* 1993; 22:13–33.
97. Moore TA, Zlotnik A. Differential effects of flk-2/flt-3 ligand and stem cell factor on murine thymic progenitor cells. *J Immunol* 1997; 158:4187–4192.
98. Tjonnfjord GE, Veiby OP, Steen R, Egeland T. T lymphocyte differentiation in vitro from adult human prethymic $CD34^+$ bone marrow cells. *J Exp Med* 1993; 177:1531–1539.
99. Molineux G, Migdalska A, Szmitkowski M, Zsebo K, Dexter TM. The effects on hematopoiesis of recombinant stem cell factor (ligand for c-kit) administered in vivo to mice either alone or in combination with granulocyte colony-stimulating factor. *Blood* 1991; 78:961–996.
100. Andrews RG, Knitter GN, Bartelmez SH, et al. Recombinant human stem cell factor, a c-*kit* ligand, stimulates hematopoiesis in primates. *Blood* 1991; 78:1975–1980.
101. Laky K, Lefrancois L, Puddington L. Age-dependent intestinal lymphoproliferative disorder due to stem cell factor receptor deficiency: parameters in small and large intestine. *J Immunol* 1997; 158:1417–1427.
102. Wang T, Langley KE, Gourley WK, Klimpel GR. Stem cell factor (SCF) can regulate the activation and expansion of murine intraepithelial lymphocytes. *Cytokine* 2000; 12:272–280.
103. Woodward J, Jenkinson E. Identification and characterization of lymphoid precursors in the murine intestinal epithelium. *Eur J Immunol* 2001; 31:3329–3338.
104. Murray AM, Simm B, Beagley KW. Cytokine gene expression in murine fetal intestine: potential for extrathymic T cell development. *Cytokine* 1998; 10:337–345.
105. Wang T, Alam R, Langley KE, Klimpel GR. Stem cell factor and IL-2 act synergistically in inducing intraepithelial lymphocyte proliferation and cytokine production: upregulation of the IL-2 receptor γ-chain and signaling via JAK-3. *Cell Immunol* 2000; 205:62–71.
106. Payne KJ, Medina KL, Kincade PW. Loss of c-kit accompanies B-lineage commitment and acquisition of CD45R by most murine B-lymphocyte precursors. *Blood* 1999; 94:713–723.
107. Borge O, Alolfsson J, Mörtensson A, Mörtensson I-L, Jacobsen SEW. Lymphoid-restricted development from multipotent candidate murine stem cells: distinct and complementary functions of the c-kit and flt3-ligands. *Blood* 1999; 94:3781–3790.

108. McNiece IK, Langley KE, Zsebo KM. The role of recombinant stem cell factor in early B cell development. Synergistic interaction with IL-7. *J Immunol* 1991; 146:3785–3790.
109. Rolink A, Streb M, Nishikawa S-I, Melchers F. The c-kit-encoded tyrosine kinase regulates the proliferation of early pre-B cells. *Eur J Immunol* 1991; 21:2609–2612.
110. Miller JS. The biology of natural killer cells in cancer, infection, and pregnancy. *Exp Hematol* 2001; 29:1157–1168.
111. Fehniger TA, Caligiuri MA. Ontogeny and expansion of natural killer cells: clinical implications. *Int Rev Immunol* 2001; 20:503–534.
112. Shibuya A, Nagayoshi K, Nakamura K, Nakauchi H. Lymphokine requirement for the generation of natural killer cells from CD34+ hematopoietic progenitor cells. *Blood* 1995; 85:3538–3546.
113. Muench MO, Humeau L, Paek B, et al. Differential effects of interleukin-3, interleukin-7, interleukin-15, and granulocyte-macrophage colony-stimulating factor in the generation of natural killer and B cells from primitive human fetal liver progenitors. *Exp Hematol* 2000; 28:961–973.
114. Seaman WE, Talal N. Natural killing by spleen cells from W/W^v and Sl/Sl^d anemic mice. *Exp Hematol* 1981; 9:691–696.
115. Williams NS, Klem J, Puzanov IJ, Sivakumar PV, Bennett M, Kumar V. Differentiation of NK1.1+, Ly49+ cells from flt3+ multipotent marrow progenitor cells. *J Immunol* 1999; 163:2648–2656.
116. Miller SC, Fleming WH, Zsebo KM, Weissman IL. The in vivo effects of steel factor on natural killer lineage cells in murine spleen and bone marrow. *Nat Immun* 1993; 12:293–301.
117. Hart D. Dendritic cells: unique leukocyte populations which control the primary immune response. *Blood* 1997; 90:3245–3287.
118. Bell D, Young JW, Banchereau J. Dendritic cells. *Adv Immunol* 1999; 72:255–324.
119. Zhang Y, Wang J, Ogata M, Hashimoto S, Onai N, Matsushima K. Development of dendritic cells in vitro from murine fetal liver-derived lineage phenotype-negative c-kit(+) hematopoietic progenitor cells. *Blood* 2000; 95:138–146.
120. Jackson SH, Alicea C, Owens JW, Eigsti CL, Malech HL. Characterization of an early dendritic cell precursor derived from murine lineage-negative hematopoietic progenitor cells. *Exp Hematol* 2002; 30:430–439.
121. Galli SJ. Mast cells and basophils. *Curr Opin Hematol* 2000; 7:32–39.
122. Wedemeyer J, Tsai M, Galli SJ. Roles of mast cells and basophils in innate and acquired immunity. *Curr Opin Immunol* 2000; 12:624–631.
123. Malaviya R, Abraham SN. Clinical implications of mast cell-bacteria interaction. *J Mol Med* 1998; 76:617–623.
124. Austen KF, Boyce JA. Mast cell lineage development and phenotypic regulation. *Leuk Res* 2001; 25:511–518.
125. Ulich TR, del Castillo J, Yi ES, et al. Hematologic effects of stem cell factor in vivo and in vitro in rodents. *Blood* 1991; 78:645–650.
126. Supajatura V, Ushio H, Nakao A, Okumura K, Ra C, Ogawa H. Protective roles of mast cells against enterobacterial infection are mediated by Toll-like receptor 4. *J Immunol* 2001; 167:2250–2256.
127. Maliviya R, Gao Z, Thankavel K, van der Merwe PA, Abraham SN. The mast cell tumor necrosis factor α response to FimH-expressing *Escherichia coli* is mediated by the glycosylphosphatidylinositol-anchored molecule CD48. *Proc Natl Acad Sci USA* 1999; 96:8110–8115.
128. Arock M, Ross E, Lai-Kuen R, Averlant G, Gao Z, Abraham SN. Phagocytic and tumor necrosis factor alpha response of human mast cells following exposure to gram-negative and gram positive bacteria. *Infect Immun* 1998; 66:6030–6034.
129. Saito H, Ebisawa M, Tachimoto H, et al. Selective growth of human mast cells induced by Steel factor, IL-6, and prostaglandin E2 from cord blood mononuclear cells. *J Immunol* 1996; 157:343–350.
130. Ochi H, Hirani WM, Yuan Q, Friend DS, Austen KF, Boyce JA. T helper cell type 2 cytokine-mediated comitogenic responses and CCR3 expression during differentiation of human mast cells in vitro. *J Exp Med* 1999; 190:267–280.
131. Yuan Q, Gurish MF, Friend DS, Austen KF, Boyce JA. Generation of a novel stem cell factor-dependent mast cell progenitor. *J Immunol* 1998; 161:5143–5146.
132. Gagari E, Tsai M, Lantz CS, Fox LG, Galli SJ. Differential release of mast cell interleukin-6 via c-kit. *Blood* 1997; 89:2654–2663.
133. Tsai M, Wedemeyer J, Ganiatsas S, Tam S-Y, Zon LI, Galli SJ. *In vivo* immunological function of mast cells derived from embryonic stem cells: an approach for the rapid analysis of even embryonic lethal mutations in adult mice *in vivo*. *Proc Natl Acad Sci USA* 2000; 97:9186–9190.

134. Emerson SG. Ex vivo expansion of hematopoietic precursors, progenitors, and stem cells: the next generation of cellular therapeutics. *Blood* 1996; 87:3082–3088.
135. Gothot A, vander Loo JCM, Clapp DW, Srour EF. Cell cycle-related changes in repopulating capacity of human mobilized peripheral blood CD34+ cells in non-obese diabetic/severe combined immune-deficient mice. *Blood* 1998; 92:2641–2649.
136. Glimm H, Oh I-H, Eaves CJ. Human hematopoietic stem cells stimulated to proliferate in vitro lose engraftment potential during their $S/G_2/M$ transit and do not reenter G_0. *Blood* 2000; 96:4185–4193.
137. Dunbar CE, Takatoku M, Donahue RE. The impact of ex vivo cytokine stimulation on engraftment of primitive hematopoietic cells in a non-human primate model. *Ann NY Acad Sci* 2001; 938:236–244.
138. Kollet O, Spiegel A, Peled A, et al. Rapid and efficient homing of human $CD34^+CD38^{-/low}CXCR4^+$ stem and progenitor cells to the bone marrow and spleen of NOD/SCID and NOD/SCID/B2m*null* mice. *Blood* 2001; 97:3283–3291.
139. Reiffers J, Cailliot C, Dazey B, Attal M, Caraux J, Boiron J-M. Abrogation of post-myeloablative chemotherapy neutropenia by ex-vivo expanded autologous CD34-positive cells. *Lancet* 1999; 354:1092–1093.
140. Paquette RL, Dergham ST, Karpf E, et al. Ex vivo expanded unselected peripheral blood: progenitor cells posttransplantation neutropenia, thrombocytopenia, and anemia in patients with breast cancer. *Blood* 2000; 96:2385–2390.
141. McNiece I, Jones R, Bearman SI, et al. Ex vivo expanded peripheral blood progenitor cells provide rapid neutrophil recovery after high-dose chemotherapy in patients with breast cancer. *Blood* 2000; 96:3001–3007.
142. Kohn DB. The current status of gene therapy using hematopoietic stem cells. *Curr Opin Pediatr* 1995; 7:56–63.
143. Havega M, Hoogerbrugge P, Valerio D, van Es HHG. Retroviral stem cell gene therapy. *Stem Cells* 1997; 15:162–179.
144. Heim DA, Dunbar CE. Hematopoietic stem cell gene therapy: towards clinically significant gene transfer efficiency. *Immunol Rev* 2000; 178:29–38.
145. Movassagh M, Caillot L, Baillou C, Guigon M, Lemoine FM. Optimization of the cycling of clonogenic and primitive cord blood progenitors by various growth factors. *Stem Cells* 1997; 16:214–222.
146. Jiang Y, Prosper F, Verfaille CM. Opposing effects of engagement of integrins and stimulation of cytokine receptors on cell cycle progression of normal human hematopoietic progenitors. *Blood* 2000; 95:846–854.
147. Hennemann B, Conneally E, Pawliuk R, et al. Optimization of retroviral-mediated gene transfer to human NOD/SCID mouse repopulating cord blood cells through a systematic analysis of protocol variables. *Exp Hematol* 1999; 27:817–825.
148. Crooks GM, Kohn DB. Growth factors increase amphotropic retrovirus binding to human CD34+ bone marrow progenitor cells. *Blood* 1993; 82:3290–3297.
149. Fleming WH, Alpern EJ, Uchida N, Ikuta K, Weissman IL. Steel factor influences the distribution and activity of murine hematopoietic stem cells *in vivo*. *Proc Natl Acad Sci USA* 1993; 90:3760–3764.
150. Mauch P, Lamont C, Neben TY, Quinto C, Goldman SJ, Witsell A. Hematopoietic stem cells in the blood after stem cell factor and interleukin-11 administration: evidence for different mechanisms of mobilization. *Blood* 1995; 12:4674–4680.
151. Bodine DM, Seidel NE, Zsebo KM, Orlic D. In vivo administration of stem cell factor to mice increases the absolute number of pluripotent hematopoietic stem cells. *Blood* 1993; 82:445–455
152. Harrison DE, Zsebo KZ, Astle CM. Splenic primitive hematopoietic stem cell (PHSC) activity is enhanced by steel factor because of PHSC proliferation. *Blood* 1994; 83:3146–3151.
153. Iscove NN, Nawa K. Hematopoietic stem cells expand during serial transplantation *in vivo* without apparent exhaustion. *Curr Biol* 1997; 7:805–808.
154. de Haan G, Dontje B, Nijhof W. Concepts of hematopoietic cell amplification. Synergy, redundancy and pleiotropy of cytokines affecting the regulation of erythropoiesis. *Leuk Lymph* 1996; 22:385–394.
155. Bodine DM, Seidel NE, Orlic D. Bone marrow collected 14 days after in vivo administration of granulocyte colony-stimulating factor and stem cell factor to mice has 10-fold more repopulating ability than untreated bone marrow. *Blood* 1996; 88:89–97.
156. Molineux G, Migdalska A, Haley J, Evans GS, Dexter TM. Total marrow failure induced by pegylated stem-cell factor administered before 5-fluorouracil. *Blood* 1994; 83:3491–3499.
157. Jin L, Neff T, Blau AC. Marrow sensitization to 5-fluorouracil using the ligands for flt-3 and c-kit. *Exp Hematol* 1999; 27:520–525.

158. de Haan G, Dontje B, Nijhof W, Loeffler M. Effects of continuous stem cell factor administration on normal and erythropoietin-stimulated murine hemopoiesis: experimental results and model analysis. *Stem Cells* 1995; 13:65–76.
159. McNiece IK, Briddell RA, Yan XQ, et al. The role of stem cell factor in mobilization of peripheral blood progenitor cells. *Leuk Lymph* 1994; 15:405–409.
160. Lacerna L Jr, Sheridan WP, Basser R, et al. Stem cell factor. In: Ho AD, Haas R, Champlin RE, eds., *Hematopoietic Stem Cell Transplantation.* New York: Marcel Dekker. 2000:31–46.
161. Zsebo KM, Smith KA, Hartley CA, et al. Radioprotection of mice by recombinant rat stem cell factor. *Proc Natl Acad Sci USA* 1992; 89:9464–9468.
162. Leigh BR, Webb S, Hancock SL, Knox SJ. Stem cell factor enhances the survival of irradiated human bone marrow maintained in SCID mice. *Stem Cells* 1994; 12:430–435.
163. Down JD, de Haan G, Dillingh JH, Dontje B, Nijhof W. Stem cell factor has contrasting effects in combination with 5-fluorouracil or total-body irradiation on frequencies of different hematopoietic subsets and engraftment of transplanted bone marrow. *Radiat Res* 1997; 147:680–685.
164. de Haan G, Dontje B, Engel C, Loeffler M, Nijhof W. Prophylactic pretreatment of mice with hematopoietic growth factors induces expansion of primitive cell compartments and results in protection against 5-fluorouracil-induced toxicity. *Blood* 1996; 87:4581–4588.
165. Patchen ML, Fischer R, Schmauder-Chock EA, Williams DE. Mast cell growth factor enhances multilineage hematopoietic recovery in vivo following radiation-induced aplasia. *Exp Hematol* 1994; 22:31–39.
166. Steinshamn S, Bergh K, Waage A. Effects of stem cell factor and granulocyte colony-stimulating factor on granulocyte recovery and *Candida albicans* infection in granulocytopenic mice. *J Infect Dis* 1993; 168:1444–1448.
167. Du XX, Keller D, Maze R, Williams DA. Comparative effects of in vivo treatment using interleukin-11 and stem cell factor on reconstitution in mice after bone marrow transplantation. *Blood* 1993; 82:1016–1022.
168. Linnekin D. Early signaling pathways activated by c-kit in hematopoietic cells. *Int J Biochem Cell Biol* 1999; 31:1053–1074.
169. Lee Y, Mantel C, Anzai N, Braun SE, Broxmeyer HE. Transcriptional and ERK1/2-dependent synergistic upregulation of $p21^{cip1/waf1}$ associated with steel factor synergy in MO7e. *Biochem Biophys Res Commun* 2001; 280:675–683.
170. Sui Z, Krantz SB, Zhao Z. Synergistic activation of MAP kinase (ERK1/2) by erythropoietin and stem cell factor is essential for expanded erythropoiesis. *Blood* 1998; 92:1142–1149.
171. Duarte RF, Frank DA. SCF and G-CSF lead to the synergistic induction of proliferation and gene expression through complementary signaling pathways. *Blood* 2000; 96:3422–3430.
172. Tamir A, Petrocelli T, Stetler K, et al. Stem cell factor inhibits erythroid differentiation by modulating the activity of G1-cyclin-dependent kinase complexes: a role for p27 in erythroid differentiation coupled G_1 arrest. *Cell Growth Differ* 2000; 11:269–277.
173. Sui X, Krantz SB, Zhao ZJ. Stem cell factor and erythropoietin inhibit apoptosis of human erythroid progenitor cells through different signalling pathways. *Br J Haematol* 2000; 110:63–70.
174. Nishio M, Oda A, Koizumi K, et al. Stem cell factor prevents Fas-mediated apoptosis of human erythroid precursor cells with Src-like kinase dependency. *Exp Hematol* 2001; 29:19–29.
175. Chung I-J, Dai C, Krantz SB. Stem cell factor increases the expression of FLIP that inhibits IFNγ-induced apoptosis in human erythroid progenitor cells. *Blood* 2003; 101:1324–1328.
176. Blume-Jensen P, Janknecht R, Hunter T. The kit receptor promotes cell survival via activation of PI 3-kinase and subsequent Akt-mediated phosphorylation of Bad on Ser136. *Curr Biol* 1998; 8:779–782.
177. Wu H, Klingmüller U, Besmer P, Lodish HF. Interaction of the erythropoietin and stem-cell-factor receptors. *Nature* 1995; 377:242–246.
178. Jacobs-Helber SM, Penta K, Sun Z, Lawson A, Sawyer ST. Distinct signaling from stem cell factor and erythropoietin in HCD57 cells. *J Biol Chem* 1997; 272:6850–6853.
179. Kapur R, Majumdar M, Xiao X, McAndrews-Hill M, Schindler K, Williams DA. Signaling through the interaction of membrane-restricted stem cell factor and *c-kit* receptor tyrosine kinase: genetic evidence for a differential role in erythropoiesis. *Blood* 1998; 91:879–889.
180. Wu H, Klingmüller U, Acurio A, Hsiao JG, Lodish HF. Functional interaction of erythropoietin and stem cell factor receptors is essential for erythroid colony formation. *Proc Natl Acad Sci USA* 1997; 94:1806–1810.

181. Scott CL, Robb L, Papaevangeliou B, Mansfield R, Nicola NA, Begley CG. Reassessment of interactions between hematopoietic receptors using common beta-chain and interleukin-3–specific receptor beta-chain–null cells: no evidence of functional interactions with receptors for erythropoietin, granulocyte colony-stimulating factor, or stem cell factor. *Blood* 2000; 96:1588–1590.
182. Kunisada T, Lu S-Z, Yoshida H, et al. Murine cutaneous mastocytosis and epidermal melanocytosis induced by keratinocyte expression of transgenic stem cell factor. *J Exp Med* 1998; 187:1565–1573.
183. Miyazawa K, Williams DA, Gotoh A, Nishimaki J, Broxmeyer HE, Toyama K. Membrane-bound steel factor induces more persistent tyrosine kinase activation and longer life span of *c-kit* gene-encoded protein than its soluble form. *Blood* 1995; 85:641–649.
184. Kapur R, Chandra S, Cooper R, McCarthy J, Williams DA. Role of p38 and ERK MAP kinase in proliferation of erythroid progenitors in response to stimulation by soluble and membrane isoforms of stem cell factor. *Blood* 2002; 100:1287–1293.
185. Bedell MA, Copeland NG, Jenkins NA. Multiple pathways for Steel regulation suggested by genomic and sequence analysis of the murine Steel gene. *Genetics* 1996; 142:927–934.
186. Taylor WE, Najmabadi H, Strathearn M, et al. Human stem cell factor promoter deoxyribonucleic acid sequence and regulation by cyclic 3′,5′-adenosine monophosphate in a Sertoli cell line. *Endocrinology* 1996; 137:5407–5414.
187. Dahlen DD, Lin NA, Liu Y-C, Broudy VC. Soluble c-kit receptor blocks stem cell factor bioactivity in vitro. *Leuk Res* 2001; 25:413–421.
188. Akin C, Schwartz LB, Kitoh T, et al. Soluble stem cell factor receptor (CD117) and IL-2 receptor alpha chain (CD25) levels in the plasma of patients with mastocytosis: relationships to disease severity and bone marrow pathology. *Blood* 2000; 96:1267–1273.
189. Metcalfe DD, Akin C. Mastocytosis: molecular mechanisms and clinical disease heterogeneity. *Leuk Res* 2001; 25:577–582.
190. Gommerman JK, Rottapel R, Berger SA. Phosphatidyl 3-kinase and Ca^{2+} influx dependence for ligand-stimulated internalization of the c-kit receptor. *J Biol Chem* 1997; 272:30519–30525.
191. Broudy VC, Lin NL, Liles WC, et al. Signaling via Src family kinases is required for normal internalization of the receptor c-kit. *Blood* 1999; 94:1979–1986.
192. Krosl G, He G, Lefrancois M, et al. Transcription factor SCL is required for c-kit expression and c-Kit function in hemopoietic cells. *J Exp Med* 1998; 188:439–450.
193. Vitelli L, Condorelli G, Lulli V, et al. A pentamer transcriptional complex including tal-1 and retinoblastoma protein downmodulates c-kit expression in normal erythroblasts. *Mol Cell Biol* 2000; 20:5330–5342.
194. Lécuyer E, Herblot S, Saint-Denis M, et al. The SCL complex regulates c-kit expression in hematopoietic cells through functional interaction with Sp1. *Blood* 2002; 100:2430–2440.
195. Heinrich MC, Blanke CD, Druker BJ, Corless CL. Inhibition of KIT tyrosine kinase activity: a novel molecular approach to the treatment of KIT-positive malignancies. *J Clin Oncol* 2002; 20:1692–1703.
196. Natali PG, Nicotra MR, Winkler AB, Cavaliere R, Bigotti A, Ullrich A. Progression of human cutaneous melanoma is associated with loss of expression of c-kit proto-oncogene receptor. *Int J Cancer* 1992; 52:197–201.
197. Natali PG, Nicotra MR, Sures I, Mottolese M, Botti C, Ullrich A. Breast cancer is associated with loss of the c-kit oncogene product. *Int J Cancer* 1992; 52:713–717.
198. van Oosterom AT, Judson IR, Verweij J, et al. Update of phase I study of imatinib (STI571) in advanced soft tissue sarcomas and gastrointestinal stromal tumors: a report of the EORTC Soft Tissue and Bone Sarcoma Group. *Eur J Cancer* 2002; 38:S83–S87.
199. Demetri GD, von Mehren M, Blanke CD, et al. Efficacy and safety of imatinib mesylate in advanced gastrointestinal stromal tumors. *N Engl J Med* 2002; 347:472–480.
200. Huang S, Luca M, Gutman M, et al. Enforced c-kit expression renders highly metastatic human melanoma cells susceptible to stem cell factor-induced apoptosis and inhibits their tumorigenic and metastatic potential. *Oncogene* 1996; 13:2339–2347.
201. Bar-Eli M. Gene regulation in melanoma progression by the AP-2 transcription factor. *Pigment Cell Res* 2001; 14:78–85.
202. Nadal-Ginard B, Kajstura J, Leri A, Anversa P. Myocyte death, growth, and regeneration in cardiac hypertrophy and failure. *Circ Res* 2003; 92:139–150.
203. Jackson KA, Majka SM, Wulf GG, Goodell MA. Stem cells: a minireview. *J Cell Biochem Suppl* 2002; 38:1–6.
204. Tisdale JF Jr, Dunbar CE. Plasticity and hematopoiesis: Circe's transforming potion? *Curr Opin Hematol* 2002; 9:268–273.

9 Hematopoietic Growth Factors

Preclinical Studies of Myeloid and Immune Reconstitution

Ann M. Farese, MS, MT (ASCP)
and Thomas J. MacVittie, PhD

CONTENTS

1. INTRODUCTION

The ability to deliver the prescribed dose of chemotherapy and/or radiation therapy remains problematic owing to associated hematopoietic toxicities, which include neutropenia and thrombocytopenia. Additionally, immune suppression, both acute and delayed, is a consequence of cytotoxic therapy, especially in response to dose intensification, schedule compression, or myeloablative conditioning for stem cell transplantation. New strategies applied to current hematopoietic growth factors (HGFs) as well as new HGFs will be required to manage effectively the cytopenia and consequences associated with chemotherapy employed in an effort to realize its full therapeutic value.

A number of recent HGFs have demonstrated significant potential of moving from "bench to bedside." The c-kit and flt-3 ligands were cloned in the early 1990s *(1–6)*. Both ligands had unique and redundant biologic effects on hematopoietic stem cells (HSCs), and it was anticipated that these growth factors would stimulate in vivo regeneration of chemotherapy or radiation-depleted HSCs *(7)*. Thrombopoietin (TPO), the physiologic regulator of platelet production, had been cloned *(8–12),* and the preclinical

From: *Cancer Drug Discovery and Development*
Hematopoietic Growth Factors in Oncology: Basic Science and Clinical Therapeutics
Edited by: G. Morstyn, M. Foote, and G. J. Lieschke © Humana Press Inc., Totowa, NJ

Table 1
Growth Factors Associated With Treatment of Therapy-Induced Cytopenia

Thrombocytopenia
Megakaryocyte growth and development factor (MGDF)
Thrombopoietin (TPO)
Interleukin-11 (IL-11)
Promegapoietin (PMP) (mpl-L/IL-3 chimeric)
TPO peptide mimetic
Granulocytopenia
Granulocyte colony-stimulating factor (G-CSF; filgrastim)
Granulocyte-macrophage colony-stimulating factor (GM-CSF; sargramostim, molgramostim)
Pegfilgrastim
Myelopoietins (leridistim; IL-3/G-CSF chimeric)
Peg-leridistim
Progenipoietins (Flt-3/G-CSF chimeric)
PEG-G-CSF (nartograstim)

database in support of its translational potential was consistent and substantial *(13–18)*. Interleukin-11 (IL-11), with a modest preclinical database, continued through clinical trials and was approved by the Food and Drug Administration (FDA) for prevention of chemotherapy-induced thrombocytopenia *(19,20)*. Additionally, new chimeric growth factor receptor agonists had been engineered, and second-generation variations of granulocyte colony-stimulating factor (G-CSF) and erythropoietin (EPO) were being evaluated in preclinical studies *(21–28)*. A new generation of small peptide and nonpeptidyl agonists of growth factor receptors and synthesized growth factor receptor-associated peptides was being investigated in early preclinical studies *(29–35)*. It appeared that control of treatment-associated myelosuppression, neutropenia, and thrombocytopenia was within reach. However, the translation from preclinical effectiveness in animal models to successful clinical trials has proved difficult and elusive for many new growth factors (Table 1).

2. THROMBOCYTOPOIETIC GROWTH FACTORS: TPO, PEG-MGDF, IL-11, AND PROMEGAPOIETIN

Clearly, the growth factor with the greatest potential for the treatment of thrombocytopenia is TPO. The thrombopoietic potential of the two mpl ligands (recombinant human [rHu] TPO, the full-length glycosylated molecule; and megakaryocyte growth and development factor, a nonglycosylated, polyethylene glycol-derived and truncated form of the full-length molecule [PEG-rHuMGDF]) being evaluated in clinical trials was evident early from the consistent and substantial amount of preclinical in vitro and in vivo data in both rodent and nonhuman primate models of myelosuppression *(13–18,36–41)*. Evaluation of the mpl ligands (PEG-rHuMGDF, rHuTPO) in nonhuman primate models of radiation-induced myelosuppression showed that it significantly lessened the degree and duration of thrombocytopenia and also improved myelopoietic and erythropoietic recovery *(17,18)*.

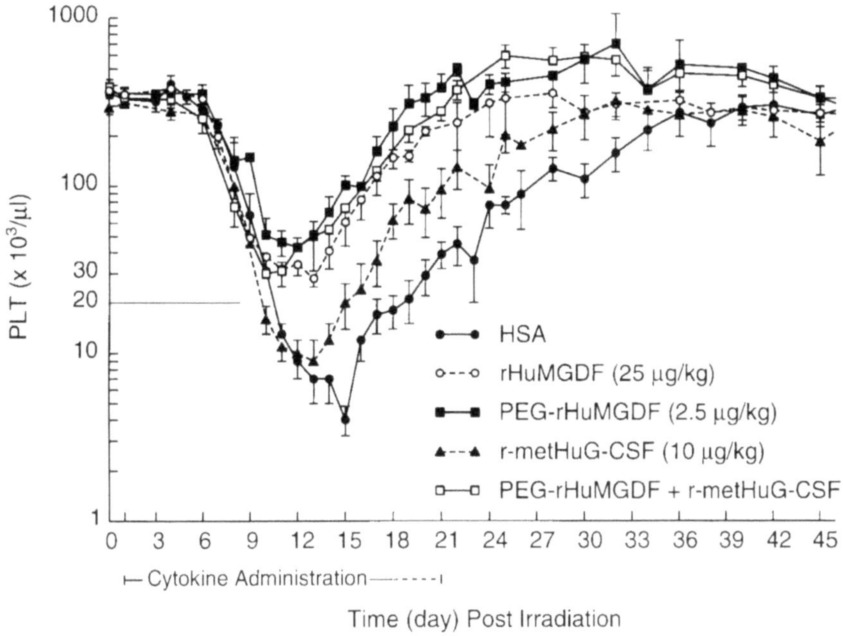

Fig. 1. Effects of cytokine administration on peripheral blood platelets (PLT) in irradiated primates. The PLT observed in irradiated rhesus macaques after recombinant human megakaryocyte growth and development factor (rHuMGDF), pegylated (PEG)-rHuMGDF, recombinant human methylated granulocyte colony-stimulating factor (r-metHuG-CSF), PEG-rHuMGDF combined with r-metHuG-CSF, or human serum albumin (HSA) administration. Cytokines or control protein were administered subcutaneously from d 1–18 post exposure. Data represent mean ± SEM of the absolute PLT for the cytokine or HSA-treated animals. (Reprinted with permission from ref. *17*.)

Farese et al. *(17)* first reported the therapeutic efficacy of PEG-rHuMGDF both alone and in combination with rHuG-CSF in a rhesus macaque model of severe radiation-induced myelosuppression. In that study, PEG-rHuMGDF showed an approx 10-fold increase in biologic activity relative to the nonpegylated MGDF. Both forms of the truncated MGDF, however, significantly improved all platelet-related parameters indicative of enhanced thrombopoiesis: platelet nadir, duration of thrombocytopenia, recovery time to a platelet count of >20 × 10^9/L, and number of whole blood transfusions (Fig. 1). It was of interest that PEG-rHuMGDF, co-administered with rHuG-CSF, significantly improved all platelet-related parameters relative to PEG-rHuMGDF monotherapy while significantly enhancing neutrophil recovery relative to rHuG-CSF monotherapy. Wagemaker's group noted comparable responses when evaluating the full-length mpl ligand rHuTPO, in a similar model of sublethally irradiated rhesus macaques *(18,38)*. In another series of studies, the truncated version of mpl ligand was evaluated as monotherapy and in combination with the high-affinity IL-3 receptor agonist called daniplestim in irradiated rhesus macaques *(39)*. Whereas the truncated form of mpl ligand was effective in significantly enhancing recovery of all platelet parameters, the combination of daniplestim plus mpl ligand further improved the stimulatory effect of cytokine monotherapy in this model of severe, radiation-induced myelosuppression (Fig. 2).

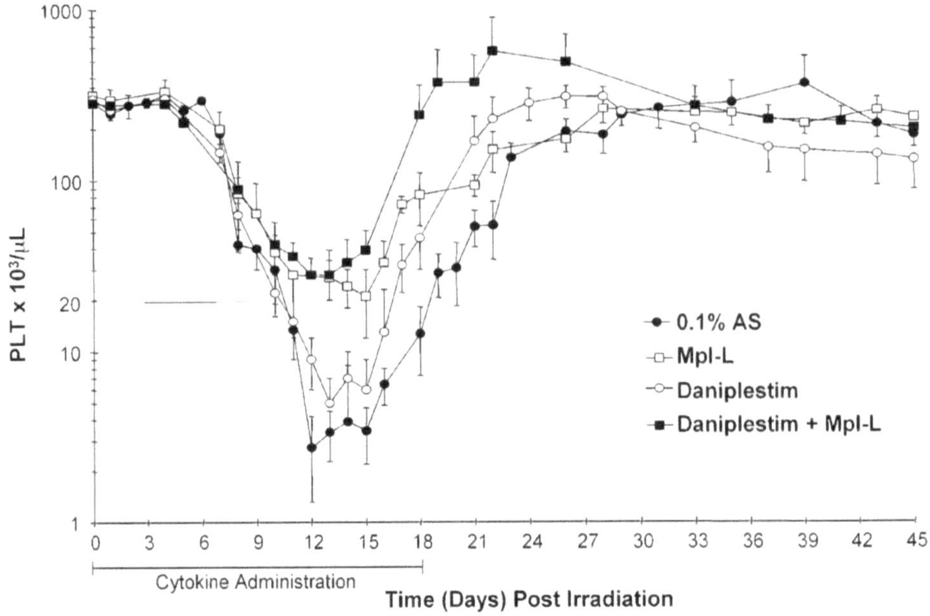

Fig. 2. Effects of cytokine administration on peripheral blood platelets (PLT) in 600-cGy X-irradiated nonhuman primates. The PLT were observed prior to and after treatment with control protein (0.1% autologous serum [AS]), daniplestim alone, mpl ligand (Mpl-L) alone, or combined daniplestim/Mpl-L. Cytokines or control protein were administered subcutaneously from d 1–18 post exposure. Data represent mean values (± SE). (Reprinted with permission from ref. *39.* © AlphaMed Press.)

The treatment efficacy of PEG-rHuMGDF and rHuTPO was further underscored by several studies that examined the timing of growth factor administration relative to a cytotoxic insult *(15,38,40)*. Whereas convention dictated the consecutive, daily administration of rHuG-CSF or recombinant human granulocyte colony-stimulating factor (rHuGM-CSF), it was shown that a single injection of PEG-rHuMGDF or rHuTPO at an early time (1–24 h) after irradiation is able to improve recovery from thrombocytopenia effectively in a manner equivalent to conventional daily administration of either mpl ligand *(16,41)*. Shibuya et al. *(15)* showed that a single injection of PEG-rHuMGDF, 1 h after sublethal irradiation of mice, effectively improved multilineage cell recovery in addition to marrow-derived, committed, and primitive hematopoietic progenitors. Neelis et al. *(38)* further defined the clinical potential of rHuTPO by investigating the efficacy of single-dose administration with co-administration of either rHuG-CSF or rHuGM-CSF in sublethally irradiated rhesus macaques (Fig. 3). As previously noted, there were no adverse effects of the co-administered cytokines, and a single administration of rHuTPO within hours of irradiation was sufficient to prevent thrombocytopenia *(15–18,38)*. Additionally, the single administration of rHuTPO significantly improved the performance of rHuG-CSF and rHuGM-CSF in alleviating severe neutropenia *(38)*. Remarkably, the single, low dose of rHuTPO or PEG-rHuMGDF administered within 24 h of exposure was as effective as conventional daily administration of the cytokine for 14–21 d in stimulating thrombopoiesis and recovery of platelets.

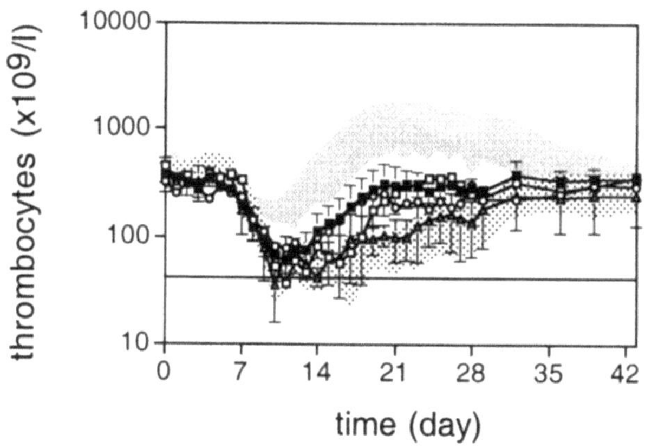

Fig. 3. Thrombocyte counts after 5 Gy TBI (d 0) for monkeys treated with TPO 5 μg (filled squares, $n = 4$) TPO 50 μg (open squares), TPO 0.5 μg (circles, $n = 2$), and concurrent placebo treatment (triangles, $n = 4$). The lower shaded area represents the mean (± SD) of four monkeys treated with human TPO for 21 d after irradiation. Data represent the arithmetic mean (± SD) of the various treatment groups. The horizontal line defines the level of thrombocytopenia (40×10^9/L) below which thrombocyte transfusions are given. (Reprinted with permission from ref. *38*. © American Society of Hematology.)

The magnitude of the thrombocytopoietic response was significantly affected by the time interval between PEG-rHuMGDF and radiation exposure. Delaying the initiation of PEG-rHuMGDF treatment remarkably reduced its therapeutic effects. A single injection of PEG-rHuMGDF at 60 h after irradiation of mice reduced its effect on platelet recovery to that of the control cohort *(15)*, whereas the initiation of consecutive daily injections of PEG-rHuMGDF 5 d after irradiation in rhesus macaques improved platelet recovery relative to control-treated cohorts but diminished its effect from that noted with initiation of treatment on d 1 *(41)*. It is apparent that treatment, to be effective, must be initiated early (within 24 h) after the cytotoxic insult. These results are consistent with studies demonstrating that treatment efficacy of rHuG-CSF, pegfilgrastim, IL-6, or IL-11 is most effective when initiated early after irradiation *(42–45)*. These data suggested that although abbreviated single or every-other-day administration schedules may be effective, PEG-rHuMGDF or rHuTPO must be initiated early after a cytotoxic insult.

A singular disappointment in the preclinical development of the mpl ligands was their lack of therapeutic efficacy when administered subsequent to autologous bone marrow transplantation (AuBMT) in nonhuman primates or canines. Neither rHuTPO nor PEG-rHuMGDF, administered daily at a standard dose (2.5–10 μg/kg/d) for several weeks after transplant, prevented thrombocytopenia consequent to myelosuppressive conditioning for AuBMT, nor did it stimulate regeneration of platelets to normal values (Fig. 4) *(46–49)*. These results are consistent with the clinical trial experience *(50–54)*. Conventional doses and schedule of administration of rHuTPO or PEG-rHuMGDF were ineffective in demonstrating meaningful benefit after stem cell transplantation. The preclinical and clinical experience suggests that control of cytotoxic therapy-associated thrombocytopenia would be dependent on defining optimal dose and schedule for specific myelotoxic regimens. Based on mathematical modeling of PEG-rHuMGDF

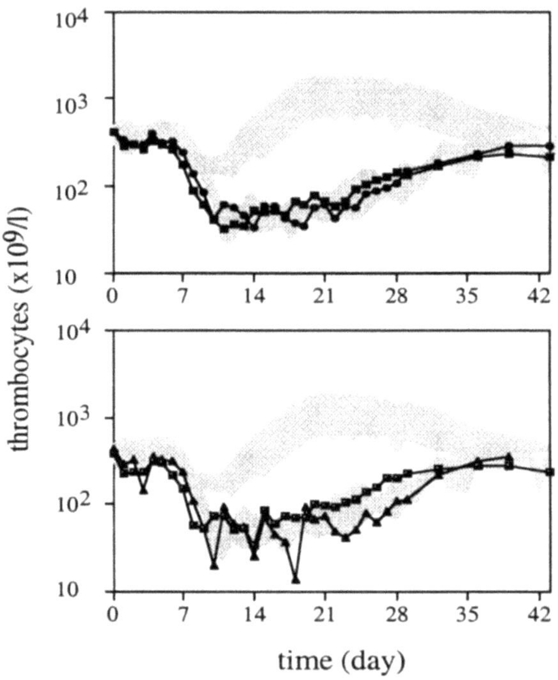

Fig. 4. Comparison of the effect of TPO after transplantation of purified stem cells and unfractionated bone marrow. In the upper panel the mean thrombocyte counts of four TPO-treated stem cell-transplanted monkeys (closed squares) and three placebo-treated stem cell-transplanted monkeys (closed circles) are plotted. The lower panel displays the mean of two TPO-treated unfractionated marrow-transplanted monkeys (half-closed squares) and the unfractionated marrow-transplanted control monkey (closed triangles). The dose and route of TPO were the same for all monkeys (10 µg/kg/d, sc, d 1–21). The shaded areas represent means ± SDs of thrombocyte levels of 5-Gy irradiated monkeys after TBI: the lower shaded area represents eight placebo-treated controls, and the upper one four TPO-treated monkeys. (Reprinted with permission from ref. *46*. © 1997, with permission from Elsevier.)

pharmacokinetics and pharmacodynamics, Farese et al. examined the relative efficacy of administering PEG-rHuMGDF in several regimens to rhesus macaques receiving AuBMT *(47,55)*. Conventional, consecutive, daily administration of PEG-rHuMGDF initiated within 24 h of AuBMT failed to enhance platelet recovery. PEG-rHuMGDF when administered either before (d –9 to d –5), or after (daily injections initiated on d 1 after AuBMT) or in an abbreviated schedule with high doses administered at d 1 and d 3 after AuBMT, significantly lessened the duration of thrombocytopenia (Fig. 5). These data confirmed predictions from pharmacokinetic/pharmacodynamic modeling that thrombocytopenia can be prevented after AuBMT using the appropriate dose and schedule of PEG-rHuMGDF.

2.1. IL-11

The preclinical pharmacology associated with rHuIL-11 administration to rodent and nonhuman primate models of modest, chemotherapy-induced thrombocytopenia showed consistent stimulation of platelet recovery relative to control cohorts

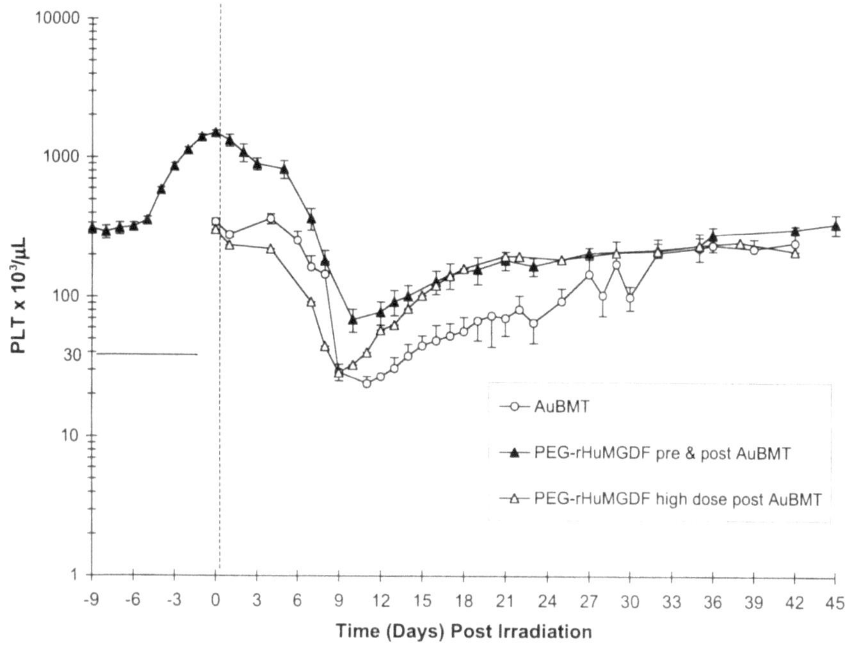

Fig. 5. Effect of PEG-rHuMGDF on platelet (PLT) recovery after autologous bone marrow transplantation (AuBMT). Mean peripheral PLT × 10^3/µL (± SEM) in rhesus monkeys after myeloablation and AuBMT with either no cytokine treatment (AuBMT, $n = 9$) or pegylated recombinant human megakaryocyte growth and development factor (PEG-rHuMGDF) administration before and after transplant (2.5 µg/kg/d, from d –9 to d –5 and d 1 post AuBMT until platelet counts reached 200,000/µL (PEG-rHuMGDF pre and post AuBMT, $n = 4$) or high-dose PEG-rHuMGDF administration (300 µg/kg/d) on d 1 and d 3 only post AuBMT (high-dose PEG-rHuMGDF post AuBMT, $n = 5$). (Reprinted with permission from ref. *47*. © AlphaMed Press.)

(42,56–58). In carboplatin-treated rhesus macaques, rHuIL-11 administered within 24 h after cessation of chemotherapy significantly reduced the depth of the platelet nadir and significantly accelerated platelet recovery compared with the control-treated group *(58)*. Mean platelet counts were <50 × 10^9/L for 2 d relative to 5.5 d for the rHuIL-11 and control-treated cohorts, respectively. An additional study in cynomolgous macaques subjected to nimustine (ACNU)-induced thrombocytopenia confirmed that rHuIL-11 therapy initiated within 24 h of ACNU and continued for 21 d could successfully improve platelet nadir and recovery time compared with the control cohort *(57)*. Leonard et al. *(42)* showed that the increased platelet recovery was markedly affected by the interval between chemotherapy and rHuIL-11 administration. Only when rHuIL-11 was injected within 24 h after chemotherapy were the platelet-related parameters improved. Longer delays in platelet recovery were noted with increasing intervals between chemotherapy and rHuIL-11 administration. Furthermore, the most effective administration schedule required 14 d of consecutive administration. A more modest effect of IL-11 therapy was observed after treatment of sublethally irradiated canines *(59)*. Irradiated dogs were treated with rHuIL-11 starting within 2 h of irradiation and continued for 28 d. The rHuIL-11-treated cohort

had decreased platelet counts (<150 × 10^9/L) for a median of 24 d, compared with 28 d for the control group. Although there was a modest trend toward accelerated recovery, the results were not significant.

Collins et al. *(60)*, in an interesting abstract report, described the combination of rHuIL-11 with recombinant murine TPO (rMuTPO) in a murine model of carboplatin/irradiation-induced myelosuppression. Mice were treated with rHuIL-11 for 10 consecutive days, or rMuTPO every other day, for 10 d as monotherapy or the combination of rHuIL-11 and rMuTPO in their respective regimens. Although the respective monotherapy improved both platelet nadir and recovery, co-administration significantly improved the platelet parameters and completely abrogated the carboplatin/irradiation-induced thrombocytopenia. The combined rHuIL-11/rMuTPO treatment prevented severe anemia and stimulated a marked increase in marrow-derived megakaryocyte progenitors. These data suggested that combined IL-11 and TPO, administered in the schedule described, can significantly improve platelet recovery after myelosuppression. rHuIL-3 has also been combined with rHuIL-11 in a demonstration of hematopoietic synergy in rodent models of severe myelosuppression or bone marrow transplantation *(61)*. The combined therapy enhanced platelet recovery and increased survival of lethally irradiated mice. The pharmacology associated with IL-11 administration suggested that in myelosuppressed patients, treatment with rHuIL-11 must be initiated within 24 h of chemotherapy and maintained for an adequate duration for optimal efficacy in preventing severe thrombocytopenia.

2.2. Chimeric Growth Factor Receptor Agonist (Promegapoietin)

Subsequent to cloning of the mpl ligands, a family of novel, engineered, chimeric cytokine receptor agonists for the IL-3 and mpl receptor called promegapoietin (PMP) was developed *(62)*.

PMP showed significant therapeutic efficacy for restoration of platelets in preclinical models of irradiation-induced myelosuppression in a manner comparable to that noted for PEG-rHuMGDF and rHuTPO. It was shown that, similar to PEG-rHuMGDF or rHuTPO, a single dose of PMP administered within 1–2 h after exposure was comparable in therapeutic efficacy to the conventional daily administration of PMP in enhancing thrombopoietic recovery from severe radiation-induced myelosuppression (Fig. 6) *(22)*. PMP was evaluated in four administration schedules: daily for 18 d; 9 doses every other day for 3 wk; a single high dose at 20 h; or a single high dose 2 h after 600-cGy total body irradiation in the rhesus macaque. PMP, irrespective of administration schedule, significantly improved all platelet-related parameters, thrombocytopenia was eliminated, severity of platelet nadirs was significantly improved, and duration of thrombocytopenia was significantly reduced relative to the control-treated cohort. Consequently, all PMP-treated cohorts were transfusion-independent *(22)*. These results provided a clear rationale for the clinical evaluation of promegapoietin and its potential for increased efficacy owing to the IL-3 component of the chimeric molecule.

3. GRANULOPOIETIC GROWTH FACTORS: MYELOPOIETINS, PROGENIPOIETIN, PEG-LERIDISTIM, AND PEGFILGRASTIM

The granulopoietic cytokines rHuG-CSF and rHuGM-CSF remain the standard of treatment for cytotoxic therapy-induced neutropenia *(63–67)*. Although effective in

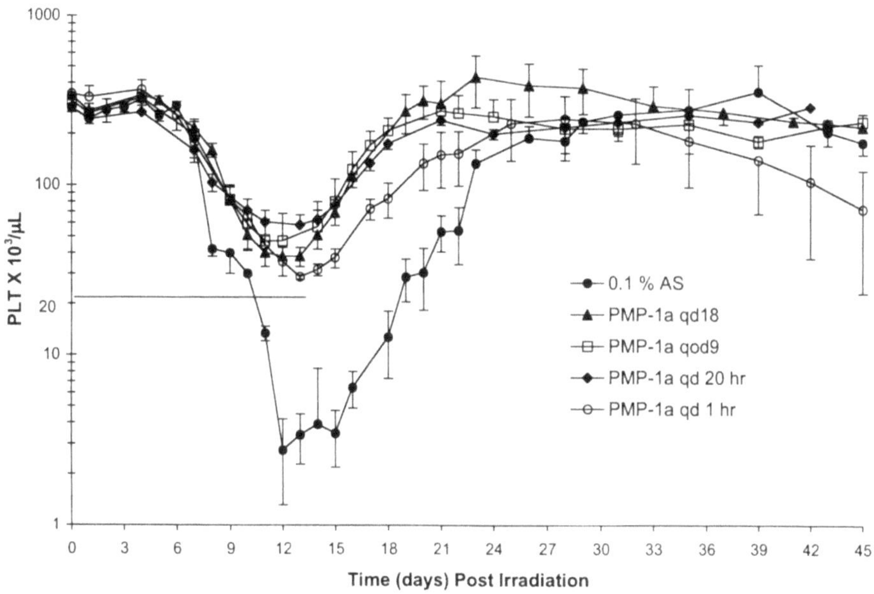

Fig. 6. Effects of promegapoietin (PMP)-1a administration in four different schedules on peripheral blood platelets (PLT) in 600-cGy X-irradiated nonhuman primates. The PLT were observed before and after treatment with control protein (0.1% autologous serum, n = 11), or PMP-1a administered: (1) qd for 18 d; (2) qod for 9 injections (qod 9, n = 4); (3) qd one time at 20 h (qd 20 h, n = 4); and (4) qd one time at 1 h post TBI (qd 1 h, n = 3). Data represent the mean values (± SE). (Reprinted with permission from ref. *22*. © AlphaMed Press.)

conventional daily administration schedules, the repetitive administration has drawbacks in the multiple-cycle, chemotherapy setting. Multiple daily injections of colony-stimulating factors are inconvenient to patients and support staff, promote noncompliance and potential for missed doses, and negatively impact the patient's quality of life. The modest pharmacokinetic parameters of filgrastim necessitate daily administration to modulate the chemotherapy-induced neutropenia. An abbreviated administration schedule with therapeutic efficiency equivalent to conventional, every-day administration, would be favorable in the clinical setting.

3.1. Chimeric Growth Factor Receptor Agonists: Myelopoietins, Leridistem, and Peg-Leridistim

3.1.1. Myelopoietin

Myelopoietins are a family of proteins that are dual receptor agonists of the human IL-3 and G-CSF receptor complexes. Two members of the myelopoietin family, myelopoietin SC-68420 and leridistim, have been evaluated for their ability to enhance hematopoietic recovery in a nonhuman primate model of radiation-induced myelosuppression *(21,68)*. Myelopoietin (SC-68420) was initially shown to effectively stimulate bone marrow regeneration (clonogenic activity) and neutrophil recovery when administered daily, subcutaneously, in a twice-a-day or once-a-day schedule beginning on d 1 after irradiation and continued for 18–23 d *(21)*. Myelopoietin, regardless of administration schedule, significantly reduced the mean duration of neutropenia and improved the neutrophil nadir and time to recovery of neutrophils to an ANC $> 0.5 \times 10^9$/L relative to the control-treated cohort. Thus myelopoietin (SC-68240) administered daily was as effective as a twice-a-day schedule for enhancing neutrophil recovery after high-dose radiation-induced myelosuppression.

3.1.2. Leridistim

These results prompted further evaluation of another structurally distinct member of the myelopoietin family, leridistim.

Leridistim was evaluated in a more abbreviated schedule, lower dose, and intravenous vs subcutaneous administration route *(68)*. Animals were irradiated on d 0 and then received, on d 1, leridistim sc in an abbreviated, every-other-day schedule at 200 μg/kg or daily at 50 μg/kg; or iv, daily or every-other-day schedules at 200 μg/kg/injection. Other experimental cohorts received filgrastim in an every-other-day schedule at 100 μg/kg/injection or autologous serum (daily). Leridistim was administered until an absolute neutrophil count (ANC) $\geq 3 \times 10^9$/L was attained (range: 13–18 d). Leridistim administered subcutaneously in an alternate-day schedule significantly enhanced neutrophil recovery. The abbreviated, every-other-day schedule administered subcutaneously was as effective as the conventional daily or twice-a-day schedule used to assess myelopoietin (SC-68240), in the same animal model (Table 2) *(21)*. This response was of interest considering the ineffective results of leridistim's component growth factors, IL-3 and G-CSF, when administered in schedules less than twice a day or daily, respectively. Filgrastim (100 μg/kg) administered in an sc, every-other-day schedule did not significantly enhance neutrophil-related parameters *(68)*. On the other hand, filgrastim administered in a conventional daily, schedule either alone or in combination with daniplestim (an IL-3 receptor agonist) effectively enhanced neutrophil recovery in two similar models of radiation-induced myelosuppression *(17,18,69)*. It was hypothesized that since IL-3 receptors are present on $CD34^+$ cell subsets purified from human and rhesus marrow *(70,71)*, the IL-3 component in leridistim could contribute to the enhanced granulopoietic response by priming progenitor cells for subsequent stimulation by endogenous growth factors released within the radiation-damaged marrow microenvironment *(72,73)* as well as by exerting trophic or survival-promoting effects on responsive progenitors *(74–77)*. These data suggested that if the appropriate dose and schedule could be achieved in clinical trials, leridistim would be an effective therapeutic for drug-induced myelosuppression.

3.1.3. Peg-Leridistim

Leridistim was subsequently pegylated using a 30-kDa polyethylene glycol moiety attached to the *Escherichia coli*-derived leridistim. Peg-leridistim was subjected to pharmacokinetic and pharmacodynamic analysis before evaluating biologic efficacy in a rhesus model of radiation-induced myelosuppression. The pharmacokinetic parameters assessed after the administration of a single, subcutaneous bolus to normal rhesus monkeys indicated that pegylation effectively enhanced overall relative exposure (area under the concentration curve [AUC]) by delaying the time (T_{max}) to, as well as the level of, the observed maximum plasma concentration (C_{max}), while also effectively doubling the elimination half-life ($T_{1/2}$). The net result was a reduction in overall rate of clearance by nearly 20-fold *(78)*. The pharmacokinetic analysis of peg-leridistim in

Table 2
Neutrophil-Related Parameters in Sublethally X-Irradiated Rhesus Monkeys Treated With Leridistim: Duration, Nadir, Time to Recovery, and Clinical Support[a]

Treatment (dose, route, schedule)	*Duration (d) of neutropenia*	*ANC nadir (L^{-1})*	*Time to recovery (d)*	*Antibiotic support (d)*
Control 0.1% AS, sc, qd	19.1 ± 2.3	16 ± 6	24.5 ± 2.2	19.6 ± 1.7
Leridistim				
50 µg/kg, sc, qd	3.3 ± 1.6*	400 ± 100*	11.0 ± 2.4*	8.0 ± 2.2*
200 µg/kg, sc, qod	1.0 ± 0.6*	601 ± 100*	4.1 ± 2.2*	5.8 ± 1.0*
200 µg/kg, iv, qd	2.7 ± 1.8*	442 ± 227*	7.0 ± 4.4*	4.3 ± 3.0*
200 µg/kg, iv, qod	9.0 ± 1.7**	63 ± 30**	16.3 ± 1.2**	14.7 ± 0.3
G-CSF				
100 µg/kg, sc, qod	14.2 ± 1.9	10 ± 4	19.4 ± 1.7	17.8 ± 1.8
SC-64820, myelopoietin				
200 µg/kg, sc, qd[b]	2.8 ± 1.4	435 ± 200	8.3 ± 3.5	8.3 ± 1.3

ABBREVIATION: ANC, absolute neutrophil count; G-CSF, granulocyte colony-stimulating factor.

[a] Monkeys received total body irradiation (250 kVp) to 600 cGy with X-radiation and were treated subcutaneously (sc) with control protein, autologous serum (AS) (n = 9) or leridistim at 200 µg/kg/d, every other day (qod) (n = 8), or 50 µg/kg/d, daily (qd) (n = 7) or intravenously (iv) with leridistim at 200 µg/kg/d either qd or qod, n = 3 per cohort according to protocol. The duration of neutropenia is defined as days of absolute neutrophil count (ANC) $< 0.5 \times 10^9$/L and thrombocytopenia is defined as days of platelets $< 20 \times 10^9$/L. Time to recovery is the number of days required for the ANC to reach $\geq 0.5 \times 10^9$/L and platelets to reach $\geq 20 \times 10^9$/L. Data represent mean values ± SEM.

[b] Previous Dataset: published study showing effects of SC-68420, myelopoietin, administered daily (qd) subcutaneously at 200 µg/d in the same 600 cGy X-irradiation model *(21)*. This study showed that sc, qd, and bid administration were equivalent in bioeffect.

* Statistically different from AS-treated controls ($p < 0.01$).

** Statistically different from AS-treated controls ($p < 0.05$).

irradiated monkeys suggested that the net effect was a slowing of the receptor-mediated clearance as neutrophil counts decreased and an effective enhancement of the observed elimination half-life ($t_{1/2}$) from 7–8 h to 33 h.

Peg-leridistim was evaluated as a single- or two-dose regimen separated by 4 or 7 d, to significantly improve neutrophil recovery after radiation-induced myelosuppression (Fig. 7) *(78)*. Two groups received Peg-leridistim or leridistim at a dose of 600 µg/kg on d 1, and two other groups received Peg-leridistim at 200 µg/kg on d 1 and d 4 or 7. This study showed that all Peg-leridistim treatment schedules significantly improved all neutrophil-related parameters after irradiation compared with the control-treated cohort and were equivalent in effect when compared among themselves. Furthermore, the Peg-leridistim-induced improvement in neutrophil regeneration was equivalent to that noted with leridistim or myelopoietin administered in the conventional daily or every-other-day schedule *(21,68)*. Therefore, the single injection of Peg-leridistim was equivalent in effect to the double injection of Peg-leridistim and leridistim administered twice a day, daily, or every other day over 18–23 d after irradiation.

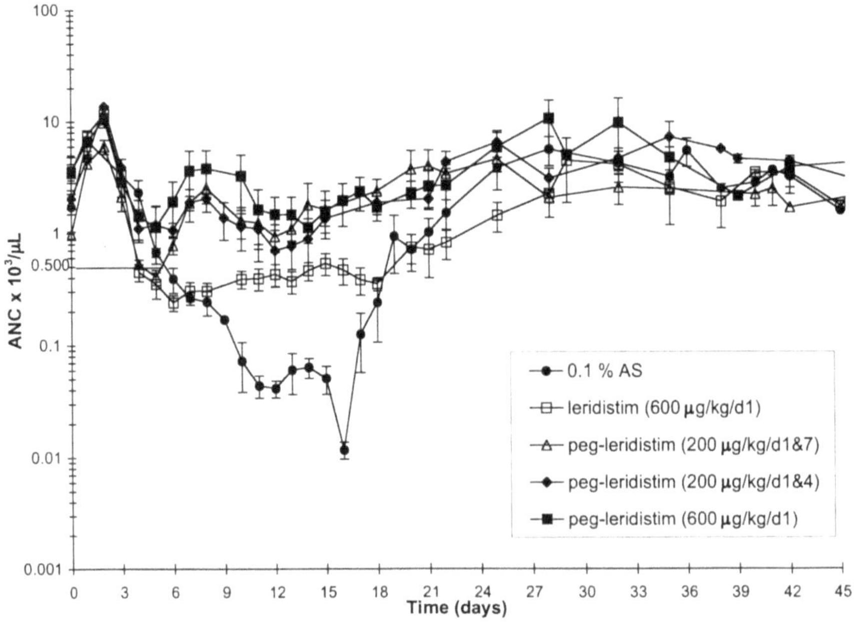

Fig. 7. Effect of leridistim and peg-leridistim on peripheral blood absolute neutrophil counts (ANC) in 600-cGy X-irradiated rhesus macaques. Animals were administered either leridistim (n = 4) or peg-leridistim (n = 5) at 600 µg/kg on d 1, or peg-leridistim on d 1 and d 4 (n = 4), or d 1 and d 7 (n = 4) at 200 µg/kg/d, or control autologous serum (AS) (n = 7). Values are mean ± SE. (Reprinted with permission from ref. *78*. © AlphaMed Press.)

3.2. Pegfilgrastim

Pegfilgrastim, a new form of filgrastim, has been manufactured by the covalent attachment of a 20-kDa polyethylene glycol moiety to the amino terminus of *E. coli*-derived filgrastim. Recent studies in a rodent model of 5-fluorouracil (5-FU)-induced myelosuppression showed improved neutrophil recovery after a single dose of pegfilgrastim *(79)*. Hartley et al. *(80)* extended these studies and evaluated the timing of pegfilgrastim administration relative to chemotherapy. Pegfilgrastim was administered at various times, either before or after treatment of mice with cyclophosphamide. Preadministration of pegfilgrastim was relatively ineffective, whereas pegfilgrastim injected early (on d 1 after chemotherapy) appeared to be the most effective in delaying the severity and duration of neutropenia. Further delaying the single-dose administration of pegfilgrastim lessened its effectiveness.

Recent preclinical studies from our laboratory underscored the therapeutic potential of the pegylated form of filgrastim *(24,26)*. A single dose of pegfilgrastim was effective in improving neutrophil recovery in nonhuman primate models of myelosuppression or AuBMT subsequent to high-dose radiation conditioning. Neutrophil recovery, after a single injection of pegfilgrastim (300 µg/kg), was equivalent to conventional daily dosing (10 µg/kg) with filgrastim, whereas when pegfilgrastim was administered as two doses on d 1 and d 7 after irradiation, neutrophil recovery was significantly improved relative to filgrastim after radiation-induced myelosuppression *(26)*. One dose

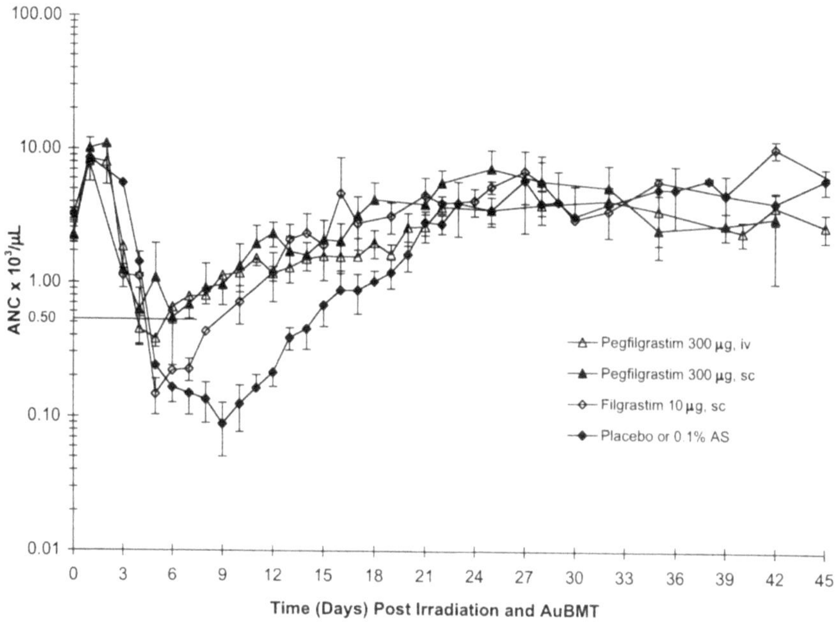

Fig. 8. Effect of pegfilgrastim administration on peripheral blood absolute neutrophil counts (ANC) recovery after 920-cGy X-irradiation and autologous bone marrow transplantation (AuBMT) in rhesus macaques. ANC recovery was observed in animals administered pegfilgrstim at 300 μg/kg iv (*n* = 4) or sc (*n* = 3), or filgrastim at 10 μg/kg daily (*n* = 4) via sc administration until the ANC reached 3,000/μL (range 12–17 d), or control autologous sera on d 1–18 (*n* = 13) after irradiation and AuBMT. Values are means ± SEM. (Reprinted with permission from ref. *24*.)

of pegfilgrastim (300 μg/kg) also significantly improved neutrophil recovery relative to conventional filgrastim treatment after AuBMT (Fig. 8) *(24)*. These results were consistent with prospective modeling and simulations based on pharmacokinetic and pharmacodynamic analysis in normal animals and early phase 1 clinical trials *(81,82)*.

3.3. Progenipoietins

Progenipoietins (ProGPs) are another class of engineered proteins containing both fetal liver tyrosine kinase-3 (flt-3) and G-CSF receptor agonist activities *(27)*. Initial in vitro and in vivo studies suggested that the ProGP family of dual receptor agonists were potent HGFs, combining the synergistic potential of flt-3 ligand and G-CSF in a single molecule. In vitro, the ProGP molecules bound to flt-3 ligand and G-CSF receptors with approximately the same equilibrium dissociation constants as the native ligands and can bind both flt-3 and G-CSF receptors simultaneously, promote the proliferation of flt-3- and G-CSF-responsive cell lines, and stimulate growth of clonogenic colony-forming cells with potency greater than the combination of flt-3 and G-CSF *(27)*. A series of in vivo studies in normal mice confirmed the hematopoietic potential of these molecules to include the mobilization of significant numbers of dendritic cells into peripheral blood and spleen *(27)*. These early results suggested the continued evaluation of selected progenipoietins in an effort to decipher their therapeutic utility in enhancing myeloid and immune reconstitution after radiation-induced myelosuppression.

Structurally distinct members of the progenipoietins, ProGP-1, -2, and -4 were evaluated for their ability to stimulate hematopoietic recovery in a well-codified model of radiation-induced myelosuppression in the rhesus macaque *(23,25)*. The ProGPs were assessed in a conventional daily administration and in an abbreviated, every-other-day schedule, beginning on d 1 after irradiation and continuing until the ANC was $>3 \times 10^9$/L (range: 12–14 d). ProGP-1, -2, and -4, at all doses and administration schedules, significantly improved neutrophil nadirs, duration of neutropenia, and time to recovery of ANC to $>0.5 \times 10^9$/L. Additionally, the number of days in which antibiotic support was required were significantly reduced relative to the control cohort. Control, neutropenic nadirs were improved from a range of 8–16/µL to 350–413/µL, and neutropenic durations (days of ANC $< 0.5 \times 10^9$/L) were improved from approx d 16 in controls to <d 2 after ProGP administration. The ProGP molecules can effectively stimulate recovery of neutrophils in high-dose, irradiated rhesus macaques and therefore may have had an important role in the clinical setting for management of the myelosuppressed host.

4. CYTOKINE-BASED TREATMENT FOR IMMUNE RECONSTITUTION: IL-7, KERATINOCYTE GROWTH FACTOR

Acute hematopoietic toxicity remains as a dose-limiting factor consequent to intensive chemotherapy and/or preparative regimens for stem cell transplantation. Growth factor therapy using filgrastim, pegfilgrastim, rHuGM-CSF, or rHuIL-11 has provided a measure of support for acute myelosuppression *(19,20,65–67,83–88)*. No effective treatment is available for prolonged T-lymphocyte deficiencies associated with cytotoxic therapy and stem cell transplantation.

Immune suppression, as profound cytotoxicity to the T-cell compartment, is a common problem associated with high-dose chemotherapy, myeloablative conditioning for stem cell transplantation, and human immunodeficiency virus (HIV) infection *(89–93)*. Significant delay in regeneration of CD4 T cells, impaired function of newly generated CD8 T cells, marked imbalance in the CD4/CD8 ratio and a limited T-cell receptor (TCR) repertoire leave the patient at risk for infectious complications and viral disease. Therefore, new therapeutic strategies are required that can promote the naive, thymic-dependent, T-cell regeneration that is essential for long-term immune reconstitution.

Several growth factors, including IL-2, -4, -7, and -17, c-kit ligand, flt-3 ligand, and thymic stromal lymphopoietin, are associated with T-cell differentiation and proliferation *(94–100)*. Of these cytokines, IL-7, produced by both thymic and marrow stroma *(101)*, acts at a later stage in development and is a requisite factor in lymphopoiesis *(98–103)*. The pleiotropic c-kit ligand and flt-3 ligand act at the very early stages of hematopoietic and lymphoid development. c-kit ligand has been shown to recruit candidate murine stem cells, whereas flt-3 ligand appears to be essential in the development of these cells toward lymphoid-restricted progenitors in vivo *(7)* and in vitro *(94,104–106)*. Furthermore, flt-3 ligand, through its action on dendritic cell expansion, may augment antigen-driven peripheral T-cell homeostasis *(107–109)*. Fry et al., using flt-3 ligand in rodent models of bone marrow transplant in both thymectomized and euthymic recipients, suggested that it is capable of enhancing both thymic-independent and thymopoietic homeostatic pathways for T-cell restoration *(107,110)*.

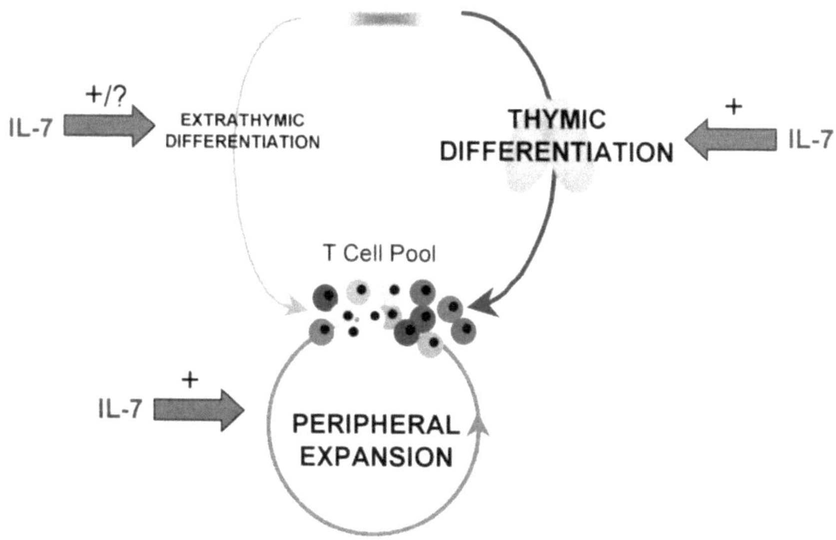

Fig. 9. Modulation of T-cell regenerative pathways by interleukin-7 (IL-7). After T-cell depletion, regeneration of the peripheral T-cell pool can occur through multiple mechanisms. (Reprinted with permission from ref. *116*. © American Society of Hematology.)

4.1. IL-7

IL-7 administration increased the rate of T-cell immune reconstitution in murine models of AuBMT and/or chemotherapy-induced cytotoxicity *(111–115)*. Bolotin et al. *(114)* showed that relative to controls, bone marrow-transplanted mice treated with rHuIL-7 had more rapid normalization of thymic cellularity, normal proportions of thymic cellular subsets, peripheral $CD4^+$ cells, and improved antigen-specific T- and B-cell function. Mackall and colleagues *(116)* extended these studies to show that rHuIL-7 administration exerts its beneficial effect on immune reconstitution by increased thymopoiesis and a direct increase in the magnitude of antigen-driven peripheral expansion (Fig. 9) *(116)*. Thus, treatment with rHuIL-7 enhances thymopoiesis after chemotherapy or myeloablative transplant conditioning as well as antigen-driven T-cell expansion in T-cell depleted or thymic-deficient hosts *(111–117)*.

A cautionary note should be applied considering the use of rHuIL-7 therapy in the context of graft-vs-host disease (GvHD) after allogeneic stem cell transplant. Pharmacologic doses of rHuIL-7 may have potent effects on mature T cells *(115,117)*. rHuIL-7 treatment may induce peripheral T cell expansion and effectively enhance the response of mature T cells to alloantigen. These consequences may well predict enhancement of GvHD and graft rejection. Mackall's group used a murine model of parent stem cells into F1 progeny to study the effect of rHuIL-7 on immune reconstitution and GvHD after allogeneic bone marrow transplant (AlloBMT). In this model, administration of rHuIL-7 lowered the threshold dose of T cells required to induce clinical signs of GvHD as well as lethal GvHD. rHuIL-7 administration was associated with a greater degree of inflammation and tissue damage at all T-cell doses used. It was observed, however, that in a setting of AlloBMT in T-cell-depleted hosts, rHuIL-7 therapy enhanced thymic function, although not to the degree noted with treatment of syngeneic bone marrow recipients. This study stands in contrast to that reported by Alpodogan et al. *(118)*, in which post-transplant administration of rHuIL-7 to recipients of AlloBMT enhanced lymphoid reconstitution without aggravating GvHD. It was noted that the alloreactive donor-derived T-cells from the AlloBMT recipients expressed few IL-7 receptors. Resolution of these disparate results will require further examination of the respective variations in IL-7 dose and time and duration of IL-7 administration.

4.2. Keratinocyte Growth Factor

Keratinocyte growth factor (KGF), a member of the acidic fibroblast growth factor (FGF-7) family, is produced by fibroblasts and mesenchymal cells and acts on a wide range of epithelial-derived cells that express a unique splice variant of the FGFR2 receptor *(119–122)*. Mice that are lacking either FGF-10 or FGFR2 splice variant have significant defects in thymopoiesis, hypoplastic thymic tissue, and impaired thymic epithelial cell development *(121,123)*. Additionally, KGF has been shown to protect epithelial cells from chemotherapy- or radiation-induced injury *(124,125)*. Subsequent studies demonstrated that pretreatment of mice with rHuKGF ameliorated GvHD and manifestations of idiopathic pneumonia after intensive chemotherapy-induced conditioning and AlloBMT *(126–128)*. Pretreatment with rHuKGF reduced GvHD-induced weight loss and mortality as well as lesions in the skin and lungs of the long-term survivors *(126)*. Krijanovsky et al. *(129)* showed that rHuKGF given before and after AlloBMT ameliorated GvHD while preserving the graft-versus-leukemia (GvL) properties of the graft. Blazar's group *(130)* extended these early studies and further demonstrated that rHuKGF reduced GvHD, by mechanisms independent of repair of the conditioning-induced injury. Murine GvHD could be ameliorated in the absence of conditioning in SCID recipients of allogenic T cells. rHuKGF could be administered before (3-d course) or after (7-d course) T-cell transfer with no difference in survival, although the post-treatment schedule promoted higher body weights.

Blazar and Weinberg further extended these studies by determining the ability of rHuKGF pretreatment to enhance immune reconstitution through its restorative/protective effect on thymic epithelial cells and consequent production of intrathymic IL-7 *(131)*. In this report, the rHuKGF-treated recipients showed enhanced thymopoiesis and increased numbers of functional peripheral T cells. Furthermore, rHuKGF pretreatment increased thymopoietic capacity of mice after congenic or AlloBMT and after any of five conditioning regimens that differed in radiation dose or cytotoxic therapy. It was noted previously that rHuKGF treatment decreased the incidence and severity of GvHD in murine allogeneic recipients, most likely by decreasing the degree of epithelial cell damage associated with GvHD *(130)*. It is not apparent in the work by Min et al. *(131)* that rHuKGF administration could prevent GvHD-induced thymic injury, since overt GvHD did not develop in their model.

4.3. What's New: Ligand Receptor-Associated Peptides and Ligand Mimetics

A new series of synthesized peptides has been described. These peptides are identical to an extracellular domain of the selected growth factor/hormone receptor and are distant from the ligand-binding site *(34,132)*. This peptide activates the receptor signal transduction pathway in the absence of the natural ligand. Naranda et al. *(34)* reported on the synthesis of a peptide that activates the EPO receptor domain in the absence of EPO. Furthermore, neither the peptide nor EPO altered the affinity of the other for the receptor; thus the peptide does not bind to the EPO binding site. In vivo activity in this regard was demonstrated in a rodent model of carboplatin-induced anemia. Administration of the EPO receptor peptide, in the absence of exogenously administered EPO, significantly improved the hematocrit value relative to the control cohort.

These investigators have recently synthesized another peptide that binds to a portion of the extracellular domain of the human TPO receptor, c-mpl (Dr. Lennart Olsson, personal communication). As noted with the EPO receptor peptide, this peptide binds to c-mpl elsewhere than at the TPO binding site; therefore peptide and growth factor may act together for additive or synergistic activity. Preclinical experiments in rodent models of chemotherapy-induced thrombocytopenia have shown the TPO receptor peptide to be as efficient as recombinant TPO in enhancing platelet recovery. It was also conveyed that the TPO receptor peptide can act in synergy with administered TPO or with the endogenous TPO released *in situ* during periods of thrombocytopenia.

These peptides differ from the previously described EPO mimetics and peptide agonists of the TPO receptor c-mpl *(29–33)*. The mimetic peptides bind and compete with the natural ligand for the binding site. In the case of agonists for c-mpl, dimeric peptides were constructed that had greater affinity and potency than the monomeric peptide. The peptide dimer stimulated proliferation of megakaryocyte progenitors and maturation of megakaryocytes from human bone marrow *(29)*.

Recently, a nonpeptidyl small molecule that is capable of activating the G-CSF receptor signal transduction pathway, both in vitro and in vivo, has been reported *(133)*. Tian et al. *(133)* have described the identification of this molecule (SB247464), which binds to the extracellular domain of the G-CSF receptor that is distinct from the G-CSF binding site. This G-CSF mimic stimulated granulocyte colonies from murine bone marrow and significantly increased neutrophil counts when administered on a daily basis to normal mice.

To the best of our knowledge, these growth factor mimetics and peptide receptor agonists have not been further evaluated in animal models of chemotherapy or radiation-induced myelosuppression.

5. SUMMARY

The potential for effective therapeutic treatment of chemotherapy-induced neutropenia and thrombocytopenia was high. In preclinical models, a single injection of either mpl ligand (PEG-rHuMGDF or rHuTPO) was effective in ameliorating radiation-induced thrombocytopenia. The new-generation pegylated forms of filgrastim and leridistim showed that a single injection has therapeutic efficacy equivalent to respective, conventional daily dosing. The potential for single injections of a mpl ligand and a pegylated form of G-CSF to control the thrombocytopenia and neutropenia observed in the oncology setting was evident. However, PEG-rHuMGDF, promegapoietin, leridistim, and progenipoietin have been removed from human trials, and development of Peg-leridistim has been stopped. At this writing, TPO remains in clinical trials within the United States, although the optimum schedule appears to require prophylactic administration in dose-intensive chemotherapy regimens. PEG-rHuMGDF remains in clinical trials but only in Japan, China, Korea, and Taiwan. rHuIL-11, although approved for treatment of thrombocytopenia, is not without side effects that may ultimately limit its use in the clinical community. Pegfilgrastim has been approved by the FDA. The ability to administer a single injection that elicits an response equivalent to multiple daily injections will be a welcome addition to the clinical management of neutropenia. To conclude, although a number of new hematopoietic growth factors have been developed within the last decade, only two, rHuIL-11 and pegfilgrastim, have been approved by the FDA.

REFERENCES

1. Huang E, Nocka K, Beier DR, et al. The hematopoietic growth factor KL is encoded at the SI locus and is the ligand of the c-kit receptor, the gene product of the W locus. *Cell* 1990; 63:225–233.
2. Hannum C, Culpepper J, Campbell D, et al. Ligand for FLT3/FLK2 receptor tyrosine kinase regulates growth of haematopoietic stem cells and is encoded by variant mRNAs. *Nature* 1994; 368:643–648.
3. Martin FH, Suggs SV, Langley KE, et al. Primary structure and functional expression of rat and human stem cell factor DNAs. *Cell* 1990; 63:203–211.
4. Williams DE, Eisenman J, Baird A, et al. Identification of a ligand for the c-kit proto-oncogene. *Cell* 1990; 63:167–174.
5. Lyman SD, James L, Vanden Bos T, et al. Molecular cloning of a ligand for the flt3/flk-2 tyrosine kinase receptor: a proliferative factor for primitive hematopoietic cells. *Cell* 1993; 75:1157–1167.
6. Lyman SD, James L, Johnson L, et al. Cloning of the human homologue of the murine flt3 ligand: a growth factor for early hematopoietic progenitor cells. *Blood* 1994; 83:2795–2801.
7. Lyman SD, Jacobsen SEW. c-kit ligand and flt3 ligand: stem/progenitor cell factors with overlapping yet distinct activities. *Blood* 1998; 91:1101–1134.
8. Bartley T, Bogenberger J, Hunt P, et al. Identification and cloning of a megakaryocyte growth and development factor that is a ligand for the cytokine receptor Mpl. *Cell* 1994; 77:1117–1124.
9. Lok S, Kaushansky K, Holly RD, et al. Cloning and expression of murine thrombopoietin cDNA and stimulation of platelet production in vivo. *Nature* 1994; 369:565–568.
10. Kuter DJ, Beeler DL, Rosenberg RD. The purification of megapoietin: a physiological regulator of megakaryocyte growth and development production. *Proc Natl Acad Sci USA* 1994; 91:11104–11108.
11. de Sauvage FJ, Hass PE, Spencer SD, et al. Stimulation of megakaryocytopoiesis and thrombopoiesis by the c- Mpl ligand. *Nature* 1994; 369:533–538.
12. Wendling F, Maraskovsky E, Debili N, et al. c-Mpl ligand is a humoral regulator of megakaryocytopoiesis. *Nature* 1994; 369:571–574.
13. Gurney AL, Carver-Moore K, de Sauvage FJ, et al. Thrombocytopenia in c-mpl deficient mice. *Science* 1994; 265:1445–1447.
14. Borge OJ, Ramsfjell V, Cui L, et al. Ability of early acting cytokines to directly promote survival and suppress apoptosis of human primitive CD34+CD38– bone marrow cells with multilineage potential at the single-cell level: key role of thrombopoietin. *Blood* 1997; 90:2282–2292.
15. Shibuya K, Akahori H, Takahashi K, et al. Multilineage hematopoietic recovery by a single injection of pegylated recombinant human megakaryocyte growth and development factor in myelosuppressed mice. *Blood* 1998; 91:37–45.
16. Thomas GR, Thibodeaux H, Erret CJ, et al. In vivo biological effects of various forms of thrombopoietin in a murine model of transient thrombocytopenia. *Stem Cells* 1996; 14:246–255.
17. Farese AM, Hunt P, Grab LB, et al. Combined administration of recombinant human megakaryocyte growth and development factor and granulocyte colony-stimulating factor enhances multilineage hematopoietic reconstitution in nonhuman primates after radiation-induced marrow aplasia. *J Clin Invest* 1996; 97:2145–2151.
18. Neelis KJ, Dubbelman YD, Qingliang L, et al. Simultaneous administration of TPO and G-CSF after cytoreductive treatment of rhesus monkeys prevents thrombocytopenia, accelerates platelet and red cell reconstitution, alleviates neutropenia, and promotes the recovery of immature bone marrow cells. *Exp Hematol* 1997; 25:1084–1093.

19. Isaacs C, Robert NJ, Bailey FA, et al. Randomized placebo-controlled study of recombinant human interleukin-11 to prevent chemotherapy-induced thrombocytopenia in patients with breast cancer receiving dose-intensive cyclophosphamide and doxorubicin. *J Clin Oncol* 1997; 15:3368–3377.
20. Tepler I, Elias L, Smith WI, et al. A randomized placebo-controlled trial of recombinant human interleukin-11 in cancer patients with severe thrombocytopenia due to chemotherapy. *Blood* 1996; 87:3607–3614.
21. MacVittie T, Farese AM, Smith WG, et al. Myelopoietin, an engineered chimeric IL-3 and G-CSF receptor agonist, stimulates multilineage hematopoietic recovery in a nonhuman primate model of radiation-induced myelosuppression. *Blood* 2000; 95:837–845.
22. Farese AM, Smith WG, Giri JG, et al. Promegapoietin-1a, an engineered chimeric IL-3 and Mpl-L receptor agonist, stimulates hematopoietic recovery in conventional and abbreviated schedules following radiation-indiced myelosuppression in nonhuman primates. *Stem Cells* 2001; 19:329–338.
23. MacVittie TJ, Farese AM, Lind LB, et al. Progenipoietin-G stimulates hematopoietic recovery following myelosuppression [abstract]. *Blood* 1997; 90:581.
24. Farese AM, Yang B-B, Roskos L, et al. Pegfilgrastim, a sustained form of filgrastim, significantly improves neutrophil recovery after marrow transplantation in rhesus macques. *Bone Marrow Transplant* 2003; 32:399–404.
25. Farese AM, MacVittie TJ, Dacquel-Smith L, et al. Progenipoietins, chimeric agonists of FLT-3 and the G-CSF receptors, stimulate multilineage hematopoietic recovery in myelosuppressed nonhuman primates [abstract]. *Blood* 1998; 92:507.
26. Farese AM, Roskos L, Stead RB, et al. r-metHuG-CSF-SD/01 (SD/01) significantly improves neutrophil recovery in myelosuppressed non human primates [abstract]. *Blood* 1999; 94:49.
27. Streeter PR, Minster NI, Kahn LE, et al. Progenipoietins: biological characterization of a family of dual agonists of fetal liver tyrosine kinase-3 and the granulocyte colony-stimulating factor receptor. *Exp Hematol* 2001; 29:41–50.
28. Macdougall IC. Novel erythropoiesis stimulating protein [abstract]. *Semin Nephrol* 2000; 4:375–381.
29. Dower WJ, Cwirla SE, Balasubramanian P, et al. Peptide agonists of the thrombopoietin receptor. *Stem Cells* 1998; 16:21–29.
30. Wrighton NC, Farrell FX, Chang R, et al. Small peptides as potent mimetics of the protein hormone erythropoietin. *Science* 1996; 273:458–463.
31. Cwirla SE, Balasubramanian P, Duffin DJ, et al. Peptide agonist of the thrombopoietin receptor as potent as the natural cytokine. *Science* 1997; 276:1699.
32. Livnah O, Stura EA, Johnson DL, et al. Functional mimicry of a protein hormone by a peptide agonist: the EPO receptor complex at 2.3 Å. *Science* 1996; 273:464–471.
33. Kimura T, Kaburaki H, Miyamoto S, et al. Discovery of a novel thrombopoietin mimic agonist peptide. *J Biochem* 1997; 122:1046–1051.
34. Naranda T, Wong K, Kaufman RI, et al. Activation of erythropoietin receptor in the absence of hormone by a peptide that binds to a domain different from the hormone binding site. *Proc Natl Acad Sci USA* 1999; 96:7569–7574.
35. de Serres M, Yeager RL, Dillberger JE, et al. Pharmacokinetics and hematological effects of the PEGylated thrombopoietin mimetic GW395058 in rats and monkeys after intravenous or subcutaneous administration. *Stem Cells* 1999; 17:316–326.
36. Hokom MM, Lacey D, Kinsler O, et al. Pegylated megakaryocyte growth and development factor abrogates the lethal thrombocytopenia associated with carboplatin and irradiation in mice. *Blood* 1995; 86:4486–4492.
37. Grossman A, Lenox J, Ren HP, et al. Thrombopoietin accelerates platelet, red blood cell, and neutrophilic recovery in myelosuppressed mice. *Exp Hematol* 1996; 24:1238–1246.
38. Neelis KJ, Hartong SCC, Egeland T, et al. The efficacy of single-dose administration of thrombopoietin with coadministration of either granulocyte/macrophage or granulocyte colony-stimulating factor in myelosuppressed rhesus monkeys. *Blood* 1997; 90:2565–2573.
39. Farese A, MacVittie TJ, Lind LB, et al. The combined administration of daniplestim and MpL ligand augments the hematopoietic reconstitution observed with single cytokine administration in a nonhuman primate model of myelosuppression. In: Murphy MJ, Kutner DJ, eds., *Thrombopoietin: From Molecule to Medicine.* Miamisburg: AlphaMed. 1998:143–154.
40. Akahori H, Shibuya A, Ozai M, et al. Effect of pegylated recombinant human megakaryocyte growth and development factor on thrombocytopenia induced by a new myelosuppressive chemotherapy regimen in mice. *Stem Cells* 1996; 14:678–689.

41. MacVittie TJ, Farese AM, Grab LB, et al . Effect of delayed administration of recombinant human megakaryocyte growth and development factor on hematopoietic reconstitution in nonhuman primates following radiation-induced marrow aplasia [abstract]. *Exp Hematol* 1995; 23:830.
42. Leonard JP, Quinto CM, Goldman SJ, et al. Recombinant human interleukin-11(rhIL-11) multilineage hematopoietic recovery in mice after a myelosuppressive regimen of sublethal irradiation and carboplatin. *Blood* 1994; 83:1499–1506.
43. Patchen ML, MacVittie TJ, Williams JL, et al. Administration of interleukin-6 stimulates multilineage hematopoiesis and accelerates recovery from radiation-induced hematopoietic depression. *Blood* 1991; 77:472–480.
44. Sureda A, Valls A, Kadar E, et al. A single dose of granulocyte colony stimulating factor modifies radiation-induced death in B6D2F1 mice. *Exp Hematol* 1993; 21:1605–1607.
45. Tanikawa S, Nose M, Yoshiro A, et al. Effects of recombinant human granuloctye colony-stimulating factor on the hematologic recovery and survival of irradiated mice. *Blood* 1990; 76:445–449.
46. Neelis KJ, Dubbelman YD, Wognum AW, et al. Lack of efficacy of thrombopoietin and granulocyte colony-stimulating factor after high dose total-body irradiation and autologous stem cell or bone marrow transplantation in rhesus monkeys. *Exp Hematol* 1997; 25:1094–1103.
47. Farese AM, MacVittie TJ, Roskos L, et al. Hematopoietic recovery following autologous bone marrow transplantation in a nonhuman primate: effect of variation of treatment schedule with Peg-rHuMGDF. *Stem Cells* 2003; 21:79–89.
48. Hartong SCC, Neelis KJ, Visser JWM, et al. Lack of efficacy of thrombopoietin and granulocyte-macrophage colony-stimulating factor after total body irradiation and autologous bone marrow transplantation in rhesus monkeys. *Exp Hematol* 2000; 28:753–759.
49. Nash RA, Takatu A, Feng Z, et al. Effect of c-mpl ligands after total body irradiation (TBI) with and without allogeneic hematopoietic stem cell transplantation: low-dose TBI does not prevent sensitization. *Bio Blood Marrow Transplant* 2002; 8:360–367.
50. Beveridge R, Schuster M, Waller E, et al. Randomized, double-blind, placebo-controlled trial of pegylated recombinant human megakaryocyte growth and development factor (PEG-rHuMGDF) in breast cancer patients (Pts) following autologous bone marrow transplantation (ABMT) [abstract]. *Blood* 1997; 90:580a.
51. Nash RA, Kurzrock R, DiPersio J, et al. A phase I trial of recombinant human thrombopoietin in patients with delayed platelet recovery after hematopoietic stem cell transplantation. *Bio Blood Marrow Transplant* 2000; 6:25–34.
52. Fields KK, Crump M, Bence-Bruckler I, et al. Use of PEG-rHuMGDF in platelet engraftment after autologous stem cell transplantation. *Blood Marrow Transplant* 2000; 26:1083–1088.
53. Wolff SN, Herzig R, Lynch J, et al. Recombinant human thrombopoietin (rhTPO) after autologous bone marrow transplantation: a phase I pharmacokinetic and pharmacodynamic study. *Bone Marrow Transplant* 2001; 27:261–268.
54. Bolwell B, Vredenburgh J, Overmoyer B, et al. Phase I study of pegylated recombinant human megkaryocyte growth and development factor (PEG-rHuMGDF) in breast cancer patients after autologous peripheral blood progenitor cell (PBPC) transplantation. *Bone Marrow Transplant* 2000; 26:141–145.
55. Roskos L, Stead R, Harker L, et al. A cytokinetic model of platelet (PLT) production and destruction following administration of PEG-rHuMGDF [abstract]. *Blood* 1997; 90:171a.
56. Du X, Williams D. Interleukin-11: review of molecular, cell biology, and clinical use. *Blood* 1997; 89:3897–3908.
57. Saitoh M, Taguchi K, Yasuda S, et al. Thrombopoietic activity of recombinant human interleukin-11 in nonhuman primates with ACNU-induced thrombocytopenia. *J Interferon Cytokine Res* 2000; 20:539–545.
58. Schlerman FJ, Bree AG, Kaviani MD, et al. Thrombopoietic activity of recombinant human interleukin 11 (rHuIL-11) in normal and myelosuppressed nonhuman primates. *Stem Cells* 1996; 14:517–532.
59. Nash RA, Siedel K, Storb R, et al. Effects of rhIL-11 on normal dogs and after sublethal radiation. *Exp Hematol* 1995; 23:389–396.
60. Collins M, Quinto C, Goldman SJ. rhIL-11 and thrombopoietin synergize to improve platelet recovery in mice treated with a combined modality regimen of carboplatin and irradiation [abstract]. *Blood* 1997; 90:758.
61. Galmiche MC, Vogel CA, Delaloye AB, et al. Combined effects of interleukin-3 and interleukin-11 on hematopoiesis in irradiated mice. *Exp Hematol* 1996; 24:1298–1306.

62. Doshi, PD, Giri JG, Abegg AL, et al. Promegapoietin, a family of chimeric growth factors, supports megakaryocyte development through activation of IL-3 and c-Mpl ligand signaling pathways. *Exp Hematol* 2003; 29:1177–1184.
63. Bishop MR, Tarantolo SR, Geller RB, et al. A randomized, double-blind trial of filgrastim (granulocyte colony-stimulating factor) versus placebo following allogeneic blood stem cell transplantation. *Blood* 2000; 96:80–85.
64. Welte K, Gabrilove J, Bronchud MH, et al. Filgrastim (r-metHuG-CSF): the first 10 years. *Blood* 1996; 88:1907–1929.
65. Morstyn G, Campbell L, Souza LM, et al. Effect of granulocyte colony stimulating factor on neutropenia induced by cytotoxic chemotherapy. *Lancet* 1988; 1:668–672.
66. Sheridan WP, Morstyn G, Wolf M, et al. Granulocyte colony-stimulating factor and neutrophil recovery after high-dose chemotherapy and autologous bone marrow transplantation. *Lancet* 1989; 2:891–895.
67. Crawford J, Ozer H, Stoller R, et al. Reduction by granulocyte-colony stimulating factor of fever and neutropenia induced by chemotherapy in patients with small-cell lung cancer. *N Engl J Med*i 1991; 325:164–170.
68. Farese AM, Casey DB, Smith WG, et al. Leridistim, a chimeric dual G-CSF and IL-3 receptor agonist, enhances multilineage hematopoietic recovery in nonhuman primate model of radiation-induced myelosuppression: effect of schedule, dose, and route of administration. *Stem Cells* 2001; 19:522–533.
69. MacVittie TJ, Farese AM, Herodin F, et al. Combination therapy of radiation-induced bone marrow aplasia in nonhuman primates using synthokine SC-55494 and recombinant human granulocyte colony-stimulating factor. *Blood* 1996; 87:4129–4135.
70. Sato N, Caux C, Kitamura T, et al. Expression and factor-dependent modulation of interleukin-3 receptor subunits on human hematopoietic cells. *Blood* 1993; 82:752–761.
71. Wognum AW, Visser TP, de Jong MO, et al. Differential expression of receptors for interleukin-3 on subsets of CD34-expressing hematopoietic cells for rhesus monkeys. *Blood* 1995; 86:581–591.
72. Wickenhauser C, Lorenzen J, Thiele J, et al. Secretion of cytokines (Interleukins-1 , -3, and -6 and granulocyte macrophage colony-stimulating factor) by normal human bone marrow megakaryocytes. *Blood* 1995; 85:685–691.
73. Aglietta M, Sanavio F, Stacchini A, et al. Interleukin-3 in vivo: kinetic of response of target cells. *Blood* 1993; 82:2054–2061.
74. Brandt JE, Bhalla K, Hoffman R. Effects of interleukin-3 and c-kit ligand on the survival of various classes of human hematopoietic progenitor cells. *Blood* 1994; 83:1507–1514.
75. Collins MK, Marvel J, Malde P, et al. Interleukin-3 protects murine bone marrow cells from apoptosis induced by DNA damaging agents. *J Exp Med* 1992; 176:1043–1051.
76. Silva A, Wyllie A, Collins MKL. p53 is not required for regulation of apoptosis or radioprotection by interleukin-3. *Blood* 1997; 89:2717–2722.
77. Collins MKL, Perkins GR, Rodriguez-Tarduchy G, et al. Growth factors as survival factors: regulation of apoptosis. *Bioessays* 1994; 16:133–138.
78. Farese AM, Casey DB, Vigneulle RM, et al. A single dose of pegylated leridistim significantly improves neutrophil recovery in sublethally irradiated rhesus macaques. *Stem Cells* 2001; 19:514–521.
79. Molineux G, Kinstler O, Briddell B, et al. A new form of filgrastim with sustained duration in vivo and enhanced ability to mobilize PBPC in both mice and humans. *Exp Hematol* 1999; 27:1724–1734.
80. Hartley C, McElroy T, Sutherland W, et al. Treatment with SD/01 relative to chemotherapy in mice [abstract]. *Exp Hematol* 2000; 7:192–193.
81. Cheung EN, Cosenza M, Lopez O, et al. Modeling of r-metHuG-CSF-SD/01 (SD/01) mediated granulopoiesis in normal animals with mathematical extrapolation to neutropenic settings [abstract]. *Blood* 1998; 92:379.
82. Roskos LK, Yang B, Schwab G, et al. Cytokinetic model of rmethHuG-CSF-SD/01 (SD/01) mediated granulopoiesis and the "self-regulation" of SD/01 elimination in non-small cell lung cancer [abstract]. *Blood* 1998; 92:507A.
83. Holmes FA, Jones SE, O'Shaughnessy J, et al. Comparable efficacy and safety profiles of once-per-cycle pegfilgrastim and daily injection filgrastim in chemotherapy-induced neutropenia: a multicenter dose-finding study in women with breast cancer. *Ann Oncol* 2002; 13:903–909.
84. Holmes FA, O'Shaughnessy JA, Vukelja S, et al. Blinded, randomized, multicenter study to evaluate single administration pegfilgrastim one per cycle versus daily filgrastim as an adjunct to chemotherapy in patients with high-risk stage II or stage III/IV breast cancer. *J Clin Oncol* 2002; 20:727–731.

85. Johnston E, Crawford J, Blackwell S, et al. Randomized dose-escalation study of SD/01 compared with daily filgrastim in patients receiving chemotherapy. *J Clin Oncol* 2000; 18:2522–2528.
86. Morstyn G, Campbell L, Lieschke G. Treatment of chemotherapy-induced neutropenia by subcutaneously administered granulocyte colony-stimulating factor with optimization of dose and duration of therapy. *J Clin Oncol* 1989; 7:1554–1562.
87. Vadhan-Raj S, Keating M, LeMaistre PL, et al. Effects of recombinant human granulocyte-macrophage colony-stimulating factor in patients with myelodysplastic syndrome. *N Engl J Med* 1987; 317:1545–1552.
88. Antman KS, Griffin JD, Elias A, et al. Effect of recombinant human granulocyte-macrophage colony-stimulating factor on chemotherapy-induced myelosuppression. *N Engl J Med* 1988; 319:593–598.
89. Mackall CL, Fleisher TA, Brown MR, et al. Lymphocyte depletion during treatment with intensive chemotherapy for cancer. *Blood* 1994; 84:2221–2228.
90. Hakim FT, Cepeda R, Kaimei S, et al. Constraints on CD4 recovery postchemotherapy in adults: thymic insufficiency and apoptotic decline of expanded peripheral CD4 cells. *Blood* 1997; 90:3789–3798.
91. Mackall CL, Fleisher TA, Brown MR, et al. Distinctions between $CD8^+$ and $CD4^+$ T-cell regeneration pathways result in prolonged T-cell subset imbalance after intensive chemotherapy. *Blood* 1997; 89:3700–3707.
92. Roux E, Dumont-Girard F, Starobinski M, et al. Recovery of immune reactivity after T-cell—depleted bone marrow transplanation depends on thymic activity. *Blood* 2000; 96:2299–2303.
93. Roux E, Helg C, Dumont-Girard F, et al. Analysis of T-cell repopulation after allogeneic bone marrow transplantation: significant differences between recipients of T-cell depleted and unmanipulated grafts. *Blood* 1996; 87:3984–3992.
94. Borge OJ, Adolfsson J, Martensson A, et al. Lymphoid-restricted development from multipotent candidate murine stem cells: distinct and complimentary functions of the c-kit and flt3-ligands. *Blood* 1999; 94:3781–3790.
95. Antonysamy MA, Thomson AW. FLT3 ligand (FL) and its influence on immune reactivity. *Cytokine* 2000; 12:87–100.
96. Hirayama F, Aiba Y, Ikebuchi K, et al. Differentiation in culture of murine primitive lymphohematopoietic progenitors toward T-cell lineage. *Blood* 1999; 93:4187–4195.
97. Sims JE, Williams DE, Morrissey PJ, et al. Molecular cloning and biological characterization of a novel murine lymphoid growth factor. *J Exp Med* 2000; 192:671–680.
98. Guest I, Uetrecht J. Bone marrow stem cell protection from chemotherapy by low-molecular-weight compunds. *Exp Hematol* 2001; 29:123–137.
99. Andrew D, Aspinall R. IL-7 and not stem cell factor reverses both the increase in apoptosis and the decline in thympoiesis seen in aged mice. *J Immunol* 2001; 166:1524–1530.
100. Hassan J, Reen DJ. Human recent thymic emigrants—Identification, expansion, and survival characteristics. *J Immunol* 2001; 167:1970–1976.
101. Geiselhart LA, Humphries CA, Gregorio TA, et al. IL-7 administration alters the CD4:CD8 ratio, increases T cell numbers, and increases T cell function in the absence of activation. *J Immunol* 2001; 166:3019–3027.
102. Schluns KS, Kieper WC, Jameson SC, et al. Interleukin-7 mediates the homeostasis of naive and memory CD8 T cells in vivo. *Nat Immunol* 2000; 1:426–432.
103. Fry TJ, Mackall CL. Interleukin-7: master regulator of peripheral T-cell homeostasis? *Trends Immunol* 2001; 22:564–571.
104. Berthro JM, Loilleux S, Chapel A, et al. CD135 (Flk2/Flt3) expression by human thymocytes delineates a possible role of Flt3-ligand in T cell precursor proliferation and differentiation. *Scand J Immunol* 2001; 51:53–61.
105. Hirayama F, Lyman SD, Clark SC, et al. The flt3 ligand supports proliferation of lymphohematopoietic progenitors and early B-lymphoid progenitors. *Blood* 1995; 85:1762–1768.
106. Sitnicka E, Bryder D, Adolfsson J, et al. FLT3 ligand is critically involved in generation of early and common lymphoid progenitors but not in the regulation of the size of the hematopoietic stem cell [abstract]. *Blood* 2000; 96:492a–492.
107. Fry TJ, Sinhn M, Thomas EK, et al. Flt3 Ligand: a potential new immunorestorative agent [abstract]. *Blood* 2001; 98:735a.
108. Mackall CL, Bare CV, Granger LA, et al. Thymic-independent T-cell regeneration occurs via antigen-driven expansion of peripheral T cells resulting in a repertoire that is limited in diversity and prone to skewing. *J Immunol* 1996; 156:4609–4616.

109. Rocha B, Boehmer H. Peripheral selection of the T cell repertoire. *Science* 1991; 251:1225–1228.
110. Haynes BF, Hale LP, Weinhold KJ, et al. Analysis of the adult thymus in reconstitution of T lymphocyte in HIV-1 infection. *J Clin Invest* 1999; 103:453–460.
111. Boerman OC, Gregorio TA, Grzegorzewski KJ, et al. Recombinant human IL-7 administration in mice affects colony-forming units-spleen and lymphoid precursor cell localization an decelerates engraftment of bone marrow transplants. *J Leukoc Biol* 1995; 58:151–158.
112. Abdul-Hai A, Or R, Slavin S, et al. Immune reconstitution by interleukin-7 after syngeneic bone marrow transplantation in mice. *Exp Hematol* 1996; 24:1416–1422.
113. Morrissey PJ, Conlon P, Braddy S, et al. Administration of IL-7 to mice with cyclophosphamide-induced lymphopenia accelerates lymphocyte repopulation. *J Immunol* 1991; 146:1547–1552.
114. Bolotin E, Smogorzewska M, Smith S, et al. Enhancement of thymopoiesis after bone marrow transplant by in vivo interleukin-7. *Blood* 1996; 88:1887–1894.
115. Mackall CL, Fry TJ, Bare C, et al. IL-7 increases both thymic-dependent and thymic-independent T-cell regeneration after bone marrow transplantation. *Blood* 2001; 97:1491–1497.
116. Fry TJ, Mackall CL. Interleukin-7: from bench to clinic. *Blood* 2002; 99:3892–3904.
117. Fry TJ, Christensen BL, Komschilies KL, et al. Interleukin-7 restores immunity in athymic T-cell—depleted hosts. *Blood* 2001; 97:1525–1533.
118. Alpdogan O, Schmaltz C, Muriglan SJ, et al. Administration of interleukin-7 after allogeneic bone marrow transplantation improves immune reconstitution without aggravating graft-versus-host disease. *Blood* 2001; 98:2256–2265.
119. Finch PW, Cunha GR, Rubin JS, et al. Pattern of keratinocyte growth factor and keratinocyte growth factor receptor expression during mouse fetal development suggests a role in mediating morphogenetic mesenchymal-epithelial interactions. *Dev Dynamics* 1995; 203:223–240.
120. Rubin JS, Osada H, Finch PW, et al. Purification and characterization of a newly identified growth factor specific for epithelial cells. *Proc Natl Acad Sci USA* 1989; 86:802–806.
121. Revest JM, Suniara RK, Kerr K, et al. Development of the thymus requires singaling through the fibroblast growth factor receptor R2IIIb. *J Immunol* 2001; 167:1954–1961.
122. Orr-Urtreger A, Bedford MT, Burakova T, et al. Developmental localization of the splicing alternatives of fibroblast growth factor receptor-2 (FGFR2). *Dev Biol* 1993; 158:475–486.
123. Ornitz DM, Xu JS, Colvin DG, et al. Receptor specificity of the fibroblast growth-factor family. *J Biol Chem* 1996; 271:15292–15297.
124. Yi ES, Williams ST, Lee H, et al. Keratinocyte growth factor ameliorates radiation- and bleomycin-induced lung injury and mortality. *Am J Pathol* 1996; 149:1963–1970.
125. Farrell CL, Bready JV, Rex KL, et al. Keratinocyte growth factor protects mice from chemotherapy and radiation-induced gastrointestinal injury and mortality. *Cancer Res* 1998; 58:933–939.
126. Panoskaltsis-Mortari A, Lacey DL, Vallera DA, et al. Keratinocyte growth factor administered before conditioning ameliorates graft-versus-host disease after allogeneic bone marrow transplantation in mice. *Blood* 1998; 92:3960–3967.
127. Panoskaltsis-Mortari A, Ingbar DH, Jung P, et al. Keratinocyte growth factor (KGF) given before conditioning decreases B7 ligand and granzyme B expression in situ and hastens lung repair post-allogeneic bone marrow transplantation (BMT) in mice. *Am J Physiol Lung Cell Mol Physiol* 2000; 278:L988–L999.
128. Haddad IY, Panoskaltsis-Mortari A, Ingbar DH, et al. Interactions of keratinocyte growth factor with a nitrating species after arrow transplantation in mice. *Am J Physiol Lung Cell Mol Physiol* 1999; 277:L391-L400.
129. Krijanovski OI, Hill GR, Cooke KR, et al. Keratinocyte growth factor separates graft-versus-leukemia effects from graft-versus-host disease. *Blood* 1999; 94:825–831.
130. Panoskaltsis-Mortari A, Taylor PA, Rubin JS, et al. Keratinocyte growth factor facilitates alloengraftment and ameliorates graft-versus-host disease in mice by a mechanism independent of repair of conditioning-induced tissue injury [abstract]. *Blood* 2000; 96:4350–4356.
131. Min D, Taylor PA, Panoskaltsis-Mortari A, et al. Protection from thymic epithelial cell injury by keratinocyte growth factor: a new approach to improve thymic and peripheral T-cell reconstitution after bone marrow transplantation. *Blood* 2002; 99:4592–4600.
132. Naranda T, Goldstein A, Olsson L. A peptide derived from an extracellular domain selectively inhibits receptor internalization: target sequences on insulin and insulin-like growth factor 1 receptors. *Proc Natl Acad Sci USA* 1997; 94:11692–11697.
133. Tian S, Lamb P, King AG, et al. A small, nonpeptidyl mimic of granulocyte-colony-stimulating factor. *Science* 1998; 281:257–259.

III Use of Hematopoietic Growth Factors in Oncology

10 Commentary on the ASCO and ESMO Evidence-Based Clinical Practice Guidelines for the Use of Hematopoietic Colony-Stimulating Factors

Richard M. Fox, MB, PhD, FRACP

CONTENTS

1. INTRODUCTION

Guidelines have been issued for the use of recombinant human granulocyte colony-stimulating factor (rHuG-CSF) and recombinant human granulocyte-macrophage colony-stimulating factor (rHuGM-CSF) *(1,2)*. The stimulus for the development of these guidelines followed the 1991 Food and Drug Administration (FDA) approval for the clinical use of rHuG-CSF and rHuGM-CSF in the United States. The uptake and use of these agents was rapid and deep. By 1994, use of colony-stimulating factors (CSFs) had expanded to 10% of some United States-based hospital budgets and, of concern, survival rate among the patients so treated did not seem to have improved. The widespread use of these agents and the subsequent economic impact stimulated the American Society of Clinical Oncology (ASCO) to publish its first clinical practice guidelines in 1994 *(3)*. These guidelines were updated in 1996 *(4)* and in 2000 (1). The European Society for Medical Oncology (ESMO) recommendations for the use of these hematopoietic growth factors (HGFs) appeared in 2001 *(2)*.

The more frequent use of these HGFs has been in either primary or secondary prevention of febrile neutropenia or the treatment of febrile neutropenia. These indications

From: *Cancer Drug Discovery and Development*
Hematopoietic Growth Factors in Oncology: Basic Science and Clinical Therapeutics
Edited by: G. Morstyn, M. A. Foote, and G. J. Lieschke © Humana Press Inc., Totowa, NJ

are independent of its use in other conditions, such as the mobilization of peripheral blood progenitor cells (PBPCs) to support high-dose chemotherapy regimes.

Febrile neutropenia has been a dose-limiting effect for a wide range of chemotherapies. The magnitude of neutropenia and infection has been related to chemotherapy intensity, although host-related and disease-related factors have a role. In general, febrile neutropenia has been treated by hospitalization and the administration of empiric antibiotic therapy, often for several days. In the initial randomized clinical trial used for FDA licensing in the United States, the observed incidence of febrile neutropenia was approx 40% *(5)*. Based on this information, a guideline for the use of CSFs was formulated and stated that with such a rate of febrile neutropenia, use of CSFs for primary prophylaxis was warranted.

The 40% rate of febrile neutropenia related to a series of patients with small-cell lung cancer (SCLC) treated with cyclophosphamide 1 g/m^2, doxorubicin 50 mg/m^2, and etoposide 120 mg/m^2 on d 1, 2, and 3 of the chemotherapy cycle. Patients were randomized to receive either rHuG-CSF or placebo after chemotherapy. The incidence of neutropenia with fever in the patients receiving placebo was 57%, and in the rHuG-CSF-treated patients it was 28%. The median duration of a neutrophil count $< 0.5 \times 10^9$/L was 6 d in the patients receiving placebo and 3 d in patients treated with rHuG-CSF; the duration of fever with neutropenia was 5 d in patients receiving placebo and 4 d in patients treated with rHuG-CSF. Patients receiving placebo had 4 d of hospitalization compared with 2 d for patients receiving rHuG-CSF. An analysis for cost effectiveness was in favor of the use of rHuG-CSF in primary prevention. It was concluded that there was a 50% reduction in the incidence of febrile neutropenia, antibiotic use, and hospitalization and that these reductions offered substantial economic as well as clinical benefit. This study was pivotal in the FDA approval process for rHuG-CSF; however, the cytotoxic doses used in the Crawford et al. *(5)* study are higher than those used in contemporary regimes.

The 2000 update of recommendations by the ASCO describes a number of the commonly used chemotherapy regimes and the reported rates of neutropenia, fever, and sepsis. The guideline note that many new chemotherapeutic agents, which include the taxanes, topoisomerase 1 inhibitors, and vinorelbine, have been used as part of these regimes in the latter part of the 1990s. The guidelines emphasize that a few of the commonly used combination drug regimes produce significant complications relating to neutropenia. The exception, of course, is when relapsed or refractory disease was being treated.

The basic thrust of the updated recommendations is that the routine use of CSFs for primary prophylaxis is not justified on the basis of cost savings with any of the current routine chemotherapy regimes. It notes that cost analyses have shown that CSFs save money when the risk of febrile neutropenia is greater than 40% but that no routine regimes have rates greater than 15%. (This excludes induction treatment of acute leukemia.) This analysis is based on economic modeling using costs of hospitalization for episodes of febrile neutropenia at US $10,000. The guidelines suggest that CSFs could be routinely used with justification if they cost substantially less.

The guidelines note that for secondary prophylaxis, the rate of febrile neutropenia could be on the order of 40% and would justify use of CSFs but suggest that dose modification would be a medically acceptable alternative on the basis that major clinical benefit of maintaining delivery of previously toxic levels of chemotherapy with CSF has not been demonstrated.

Similarly, the ESMO recommendations note that despite relatively high rates of low neutrophil counts during standard-dose chemotherapy regime (apart from acute leukemia), the rates of febrile neutropenia and other complications and mortality rates are relatively low for most standard chemotherapies. ESMO similarly concludes that these rates do not justify the routine use of HSFs.

2. SPECIFIC ISSUES

2.1. Guideline for Primary Prophylactic Administration

The ASCO guidelines note that the use of CSF has had little impact on empiric cure rate in patients with non-Hodgkin's lymphoma (NHL), SCLC, testicular cancer, or breast cancer. This finding reflects the lower incidence of febrile neutropenia in current regimes and the recognition in the 1990s that increasing chemotherapy dose intensity has not shown improvement in outcomes.

The guidelines conclude that for most chemotherapy regimes, primary administration is not recommended, but they do note that special circumstances exist. Special circumstances include patients who may be judged to be at high risk for the development of febrile neutropenia when there is demonstrated bone marrow compromise, comorbidity, extensive previous chemotherapy or radiotherapy, poor performance status, or active tissue infection.

The recommendations by ESMO are similar and suggest that the use of CSFs is reasonable only if there is a greater than 40% probability of febrile neutropenia or if the dose reduction is deemed detrimental to outcome. The ESMO guidelines similarly note that special situations exist for the use of CSF for primary prophylaxis in patients who have had previous extensive chemotherapy or radiotherapy, HIV infection, poor performance status, or chemotherapy in the presence of active infection.

2.2. Secondary Prophylactic CSF Administration

Secondary prophylactic use is defined as the use of a CSF in patients with a previous episode of febrile neutropenia to prevent subsequent episodes. ASCO guidelines for use of CSF restrict the use to a subset of patients who are more likely to benefit from such support. It is intended to allow chemotherapy dose maintenance (if this was intended to improve outcome); however, the guidelines do note that in noncurative chemotherapy, one could consider dose reduction as an alternative after an episode of febrile neutropenia. Data appear to be lacking to support the idea of dose maintenance by the use of CSF as secondary prophylaxis in noncurative tumor treatments.

Similar recommendations are made by ESMO. These guidelines warrant the use of CSF if further infections in the next treatment cycle were considered to be potentially life-threatening or if dose reduction or chemotherapy delays could compromise cure rate or disease-free or overall survival.

2.3. Use in Afebrile Neutropenic Patients

The ASCO guidelines reported that surveys in 1994 showed that some 34% of oncologists in the United States used CSF in afebrile neutropenic patients. The guidelines note that two randomized studies showed no benefits for the use of CSF in this situation. The 2000 recommendation is that routine use of CSFs in febrile neutropenia patients is inappropriate. The ESMO recommendation concurs with the ASCO guideline.

2.4. Use in Febrile Neutropenic Patients

The ASCO guideline cites eight randomized control clinical trials that collectively do not support the routine use of CSFs in uncomplicated fever and neutropenia. They do, however, indicate the potential use of CSFs in high-risk, poor-prognosis patients with febrile neutropenia, including patients with an absolute neutrophil count (ANC) < 0.1×10^9/L, uncontrolled primary disease, pneumonia, hypotension, multiorgan dysfunction, invasive fungal infection, and advanced age. Similar recommendations are made by the ESMO guidelines.

Alternative preventative approaches suggested by the guidelines include chemotherapy dose reduction or the use of less myelosuppressive chemotherapy in noncurative regimes. The guidelines do not recommend antibiotic prophylaxis.

2.5. Use in Increasing Chemotherapy Dose Intensity

The guidelines note that there is an apparent steep dose-response curve in preclinical studies but that retrospective analyses of dose-delivered intensity in the clinic suggest that bias may have been introduced. Some of the randomized trials compared lower than standard-dose chemotherapy with standard-dose chemotherapy. In the late 1990s, trials increasing dose intensity above standard levels were not shown to improve survival. The recommendation was that outside the setting of clinical trials, the use of CSFs to increase dose intensity was not justified.

2.6. CSFs as Adjuncts to Hematopoietic Progenitor Cell Transplantation

The use of CSFs to enhance the mobilization of PBPC numbers can reduce the number and cost of leukapheresis procedures. The administration of PBPCs speeds hematologic recovery. Progenitor cells generated by CSFs are used widely in both autologous and allogeneic high-dose chemotherapy therapies. The ASCO guidelines recommend the use of CSF both to mobilize progenitor cells and to stimulate the recovery period after the infusion of the progenitor cells. The ASCO recommendation for use of CSFs after infusion is based on several studies reported in 1995 and concurs with the ESMO recommendations. ESMO, however, does not recommend the use of CSF after the infusion of progenitor cells. The basis for the ESMO recommendation is not described or referenced in the guideline, and the recommendations note that this is an area for further clinical investigation.

2.7. CSFs in Patients With Acute Leukemia and Myelodysplastic Syndromes

Most patients receiving induction or consolidation therapies for acute leukemia develop febrile neutropenia. These therapies have other complications, including coagulopathy, thrombocytopenic hemorrhage, fungal infections, and amphotericin-induced renal damage. These complications are particularly more severe in older patients. The ASCOs guidelines note that several randomized clinical trials have studied the administration of CSFs in this setting and that the studies show a reduction in the time to recovery of ANC to 0.5×10^9/L within 2–6 d after administration. The ANC recovery did not influence complete response rates nor was there evidence of stimulation of leukemic growth. These trials have demonstrated a reduction in duration of hospitalization and antibiotic use, and the benefits appear to be greater in older patients. The ASCO guidelines note that studies have not yet shown significant improvement in longer term outcome. The guidelines conclude that minimal risk is associated with the use of CSFs in this situation; however, the choice of whether to use CSFs is likely to be determined by cost consideration: the cost of the use of a CSF must be balanced against possible reduction of hospitalization associated with the slightly more rapid marrow recovery, particularly in patients aged 55 yr or older. Available data do not conclusively show that use of CSFs significantly accelerates recovery of ANC to the $0.1–0.5 \times 10^9$/L necessary to protect against infection.

The ASCO recommendations contrast with the ESMO guidelines, which do not consider CSFs to be indicated for patients with acute myeloid leukemia after induction therapy, although it is suggested that they may have a role in induction therapy for patients with acute lymphoblastic leukemia.

The ASCO recommendations note that in patients with myelodysplastic syndromes complicated by neutropenia, the administration of CSFs can increase ANC. ANC decreases, however, when administration stops. The increase in ANC is associated with clinical resolution of infection. The recommendation was intermittent, i.e., as required, CSFs were given to the subset of patients with severe continuing neutropenia and recurrent episodes of infection. Often such patients have a satisfactory increase in ANC, e.g., to $>0.5 \times 10^9$/L with once- or twice-weekly injections.

2.8. CSF Use in Patients Receiving Concurrent Chemotherapy and Radiotherapy

The danger of inducing thrombocytopenia, especially when rHuGM-CSF is used, is stressed by the guidelines. In particular, adverse interactions with simultaneous mediastinal irradiation and CSF administration is noted and is generally not recommended.

3. IMPACT OF GUIDELINES

The ASCO Health Services Research Committee sought to assess patterns of CSF use before the publication of the first guideline. A questionnaire describing various clinical scenarios was mailed to oncologists and hematologists in the United States. In each scenario, the physician was asked whether he/she would prefer to use a CSF to prevent or treat neutropenia. Most physicians preferred to use CSFs for secondary prophylaxis in patients receiving chemotherapy at rates of 44–85% rather than reduce doses. Patterns of use did not differ for palliative, curative, or adjuvant chemotherapy. More than half of the physicians chose to use CSFs in the treatment of febrile neutropenia, which was not supported in subsequent guidelines. Interestingly, physicians who practiced at academic medical centers and those practicing at health maintenance organizations (HMOs) had the same opinions. Physicians at the academic or HMO centers were more likely to prefer dose reduction strategies, whereas physicians receiving a fee for service used CSFs more often. It was believed, therefore, that the guidelines would be most likely to reduce the use of CSFs for the treatment of afebrile and uncomplicated febrile neutropenia *(6)*.

A similar finding was made by a further survey by the ASCO Health Services Committee. A questionnaire was sent to oncologists and hematologists describing the clinical scenario for a 67-yr-old man with newly diagnosed *de novo* acute myeloid leukemia. Physicians were asked about their preference for adjunctive use of a CSF after induction and consolidation chemotherapy. Support for the use of a CSF was 40% after induction chemotherapy and was similar to that for not using the agent. The most important determinant of support for the use of CSF, however, was being in a fee-for-service practice, i.e., use was accompanied by financial profit to the physician practice. Support was low otherwise *(7)*.

A French group did a multicenter study of the impact of prescription guidelines on the use of CSFs *(8)*. Two hospital groups were compared: a guidelines group (seven teaching hospitals) that circulated guidelines and a control group (eight teaching hospitals) that did not circulate guidelines. Times before and after distribution of the guidelines were assessed also. Data from approx 404 patients were analyzed for the indication of postchemotherapy neutropenia. The total compliance in the first period, i.e., before the publication of the guidelines, was 44% in the control group and 51% in the guideline group, a nonsignificant difference statistically. During the second period, i.e., after the publication of the guidelines, compliance was 32% vs 60% in the two groups ($p < 0.001$). The authors concluded that prescription reference systems needed to be continually redefined according to available data and circulated widely to improve the quality of health care and to control expenses *(8)*.

Further studies of the relationship between the introduction of the ASCO guidelines and the use of CSFs were made *(9)*. The study was performed in a large, 830-bed university hospital in Paris before and after the ASCO guidelines were implemented. The guidelines were first disseminated as a continuing medical education program and then actively implemented using a CSF prescription order form summarizing the guidelines. Seven other university-associated hospitals in Paris at which the ASCO guidelines were not actively implemented comprised the control group. The main outcome measure was the proportion of prescriptions in compliance with the 1996 update of the ASCO guidelines.

Before implementation of the ASCO guidelines, compliance with guidelines was 39% at the study site and 31% at the control site ($p > 0.0.05$). Six months after dissemination and implementation of the guidelines, compliance with the ASCO guidelines increased significantly compared with baseline in the study group to 61% ($p = 0.003$). Even after the guidelines were implemented, however, compliance with guidelines for the use of CSFs as primary prophylaxis did not change significantly vs. before implementation in the study group ([12%] before implementation vs 6% after implementation [$p > 0.05$]) *(9)*.

4. EVOLVING RECOMMENDATIONS

The guidelines will need to be reviewed regularly and updated as treatment regimens change and/or new drugs are introduced. For example, cyclosphosphamide, doxorubicin, vincristine, prednisone (CHOP)-14 has been proposed as a new standard regime for patients older than 60 yr with aggressive NHL *(10)*. In this study, CHOP administration was intensified (a 14-d cycle vs a 21-d cycle) in the two-weekly regime with rHuG-CSF starting from d 4. This administration provided improved results compared with standard CHOP 21; no improvement was achieved by the addition of etoposide, in part owing to its toxicity in this population.

REFERENCES

1. Ozer H, Armitage JO, Bennett CL, et al. 2000 update of recommendations for the use of hematopoietic colony-stimulating factors: evidence based, clinical practice guidelines. *J Clin Oncol* 2000; 18:3558–3585.
2. ESMO recommendations for the application of haematopoietic growth factors (hGFs). *Ann Oncol* 2001; 12:1219–1220.

3. ASCO Ad Hoc Colony-Stimulating Factor Guidelines Expert Panel. American Society of Clinical Oncology recommendation for the use of hematopoietic colony-stimulating factors: evidence-based, clinical practice guidelines. *J Clin Oncol* 1994; 12:2471–2508.
4. ASCO Health Services Research Committee. Update of recommendations for the use of hematopoietic colony-stimulating factors: evidence-based clinical practice guidelines. *J Clin Oncol* 1996; 14:1957–1960.
5. Crawford J, Ozer H, Stoller R, et al. Reduction by granulocyte colony-stimulating factor of fever and neutropenia induced by chemotherapy in patients with small-cell lung cancer. *N Engl J Med* 1991; 325:164–170.
6. Bennett CL, Smith TJ, Weeks JC, et al. Use of hematopoietic colony-stimulating factors: the American Society of Clinical Oncology survey. *J Clin Oncol* 1996; 14:2511–2520.
7. Bennett CL, Bishop MR, Tallman MS, et al. The association between physician reimbursement in the US and use of hematopoietic colony stimulating factors as adjunct therapy for older patients with acute myeloid leukemia: results from the 1997 American Society of Clinical Oncology survey. *Ann Oncol* 1999; 10:1355–1359.
8. Gren N, Pointereau-Bellanger A, Conort O, et al. Multicenter study of the impact of prescription guidelines on the use of colony stimulating factors. *Anticancer Drugs* 2000; 11:109–115.
9. Debrix I, Tilleul P, Milleron B, et al. The relationship between introduction of American Society of Clinical Oncology guidelines and the use of colony-stimulating factors in clinical practice in a Paris university hospital. *Clin Ther* 2001; 23:1116–1127.
10. Pfreundschuh M, Trumper L, Kloess M, et al. 2-Weekly CHOP (CHOP-14): the new standard regimen for patients with aggressive non-Hodgkin's lymphoma (NHL) > 60 years of age. *Ann Oncol* 2002; 13(suppl 2):27.

11 Neutropenia and the Problem of Fever and Infection in Patients With Cancer

David C. Dale, MD

CONTENTS

1. INTRODUCTION

The role of blood neutrophils in the defense against infections is well recognized. A deficiency of neutrophils, or neutropenia, defined as an absolute neutrophil count (ANC) < 1.5×10^9/L, limits the rate at which neutrophils can accumulate at a site of tissue injury or infection. Chemotherapy can cause neutropenia and ultimately affect this defense mechanism. With severe neutropenia (an ANC < 0.5×10^9/L) the risk of serious infections increases substantially.

In patients with chemotherapy-induced neutropenia, infection is usually marked by fever that is usually defined as a body temperature of >38.3°C (101°F). The risk of fever with severe neutropenia, or febrile neutropenia (FN), increases approx 10% each day the blood neutrophil count remains < 0.5×10^9/L *(1)*. Approximately 50% of patients with chemotherapy-induced FN will have a definable bacterial infection *(2)*. The risk of bacteremia is approx 20% in patients presenting with fever and an ANC < 0.1×10^9/L *(2)*; the predicted mortality rate is approx 40%. Thus, neutropenia and FN are important clinical problems that limit the delivery of chemotherapy, cause much human suffering, and result in huge health care expenditures.

From: *Cancer Drug Discovery and Development*
Hematopoietic Growth Factors in Oncology: Basic Science and Clinical Therapeutics
Edited by: G. Morstyn, M. A. Foote, and G. J. Lieschke

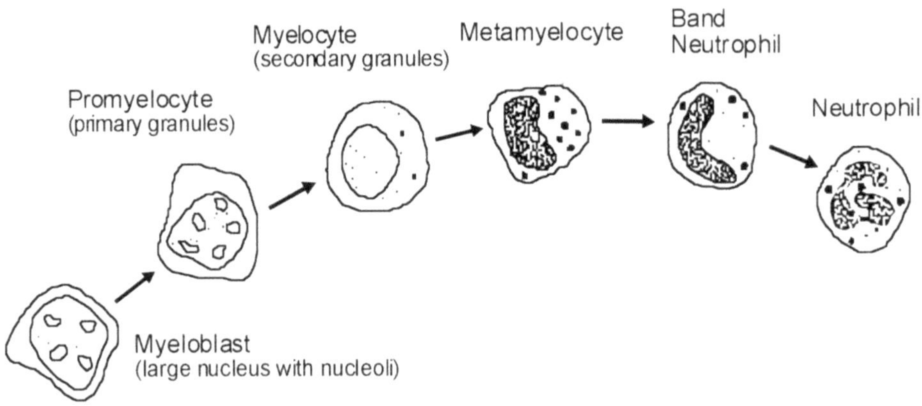

Fig. 1. Stages in neutrophil development in the bone marrow.

This chapter provides an overview of the normal production of neutrophils and the mechanism and consequences of neutropenia in patients with cancer. A summary is included of studies designed to identify factors that increase the risk of developing FN in patients receiving cancer chemotherapy. The chapter outlines current recommendations for the use of hematopoietic growth factors (HGFs), particularly recombinant human granulocyte colony-stimulating factor (rHuG-CSF), in the management of chemotherapy-induced neutropenia, and describes some important unanswered questions about managing fever and infection in patients with cancer.

2. NEUTROPHILS

Neutrophils are part of the body's innate host defense system that protects against invasion by micro-organisms found on body surfaces, particularly on the skin and in the oropharynx and gastrointestinal tract. The rapid accumulation of neutrophils at an acute injury site is the body's first response to limit infection and initiate the repair process.

2.1. Development

Neutrophils are formed in the bone marrow from hematopoietic stem cells, the same cell origin as all other blood cells. Approximately 10–14 d are needed for a hematopoietic stem cell to differentiate into a cell committed to the myeloid lineage and then proliferate and develop into a mature neutrophil (Fig. 1). During the process of neutrophil formation, approx 50% of the time is spent in the proliferative or mitotic phase, in which myeloblasts mature into promyelocytes and then myelocytes, and 50% is spent in the postmitotic phase, in which metamyelocytes mature into bands and then neutrophils. In the mitotic phase, neutrophils acquire most of their primary and secondary granules, the organelles containing the enzymes and specific microbicidal proteins that are necessary for killing bacteria and fungi. Later in development, the cells acquire actin and other critical proteins that facilitate the movement of the cells, and they accumulate the stores of glycogen necessary for the intense metabolic burst that occurs with phagocytosis and killing of bacteria. In the last stages of development, the cells acquire the surface properties and receptors of mature blood neutrophils; they lose their endoplasmic reticulum and the capacity for synthesis of proteins, and the nucleus condenses to assume the characteristic lobular shape of the mature cell. At maturity, the neutrophil is destined to either an apoptotic death in the bone marrow or blood or to disintegrate as it engages in the ingestion and killing of microbes.

2.2. *Function*

In a normal, healthy person, neutrophils are found almost exclusively in the blood and bone marrow. In the blood, some neutrophils flow in the central axial stream with erythrocytes, platelets, and other leukocytes. These neutrophils are described as being in the circulating pool. Other neutrophils are found rolling along the vascular endothelium. These neutrophils are described as being in the marginal pool. Neutrophils in the circulating pool are in a dynamic equilibrium with neutrophils in the marginal pool.

An intrinsic property of neutrophils is to adhere to foreign surfaces and at sites of inflammation. At an inflammation site, neutrophils stick to the endothelium (adherence); migrate from the circulation, squeezing out between vascular endothelial cells (diapedesis) and ingest and kill micro-organisms. Adherence is mediated by integrins and selectins on the neutrophils and their receptors on the endothelium. Migration is mediated by chemotactic factors from the tissues interacting with chemotactic receptors of the neutrophils.

3. CHEMOTHERAPY EFFECTS

The skin and mucous membranes form the primary barriers to invasion of the body by micro-organisms. The skin is normally quite impervious, and infection is almost always caused by a mechanical break or injury, including medical procedures such as intravenous catheter insertion. The oropharynx is normally coated by bacteria, most of which are regarded as of low pathogenicity. Normally, these areas are kept free of overt infection by the constant exudates of neutrophils around the teeth and at breaks in the surface integrity. In healthy persons, large numbers of neutrophils are constantly exuding to these surfaces. Interruption of the neutrophil supply, as occurs with myelotoxic chemotherapy, is often first manifest by oral pain, mouth ulcers, and inflammation of the gingivae.

Further along the gastrointestinal tract, the epithelium on the surface of the large and small intestine is constantly being renewed. The toxic effects of chemotherapy disrupt this fragile barrier; bacterial invasion can occur, particularly in patients with neutropenia. Gram-negative bacteremias associated with cancer chemotherapy usually originate from the gastrointestinal tract. The gut is also the site for emergence of resistant Gram-negative organisms after exposure to broad-spectrum antibiotics.

Although many genetic and acquired mechanisms can impair neutrophil functions, it is the quantitative deficiency of neutrophils, not a functional abnormality that is the primary defect leading to susceptibility to infection in patients with cancer. With chemotherapy-induced neutropenia, the supply of neutrophils is limited, and the number of migrating neutrophils is inadequate. Bacterial multiplication and invasion occur; if these are unchecked by antibiotics, infection and bacteremia predictably follow.

3.1. Neutropenia and the Effects of Chemotherapy

Neutropenia can occur by several mechanisms including massive use of neutrophils in the periphery (e.g., in the sepsis syndrome), redistribution of cells including accumulation in the spleen (e.g., rheumatoid arthritis and malaria), and impaired production by the bone marrow. In patients with acute myelogenous leukemia (AML), neutropenia occurs from the expansion of abnormal clone progenitor cells that lack the capacity for full myeloid development. In other hematologic malignancies, neutropenia can occur as a consequence of the disease. In most malignancies, however, neutropenia is attributable to the effects of chemotherapy that reduce myeloid cell proliferation in the bone marrow. With all myelotoxic chemotherapy, the risk of neutropenia depends on the dosing regimen and resiliency of the patient's hematopoietic system.

Our understanding of the risk of chemotherapy-induced neutropenia is based on the mechanism of action of the specific drugs and drug combinations, in vivo and in vitro studies of drug effects on hematopoietic cells, and results from clinical investigations. Of note, most of these agents cause a similar pattern of reduction in blood cell counts. Neutropenia is the most frequent dose-limiting toxicity. The usual duration of severe neutropenia after administration of a single agents or a combination of agents is approx 3–7 d, beginning approx 3–5 d after chemotherapy administration. Recovery of the bone marrow and return of blood neutrophil counts to normal often takes 3 or more wk. Exceptions include single doses of the alkylating agents that can cause myelosuppression lasting only 2–3 d (i.e., cyclophosphamide) and myelosuppression lasting several weeks or more (i.e., busulfan and BCNU [carmustine]).

Chemotherapy-induced cellular and molecular changes resulting in myeloid cell toxicity are not well understood. Currently, most malignancies are treated with combination chemotherapy, administering treatments to maximize anticancer effects and minimize toxicity. The practice of administrating chemotherapy at 3- to 4-wk intervals was derived empirically from the time normally required for myeloid recovery after administration of most chemotherapy drugs.

Understanding the myelotoxicities of combination chemotherapy regimens requires careful clinical observation and serial blood cell counts over the course of several chemotherapy cycles, usually in the setting of a randomized, controlled trial; however, methods for measuring toxicity, such as timing of blood count samples, reporting of chemotherapy doses and dose intensity, assessing temperature and patient clinical status, and recording administration of antibiotics and other therapies, are not standardized. Many randomized treatment trials, such as those for non-Hodgkin's lymphoma (NHL) and metastatic breast cancer, have not reported on myelotoxicity *(3)*. In trials reporting toxicity, wide variation is seen in the reported occurrence of neutropenia or granulocytopenia. Toxicities are also reported by grade (i.e., grades 1–4) in some studies and by absolute blood counts in others. In breast cancer trials of the combination of cyclophosphamide, methotrexate, and fluorouracil (CMF), the risk of grade 3 or 4 neutropenia varied from 1 to 78% *(3)*. This wide range was undoubtedly owing to the timing of blood counts rather than the patients' responses to therapy. In patients with breast cancer, the mean risk of developing severe neutropenia with administration of a standard CMF regimen is probably 25%.

3.2. Risk Factors for Chemotherapy-Induced Febrile Neutropenia

Infection and inflammation stimulate release of endogenous cytokines (e.g., interleukin-1 [IL-1], tumor necrosis factor [TNF], and IL-6) into the circulation. These cytokines reset the thermoregulatory center in the hypothalamus to retain heat and allow the core temperature of the body to increase. Mononuclear phagocytes are the principle producers of the endogenous cytokines that cause fever and are much less affected by chemotherapy than neutrophils. Therefore, fever is reliable as a marker of infection in patients receiving chemotherapy, including neutropenic patients.

Over the past decade, the risk of FN among patients receiving cancer therapy has received increasing attention. In 1992, Talcott and colleagues *(4)* studied 444 patients with cancer who had fever and neutropenia and were hospitalized. Clinical parameters that predicted subsequent morbidity and mortality and were easily measurable during the first 24 h of hospitalization were identified. The presence of serious comorbidities or uncontrolled cancer or the development of FN during hospitalization predicted an adverse outcome. The in-hospital mortality rate was approx 10% for patients with one of these identified risk factors. This study also identified patients with a low morbidity and mortality risk that could be managed with shorter hospitalizations and less intensive antibiotic treatments.

In a review of the risk of FN among patients with intermediate-grade NHL receiving cyclophosphamide, doxorubicin, vincristine, and prednisone (CHOP) therapy, Lyman and coworkers *(5,6)* identified several factors associated with an increased risk of neutropenia-related complications. Data for this study came from 577 patients and 224 occurrences of FN in 12 community and academic oncology practices. Age > 65 yr ($p = 0.001$), significant cardiovascular or renal disease ($p = 0.02$), baseline hemoglobin concentration < 12 g/dL ($p = 0.018$), and administration of >80% planned dose intensity ($p = 0.018$) were associated with an increased risk of neutropenia-related complications. In this study, patients not receiving prophylactic colony-stimulating factor (CSF) had a significantly greater risk of FN ($p = 0.046$) than patients receiving prophylactic CSF. In multivariate analysis, the risk of FN remained significant for age, cardiovascular and renal disease, baseline hemoglobin concentration, planned chemotherapy dose, and no CSF prophylactic treatment. No significant relationship among sex, stage of disease at initiation of therapy, or lactic dehydrogenase value was reported.

Another predictive model is based on measurement of neutrophil counts before and after the first course of chemotherapy. Silber and coworkers *(7)* first reported this model to predict FN in patients with early-stage breast cancer receiving adjuvant chemotherapy. This study and subsequent investigations *(8)* showed that patients with an ANC < 0.5×10^9/L during the first chemotherapy cycle are at increased risk of serious neutropenia-related adverse effects during subsequent chemotherapy cycles. This important finding led to the practice of secondary prophylaxis (i.e., giving growth factors, specifically rHuG-CSF, only to patients shown to be at high risk for severe neutropenia based on neutrophil data from their first cycle of treatment).

Further investigations, however, have revealed that elderly patients, and perhaps some other groups, are at high risk of FN during their first course of chemotherapy. In reviewing CHOP therapy for NHL, Lyman et al. *(6)* found that 74% of all FN episodes occurred with the first two cycles of chemotherapy. For patients ≥ 65 yr of age, the incidence of first-cycle FN was about 20%, with a gradual increase in the cumulative probability of FN over the course of treatment to approx 35%. Thus, >50% of these events occurred with the first exposure to chemotherapy. In a parallel investigation of the risk of FN in patients with breast cancer receiving adjuvant therapy, Agboola and coworkers *(9)* reported that increasing age predicted hematologic toxicity. In this report, other predictors were an ANC < 0.5×10^9/L and a first-cycle decrease in hemoglobin concentration > 1 g/dL. In addition, FN during the first chemotherapy cycle predicted FN during subsequent cycles.

An important and provocative finding in these investigations is the high proportion of overall risk of FN that is present at the beginning of treatment, which is when standard-dose chemotherapy is first given to a previously untreated patient. For years, the treatment paradigm has emphasized the progressive toxicity associated with sequential chemotherapy dosing. Direct and predictable cumulative toxicity for erythroid cells and platelets may occur, but current data suggest that myeloid cells (i.e., neutrophils and monocytes) may show inherently different responses. Careful observation of blood cell counts in patients with small-cell lung cancer (SCLC) treated with up to six cycles of cyclophosphamide, doxorubicin, and etoposide illustrated that neutrophil counts were not progressively lower with each cycle *(10)*. These results suggest that the hematopoietic tissues of the bone marrow adapt to the sequential insults of chemotherapy, just as the bone marrow adapts to produce more neutrophils in response to chronic infection. This study also illustrated the effects of rHuG-CSF treatment, which ameliorated the effects of chemotherapy, reducing the depth and duration of neutropenia.

As these studies point out, age is a consistent predictor of FN risk. It is known that blood cell counts, including neutrophil and monocyte counts, are similar in healthy young and healthy elderly patients. The functions of these cells are similar in healthy young and healthy elderly patients. Some evidence points to a decrease in the hematopoietic reserves in the elderly, as reflected by reduced numbers of CD 34^+ hematopoietic progenitor cells mobilized after stimulation with rHuG-CSF *(11)*. Results from a small, but provocative, study of patients with SCLC suggest that a reduced CD 34^+ cell response to rHuG-CSF predicts a greater risk of developing neutropenia after cancer chemotherapy *(12)*. Thus, $CD34^+$ cell counts may be a better predictor of neutropenia risk than blood neutrophil counts. Further investigation of the number and function of these progenitor cells before and during cancer chemotherapy may be helpful in developing new biologic predictors that could be used to predict patients at risk of developing neutropenia.

3.3. Pathogens Associated With Chemotherapy-Induced Neutropenia and Infection

Most infections in patients with severe neutropenia are caused by either aerobic Gram-negative bacilli, particularly *Escherichia coli, Klebsiella pneumoniae,* and *Pseudomonas aeruginosa,* or Gram-positive cocci, particularly *Staphylococcus aureus* and α-hemolytic streptococci *(2)*. In recent years, infections by *S. aureus,* including methicillin-resistant and vancomycin-resistant species, have been increasing *(13)*. Infections by anaerobic organisms are relatively uncommon, although the microaerophilic organisms of the mouth contribute to gingivitis and mucositis in patients with neutropenia. For unclear reasons, clostridial infections, including bacteremias, occur in patients with various forms of chronic neutropenia; however, clostridial blood stream infections occur infrequently in patients with chemotherapy-induced neutropenia. *Clostridia difficile,* however, is an important cause of diarrhea, abdominal pain, and fever in all patients with neutropenia, particularly after exposure to broad-spectrum antibiotics. Infections by mycobacteria including *Mycobacterium tuberculosis* are generally not a problem with conventional chemotherapy. Tunnel infections of indwelling venous catheters by atypical mycobacteria, as well as by Gram-positive cocci, are always a concern.

Over the past two decades, mycotic infections in patients with severe neutropenia have steadily increased *(14)*. Fungal infections are a greater problem with prolonged neutropenia and antibiotic administration in the setting of hematopoietic stem cell transplantation and high-dose chemotherapy than with conventional chemotherapy for solid tumors *(15)*. Predisposing factors for fungal infections include diabetes mellitus and corticosteroid treatment. Most infections are caused by *Candida* species, and an increased proportion is caused by resistant organisms *(16)*. Major morbidity and mortality continue to be associated with infections by invasive molds, especially *Aspergillus* and *Fusarium* species. By the time these invasive molds are clinically recognized with current techniques, the chance of survival is generally <50%, even with optimal therapy *(17)*.

4. TREATMENT OF CHEMOTHERAPY-INDUCED FEBRILE NEUTROPENIA

The treatment of patients with chemotherapy-induced FN is multifactorial and includes not only antibiotic and CSF therapy but also supportive measures. Observational vigilance is an important aspect in the care of patients with chemotherapy-induced neutropenia; there is no substitute for frequent observation and examination, particularly of the oropharynx, chest, and abdominal and perirectal areas. Frequent blood cell counts, blood cultures, and culture and examination of exudates and other bodily fluids in patients with fever remain the mainstay of good medical care. In addition to good skin care and oral hygiene, every effort should be made to maintain good functional status through nutritional support and exercise. Patients with cancer should be encouraged to decrease or eliminate smoking and maintain their immunization status, including influenza immunizations. Education of the patient and family, as observers of health status, is also important, particularly to recognize the occurrence of inflammation and fever and to understand the significance of changes in blood counts.

4.1. Antibiotic Therapy

Patients with FN should receive empirical, broad-spectrum antibiotic therapy. Each episode of FN must be assumed to be a potentially serious bacterial infection. Ordinarily, each episode of FN should be treated with maximal doses of intravenous antibiotics while diagnostic studies are in progress. For most patients, a brief hospital stay is also important for observation and treatment because of difficulty in determining which patients have serious infections in the physician's office or emergency room.

When there are significant obstacles to obtaining diagnostic studies, it is best to begin empirical antibiotic therapy without delay. Frequently, patients have indwelling catheters that can be the source of fever and infection. Antibiotic therapy can be initiated without removing the catheter; however, it is prudent to consider removing any intravenous device, particularly in critically ill patients *(2)*. Sepsis from a tunnel infection, often caused by *S. aureus,* is currently a major clinical problem *(18)*. If an indwelling multiple-lumen catheter is not removed, some experts recommend rotating antibiotic administration through each lumen *(2)*.

Table 1
rHuG-CSF and rHuGM-CSF Comparison

Parameter	*rHuG-CSF*	*rHuGM-CSF*
Chromosome location	17	4
Source of gene	Bladder carcinoma cell line (filgrastim), squamous carcinoma cell line (lenograstim)	Human monocyte cell line (molgramostim), T-lymphoma cell line (sargramostim)
Amino acids	174[a]	127 or 128[b]
Glycosylation	*O*-linked (lenograstim)	*N*-linked (sargramostim)
Expression system		
Generic names	Filgrastim, lenograstim, pegfilgrastim, nartograstim	Sargramostim, molgramostim

ABBREVIATIONS: rHuG-CSF, recombinant human granulocyte colony-stimulating factor; rHuGM-CSF, recombinant human granulocyte-macrophage colony-stimulating factor.

[a] Native G-CSF has two forms, 1 with 177 amino acids, which is less active than the other form with 174 amino acids; filgrastim has an N-terminal methionine.

[b] Molgramostim has 128 amino acids and sargramostim has 127 amino acids.

Data from refs. *19* and *20*.

The initial selection of empirical, broad-spectrum antibiotics for patients with FN has evolved gradually over the past 20 yr. Currently, treatment with a single antibiotic (e.g., the cephalosporin ceftazidime) is a frequently used approach in the United States *(2)*. A cephalosporin-vancomycin combination for patients presumed to have a resistant staphylococcal infections is recommended *(2)*. A third-generation cephalosporin-, antipseudomonal penicillin-, or carbapenem-aminoglycoside combination is recommended for patients with a presumed or proven resistant Gram-negative infection *(2)*. A panel of experts from the Infectious Disease Society of America has made recommendations for antibiotic therapy for neutropenic patients *(2)*.

4.2. Colony-Stimulating Factor Therapy

The CSFs are glycoproteins that regulate the proliferation, differentiation, functional activity, and survival of myeloid cells. They were discovered through their capacity to stimulate single myeloid progenitor cells to proliferate in vitro and form clusters and colonies of differentiated cells, particularly neutrophils and monocytes. Basic characteristics of the CSFs rHuG-CSF and rHuGM-CSF are outlined in Table 1.

Several characteristics of the CSFs are of great clinical importance for the management of chemotherapy-induced neutropenia and FN:

1. Both G-CSF and GM-CSF are produced endogenously by many cell types. Amounts of circulating G-CSFs increase markedly with naturally occurring and experimentally induced infections *(21,22)*. In experimental animals, a deficiency of G-CSF is associated with the development of neutropenia *(23)*. Experimental studies indicate that G-CSF is the natural regulator for the blood neutrophil count analogous to erythropoietin (EPO) and thrombopoietin (TPO). In contrast, GM-CSF concentrations are not increased with infection, and a deficiency of GM-CSF does not result in neutropenia *(24,25)*.

2. Receptors for G-CSF and GM-CSF are expressed on primitive and mature myeloid cells, including expression on mature circulating neutrophils. Exposure of neutrophils to G-CSF or GM-CSF primes mature neutrophils for an enhanced metabolic burst when they are exposed to bacteria.
3. Both G-CSF and GM-CSF promote the survival of myeloid cells at all stages in their development; thus, these CSF have an antiapoptotic effect *(26)*.
4. Studies involving normal human volunteers who received either rHuG-CSF or rHuGM-CSF for 14 d showed that rHuG-CSF is more potent than rHuGM-CSF in stimulating neutrophil production *(27,28)*
5. In vivo administration of rHuG-CSF or rHuGM-CSF increases neutrophil production and accelerates the transit time of developing cells through the bone marrow. Increases in blood neutrophil counts after cytokine administration are attributable to increased numbers of cell divisions, shortened time between divisions, accelerated transit through the postmitotic stage of development, and increased neutrophil survival in the blood *(28)*.
6. Neutrophils made in response to rHuG-CSF or rHuGM-CSF have normal, functional bacteria-killing properties *(29)*.
7. The primary HGF now used for the prevention and treatment of FN is rHuG-CSF because of its greater potency *(30)* and fewer associated adverse effects *(31)*.

Adverse effects associated with injections of rHuG-CSF are less severe than with rHuGM-CSF *(31)*. Bone pain and headache are the most common adverse effects with rHuG-CSF *(30)*. Myalgias and flu-like symptoms are the most common adverse effects with rHuGM-CSF *(30)*.

The use of rHuG-CSF concomitant with antibiotics for treating FN has been explored in several clinical trials *(32–37)*. One study, early in the development of rHuG-CSF, involved treating 218 patients with cancer who developed fever and neutropenia (neutrophil count < 1.0×10^9/L) after chemotherapy administration *(36)*. Patients were randomized to receive either rHuG-CSF 12 μg/kg daily, beginning within 12 h of initiation of a standard antibiotic treatment, or standard antibiotic treatment alone. Patients remained on study until their neutrophil count was >0.5×10^9/L and they were afebrile for 4 d. Patients who received rHuG-CSF had more rapid neutrophil recovery than those who did not receive rHuG-CSF, but there was no reduction in overall days of fever or antibiotic treatment. However, patients who were slowest to recover appeared to benefit from rHuG-CSF.

A more recent randomized, controlled trial enrolled 210 patients with a variety of solid tumors treated with standard-dose chemotherapy *(32)*. High-risk patients who developed FN were assigned to receive a standard antibiotic regimen with or without rHuG-CSF 5 μg/kg daily. High-risk patients had neutrophil counts < 0.1×10^9/L, a short latency period from previous chemotherapy, severe comorbidities, signs of sepsis, or prior inpatient status. Administration of rHuG-CSF shortened the duration of severe neutropenia and hospitalization and reduced the use of antibiotics. Results from a recent meta-analysis *(38)*, including this trial, demonstrate that the therapeutic use of rHuG-CSF for FN is probably beneficial, particularly for high-risk patients. Further investigation is needed to define the benefits of this strategy and the details for optimum management, such as the dose and duration of treatment and optimal antibiotics to use with rHuG-CSF.

Recently, pegylated rHuG-CSF (pegfilgrastim) has been introduced to simplify the management of patients developing neutropenia after chemotherapy. Pegfilgrastim has a much longer half-life than nonpegylated filgrastim, remaining in the body long enough to stimulate complete bone marrow recovery after standard-dose chemotherapy. Pegfilgrastim has otherwise similar effects as the filgrastim. Two randomized, controlled trials were conducted to establish the effectiveness of pegfilgrastim to prevent FN *(39,40)*. Interestingly, in these trials, treatment with pegfilgrastim was associated with a lower incidence of FN, although overall it stimulated a lesser neutrophil response.

5. PREVENTION OF CHEMOTHERAPY-INDUCED FEBRILE NEUTROPENIA

5.1. Antibiotic Therapy

Administration of prophylactic antibiotics to patients receiving cancer chemotherapy is controversial, but infectious disease experts discourage this practice for two principal reasons. First, prophylactic antibiotic therapy is only marginally effective and provides a very small benefit. Second, prophylactic antibiotic therapy is associated with a greater risk of resistant organism emergence. Early efforts to sterilize body surfaces with antibiotics or other measures were unsuccessful; selective decontamination with various antibiotic regimens proved unacceptable to patients and of little benefit *(2)*. Prophylaxis with trimethoprim-sulfamethoxazole is useful to prevent *Pneumocystis carinii* pneumonia, but this infection is generally an infrequent problem in patients receiving cancer chemotherapy. The quinolones, which are useful antibiotics for the treatment of Gram-negative and Gram-positive infections, have been used for prevention of infections in patients receiving cancer chemotherapy; however, the benefit is relatively small and recognized only through meta-analyses that combine results from small trials *(41–43)*. As noted previously, a disadvantage of quinolone use is the emergence of resistant organisms. Therefore, the practice of prescribing quinolones for prevention of infections in patients undergoing cancer chemotherapy is strongly discouraged.

5.2. Colony-Stimulating Factor Therapy

Results from randomized, controlled clinical trials demonstrate that filgrastim reduces the duration and severity of neutropenia after chemotherapy administration *(10,44; see* Table 2). Results from clinical trials demonstrate that rHuGM-CSF has a more limited effect than rHuG-CSF in decreasing the duration and severity of neutropenia after cancer chemotherapy administration *(45–48)*.

The incidence of FN and documented infections, use of antibiotics, and duration of hospitalization for FN are reduced in cancer patients undergoing myelotoxic chemotherapy and receiving rHuG-CSF *(10,44,49–51)*. The original trials demonstrating these effects were completed in patients with SCLC treated with cyclophosphamide, doxorubicin, and etoposide *(10,44)*. In one study, the median number of days with neutrophils $< 0.5 \times 10^9$/L was reduced from 6 to 1 d ($p < 0.001$) *(10)*. The proportion of patients developing FN was reduced from 77 to 40% ($p < 0.001$) *(10)*. The durations of hospitalization and intravenous antibiotic administration were similarly reduced. In a second, somewhat smaller, trial, the proportion of patients developing FN was also reduced by approx 50% *(44)*.

Meta-analyses have confirmed the benefits of prophylactic rHuG-CSF and extended the result of the original two pivotal trials *(6,52)*. A recent of meta-analysis included eight controlled trials involving 1144 patients, five done with filgrastim and three with lenograstim, the glycosylated form of rHuG-CSF *(6)*. Five trials were double-blind and

Table 2
Randomized Trials of rHuG-CSF to Prevent Febrile Neutropenia

Tumor	*Chemotherapy*	*FN range (%)*	*Reference*
SCLC	CAE	40–77	*10*
SCLC	CAE	26–53	*44*
NHL	VAPEC-B	23–44	*51*
NHL	VNCOP-B	8–32	*49*

ABBREVIATIONS: NHL, non-Hodgkin's lymphoma; SCLC, small-cell lung cancer; CAE, cyclophosphamide, doxorubicin, and etoposide; VAPEC-B, vincristine, etoposide, cyclophosphamide, and bleomycin; VNCOP-B, etoposide, procarbazine, cyclophosphamide, vincristine, and bleomycin; rHuG-CSF, recombinant human granulocyte colony-stimulating factor.

placebo-controlled; three trials included untreated, control patients. Administration of rHuG-CSF significantly reduced the risk of FN and documented infections; there was a trend toward a reduction in infection-related mortality.

These very convincing studies led to wide usage of rHuG-CSF, but several important questions remain:

1. Is it safe to administer rHuG-CSF concomitant with chemotherapy? The rHuG-CSF randomized, controlled trials described previously were conducted by administering rHuG-CSF the day after completion of chemotherapy. Meropol and co-workers *(53)* administered concomitant rHuG-CSF 5 µg/kg daily and 5-fluorouracil for 5 d. Patients could receive an additional 9 d of rHuG-CSF. No control group was used, but another group of patients was treated by the same protocol without rHuG-CSF. Administration of rHuG-CSF in this trial appeared to increase fluorouracil toxicity. However, results from other trials administering rHuG-CSF concomitant with other drugs including doxorubicin, cyclophosphamide, vincristine, etoposide, and carboplatin suggest that concomitant administration may be safe. Current recommendations are to administer rHuG-CSF 24 h after the completion of chemotherapy *(54)*.
2. What is the proper dose of rHuG-CSF? Almost all trials with filgrastim have used 5 µg/kg sc once daily. Lenograstim has been administered over a range of doses, but there is not sufficient evidence to suggest that a dose other than 5 µg/kg is effective to ameliorate neutropenia or prevent FN. Thus, the standard adult and pediatric dose for both filgrastim and lenograstim is 5 µg/kg daily.
3. What is the proper duration of rHuG-CSF treatment? In the pivotal trials, rHuG-CSF was administered until the neutrophil count increased to > 10×10^9/L to ensure that full hematopoietic recovery. Randomized, controlled trials have not established equal efficacy for shorter durations of treatment, but this issue has not yet been thoroughly investigated or resolved.
4. Can initiation of rHuG-CSF be delayed for a few days after chemotherapy to decrease the duration and cost of treatment? Administration of filgrastim beginning 1, 3, or 5 d after completion of cyclophosphamide, doxorubicin, and etoposide chemotherapy was studied in a small phase 2 trial *(55)*. Administration of filgrastim beginning 5 d after chemotherapy was associated with a suboptimal hematologic recovery; administration of filgrastim beginning 1 or 3 d after chemotherapy was associated with a similar degree of

hematologic recovery; however, this study was too small to establish whether delaying filgrastim treatment to d 3 after chemotherapy was associated with a reduction in the rate of occurrence of FN. Results from a randomized trial in which administration of rHuG-CSF was delayed until patients had established neutropenia, however, showed no reduction in the duration of hospitalization or antibiotic treatment *(56)*. Thus, delaying administration is not recommended.

Because all chemotherapy regimens are not associated with the same degree of neutropenia and because patients differ substantially in the resiliency of their hematopoietic tissues and chemotherapy tolerance, there have been many efforts to establish secondary prophylaxis protocols. This approach limits the use of rHuG-CSF to patients who develop neutropenia or neutropenia complications during their first cycle of chemotherapy. Evidence for the use of rHuG-CSF as secondary prophylaxis can be derived from the pivotal trial by Crawford and co-workers *(10)*. In this study, placebo recipients in the first cycle who developed FN were treated subsequently with open-label rHuG-CSF. For these patients, the rate of FN was reduced from 100% in cycle 1 to 23% in cycle 2, without a change in their chemotherapy regimen. It may be inappropriate, however, to attribute all benefit to rHuG-CSF because effects of FN, infections, or repeated chemotherapy may affect this improvement or outcome.

As noted previously, secondary prophylaxis leaves patients, particularly the elderly, at risk for the development of severe adverse effects after their first chemotherapy cycle. For this reason, prudence is needed in the use of secondary prophylaxis. As risk factors are better defined, it can be anticipated that secondary prophylaxis will be primarily used for low-risk patients.

6. CURRENT ISSUES IN THE MANAGEMENT OF NEUTROPENIA AND INFECTIONS IN PATIENTS WITH CANCER

As outlined in this chapter, the availability of rHuG-CSF has had profound medical and scientific implications. The ability of rHuG-CSF to accelerate bone marrow recovery has greatly altered the approach to chemotherapy and management of neutropenia risk in patients with cancer. The availability of rHuG-CSF has stimulated interest in understanding the physiology and regulation of neutrophil production, as well as other ways to enhance host resistance to bacterial infections. The availability of rHuG-CSF has also stimulated interest in defining host responses to cancer chemotherapy and specific factors (i.e., cellular components, cytokines, environmental factors, bone marrow recovery rate).It is relatively easy to measure the blood neutrophil counts, but cancer chemotherapy and the HGFs exert most of their effects on hematopoietic cells in the bone marrow. Better information is needed about the kinetics of recovery of primitive hematopoietic cells and their progeny in the bone marrow to guide the use of HGFs for patients receiving cancer chemotherapy. Although several new antifungal agents have recently become available, development of new antibiotics has slowed remarkably. The promise for the next decade is better supportive care through minimizing the toxicities of cancer treatments and better understanding of how to augment host defense mechanisms.

REFERENCES

1. Blackwell S, Crawford J. Filgrastim (r-metHuG-CSF) in the chemotherapy setting. In: Morstyn G, Dexter T, eds., *Filgrastim (r-metHuG-CSF) in Clinical Practice.* New York: Marcel Dekker. 1994; 103–116.
2. Hughes WT, Armstrong D, Bodey GP, et al. 2002 guidelines for the use of antimicrobial agents in neutropenic patients with cancer. *Clin Infect Dis* 2002; 34:730–751.

3. Dale DC, McCarter GC, Crawford J et al. Myelotoxicity and dose intensity of chemotherapy: reporting practices from randomized clinical trials. *J Natl Coop Cancer Network* 2003; 1:440–454.
4. Talcott JA, Siegel RD, Finberg R, Goldman L. Risk assessment in cancer patients with fever and neutropenia: a prospective, two-center validation of a prediction rule. *J Clin Oncol* 1992; 10:316–322.
5. Lyman GH, Dale DC, Crawford J, Stolshek B, Carter W, Delgado D. Risk of febrile neutropenia among patients receiving CHOP chemotherapy. *Blood* 2001; 98:231b, abstract 4642.
6. Lyman GH, Kuderer NM, Djulbegovic B. Prophylactic granulocyte colony-stimulating factor in patients receiving dose-intensive cancer chemotherapy: a meta-analysis. *Am J Med* 2002b; 112:406–411.
7. Silber JH, Fridman M, DiPaola RS, Erder MH, Pauly MV, Fox KR. First-cycle blood counts and subsequent neutropenia, dose reduction, or delay in early-stage breast cancer therapy. *J Clin Oncol* 1998; 16:2392–2400.
8. Rivera E, Erder MH, Moore TD, et al. Targeted filgrastim support in early-stage breast cancer: towards the implementation of a risk model. *Cancer* 2003; 98:222–228.
9. Agboola O, Crawford J, Dale DC, et al. Risk models for neutropenic complications associated with breast cancer adjuvant chemotherapy. *Proc Am Soc Clin Oncol* 2002; 21:66a, abstract 261.
10. Crawford J, Ozer H, Stoller R, et al. Reduction by granulocyte colony-stimulating factor of fever and neutropenia induced by chemotherapy in patients with small-cell lung cancer. *N Engl J Med* 1991; 325:164–170.
11. Chatta GS, Price TH, Allen RC, Dale DC. Effects of in vivo recombinant methionyl granulocyte colony-stimulating factor on the neutrophil response and peripheral blood colony-forming cells in healthy young and elderly adult volunteers. *Blood* 1994; 84:2923–2929.
12. Egusa Y, Fujiwara Y, Syaharuddin E, Sumiyoshi H, Isobe T, Yamakido M. Mobilization of peripheral blood stem cells in patients with advanced thoracic malignancies after irinotecan (CPT-11) administration. *Anticancer Res* 1998; 18:481–488.
13. Zinner SH. Changing epidemiology of infections in patients with neutropenia and cancer: emphasis on gram-positive and resistant bacteria. *Clin Infect Dis* 1999; 29:490–494.
14. McNeil MM, Nash SL, Hajjeh RA, et al. Trends in mortality due to invasive mycotic diseases in the United States, 1980–1997. *Clin Infect Dis* 2001; 33:641–647.
15. De Pauw BE. Practical modalities for prevention of fungal infections in cancer patients. *Eur J Clin Microbiol Infect Dis* 1997; 16:32–41.
16. Singh N. Trends in the epidemiology of opportunistic fungal infections: predisposing factors and the impact of antimicrobial use practices. *Clin Infect Dis* 2001; 33:1692–1696.
17. Rex JH, Walsh TJ, Anaissie EJ. Fungal infections in iatrogenically compromised hosts. *Adv Intern Med* 1998; 43:321–371.
18. Hachem R, Raad I. Prevention and management of long-term catheter related infections in cancer patients. *Cancer Invest* 2002; 20:1105–1113.
19. Nagata S, Tsuchiya M, Asano S, et al. Molecular cloning and expression of cDNA for human granulocyte colony stimulating factor. *Nature* 1986; 319:415–418.
20. Souza LM, Boone TC, Gabrilove J, et al. Recombinant human granulocyte colony-stimulating factor: effects on normal and leukemic myeloid cells. *Science* 1986; 232:61–65.
21. Kawakami M, Tsutsumi H, Kumakawa T, et al. Levels of serum granulocyte colony-stimulating factor in patients with infections. *Blood* 1990; 76:1962–1964.
22. Cheers C, Haigh AM, Kelso A, Metcalf D, Stanley ER, Young AM. Production of colony-stimulating factors (CSFs) during infection: separate determinations of macrophage-, granulocyte-, granulocyte-macrophage-, and multi-CSFs. *Infect Immun* 1988; 56:247–251.
23. Hammond WP, Csiba E, Canin A, et al. Chronic neutropenia. A new canine model induced by human granulocyte colony-stimulating factor. *J Clin Invest* 1991; 87:704–710.
24. Selig C, Nothdurft W. Cytokines and progenitor cells of granulocytopoiesis in peripheral blood of patients with bacterial infections. *Infect Immun* 1995; 63:104–109.
25. Cebon J, Layton JE, Maher D, Morstyn G. Endogenous haemopoietic growth factors in neutropenia and infection. *Br J Haematol* 1994; 86:265–274.
26. Begley CG, Lopez AF, Nicola NA, et al. Purified colony-stimulating factors enhance the survival of human neutrophils and eosinophils in vitro: a rapid and sensitive microassay for colony-stimulating factors. *Blood* 1986; 68:162–166.
27. Dale DC, Liles WC, Llewellyn C, Price TH. Effects of granulocyte-macrophage colony-stimulating factor (GM-CSF) on neutrophil kinetics and function in normal human volunteers. *Am J Hematol* 1998; 57:7–15.

28. Price TH, Chatta GS, Dale DC. Effect of recombinant granulocyte colony-stimulating factor on neutrophil kinetics in normal young and elderly humans. *Blood* 1996; 88:335–340.
29. Hubel K, Dale DC, Liles WC. Therapeutic use of cytokines to modulate phagocyte function for the treatment of infectious diseases: current status of granulocyte colony-stimulating factor, granulocyte-macrophage colony-stimulating factor, macrophage colony-stimulating factor, and interferon-gamma. *J Infect Dis* 2002; 185:1490–1501.
30. Dale DC. Colony-stimulating factors for the management of neutropenia in cancer patients. *Drugs* 2002; 62:1–15.
31. Milkovich G, Moleski RJ, Reitan JF, et al. Comparative safety of filgrastim versus sargramostim in patients receiving myelosuppressive chemotherapy. *Pharmacotherapy* 2000; 20:1432–1440.
32. Garcia-Carbonero R, Mayordomo JI, Tornamira MV, et al. Granulocyte colony-stimulating factor in the treatment of high-risk febrile neutropenia: a multicenter randomized trial. *J Natl Cancer Inst* 2001; 93:31–38.
33. Anaissie EJ, Vartivarian S, Bodey GP, et al. Randomized comparison between antibiotics alone and antibiotics plus granulocyte-macrophage colony-stimulating factor (*Escherichia coli*-derived) in cancer patients with fever and neutropenia. *Am J Med* 1996; 100:17–23.
34. Vellenga E, Uyl-de Groot CA, de Wit R, et al. Randomized placebo-controlled trial of granulocyte-macrophage colony-stimulating factor in patients with chemotherapy-related febrile neutropenia. *J Clin Oncol* 1996; 14:619–627.
35. Mayordomo JI, Rivera F, Diaz-Puente MT, et al. Improving treatment of chemotherapy-induced neutropenic fever by administration of colony-stimulating factors. *J Natl Cancer Inst* 1995; 87:803–808.
36. Maher DW, Lieschke GJ, Green M, et al. Filgrastim in patients with chemotherapy-induced febrile neutropenia. A double-blind, placebo-controlled trial. *Ann Intern Med* 1994; 121:492–501.
37. Riikonen P, Saarinen UM, Makipernaa A, et al. Recombinant human granulocyte-macrophage colony-stimulating factor in the treatment of febrile neutropenia: a double blind placebo-controlled study in children. *Pediatr Infect Dis J* 1994; 13:197–202.
38. Wallam M, Agboola Y, Lyman G. Meta-analysis of colony-stimulating factors to treat febrile neutropenia (FN) in patients receiving cancer chemotherapy. *Proc ASCO* 2001; 2:306b.
39. Green MD, Koelbl H, Baselga J, et al. A randomized double-blind multicenter phase III study of fixed-dose single-administration pegfilgrastim versus daily filgrastim in patients receiving myelosuppressive chemotherapy. *Ann Oncol* 2003; 14:29–35.
40. Holmes FA, O'Shaughnessy JA, Vukelja S, et al. Blinded, randomized, multicenter study to evaluate single administration pegfilgrastim once per cycle versus daily filgrastim as an adjunct to chemotherapy in patients with high-risk stage II or stage III/IV breast cancer. *J Clin Oncol* 2002; 20:727–731.
41. Engels EA, Lau J, Barza M. Efficacy of quinolone prophylaxis in neutropenic cancer patients: a meta-analysis. *J Clin Oncol* 1998; 16:1179–1187.
42. Rotstein C, Mandell LA, Goldberg N. Fluoroquinolone prophylaxis for profoundly neutropenic cancer patients: a meta-analysis. *Curr Opin Oncol* 1997; 4:S2–7.
43. Cruciani M, Rampazzo R, Malena M, et al. Prophylaxis with fluoroquinolones for bacterial infections in neutropenic patients: a meta-analysis. *Clin Infect Dis* 1996; 23:795–805.
44. Trillet-Lenoir V, Green J, Manegold C, et al. Recombinant granulocyte colony stimulating factor reduces the infectious complications of cytotoxic chemotherapy. *Eur J Cancer* 1993; 3:319–324.
45. Weaver CH, Schulman KA, Wilson-Relyea B, Birch R, West W, Buckner CD. Randomized trial of filgrastim, sargramostim, or sequential sargramostim and filgrastim after myelosuppressive chemotherapy for the harvesting of peripheral-blood stem cells. *J Clin Oncol* 2000; 18:43–53.
46. Yau JC, Neidhart JA, Triozzi P, et al. Randomized placebo-controlled trial of granulocyte-macrophage colony-stimulating-factor support for dose-intensive cyclophosphamide, etoposide, and cisplatin. *Am J Hematol* 1996; 51:289–295.
47. Bajorin DF, Nichols CR, Schmoll HJ, et al. Recombinant human granulocyte-macrophage colony-stimulating factor as an adjunct to conventional-dose ifosfamide-based chemotherapy for patients with advanced or relapsed germ cell tumors: a randomized trial. *J Clin Oncol* 1995; 13:79–86.
48. Bunn PA, Jr, Crowley J, Kelly K, et al. Chemoradiotherapy with or without granulocyte-macrophage colony-stimulating factor in the treatment of limited-stage small-cell lung cancer: a prospective phase III randomized study of the Southwest Oncology Group. *J Clin Oncol* 1995; 13:1632–1641.
49. Zinzani PL, Pavone E, Storti S, et al. Randomized trial with or without granulocyte colony-stimulating factor as adjunct to induction VNCOP-B treatment of elderly high-grade non-Hodgkin's lymphoma. *Blood* 1997; 89:3974–3979.

50. Chevallier B, Chollet P, Merrouche Y, et al. Lenograstim prevents morbidity from intensive induction chemotherapy in the treatment of inflammatory breast cancer. *J Clin Oncol* 1995; 13:1564–1571.
51. Pettengell R, Gurney H, Radford JA, et al. Granulocyte colony-stimulating factor to prevent dose-limiting neutropenia in non-Hodgkin's lymphoma: a randomized controlled trial. *Blood* 1992; 80:1430–1436.
52. Messori A, Trippoli S, Tendi E. G-CSF for the prophylaxis of neutropenic fever in patients with small cell lung cancer receiving myelosuppressive antineoplastic chemotherapy: meta-analysis and pharmacoeconomic evaluation. *J Clin Pharm Ther* 1996; 21:57–63.
53. Meropol NJ, Miller LL, Korn EL, Braitman LE, MacDermott ML, Schuchter LM. Severe myelosuppression resulting from concurrent administration of granulocyte colony-stimulating factor and cytotoxic chemotherapy. *J Natl Cancer Inst* 1992; 84:1201–1203.
54. Ozer H, Armitage JO, Bennett CL, et al. 2000 update of recommendations for the use of hematopoietic colony-stimulating factors: evidence-based, clinical practice guidelines. American Society of Clinical Oncology Growth Factors Expert Panel. *J Clin Oncol* 2000; 18:3558–3585.
55. Crawford J, Kreisman H, Garewal H, et al. The impact of filgrastim schedule variation on hematopoietic recovery post-chemotherapy. *Ann Oncol* 1997; 8:1117–1124.
56. Koumakis G, Vassilomanolakis M, Barbounis V, et al. Optimal timing (preemptive versus supportive) of granulocyte colony-stimulating factor administration following high-dose cyclophosphamide. *Oncology* 1999; 56:28–35.

12 Thrombocytopenia and Platelet Transfusions in Patients With Cancer

Lawrence T. Goodnough, MD

CONTENTS

1. INTRODUCTION

Use of intensive chemotherapy regiments in oncology and in bone marrow/progenitor cell transplantation programs has increased the demand for platelet products, particularly in patients with severe thrombocytopenia or bleeding complications. Use of apheresis platelet transfusions has also increased substantially, from 365,000 units in 1989 to 1,264,000 units in 2001 (Table 1) *(1–3)*. This increase is being driven partly by the need for alternative platelet inventories to support cardiac surgery, oncology, and peripheral blood progenitor cell (PBPC) transplantation programs and partly by use of leukoreduced platelet products *(4)*.

Emerging issues are renewing interest in platelet transfusion practices *(5)*. This review discusses the current risks associated with platelet transfusion and emerging issues in platelet transfusion therapy, including re-evaluation of the platelet threshold for prophylactic transfusion and modification of platelet transfusion dose, as well as the role of hematopoietic growth factors in platelet recovery.

2. CURRENT RISKS OF PLATELET TRANSFUSIONS

The risks for transfusion-transmitted diseases are estimated to be at an historically low rate (Table 2) *(6)*. Nucleic acid testing has substantially decreased the risk of viral infection by shortening the window of infectivity for the hepatitis C virus and the human immunodeficiency virus (HIV).

From: *Cancer Drug Discovery and Development*
Hematopoietic Growth Factors in Oncology: Basic Science and Clinical Therapeutics
Edited by: G. Morstyn, M. A. Foote, and G. J. Lieschke © Humana Press Inc., Totowa, NJ

Table 1
Transfusion of Platelets in the United States[a]

	1989	1992	1994	1997	1999	2001
Concentrates	5146	4688	3582	3396	3036	2614
Apheresis	352	607	714	940	1003	1264
	(26%)	(44%)	(54%)	(62%)	(60%)	(74%)
Total transfusions	6958	8330	7866	9037	9054	10,19[illegible]

[a] Thousands of units. One apheresis unit = 6 concentrates.

Data from refs. *1–3*.

Table 2
Some Estimated Risks of Blood Transfusion

	Estimated frequency of occurrence per million units (per actual unit)
Infections	
Viral	
Hepatitis B	5–17 (1/60,000–1/200,000)
Hepatitis C	0.5–1 (1/800,000–1/1.7 × 10^6)
HIV	1 (1/1.4–2.4 × 10^6)
Bacterial	
Red cells	2 (1/500,000)
Platelets	500 (1/2,000)
Acute hemolytic transfusion reactions	1 to 4 (1/250,000–1,000,000)
Delayed hemolytic transfusion reactions	1000 (1/1,000)

Data from ref. *6*.

2.1. HIV Transmission

Transfusion-associated HIV infection was first reported in late 1982 and early 1983. HIV antibody testing was implemented in March 1985, and over the next 5 years, only about five cases of transfusion-associated HIV infection were reported annually. In the year before testing started, 714 cases were reported *(7)*. In late 1995, blood banks began testing donors for p24 antigen to further decrease the risk of transfusion-transmitted HIV disease. In 1999, nucleic acid testing was introduced to close the window of infectivity (from infection to detection), lowering the estimated risk for HIV transmission by blood to approx 1 in 2,000,000 units *(8)*.

2.2. Post-Transfusion Hepatitis

Labeling of blood from paid donors, a practice started in 1972, and the implementation of third-generation screening tests for hepatitis B surface antigen markedly reduced transfusion-transmitted hepatitis B but were found to eliminate only about 10% of all post-transfusion hepatitis cases by 1995 *(6)*. Risk for non-A, non-B post-transfusion hepatitis was reduced when potential HIV-positive donors were excluded and was decreased again when donors were tested for the surrogate markers alanine aminotransferase (a marker for acute liver inflammation) and antibody to hepatitis B core antigen (evidence of previous hepatitis B infection) *(9)*. Even greater reductions in the risk of transmission of non-A, non-B hepatitis were described after implementation of a test for antibody to the hepatitis C virus (Table 2) *(10)*. Finally, implementation of nucleic acid testing has reduced the current estimated risk of hepatitis C transmission to approx 1 in 1,500,000 units *(8)*.

2.3. Platelet Product Contamination

Estimated risk of sepsis related to apheresis platelets is 1:2000. This risk is greater with transfusions of pooled platelet concentrates from multiple donors. Because the risk of bacterial overgrowth increases with time, the shelf life of platelets stored at 20–24°C is limited to 5 d. The organisms implicated most commonly in fatalities, in descending order, are *Staphylococcus aureus, Klebsiella pneumoniae, Serratia marcescens,* and *Staphylococcus epidermidis (6)*.

Clinical presentation of infection with bacterially contaminated platelets can range from mild fever (potentially indistinguishable from febrile, nonhemolytic transfusion reactions) to acute sepsis, hypotension, and death. Sepsis caused by transfusion of contaminated platelets is unrecognized in part because the organisms found in platelet contamination are frequently the same as those implicated in catheter-related sepsis. The overall mortality rate of identified platelet-associated sepsis is 26% *(6)*. In the clinical setting, any patient developing fever within 6 h of receiving a platelet transfusion should be evaluated, and empiric antibiotic therapy should be considered.

No widely accepted test is used to detect bacterially contaminated blood products. One promising approach is pathogen inactivation, such as the use of psoralen and ultraviolet (UV) light to sterilize blood products *(11)*. The use of this technology is associated with decreased platelet recovery and in vivo survival, however, leading to the need for increased platelet transfusions *(12,13)*.

2.4. Cytomegalovirus Infection

Cytomegalovirus (CMV) infection caused by platelet transfusions has been a substantial cause of morbidity and mortality in immunocompromised patients with cancer. Patients who receive allogeneic bone marrow/progenitor cell transplantation are at risk for contracting the virus present in blood products because of cytotoxic preparative regimens, immunosupressive (cyclosporin and corticosteroid) therapy or graft-vs-host disease (GvHD) *(14)*. Up to 60% of this patient population will become infected with CMV, and 50% will have CMV disease if no pre-emptive therapy is given. The risk of CMV infection ranges between 28 and 57% for patients receiving a bone marrow transplant and who are seronegative and receive standard blood products *(15)*. Even with CMV-negative blood products, CMV seroconversion has been reported in 1–4% of CMV-negative donor-recipient transplant patients *(16)*. A recent analysis of our own program identified CMV viremia in only 2.5% (1 of 39) of CMV-negative donor-recipient pairs undergoing allogeneic PBPC transplantation *(17)*. Our analysis included 59 patients undergoing allogeneic PBPC transplantation in an investigational study of prophylactic granulocyte infusions from stem cell donors. Notably, results showed that CMV-positive granulocytes did not alter the risk of viremia compared with CMV-negative granulocytes (34.5% vs 26.6% incidence of CMV viremia, respectively [95% CI 0.47–4.41]).

CMV infection and CMV disease are much less common than other virally transmitted diseases in patients undergoing conventional chemotherapy or autologous bone marrow/progenitor cell transplantation *(18)* and are not a significant clinical problem except with CD34+-selected or T-cell depleted progenitor cell transplantations *(19)*.

A randomized, controlled clinical trial *(15)* in patients receiving allogeneic bone marrow transplants compared CMV-seronegative blood products with unscreened blood products that were subjected to bedside leukofiltration. Four (1.3%) of 252 patients in the CMV-seronegative cohort developed CMV infection, with no CMV disease or fatalities; 6 (2.4%) of 250 patients who had bedside leukofiltration developed CMV disease, and 5 of these patients died. Patients who had leukofiltration had an increased probability of developing CMV disease by d 100 (2.4% vs 0%, $p = 0.03$). Even when investigators eliminated CMV infections occurring within 21 d of transplantation, two patients in the leukofiltration cohort and none in the seronegative cohort died of CMV disease *(20)*. The investigators' conclusions that leukoreduced blood products are CMV-safe remain controversial *(21)*. In a consensus conference held by the Canadian Blood Service *(20)*, 7 of 10 panelists concluded that patients considered at risk for CMV disease should receive CMV-negative products, even when blood components are leukoreduced.

3. UNIVERSAL LEUKOREDUCTION

A debate over the merits of universal leukoreduction (cellular components with $<5 \times 10^6$ leukocytes) has focused on several potentially important clinical effects, including transfusion-related alloimmunization to platelets (TRAP), febrile-associated transfusion reactions (FATR), and transfusion-related immunomodulation (TRIM). Both leukoreduced and nonleukoreduced blood components remain Food and Drug Administration (FDA)-approved *(22)*.

The percentages of red cell transfusions remained static in the United States between 1994 and 1999 (17.6 and 20%, respectively), despite commercial promotion of leukocyte-depletion filters during this period *(4)*. For the first 9 mo of 1999, 13% of total red cell transfusions at our hospital were leukoreduced; our own indications for leukoreduction reflect those published previously (Table 3) *(23)*.

FATR occur in only 0.5% of patients receiving red blood cell transfusions, and of these, 18 and 8% of patients experience a second or third FATR, respectively *(24)*. Approximately 18% of all platelet transfusions are associated with FATR *(24)*, although the prevalence of platelet-associated FATR can be as high as 30% in frequently transfused populations, such as patients with cancer. Reactions characterized as severe occur in only 2% of platelet transfusions *(25)*, and bedside leukofiltration has not reduced the overall prevalence of FATR *(26)*. Bedside leukoreduction filters can cause significant hypotensive events by activating the bradykinin/kininogen systems, particularly in patients taking angiotensin-converting enzyme (ACE) inhibitors *(22)*. Universal prestorage leukoreduction for red blood cell transfusion has not been shown to change the incidence of transfusion reactions *(27)* or other clinical outcomes such as in-hospital mortality, duration of hospitalization after transfusion, and total hospital costs *(28)*.

TRAP was studied in a multicenter trial of patients newly diagnosed with leukemia *(25)*. The study found that clinical platelet refractoriness associated with human leukocyte antigen (HLA) seropositivity was reduced from 13% in patients who received transfusions of unprocessed platelet concentrates compared with 3–5% in patients who received leukoreduced apheresis platelets, leukoreduced platelet concentrates, or psoralen/UV-B treated platelets. Although this difference is statistically significant, no clinically impor-

Table 3
Indications for Leukocyte Reduced Blood Components

Established indications	
	Prevention of recurrent nonhemolytic febrile transfusion reactions to red blood cell transfusions
	Prevention or delay of alloimmunization to leukocyte antigens in selected patients who are candidates for transplantation or transfusion on a long-term basis
Indications under review	
	Prevention of the platelet-refractory state caused by alloimmunization
	Prevention of recurrent febrile reactions during platelet transfusions
	Prevention of cytomegalovirus transmission by cellular blood components
Not indicated for	
	Prevention of transfusion-associated graft-versus-host disease
	Prevention of transfusion-related acute lung injury due to the passive administration of antileukocyte antibody
	Patients who are expected to have only limited transfusion exposure
	Acellular blood components (for example, fresh frozen plasma, cryoprecipitate)

Data from ref. *23*.

tant differences were found between the patient cohorts in prevalence of transfusion reactions, hemorrhagic events, length of hospital stay, number of platelet transfusions, number of red blood cell transfusions, or mortality.

TRIM was cited as clinically important in patients undergoing renal transplantation and in women who have had multiple miscarriages *(29)*. A multicenter, controlled study found no evidence of such an effect, however, and the authors recommended against allogeneic mononuclear infusions as a treatment for unexplained, recurrent miscarriage *(30)*. Similarly, patients who received transfusions before renal transplantation had superior 1-yr renal allograft survival compared with patients who did not receive transfusions *(31)*. When data from patients who did not receive transfusions before surgery were analyzed for blood transfused at the time of transplantation surgery, 1-yr renal allograft survival was not effected. Only a few prospective studies have been done to clarify the potential immunomodulatory effects of allogeneic transfusion in other settings *(32)*. Indications for leukoreduction published in a review in 1992 *(21)* are listed in Table 3; these guidelines continue to be applicable since the completion of a controlled, prospective clinical trial *(28)* that found no benefit from universal leukoreduction *(22)*.

4. PLATELET TRANSFUSION PRACTICES

4.1. Threshold for Transfusion

Several studies have evaluated prophylactic platelet transfusion thresholds for patients with thrombocytopenia because of myelosuppressive therapy. Most patients undergoing progenitor cell transplantation received prophylactic platelet transfusions when their platelet counts were 10–20 $\times 10^9$/L, indicating that a threshold of 20 $\times 10^9$/L was most common *(33)* (Fig. 1). Only 9% of hemorrhagic events reported in this study occurred when platelet counts were <10 $\times 10^9$/L.

Two prospective, randomized studies evaluated the relative merits of platelet transfusion thresholds of 10–20 $\times 10^9$/L for patients with leukemia receiving chemotherapy

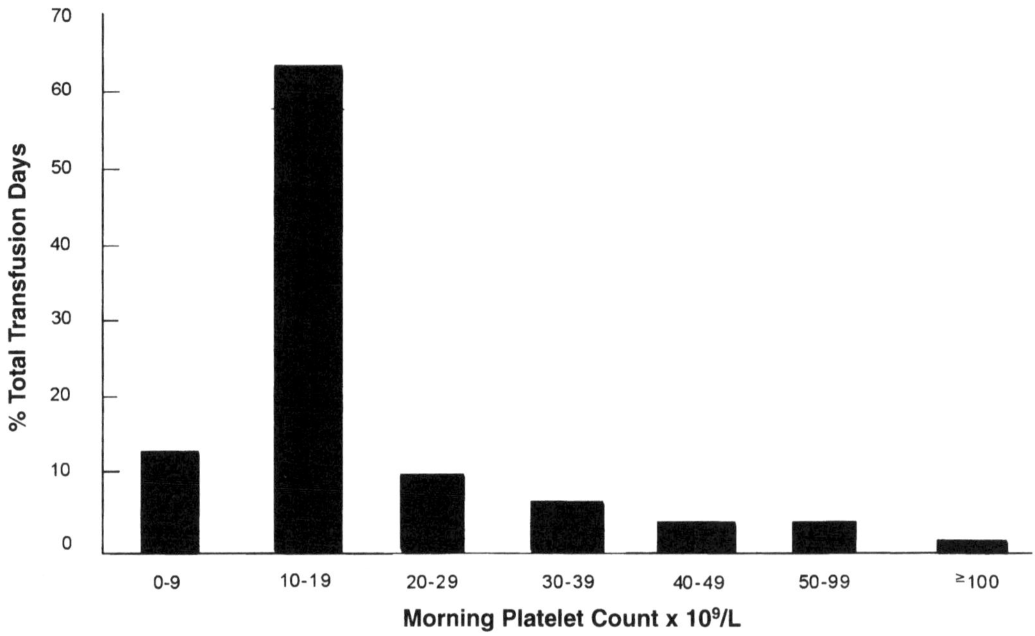

Fig. 1. Percentage of patient days in which platelet transfusions were administered to patients with a range of morning platelet counts. In a multicenter study of patients undergoing autologous (n = 456) or allogeneic (n = 335) hematopoietic stem cell transplantation, nearly two-thirds of patients received prophylactic platelet transfusion when platelet counts were between 10 and 20×10^9/L.

(34,35). Lower transfusion threshold is associated with 22% fewer platelet transfusions *(34)*. In an analysis of hemorrhagic complications, number of red blood cell transfusions, duration of hospital stay, and mortality, no differences were seen between the two thresholds. In a second study, a platelet threshold of 10×10^9/L was safe and effective compared with the 20×10^9/L threshold *(35)*. Of 105 patients in this study, 2 (1.9%) died of hemorrhagic complications, each with a platelet count $>30 \times 10^9$/L at the time of death.

4.2. Dose

Standards of the American Association of Blood Banks require that 75% of apheresis products contain $>3 \times 10^{11}$ platelets and that 75% of platelet concentrates contain $>5.5 \times 10^{10}$ platelets *(36)*; however, no consensus exists for a standardized platelet dose. Table 4 presents the platelet doses used in several recent studies and shows the broad range of platelet doses used. In an evaluation of our own hospital-based apheresis program, 32% of products contained $3–4 \times 10^{11}$ platelets and 32% of products contained $4–5 \times 10^{11}$ platelets *(37)*. Leukoreduction of apheresis platelets or platelet concentrates results in approx 20% loss of platelets *(25)*.

Mathematical modeling has suggested that low-dose platelet therapy would be more beneficial in patients with thrombocytopenia who are receiving prophylactic platelet transfusions *(38)*. The relationship between patient platelet count and in vivo platelet survival is illustrated in Fig. 2 *(39)*. A fixed platelet requirement for hemostasis is estimated to be 7.1×10^9/L/d, and platelet consumption above this threshold is mainly a result of

Table 4
Platelet Doses Used in Studies

Study	*Platelet dose* ($\times 10^{11}/mm^3$)
TRAP study *(25)*	
Six unmodified pooled platelet concentrates	4.5–1.2[a]
Six F-PC filtered units[b]	3.7–1.1[a]
One F-AP filtered unit[c]	3.7–1.3[a]
Goodnough et al. *(37)*	
One apheresis unit	4.2–1.1[a]
Rubella et al. *(34)*	
Apheresis	2.8 (1.1–5.9)[d]
Pooled concentrates	2.2 (1.4–5.0)[d]

[a] Median–SD.

[b] F-PC filtered, pooled platelet concentrates from random donors.

[c] F-AP filtered platelets obtained by apheresis from single random donors.

[d] Median (range).

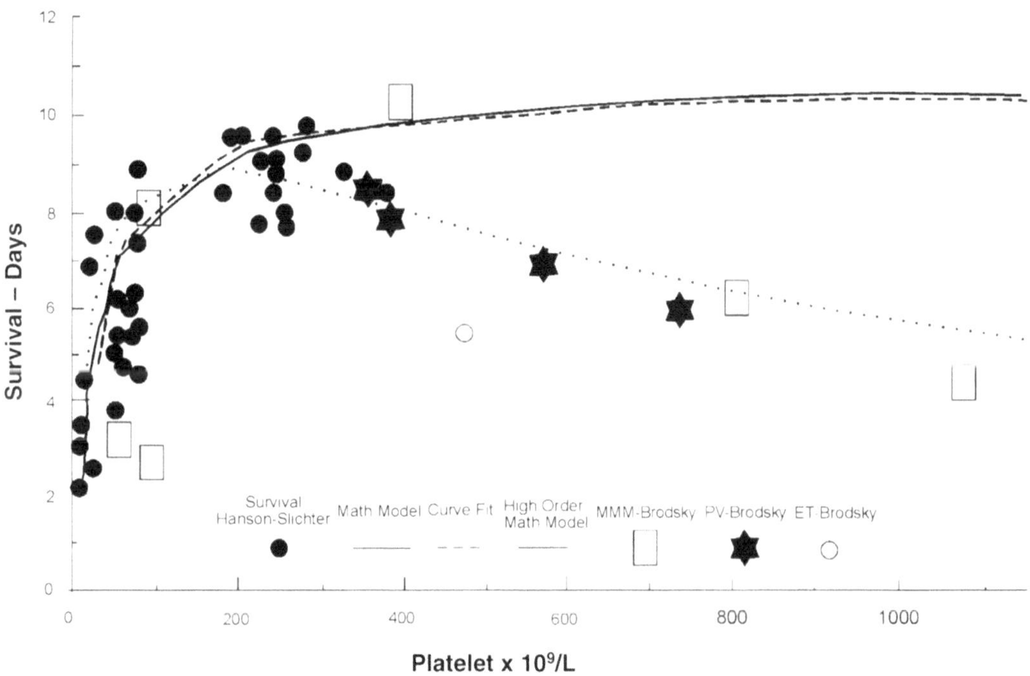

Fig. 2. The relationship between patient platelet count and in vivo platelet survival. Survival data are points obtained from normal individuals and patients with hypoplastic or aplastic marrows *(18)* and patients with myeloproliferative disease.

platelet senescence. For patients who become thrombocytopenic owing to myeloablative therapy, platelet survival decreases with increasing severity of thrombocytopenia. Thus, platelet survival is 5–7 d in patients with platelet counts in the normal range, but only 1–2 d in patients with platelet counts of 10–20 × 10^9/L—levels at which most patients with thrombocytopenia are maintained to prevent hemorrhage.

A mathematical model predicts that low-dose platelet therapy provides a 22% decrease in donor exposures (and total number of platelets) while maintaining patients at a platelet threshold >10 × 10^9/L *(38)*, even with a shorter transfusion-free interval and a greater daily relative risk of receiving additional transfusions *(40)*.

A randomized clinical trial addressed the issue of high-dose platelet therapy *(41)*. Standard, high, and very high platelet doses (4.6 × 10^{11}, 6.5 × 10^{11}, and 8.9 × 10^{11} platelets, respectively) were administered to patients receiving prophylactic platelet transfusions. The high-dose and very high-dose cohorts had greater incremental increases in platelet count and prolonged time to next transfusion than the standard-dose cohort. Interestingly, the platelet half-life estimate (i.e., slopes) for the patient cohorts was not different for post-transfusion platelet counts ranging from approx 50–110 × 10^9/L (Fig. 3). These data suggest that the in vivo platelet life span of transfused platelets cannot be normalized in this setting, even at higher platelet counts. Further studies of platelet transfusion dosage strategies are needed.

4.3. Patient Response

Patient response to platelet transfusion varies. When data from patients with thrombocytopenia undergoing hematopoietic progenitor cell transplantation were analyzed for platelet-corrected count increments after transfusion, a bell-shaped or polynomial distribution was found (Fig. 4), and patient-specific factors accounted for this distribution *(42)*. Factors usually associated with response to platelets (e.g., history of previous transfusion, pregnancy, presence of HLA or platelet-specific antibodies) did not significantly correlate with corrected count increments. These findings suggest that administration of leukoreduced platelets is not clinically important in prevention of platelet refractoriness in patients undergoing progenitor cell transplantation *(38)*.

In summary, platelet transfusion dose is variable, and patient responses to transfusion vary. Furthermore, patients with thrombocytopenia can be maintained safely at prophylactic transfusion thresholds of 10 × 10^9/L. Finally, the likelihood of hemorrhagic complications correlates poorly with degree of thrombocytopenia in patients undergoing myeloblative chemotherapy. These findings, the results of the TRAP study *(25)* and our own observations, indicate that the use of specialized products (apheresis platelets and leukoreduced platelets) needs to be reassessed in the context of emerging technologies.

5. HEMATOPOIETIC GROWTH FACTOR

A number of hematopoietic growth factors with activity on platelet growth and differentiation have been identified. Some of these factors have been cloned and expressed and include the interleukins (recombinant human interleukin [rHuIL]), particularly rHuIL-11, pegylated megakaryocyte growth and development factor (PEG-rHuMGDF), and thrombopoietin (rHuTPO). A good review of thrombopoietins can be found in Kuter et al. *(43)* and Kuter and Begley *(44)*.

5.1. rHuIL-11

rHuIL is a pleitropic cytokine that can stimulate the production of platelets. Like IL-6, IL-11 has effects on hepatocytes, preadiopocytes, neuronal cells, and immunoglobulin-producing B cells *(45,46)*. IL-11 acts during the later stages of differentiation of megakaryocytes and increases megakaryocyte size, ploidy, and the amount of acetyl-

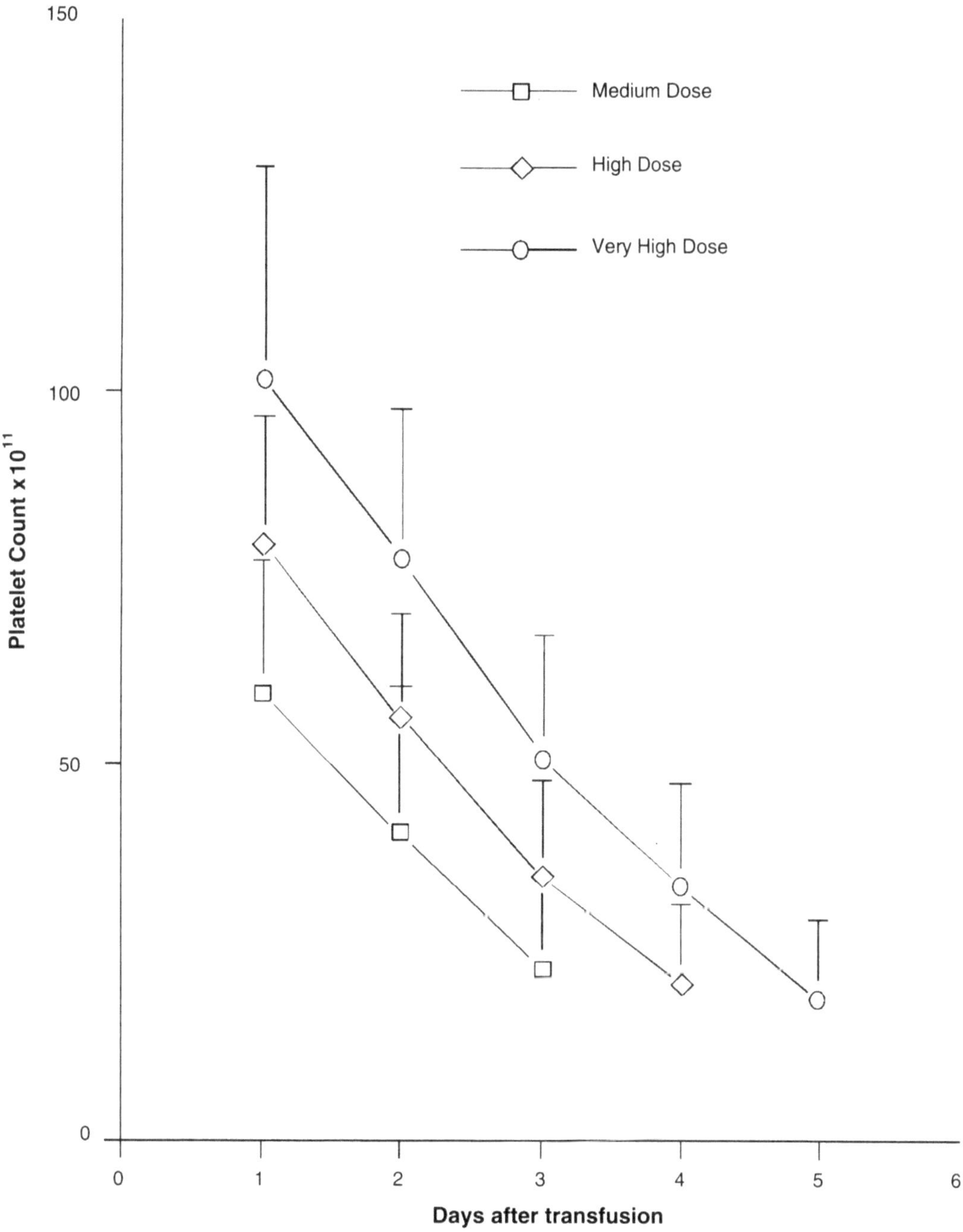

Fig. 3. The relationship between patient platelet count and in vivo platelet survival. Survival data are points obtained from normal individuals and patients with hypoplastic or aplastic marrows *(18)* and patients with myeloproliferative disease.

choline in the mouse *(47)* as well as size and ploidy in humans *(48)*. IL-6 has modest effects on megakaryocyte and platelet production *(44)* but nevertheless has shown clinical utility in increasing platelet counts and accelerating platelet recovery after chemotherapy *(49,50)*.

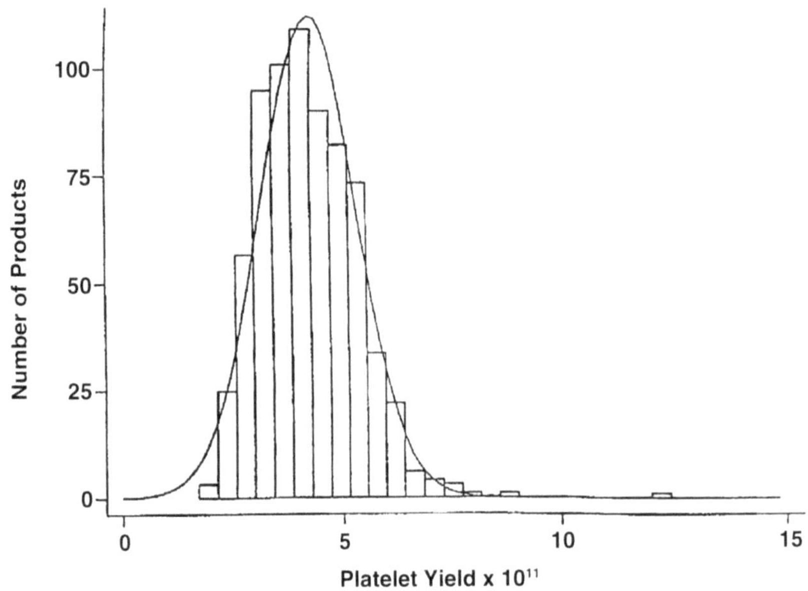

Fig. 4. Distribution of 16-h corrected count increments for 439 platelet transfusions in 42 stem cell transplantation recipients.

Administration of rHuIL-11 has been associated with several adverse effects, including fluid retention, anemia, and general malaise *(49–51)*. It has been approved for marketing for the treatment of cancer chemotherapy-related severe thrombocytopenia.

5.2. rHuTPO and PEG-*HuMGDF*

Unlike rHuIL-11, rHuTPO and PEG-rHuMGDF are Mpl ligands. Endogenous TPO is the primary physiologic regulator of megakaryocyte and platelet development. rHuTPO and PEG-rHuMGDF are recombinant forms of the c-Mpl ligand, and both were shown to be effective stimulators of megakaryocyte growth and platelet production. rHuTPO has an amino acid sequence identical to that of the native TPO sequence, is glycosylated, and is produced in mammalian cells *(44)*. Its molecular weight is 90 kDa, less than the native TPO molecule, which is 95 kDa *(44)*. PEG-rHuMGDF is not glycosylated and is produced in bacterial cells *(44)*. PEG-rHuMGDF comprises the receptor-binding, 163-amino acid terminal end of the native TPO molecule and is conjugated to a 20-kDa polyethylene glycol molecule; it has the same biologic activity as the native molecule *(52)*.

Initial clinical studies with PEG-rHuMGDF showed increased platelet counts, confirming the preclinical studies *(53–55)*. The rare but potentially serious adverse of antibody formation to MGDF leading to severe and potentially chronic thrombocytopenia, however, terminated the clinical program. Analysis of all aspects of this drug development suggest that the ideal candidate for a platelet mobilizer would be one that mimics the endogenous protein but does induce antibody formation.

REFERENCES

1. Wallace EL, Churchill WH, Surgenor DM, et al. Collection and transfusion of blood and blood components in the United States, 1992. *Transfusion* 1995; 35:802–812.
2. Wallace EL, Churchill WH, Surgenor DM, Cho GS, McGurk S. Collection and transfusion of blood and blood components in the United States, 1994. *Transfusion* 1998; 38:625–636.
3. National Blood Data Resource Center. Comprehensive Report on Blood Collection and Transfusion in the United States in 2001. Bethesda, MD: National Blood Data Resource Center. 2003.
4. Pall Corp. Demand leukocyte-depleted blood for more complete patient protection. *Ann Thorac Surg* 1997; 60:A20–A21.
5. Despotis GJ, Goodnough LT, Dynis M, Baorto D, Spitzngel E. Adverse events in platelet apheresis donors: a multivariate analysis in a hospital-based program. *Vox Sang* 1999; 77:24–32.
6. Goodnough LT, Brecher ME, Kanter MH, Aubuchon JP. Transfusion medicine, first of two parts—blood transfusion. *N Engl J Med* 1999; 340:438–447.
7. Selik RM, Ward JW, Buehler JW. Trends in transfusion-associated acquired immune deficiency syndrome in the United States, 1982–1991. *Transfusion* 1993; 33:890–893.
8. Dodd RY, Notari ED, Stramer SL. Current prevalence and incidence of infectious markers and estimated window-period risk in the American Red Cross donor population. *Transfusion* 2002; 42:975–979.
9. Stevens CE, Aach RD, Hollinger FB, et al. Hepatitis B virus antibody in blood donors and the occurrence of non-A, non-B hepatitis in transfusion recipients. An analysis of the Transfusion-Transmitted Viruses Study. *Ann Intern Med* 1984; 101:733–738.
10. Alter HJ, Purcell RH, Shih JW, et al. Detection of antibody to hepatitis C virus in prospectively followed transfusion recipients with acute and chronic non-A and non-B hepatitis. *N Engl J Med* 1989; 321:1494–1500.
11. Lin L, Cook DN, Wiesehahn GP, et al. Photochemical inactivation of viruses and bacteria in platelet concentrates by use of a novel psoralen and long-wavelength ultraviolet light. *Transfusion* 1997; 37:423–35.
12. Corash L, Behrman B, Rheinschmidt M, et al. Post-transfusion viability and tolerability of photochemically treated platelet concentrates. *Blood* 1997; 90:267a.
13. McCullough J, Vesole D, Benjamin RJ, Slichter S, Pineda A, Snyder E, et al. Pathogen-inactivated platelets using Helinx™ Technology are hemostatically effective in the thrombocytopenia patient. *Blood* 2001; 98:45A.
14. Sayers MH, Anderson KC, Goodnough LT, et al. Reducing the risk for transfusion-transmitted cytomegalovirus infection. *Ann Intern Med* 1992; 116:55–62.
15. Bowden RA, Slichter SJ, Sayers M, et al. A comparison of filtered leukocyte reduced and cytomegalovirus (CMV)-seronegative blood products for the prevention of transfusion-associated CMV infection after marrow transplant. *Blood* 1995; 86:3598–3603.
16. Rubie H, Attal M, Campardou AM, et al. Risk factors for cytomegalovirus in BMT recipients transfused exclusively with seronegative blood products. *Bone Marrow Transplant* 1993; 11:209–214.
17. Vij R, Adkins D, Brown R, et al. Risk factors for cytomegalovirus (CMV) viremia post related donor allogeneic peripheral blood stem cell transplantation. *Blood* 1999; 94:374b.
18. Wingard JR, Sostrin MB, Vriessendorp HM, et al. Interstitial pneumonitis following autologous bone marrow transplantation. *Transplantation* 1988; 46:61–65.
19. Holmberg LA, Boeckh M, Hooper H, et al. Increased incidence of cytomegalovirus disease after autologous CD34-selected peripheral blood stem cell transplantation. *Blood* 1999; 94:4029–4035.
20. Laupacis A, Brown J, Costello B, et al. Prevention of posttransfusion CMV in the era of leukoreduction: a consensus statement. *Transfusion* 2001; 41:560–569.
21. Landaw EM, Kanter M, Petz LD. Safety of filtered leukocyte-reduced blood products for prevention of transfusion-associated cytomegalovirus infection. *Blood* 1996; 87:4910.
22. Goodnough LT. The case against universal WBC (and for the practice of evidence-based medicine). *Transfusion* 2000; 40:1522–1527.
23. Lane TA, Anderson KC, Goodnough LT, et al. Leukocyte reduction in blood component therapy. *Ann Intern Med* 1992; 117:151–162.
24. Menitove JE, McElligott MC, Aster RH. Febrile transfusion reaction: what blood component should be given next? *Vox Sang* 1982; 42:318–321.
25. The Trial to Reduce Alloimmunization to Platelets Study Group. Leukocyte reduction and ultraviolet B irradiation of platelets to prevent alloimmunization and refractoriness to platelet transfusions. *N Engl J Med* 1997; 337:1861–1869.

26. Goodnough LT, Riddell J, Lazarus H, et al. Prevalence of platelet transfusion reactions before and after implementation of leukocyte-depleted platelet concentrates by filtration. *Vox Sang* 1993; 65:103–107.
27. Uhlman EJ, Isriggs E, Walhermfechtel M, Goodnough LT. Pre-storage universal WBC of RBC units does not affect the incidence of transfusion reactions. *Ttransfusion* 2001; 41:997–1000.
28. Dzik WH, Anderson JK, O Neill EM, Assmann SF, Kalish LA, Stowell CP. A prospective, randomized trial of universal WBC reduction. *Transfusion* 2002; 42:1114–1122.
29. Blajchman MA. Transfusion-associated immunomodulation and universal white cell reduction: are we putting the cart before the horse? *Transfusion* 1999; 39:665–670.
30. Ober C, Karrison T, Odem RR, et. al. Mononuclear-cell immunization in prevention of recurrent miscarriages: a randomized trial. *Lancet* 1999; 354:365–369.
31. Opelz G, Terasaki PI: Improvement of kidney-graft survival with increased numbers of blood transfusions. *N Engl J Med* 1978; 299:799–803.
32. Vamvakas EC. Transfusion-associated cancer recurrence and postoperative infection: meta-analysis of randomized, controlled clinical trials. *Transfusion* 1996; 36:175–186.
33. Bernstein SH, Nadermanee AP, Vose JM, et al. A multicenter study of platelet recovery and utilization in patients after myeloablative therapy and hematopoietic stem cell transplantation. *Blood* 1998; 91:3509–3517.
34. Rebulla P, Finazzi G, Marangoni F, et al. The threshold for prophylactic platelet transfusions in adults with acute myeloid leukemia. *N Engl J Med* 1997; 337:1870–1875.
35. Wandt H, Frank M, Ehninger G, et al. Safety and cost effectiveness of a 10×10^9/L trigger: a prospective comparative trial in 105 patients with acute myeloid leukemia. *Blood* 1998; 91:3601–3606.
36. Menitove JE, ed. *Standards for Blood Banks and Transfusion Services.* Bethesda, MD: American Association of Blood Banks. 1999.
37. Goodnough LT, Ali S, Despotis GJ, Dynis M, DiPersio JF. Economic impact of donor platelet count and platelet yield in apheresis products: relevance for emerging issues in platelet transfusion therapy. *Vox Sang* 1999; 76:43–49.
38. Hersh JK, Hom EG, Brecher ME. Mathematical modeling of platelet survival with implications for optimal transfusion practice in the chronic platelet transfusion dependent patient. *Transfusion* 1998; 38:637–644.
39. Hanson SR, Slichter SJ. Platelet kinetics in patients with bone marrow hypoplasia: evidence for fixed platelet requirements. *Blood* 1985; 66:1105–1109.
40. Klumpp TR, Herman JH, Gaughan JP, et al. Clinical consequences of alterations in platelet transfusion dose: a prospective, randomized double-blind trial. *Transfusion* 1999; 39:674–681.
41. Norol F, Bierling P, Roudot-Throvac F, et al. Platelet transfusion: a dose-response study. *Blood* 1998; 92:1448–1453.
42. Ishida A, Handa M, Wakui M, Okamota S, Kamakuva M, Ikeda Y. Clinical factors influencing post-transfusion platelet increment in patients undergoing hematopoietic pregenitor cell transplantation—a prospective analysis. *Transfusion* 1998; 38:839–847.
43. Kuter DJ, Hunt P, Sheridan W, Zucker-Franklin D. *Thrombopoiesis and Thrombopoietins. Molecular, Cellular, Preclinical, and Clinical Biology.* Totowa, NJ: Humana. 1997.
44. Kuter DJ, Begley CG. Recombinant human thrombopoietin: basic biology and evaluation of clinical studies. *Blood* 2002; 100:3457–3469.
45. Paul SR, Bennett F, Calvetti JA, et al. Molecular cloning of a cDNA encoding interleukin 11, a stromal cell-derived lymphopoietic and hematopoietic cytokine. *Proc Natl Acad Sci USA* 1990; 87:7512–7516.
46. Yin TG, Schendel P, Yang YC. Enhancement of in vitro and in vivo antigen-specific antibody responses by interleukin 11. *J Exp Med* 1992; 175:211–216.
47. Burnstein SA, Mei RL, Hentthron J, Friese P, Turner K. Leukemia inhibitory factor and interleukin-11 promote maturation of murine and human megakaryocytes in vitro. *J Cell Physiol* 1992; 153:305–312.
48. Teramura M, Kobayashi S, Hoshino S, Oshimi K, Mizoguchi H. Interleukin-11 enhances human megakaryocytopoiesis in vitro. *Blood* 1992; 79:327–331.
49. Gordon MS, McCaskill-Stevens WJ, Battiato LA, et al. A phase I trial of recombinant human interleukin-11 (Neumega rhIL-11 growth factor) in women with breast cancer receiving chemotherapy. *Blood* 1996; 87:3615–3624.
50. Vredenburgh JJ, Hussein A, Fisher D, et al. A randomized trial of recombinant human interleukin-11 following autologous bone marrow transplantation with peripheral blood progenitor cell support in patients with breast cancer. *Biol Blood Marrow Transplant* 1998; 4:134–141.

51. Tepler I, Elias L, Smith JW, et al. A randomized placebo-controlled trial of recombinant human interleukin-11 in cancer patients with severe thrombocytopenia due to chemotherapy. *Blood* 1996; 87:3607–3614.
52. Hokom MM, Lacey D, Kinstler O, et al. Pegylated megakaryocyte growth and development factor abrogates the lethal thrombocytopenia associated with carboplatin and irradiation in mice. *Blood* 1995; 86:4486–4492.
53. Basser RL, Rasko JE, Clarke K, et al. Thrombopoietic effects of pegylated recombinant human megakaryocyte growth and development factor (PEG-rHuMGDF) in patients with advanced cancer. *Lancet* 1996; 348:1279–1281.
54. Basser RL, Rasko JEJ, Clarke K, et al. Randomized, blinded, placebo-controlled phase I trial of pegylated recombinant human megakaryocyte growth and development factor with filgrastim after dose-intensive chemotherapy in patients with advanced cancer. *Blood* 1997; 89:3118–3128.
55. Fanucchi M, Glaspy J, Crawford J, et al. Effects of polyethylene glycol-conjugated recombinant human megakaryocyte growth and development factor on platelet counts after chemotherapy for lung cancer. *N Engl J Med* 1997; 336:404–409.

13 Hematopoietic Growth Factors in Lung Cancer

Johan F. Vansteenkiste, MD, PhD
and Christophe A. Dooms, MD

CONTENTS

1. USE OF CSFS FOR RBC SUPPORT

1.1. Introduction

Anemia is a common clinical problem in patients with lung cancer. Many patients with lung cancer exhibit anemia at diagnosis that may be aggravated by disease-specific therapy, which is often platinum-based. Many patients with lung cancer are symptomatic *(1)*. In these patients, anemia may cause or aggravate shortness of breath and fatigue. Fatigue is the most often reported symptom in cancer patients receiving chemotherapy and has profound consequences on quality of life (QOL) *(2)*. Anemia can be responsible for delay or reduction of cytotoxic treatment, and it is an independent negative prognostic factor of disease outcome *(3,4)*.

The impact of anemia in patients with lung cancer is largely underestimated by the medical community. Despite substantial evidence that treatment of anemia reduces the number of transfusions (and the associated risks) and improves QOL, many clinicians still only treat with red blood cell (RBC) transfusions if their patients' hemoglobin (Hb) concentration decreases to 8.0 g/dL *(5)*.

This section reviews the incidence as well as the effects on functional status, QOL, and effect on disease outcome of anemia in patients with lung cancer. The different treatment strategies, including transfusion and use of recombinant human erythropoietin (rHuEPO) and darbepoetin alfa, are highlighted, with a special focus on the (few) studies in homogeneous lung cancer cohorts. Finally, some guidelines for the use of RBC-stimulating cytokines in the clinical approach to patients with lung cancer are given.

From: *Cancer Drug Discovery and Development*
Hematopoietic Growth Factors in Oncology: Basic Science and Clinical Therapeutics
Edited by: G. Morstyn, M. A. Foote, and G. J. Lieschke © Humana Press Inc., Totowa, NJ

1.2. Causes of Anemia in Patients

Anemia in patients with lung cancer has a multifactorial etiology *(6)*. Contributing factors are the anemia of chronic disorders, concomitant postobstructive respiratory infections, tumor-induced autoimmune hemolysis, and bone marrow invasion or dysfunction caused by the tumor. These patients can also have iron, folate, or vitamin B_{12} deficiency, as well as blood loss from tumor erosion.

Endogenous EPO is of particular interest, since anemic cancer patients have been shown to have inappropriately low amounts of circulating EPO for their degree of anemia, reflecting a perturbation in this homeostatic mechanism, with loss of the normally expected inverse linear relation between serum EPO and Hb concentrations *(7,8)*. In a study with a very homogenous group of chemotherapy- and radiotherapy-naive patients with lung cancer, analysis of serum EPO and soluble transferrin receptor suggested that impaired erythroid marrow response to EPO and a relative inadequacy of EPO production were important mechanisms in the chronic anemia of lung cancer *(9)*. Both phenomena are probably owing to the production of inflammatory cytokines such as tumor necrosis factor (TNF) *(10)*.

The EPO response and RBC production is further decreased in cancer patients receiving chemotherapy, both cisplatin-based or other *(7)*. In patients with lung cancer more specifically, erythropoiesis can be greatly affected. Indeed, cisplatin-based chemotherapy is the standard of care for many patients with this disease *(11,12)*. Platinum-based chemotherapy causes anemia not only by the mechanisms listed above, but also by its direct effect on the renal tubules, which leads to a decrease in the production of EPO *(13)*. Patients with locally advanced nonsmall-cell lung cancer (NSCLC) or limited disease small-cell lung cancer (SCLC) will be even more prone to the development of anemia, since state-of-the-art therapy for these patients consists of a combination of platinum-based chemotherapy together with radiation, thereby further increasing the risk of myelosuppression *(14,15)*.

1.3. Incidence of Anemia in Patients

The prevalence of pretreatment anemia varies across different solid tumor types. In an anemia audit, up to 60% of patients with lung cancer had Hb values < 11 g/dL, a considerably higher prevalence than in patients with colorectal or breast cancer (10–20%). Consequently, approx 40% of patients with lung cancer needed blood transfusions, compared with only about 20% of patients with breast cancer *(16)*. The proportion of patients with anemia increases over the course of treatment.

The problem of anemia in patients undergoing chemotherapy has been reviewed for NSCLC *(17)* and for cancer in general *(18)*. A larger variation in both mild-to-moderate anemia (Hb concentration > 8.0 g/dL) in 8–100% of patients with lung cancer and severe anemia (Hb concentration < 8.0 g/dL) in 0–55% was reported. In a retrospective analysis including 128 patients with lung cancer, chemotherapy significantly decreased Hb concentrations compared with pretreatment values, with a significantly more prominent decline in cisplatin-based regimens compared with non-cisplatin combinations ($p < 0.001$). The incidence of anemia was equivalent in NSCLC or SCLC, if it was treated with cisplatin and etoposide, and severe anemia did not exceed 15% *(19)*. In another retrospective study, an inverse correlation ($p < 0.05$) between the total dose of cisplatin and the lowest Hb value was documented

Table 1
Anemia Rates Reported in Large Prospective Randomized Nonsmall-Cell Lung Cancer Chemotherapy Trials

	All grades (%)	*Grades 3 + 4 (%)*	*Ref.*
Older cisplatin-based chemotherapy			
Cisplatin-vindesine	66	3–6	*25,26*
Cisplatin-etoposide	66–73	3–15	*21–24*
Cisplatin-vindesine-ifosfamide	64	9	*27*
Cisplatin-vindesine-mitomycin C	47–57	4–6	*24,29*
Cisplatin-ifosfamide-mitomycin C	NR	25	*28*
Modern single-agent chemotherapy			
Gemcitabine	57–67	2–7	*22,23,25*
Docetaxel	NR	5	*30*
Paclitaxel	NR	3	*31*
Vinorelbine	52–84	1	*32–34*
Modern platinum-based regimens			
Cisplatin-gemcitabine	NR	6–31	*21,28,35–38*
Cisplatin-docetaxel	76	7–15	*37,39,40*
Cisplatin-paclitaxel	95	9–13	*37,41*
Cisplatin-vinorelbine	NR	2–49	*29,35,38,40,42,43*
Carboplatin-docetaxel	NR	10	*40*
Carboplatin-paclitaxel	80–94	5–16	*37,38,41,42,44,45*
Carboplatin-gemcitabine	46	2–5	*46,47*
Platinum-free regimens			
Gemcitabine-docetaxel	NR	2	*39*
Gemcitabine-paclitaxel	91	2–13	*44,45*
Gemcitabine-vinorelbine	72	4	*32*

NR, not reported.

(20). This finding further stresses the hypothesis that the high incidence and severity of anemia in patients with lung cancer can be explained by the use of cisplatin-based therapies.

1.3.1. Incidence of Anemia According to the Chemotherapy Regimen Used

Older cisplatin-based regimens such as cisplatin, mitomycin, and vindesine; cisplatin and etoposide; or cisplatin and teniposide induce grade 2+ anemia in 64, 46, and 83% of patients, respectively, with grade 3–4 anemia occurring in 29, 15, and 24% of the patients, respectively. With newer chemotherapy schedules such as cisplatin and gemcitabine or carboplatin and paclitaxel, anemia is common as well, and up to 30% of the patients may need blood transfusions *(17)*.

An overview of anemia rates as reported in different cohorts of some large prospective randomized chemotherapy trials for patients with NSCLC is presented in Table 1. In some of these trials, the data on anemia are rather scarce; in most, the data on transfusion rates are lacking. With the older cisplatin-based regimens *(21–29)*, the incidence of anemia varies from 36% *(24)* to 73% *(23)*, with 3–25% of the patients experiencing severe (grade 3–4) anemia. When using monotherapy with a new agent *(22,23,25,30–34)*,

Table 2
Factors Predictive of the Development of Severe Anemia

Generally accepted factors
Baseline hemoglobin (Hb) < 10.0 g/dL *(6,20,48)*
Prior anticancer treatment
Performance status *(49)*
Age *(20)*
Other factors
Baseline Hb < 12.0 g/dL *(49)*
Pretreatment weight loss *(20)*
Baseline lymphocytes < 0.7×10^9/L *(49)*

overall anemia rates vary from 52% *(32)* to 84% *(34),* but severe anemia is rare (0–7%). With the newer platinum-based chemotherapies *(21,28,29,35–47),* the incidence of anemia varies from 38% *(29)* to 95% *(41),* with 3% to as much as 31% of the patients experiencing severe (grade 3–4) anemia. In one study with the combination of cisplatin and vinorelbine, a severe anemia rate as high as 49% was reported *(43).* The experience with more recent non-platinum-based regimens is more limited *(32,39,44,45),* but the available data suggest a high overall anemia rate varying from 72% *(32)* to 91% *(44)* and a rather low incidence of severe anemia (2–4%, except for one study with 13% *[44]*).

In summary, mild or moderate anemia is a common problem in all patients with lung cancer treated with chemotherapy. Severe anemia is more prominent in platinum-based regimens, and the incidence has not decreased in the newer combinations compared with the older ones. The rate of severe anemia is low, however, in chemotherapies with a new single agent or a platinum-free combination of two agents.

1.3.2. Predictive Factors

Because of the high incidence of anemia in patients with lung cancer, rHuEPO is an important supportive measure in lung cancer chemotherapy. rHuEPO, however, is able to correct anemia and reduce the number of blood transfusions in only 50–60% of these patients. Because the use of rHuEPO is limited by its cost, attempts have been made to identify the patients at risk of developing severe anemia (Table 2), as they are more likely to benefit from rHuEPO therapy.

Baseline Hb concentrations and previous anticancer treatment, especially large-field radiotherapy or long-term myelosuppressive chemotherapy, are well-known predictive factors. In a retrospective study in patients with SCLC, the relation between baseline Hb concentration and risk of transfusion was analyzed *(48).* Patients who experience a 2.0-g/dL decrease in their Hb value during chemotherapy need a transfusion in 49% of the cases if they had a baseline Hb concentration of 15.0 g/dL. This rate was 86% if they started with a baseline Hb concentration of 13.0 g/dL, and 98% if they started with a baseline Hb concentration of 11.0 g/dL. The proportion of patients receiving transfusions increased markedly if the pretreatment Hb concentration was <10.0 g/dL *(6).* A relationship with pretreatment loss of weight and older age has been made *(20).* Elderly patients have decreased bone marrow reserve and therefore a tendency toward anemia.

A risk model for chemotherapy-induced severe anemia requiring transfusion was proposed by Ray-Coquard et al. *(49).* In a multivariate analysis with 1051 patients, a baseline Hb <12.0 g/dL, a performance status >1, and a baseline lymphocyte count <0.7 × 10^9/L were found to be of independent value. Based on these findings, a score of probability of RBC transfusion was constructed that might help select appropriate candidates for prophylactic rHuEPO treatment.

In a pharmacokinetic study of patients with head-and-neck cancer treated with cisplatin-based chemotherapy, the ultrafilterable cisplatin concentration was predictive for Hb loss *(50)*. Although this method is of theoretical interest, it is difficult to apply in clinical practice.

1.4. Effects of Anemia on Functional Status and Quality of Life

A large proportion of patients with advanced lung cancer are symptomatic *(1)*. Although it has been shown that cisplatin-based chemotherapy improves the median survival time in a significant way *(51)*, the overall gain is modest. In a recent review of >20 yr of randomized phase 3 trials in North American patients with advanced NSCLC, the very sobering conclusion was that only 5/33 trials showed a significant difference in median survival for the new treatment cohort, rarely > 2 mo *(52)*. Many of those involved in the care of patients with lung cancer agree that clinical benefit for the patient should be a primary endpoint of both clinical care and clinical research *(25,53)*. Anemia and its consequences are important issues in this respect.

Anemia may cause symptoms or aggravate the existing symptom burden of patients with lung cancer. Fatigue, shortness of breath (often already present owing to smoking-related comorbidity or to the tumor itself), dizziness, lack of energy, weakness, impaired cognitive function, psychological health, or sexual function, and disturbance of sleep are characteristic symptoms *(54)*. Patients with recently diagnosed advanced lung cancer report that fatigue is the most distressing symptom of their disease *(55)*. The sum of these symptoms compromises the patients' ability to function normally, to work, and to interact socially *(56)*.

1.4.1. Consequences of Anemia

Fatigue is the most often reported symptom in cancer patients receiving chemotherapy and has profound consequences on QOL *(2)*. Approximately 50% of patients with inoperable NSCLC report severe fatigue *(57)*.

Cella *(58)* developed the Functional Assessment of Cancer Therapy (FACT) QOL tool and the modules FACT-F (fatigue) or FACT-An (anemia). Based on these tools, the difficult relationships among anemia, fatigue, and QOL can be studied more precisely *(58)*. Results of these studies show that even mild (Hb concentration 10.0–12.0 g/dL) or moderate (Hb concentration 8–10 g/dL) anemia, present in most chemotherapy-treated patients with lung cancer, is associated with fatigue and impaired QOL.

The impact of anemia is largely underestimated by the medical community. Despite substantial evidence that treatment of anemia improves the QOL, many clinicians still only treat with RBC transfusions if their patients' Hb concentration decreases to 8.0 g/dL *(5)*. When patients discuss fatigue with their doctor, approx 77% are told that fatigue is something to be endured, and 40% are told that nothing can be done about this symptom *(59)*. Clinicians continue to believe that patients without severe anemia (Hb concentration not <8.0 g/dL) should endure this condition without treatment. For that reason, ongoing research in the field of QOL and its relationship with Hb concentrations, patient well-being, and symptom control are of major importance *(18)*.

1.4.2. Effect of Anemia Treatment on Functional Status and Quality of Life

Although chemotherapy-induced fatigue often results from multiple factors, anemia represents a common and treatable etiology, because of the clear evidence of relationship among low Hb concentration, fatigue, and poor QOL *(60)*. Different placebo-controlled and open-label studies have convincingly shown that an increase in Hb concentration caused by rHuEPO treatment significantly improves QOL and that this improvement is independent of tumor response *(61–65)*. In one large, open-label study involving 2289 patients (24% with lung cancer), the patient-rated scores for mean energy level, activity, and overall QOL were significantly ($p < 0.01$) better than at baseline after 16 wk of rHuEPO treatment *(63)*.

Crawford et al. *(66)* analyzed the incremental change in QOL associated with Hb concentration increase (1.0-g/dL increments), based on the patient data from two large community studies *(62,63)*, including a total of 4382 patients. They found a direct relationship between Hb concentration increase during rHuEPO treatment and QOL improvement across the clinically relevant Hb concentration range of 8.0–14.0 g/dL, with a maximal incremental gain in QOL with Hb concentrations between 10.0 and 12.0 g/dL (and not with concentrations between 7.0 and 10.0 g/dL, as can be achieved with transfusion). This finding means that it is worthwhile to treat patients with mild or moderate anemia; in fact, these patients benefit more from rHuEPO treatment than those with severe anemia. This issue becomes more and more important, since improved cancer therapy has increased the number of patients surviving with their cancer as a chronic illness.

1.5. Effect of Anemia on Disease Outcome

A Hb concentration >11.0 g/dL was a significantly ($p = 0.001$) favorable prognostic factor in a large retrospective analysis of 2531 patients with advanced NSCLC *(67)*. The relationship between anemia and survival was examined in a review of 60 papers, 25% of which were about lung cancer *(3)*. The relative risk of death of anemic patients with lung cancer increases by 19% (95% confidence interval (CI): 10–29). This effect is present regardless of whether the patients are treated with chemotherapy, radiotherapy, or surgery *(4)*. An important additional question is whether this effect is because the lower Hb values are a sign of more advanced disease, or whether the anemia compromises anticancer treatment and thereby survival. In the last scenario, treatment of anemia might improve disease control and outcome. Several theoretical arguments (the role of tumor hypoxia in resistance to therapy *[68]*) and patient data, in the fields of both radiotherapy (especially for head-and-neck and gynecologic cancers) and chemotherapy, suggest the last direction *(61,69,70)*.

The possible relationship between increased Hb values and survival was explored in a recent randomized, double-blind, trial of rHuEPO vs. placebo in 375 anemic patients with solid or nonmyeloid tumors receiving nonplatinum chemotherapy *(61)*. The study was not designed or powered for survival analysis, but the trend toward better survival ($p = 0.13$ univariate; $p = 0.05$ multivariate) for the rHuEPO-treated patients was nonetheless noteworthy.

1.6. Treatment of Lung Cancer-Associated Anemia

1.6.1. Transfusions

Historically, treatment options for patients with lung cancer who develop severe or symptomatic anemia were primarily limited to RBC transfusions. In fact, most physicians still do not treat, unless with RBC transfusion, in case of severe anemia *(5)*.

Although RBC transfusion is the most rapid correction, especially useful in patients with severe or life-threatening anemia, several risks are associated with it, including acute transfusion reactions and transmission of infectious agents *(71,72)*. Furthermore, the limited availability and the cost of transfusion products limit their use. Finally, there is the concern of decreased immunosurveillance of tumors by the recipient of allogeneic transfusion. A negative impact on outcome has been described in some but not all surgical series examining this issue in lung cancer *(73)* and other cancer types *(74,75)*.

1.6.2. rHuEPO

Another treatment option for the management of anemia is the administration of rHuEPO. The Food and Drug Administration (FDA) approved rHuEPO in 1989 for anemia of chronic renal failure. Early randomized trials with rHuEPO in cancer- and chemotherapy-related anemia showed that rHuEPO therapy was associated with up to 50% reduction in the number of RBC transfusions, with, however, a lag in the clinical effect, as the reduction in needed transfusions reached statistical significance only if transfusions during the first month of therapy were excluded from analysis *(64,76,77)*. A similar effect was shown for patients with lung cancer, in whom the time to Hb response (i.e., increase in 2.0 g/dL) was a mean of 54 d *(63)*. Later studies confirmed that rHuEPO, administered three times per week at a dose of 150 U/kg, increases Hb concentrations, decreases the number of required RBC transfusions, and improves QOL, regardless of tumor type or chemotherapy *(61–63,78)*.

The clinical experience with rHuEPO was reviewed in a recent meta-analysis *(79)*. rHuEPO decreased the proportion of transfused patients by 9–45% if started at a mean baseline Hb concentration of ≤10.0 g/dL or by 7–47% if started at 10.0–12.0 g/dL, and 7–39% if started at ≥12.0 g/dL. QOL data were insufficient for meta-analysis. Only studies in which rHuEPO was started at a mean baseline Hb concentration of ≤10.0 g/dL had statistically significant differences in QOL. In the data reviewed, insufficient QOL data were available to justify the start of rHuEPO before the Hb decreased to nearly 10.0 g/dL.

To our knowledge, only two prospective, randomized studies specifically addressed the use of rHuEPO in patients with lung cancer *(80,81)*. The first was an open label multicenter study designed to evaluate the efficacy and safety of rHuEPO in the prevention of the decline in Hb concentration, and in reduction of transfusion requirements, in nonanemic patients with SCLC scheduled to receive four to six cycles of platinum-based chemotherapy (Table 3) *(80)*. Of the 130 patients, 44 had 300 U/kg rHuEPO three times a week, 42 had rHuEPO 150 U/kg three times a week, and 44 had chemotherapy only. Significantly fewer rHuEPO-treated patients developed anemia (Hb concentration <10.0 g/dL) during their chemotherapy (300 U/kg: 39%; 150 U/kg: 48%; untreated: 66%; $p < 0.05$; Fig. 1). The percentage of patients requiring transfusion was 20% in the 300-U/kg cohort ($p < 0.001$), 45% in the 150-U/kg cohort ($p < 0.05$), and 59% in the untreated cohort (Fig. 2). QOL was assessed by three questions (energy level, daily activity, overall QOL) answered by the patients on a 100-mm visual analog scale and by World Health Organization (WHO) performance status. No substantial differences in QOL was seen across cohorts, which was probably owing to the liberal policy toward transfusion in all groups, resulting in similar mean Hb concentrations in the three cohorts at the end of study period.

The second study was very small and dealt with 72 patients with NSCLC treated with cisplatin-based chemotherapy *(81)*. They were randomly assigned to either 100 U/kg or

Table 3
Randomized Phase 3 Studies on the Use of Red Blood Cell Colony-Stimulating Factors in Platinum-Treated Patients with Lung Cancer

Study	*Patients (No.)*	*Hb response (%)*	*Transfusions (% of pts.)*	*Transfusions (No. of units)*	*QOL*[a]
Thatcher et al. *(80)*					
No medication	44	34	59	6.1	16
rHuEPO					
3 × 150 U/kg/wk	42	52*	45*	3.8**	24*
3 × 300U/kg/wk	44	61**	20***	2.1***	11
Vansteenkiste et al. *(88)*					
Placebo	161	18	52	1.92	19
Darbepoetin alfa	159	48***	27***	0.67***	32*
1 × 2.25 µg/wk					

ABBREVIATION: rHuEPO, recombinant human erythropoietin.

[a] In ref. *80* expressed as % change vs. baseline on a visual analog scale for the question "How do you rate your overall quality of life (QOL)?"; in ref. *88* expressed as the proportion of patients with at least a 25% improvement from baseline on the Functional Assessment of Cancer Therapy Fatigue scale (FACT-F).

* Significance vs control cohort $p < 0.05$.

** Significance vs control cohort $p < 0.01$.

*** Significance vs control cohort $p < 0.001$.

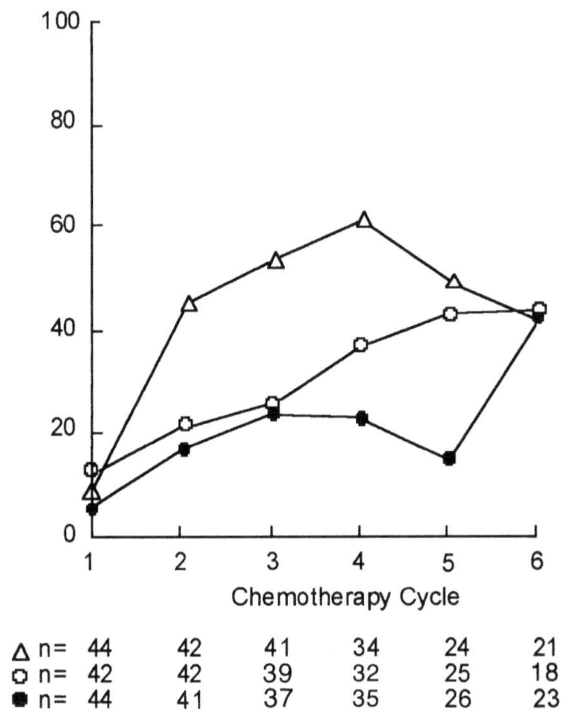

Fig. 1. Comparison of the percentage of patients becoming anemic (Hb < 10 g/dL) during platinum-based chemotherapy for small-cell lung cancer. Open triangles, untreated; open circles, rHuEPO 150 U/kg; closed circles, rHuEPO 300 U/kg. (Reprinted from ref. *80*.)

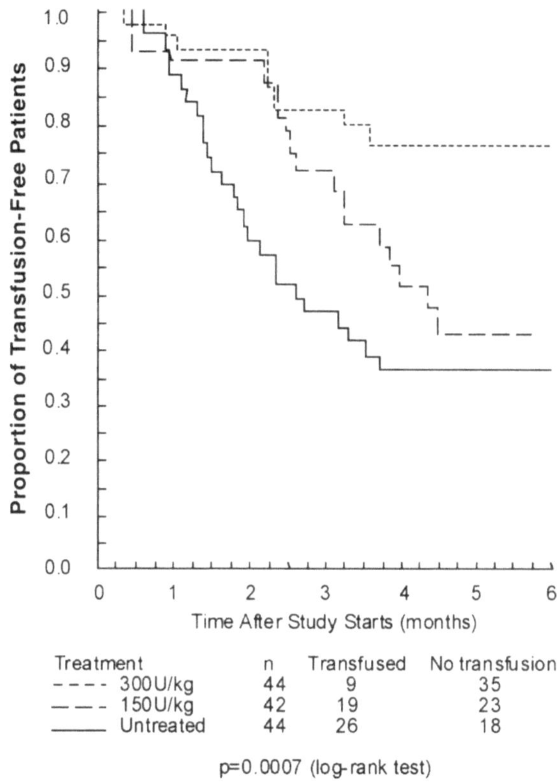

Fig. 2. Transfusion-free times during platinum-based chemotherapy for small-cell lung cancer. Dotted line, rHuEPO 300 U/kg; dashed line, rHuEPO 150 U/kg; solid line, untreated. (Reprinted from ref. *80.*)

200 U/kg of rHuEPO or placebo, administered three times a week for 6 wk. Based on only 53 evaluable patients, it was concluded that the Hb concentrations at the nadir after the second cycle of chemotherapy were significantly better in the rHuEPO-treated groups. Conclusions from this study are limited owing to the low number of evaluable patients per cohort and the short period of treatment.

1.6.3. Darbepoetin Alfa

Although rHuEPO has substantially improved our approach to anemic patients with lung cancer, several aspects of this type of treatment are still to be improved. The labeled use of rHuEPO is based on three subcutaneous injections every week. Hb response will be obtained in only 50–60% of the patients, and the time to response is 6–8 wk (54 d in patients with lung cancer in one large study *[63]*). This rather long time to response is the reason why there is a lag in the clinical effect and why the reduction in transfusion need reaches statistical significance only if transfusions during the first month of therapy are excluded from analysis *(64,76,77)*. The limited survival prospects of patients with advanced lung cancer would make a shorter time to response particularly rewarding in this group. Some of these unmet needs in our current anemia treatment are addressed by darbepoetin alfa, which represents a new generation of erythropoiesis-stimulating proteins.

Human EPO is a 46-kDa glycoprotein that contains three *N*-glycosylation sites. Both endogenous EPO and rHuEPO have varying degrees of glycosylation, sometimes by as few as 8 or as many as 14 sialic acid groups *(82)*. Darbepoetin alfa has 2 additional *N*-glycosylation sites and has up to 22 sialic acid groups.

The sialic acid content of erythropoietic proteins is directly related to their in vivo half-life and inversely proportional to their affinity to bind the EPO receptor. Preclinical research has demonstrated that the in vivo biologic activity of erythropoietic proteins depends primarily on their half-life and not on their receptor affinity *(82,83)*. Darbepoetin alfa, with its additional sialic acid groups, has an approx threefold (25.3 h vs 8 h, intravenous [iv] administration) longer serum half-life than rHuEPO in animal models and in patients with kidney disease *(84)*. Darbepoetin alfa also maintains Hb concentration as well as rHuEPO, even when administered less frequently *(84)*.

Darbepoetin alfa proved to be safe and clinically effective in early clinical studies in cancer patients undergoing chemotherapy *(85)*, when administered every 1, 2, or even 3 wk *(86)*. In one randomized phase 2 study, involving 429 patients with solid tumors receiving chemotherapy, patients were randomly assigned to darbepoetin alfa doses of 0.5–8.0 μg/kg/wk, or to a control treatment with rHuEPO at an initial dose of 150 U/kg three times weekly *(87)*. A dose of 1.5 μg/kg/week of darbepoetin alfa was active, and higher doses increased the proportion of patients with an Hb response and decreased the median time to response. These findings point at a clear dose-response relationship. Similar results were obtained with administration every 2 wk.

The pivotal randomized, double-blind, placebo controlled, phase 3 study was done in platinum-treated patients with lung cancer (Table 3) *(88)*. In the active cohort, patients received 2.25 μg/kg of darbepoetin alfa per week. This dose was based on preclinical and chronic kidney disease data *(84)*, which showed that it had similar effects as rHuEPO 150 U/kg administered three times a week, and on separate studies, in which this dose proved to be clinically effective, in patients receiving chemotherapy for both solid tumors or lymphoproliferative malignancies *(87,89)*. The dose of the study drug could be doubled at wk 7, if the Hb concentration at the beginning of wk 6 had not increased by 1.0 g/dL over the baseline.

Patients with lung cancer, who were expected to receive at least 12 additional weeks of platinum-containing chemotherapy, could be entered in the study if they were anemic (i.e., Hb concentration ≤ 11.0 g/dL), primarily because of their cancer or chemotherapy, with adequate serum folate, vitamin B_{12}, ferritin, and saturated transferrin concentrations. A total of 314 patients could be assessed for RBC transfusions and Hb response (increase of 2.0 g/dL over baseline), adverse events, antibody formation to darbepoetin alfa, hospitalizations, FACT-F score, and disease outcome.

A statistically significant and clinically meaningful reduction > 50% was observed in both the incidence of transfusions and the number of units transfused. The proportion of patients that needed transfusion was significantly lower in the darbepoetin alfa group than in the placebo group (27% vs 52%, $p < 0.001$), and this proportion was the case for the period of wk 5 until end of study, but also wk 1 until end of study (Fig. 3). They also needed fewer RBC units (mean: 0.67 vs 1.92, $p < 0.001$). The fact that the effect on the reduction of the number of required RBC transfusions was apparent even when data from the first 4 wk of therapy were included suggests that the 1-mo lag in

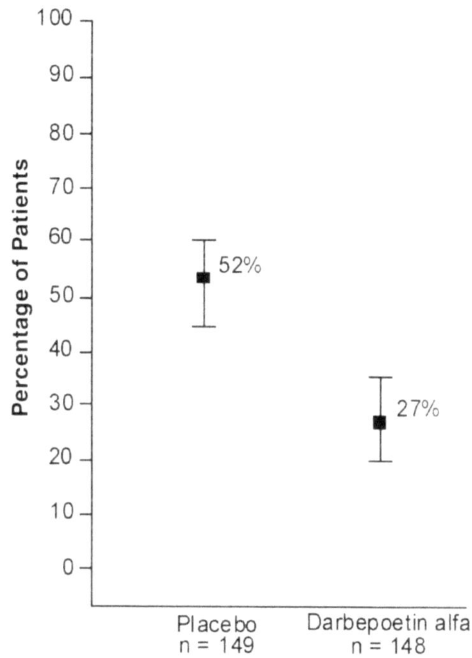

Fig. 3. Comparison of the Kaplan-Meier percentage of patients in the placebo or darbepoetin alfa groups who received a red blood cell (RBC) transfusion from wk 5 until end of study. Bars, 95%, CI, p value < 0.001. (Adapted from ref. *88*.)

the clinical effect of rHuEPO *(64,76,77)* may be surpassed with this new agent. This lag probably reflects the influence of pharmacologic doses of rHuEPO on the kinetics of erythropoiesis; such doses do not act rapidly enough to impact on the need for transfusions within the first month of treatment. The results from this study suggested that darbepoetin alfa may improve anemia management not only by less frequent administration but also by a faster onset of action. Darbepoetin alfa appeared to be safe; adverse events were similar across treatment groups, and specific items such as thrombosis or hypertension were also similar. No anti-darbepoetin alfa antibodies were detected. The patients treated with darbepoetin alfa also had better improvement in QOL. Thirty-two percent of patients in the darbepoetin alfa group showed a ≥25% improvement in FACT-F, vs only 19% in the placebo group ($p = 0.019$).

An additional interesting observation was that patients in the darbepoetin alfa group were hospitalized for 10.3±13.7 (mean±SD) d, whereas this figure was 13.0±17.7 d for the placebo group ($p = 0.13$). Although this study was not designed to identify a causal relationship between hospitalization and the use of darbepoetin alfa, it is possible that patients with higher Hb concentrations may benefit by an overall improvement in performance status that may allow for overall decreased resource utilization. The cost of drug could then be offset by a potential reduction in the duration of hospitalization and reduction in RBC transfusion.

As part of the safety evaluation, all patients who received study drug were included in an analysis of progression-free survival and overall survival. Darbepoetin alfa did

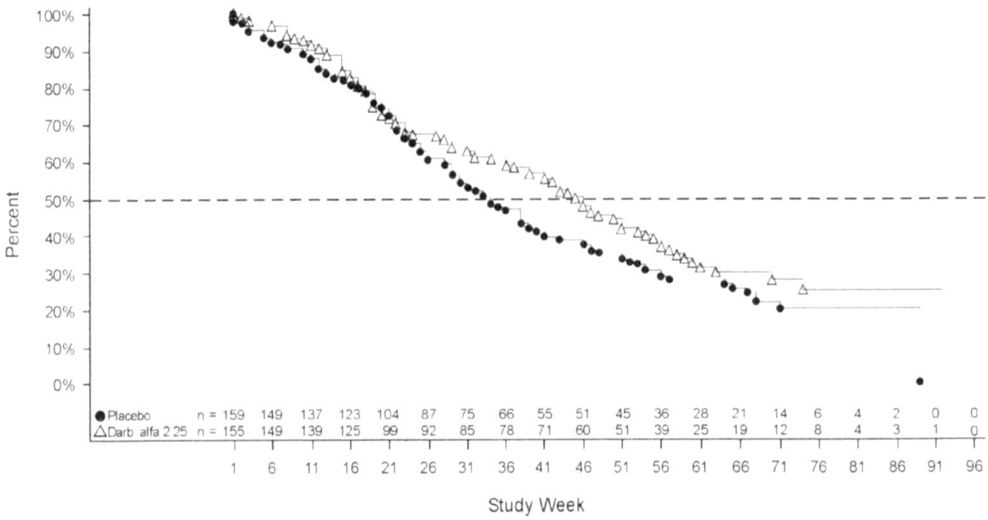

Fig. 4. Kaplan-Meier survival for placebo (closed circles) versus darbepoetin alfa patients (open triangles). The median survival time was 34 wk vs. 46 wk for patients receiving darbepoetin alfa. The number of patients at risk is shown above in the *x*-axis. (Reprinted from ref. *88.*)

not have any negative influence on survival; in contrast, the median survival time was 34 wk in the placebo group and 46 wk in the darbepoetin alfa group (Fig. 4). Although no conclusions can be drawn from this ancillary observation, these data, together with the findings in an other study *(61),* warrant further investigation of the role of anemia correction on overall treatment outcome in prospectively designed studies.

1.7. Recommendations for the Use of Erythropoietic Factors

Anemia is a problem in up to 50–60% of patients with lung cancer, especially if they are treated with platinum-based chemotherapy. Despite its well-documented profound impact on QOL, many clinicians only treat with transfusion, once severe anemia (Hb concentration < 8 g/dL) is present. Much evidence supports the use of rHuEPO for chemotherapy-induced anemia, if the Hb concentration decreases by <10 g/dL *(79).* Although recent data suggest that QOL may be preserved better if rHuEPO is started when the Hb concentration is <12 g/dL, there is at present not enough evidence to make an overall recommendation for this strategy, but rather clinical evidence in particular circumstances.

Based on randomized data, the standard prescription is 150 U/kg rHuEPO three times a week for a minimum of 4 wk *(90).* With this schedule, it takes at least 4 wk for a response to occur, and only 50–60% of patients will have an increase of Hb of 2.0 g/dL. In case of insufficient response after 4 wk, the dose may be doubled. If there is no response after 8 wk, rHuEPO should be stopped. Less robust clinical practice evidence suggests an alternative weekly dosing of 40,000 U.

Darbepoetin alfa has a threefold longer half-life than rHuEPO, which allows less frequent dosing. The benefits of less frequent administration for patients are obvious in terms of reduced injections. In addition, other benefits to patients and their caregivers include reduced time missed from work for physician visits and potentially better patient compliance. In a large randomized, placebo-controlled, phase 3 study in patients with lung cancer, using an administrations schedule of 2.25 µg/kg once weekly, darbepoetin alfa showed a statistically significant and clinically meaningful reduction > 50% in both the proportion of transfused patients and number of RBC units transfused, as well as significantly reduced fatigue *(88)*. The data suggested that darbepoetin alfa may overcome some of the limitations of rHuEPO, such as the lag time before onset of action, and may further improve our current management of cancer-related anemia.

2. USE OF CSFS FOR WBC SUPPORT

Neutropenia is a common side effect of chemotherapy for lung cancer. Neutropenia can be associated with febrile neutropenia (FN), neutropenic sepsis, which may be life-threatening, prolonged hospital admission for administration of iv antibiotics, and increased cost. Grade and duration of neutropenia have been correlated with the risk of developing sepsis.

The use of recombinant human granulocyte colony-stimulating factor (rHuG-CSF) or rHu granulocyte-macrophage colony-stimulating factor (rHuGM-CSF) was approved and recommended *(91)* based on two randomized studies in SCLC, in which their ability to reduce both the incidence and consequences of FN was demonstrated *(92,93)*.

Several studies, most in SCLC and some in NSCLC, subsequently assessed whether the use of these CSF might allow administration of higher than standard doses, sometimes even in combination with progenitor cells or autologous bone marrow support, in an attempt to improve the prognosis. This concept is most appealing for SCLC, because it is a tumor with an aggressive biology and rapidly dividing cells.

This section reviews the use of rHuG-CSF or rHuGM-CSF in lung cancer in these different settings, based on published randomized data. Finally, some guidelines for the use of white blood cell (WBC)-stimulating cytokines in the clinical approach to patients with lung cancer are given.

2.1. Small-Cell Lung Cancer

Given the systemic nature of SCLC, chemotherapy is the keystone in the treatment. Despite the high chemosensitivity of SCLC, with an objective response achieved in approx 80% of the patients, remission is in general short, and relapses are frequently chemoresistant. Treatment strategies to prolong remission have therefore dominated clinical trials for SCLC in the past decade. The use of alternating non-crossresistant chemotherapy, maintenance chemotherapy, or dose intensification strategies were examined.

Most of the studies on rHuG-CSF and rHuGM-CSF in SCLC have concentrated on the primary administration of these agents. Far fewer data exist on the use of these CSFs in secondary prophylaxis (initiation of CSF subsequent to the occurrence of chemotherapy-induced prolonged neutropenia or FN in a previous cycle) or in the therapeutic setting (treatment of established neutropenia with or without fever).

The studies focusing on the primary administration are listed in Table 4. One group of these studies examined the question of whether the use of CSFs could reduce the incidence and consequences of chemotherapy-induced neutropenia, thereby improving

Table 4
Randomized Studies Focusing on the Primary Administration of White Blood Cell Colony-Stimulating Factors in Small-Cell Lung Cancer

						Effect		*Effect*	
Ref.	*CSF*	*ED (%)*	*Primary endpoint*	*Attempt to DI*	*Effect on DI*	*Toxicity*	*FN*	*MST*	*2YS*
92	G	72	FN	No	NA	↓	↓	None	NA
93	G	64	FN	No	↑	↓	↓	None	NA
94	G	55	FN	No	↑	↓	↓	None	None
95	GM	66	N	No	↑	None	None	None	NA
96	GM	0	N	No	↓	↑	NA	None	NA
98	G	32	DI	↑ DD	None	↓	NA	NA	NA
99	G	8	DI/FN	↑ DD	↑	↑	None	None	↑
100	G	100	DI	↑ DD	↑	↓	NA	↑	↑
101	G	100	DI	↑ DD	↓	↑	NA	None	None
102	G	11	Survival	↑ DD	↑	↓	NA	None	↑
103	GM	100	Survival	↑ DS	↓	↑	None	↓	↓
104	GM	40	FN/DI	↑ DD	↑	None	None	↑	↑
105	GM	92	Survival	↑ DD	↑	↑	NA	None	None
106	G	43	Survival	↑ DS/DD	↑	↑	None	None	None

ABBREVIATIONS: CSF, colony-stimulating factor; G, granulocyte; GM, granulocyte-macrophage; ED, extensive disease; FN, febrile neutropenia; N, neutropenia; DI, dose Intensity; DD, dose density; DS, dose size; NA, not available; MST, median survival time; 2YS, 2-yr survival.

the acceptability of chemotherapy by reducing clinical infections *(92–96)*. In these studies, the incidence of FN or neutropenia is the primary endpoint. Before the advent of rHuG-CSF and rHuGM-CSF, the problem of neutropenia was tackled by reduction and/or delay of the cytotoxic treatment, which may compromise the prognosis. This was shown in a randomized study done in patients with limited SCLC, in which patients were randomly assigned to what is now considered to be a rather low dose of cisplatin, cyclophosphamide, doxorubicin, and etoposide or to a regimen with a 20% increased dose of cisplatin and a 25% increased dose of cyclophosphamide, in the first cycle only *(97)*. This relatively small difference in dose resulted in a statistically significant survival benefit for the last group (2-yr survival 43% vs 26%, $p = 0.02$).

Another group of studies examined whether the use of CSFs might allow an increase in dose intensity, to improve the prognosis *(98–106)*. Dose intensity is defined as the dose per m^2 per week. This dose can be increased either by increasing the dose itself (increase in dose size), by shortening the interval between cycles (increase in dose density), or both. In these strategies, the most common dose-limiting toxicity is neutropenia and its resultant potentially life-threatening infectious complications. It is clear that increasing the dose of a standard chemotherapy regimen or the administration of intensive weekly regimens require CSF support to avoid increased, sometimes unacceptable, toxicity. These trials have the possibility of administering an increased dose of chemotherapy or survival as primary endpoint.

Table 5
Randomized Studies on the Primary Use of White Blood Cell Colony-Stimulating Factors in Standard-Dose Chemotherapy for Small-Cell Lung Cancer

Ref.	*No.*	*Chemo*	*Cohort*	*Infectious episode (% pts.)*	*Dose reduced (% pts.)*	*Neutropenia duration (d)*	*Infection duration (d)*	*RR (%)*	*MST (mo)*
92	211	CDE[a]	C	77		6	5	80	12.2
			G	40	NA	1	4	72	11.4
				$p < 0.001$		$p < 0.001$	NS	NS	NS
93	130	CDE[a]	C	53	61	10		87	9.5
			G	26	29	3	NA	79	8.9
				$p < 0.002$	$p < 0.001$	$p < 0.001$		NS	NS
94	280	CDE[b]	C	54	28		8	80	9.8
			G	37	17	NA	7	76	11.2
				$p = 0.004$	$p < 0.001$		NS	NS	NS
95	283	CDE[c]	C	27				86	10
			GM 5/10/20	25/22/36	NA	NA	NA	58	10
				NS				NS	NS
96	215	CiE +	C	27	85[e]			85	17
		RT[d]	GM	42	75[e]	NA	NA	74	14
				$p = 0.03$	$p < 0.03$			NS	NS

ABBREVIATIONS: C, control arm; G, arm with granulocyte CSF; GM, arm with granulocyte-macrophage CSF; NA, not available; RR, response rate; MST, median survival time.

[a] CDE, cyclophosphamide 1 g/m^2 and doxorubicin 50 mg/m^2 on d 1, etoposide 120 mg/m^2 on d 1–3; G, G-CSF 230 µg/m^2/d on d 4–18.

[b] CDE, cyclophosphamide 1 g/m^2 and doxorubicin 45 mg/m^2 on d 1, etoposide 100 mg/m^2 on d 1–3; G, G-CSF 150 µg/m^2/d on d 4–13.

[c] CDE, cyclophosphamide 1g/m^2 and doxorubicin 40 mg/m^2 on d 1, etoposide 80 mg/m^2 on d 1–3; GM-CSF at 5,10, or 20 µg/kg on d 4–13.

[d] CiE+RT, cisplatin 25 mg/m^2 and etoposide 60 mg/m^2 on day 1–3; GM-CSF 250 µg/m^2; chest radiotherapy 45 Gy.

[e] In this study, expressed as % of planned dose.

2.1.1. Primary Use of CSFs in Support of Standard-Dose Chemotherapy for SCLC

The use of rHuG-CSF in a standard three-weekly regimen of cyclophosphamide-doxorubicin-etoposide (CDE) chemotherapy has been investigated in three large, randomized, placebo-controlled phase 3 trials, in which incidence of chemotherapy-induced infection was the primary endpoint. In two of these studies, a significant reduction of the incidence of FN in the rHuG-CSF cohort was observed, 77% in the placebo groups compared with 40% in the rHuG-CSF group ($p < 0.001$) in one study, and 53% vs 26% in the other study ($p < 0.002$) *(92,93)* (Table 5). Secondary endpoints such as the incidence and median duration of grade 4 neutropenia and the number of hospitalization days were also significantly reduced by 50% in the rHuG-CSF group in both trials. This reduction resulted in significantly less chemotherapy delays and dose reductions in one study *(93)*. Tumor response rate and survival were not significantly different across groups. The third randomized trial, in which a lower dose of rHuG-CSF was administered for a shorter period, had similar findings regarding the primary endpoint but did not show a reduction in the duration of neutropenia *(94)*.

The use of rHuGM-CSF in standard chemotherapy for SCLC has been less beneficial on the incidence of FN than rHuG-CSF. In one randomized trial, 283 patients with SCLC were treated with CDE chemotherapy without or with rHuGM-CSF at different dose levels (5, 10, or 20 μg/kg) *(95)*. rHuGM-CSF at 5 or 10 μg/kg significantly reduced chemotherapy-induced neutropenia and the duration of neutropenia in cycle 1. However, the incidence of FN in cycle 1 was not significantly changed, except for a favorable trend in the subgroup of rHuGM-CSF 10 μg/kg. In later cycles, the neutropenia nadirs were equivalent in all groups. rHuGM-CSF at dosages of 5 μg/kg (cycles 2 and 3) and 10 μg/kg (cycles 1–4) were able to increase significantly the amount of planned chemotherapy administrations and thus dose intensity, but this may have led to an observed significantly higher incidence of thrombocytopenia. Nevertheless, response rate and median survival time were not improved in the rHuGM-CSF cohort. The second randomized trial failed to demonstrate any benefit of rHuGM-CSF in 215 patients with limited SCLC receiving concomitant chemoradiotherapy (cisplatin-etoposide) with or without rHuGM-CSF *(96)*. rHuGM-CSF reduced the number of infectious episodes, but significantly more patients had life-threatening thrombocytopenia, more hospitalization days, more iv antibiotic administration, more nonhematologic toxicity, and more toxic deaths (nine vs one; $p < 0.01$) in the rHuGM-CSF group compared with placebo. The total dose of chemotherapy given across all six cycles was significantly smaller in the rHuGM-CSF group. It was concluded that concurrent use of rHuGM-CSF plus chemotherapy and daily radiotherapy should be avoided, as co-administration of rHuGM-CSF and radiotherapy might accelerate stem cell exhaustion.

2.1.2. Primary Use of CSF for Dose Intensification for SCLC

In a small, prospective, randomized trial, 40 patients were treated with weekly courses of dose-dense cisplatin and etoposide alternating with ifosfamide and doxorubicin, with or without rHuG-CSF *(98)* (Table 6). Although significantly less grade 3–4 neutropenia and dose reductions owing to neutropenia occurred in the rHuG-CSF group, this result did not contribute to a reduction in FN or an increase in received dose intensity compared with the control group. The small sample size precludes outcome analysis.

Sixty-five patients with SCLC received chemotherapy with vincristine, ifosfamide, carboplatin, and etoposide (VICE) with or without rHuG-CSF at a treatment interval determined by hematologic recovery in a slightly larger randomized trial *(99)*. Dose intensity and incidence of FN were the primary endpoints. In both treatment groups, the received dose intensity was significantly higher than that in the standard 4-weekly VICE regimen of that center. In contrast to studies with standard CDE chemotherapy supported by rHuG-CSF, incidence of FN was not reduced in rHuG-CSF-supported, accelerated VICE chemotherapy. This finding may be explained by the high percentage of patients with limited disease in this study compared with other studies, as well as the higher dose intensity in the rHuG-CSF group. Survival analysis was an additional endpoint and showed no significant difference in median survival but a significantly better 2-yr survival rate for rHuG-CSF group.

Table 6
Randomized Studies on the Primary Use of White Blood Cell Colony-Stimulating Factors to Increase Dose Intensity of Chemotherapy for Small-Cell Lung Cancer

Ref.	*No.*	*Chemo*	*Cohort*	*FN (% pts.)*	*Toxic deaths*	*DI*	*RR (%)*	*MST (mo)*	*2YS (%)*
98	40	CE/ID[a]	C		2	0.82	71		
			G	NA	0	0.84	74	NA	NA
					NS	NS	NS	NS	
99	65	VICE[b]	C	65	1	1.18	94	15	15
			G	70	6	1.25	93	16	32
				NS		$p = 0.03$	NS	NS	S
100	63	CODE[c]	C		4	0.72	84	7.2	6.5
			G	NA	4	0.84	97	13.3	31.3
					NS	$p = 0.03$	*NS*	$p = 0.004$	*S*
101	227	CE/COD[d]	C	9		0.82	77	10.9	8.5
		CODE	I + G	19	NA	0.72	84	11.6	11.7
				$p = 0.031$		$p = 0.001$	NS	NS	NS
102	403	CDE[e]	C			1.00	79	11	8
			I + G	NA	NA	1.32	78	12	13
						NA	NS	NS	*S*
103	125	CDE-C[f]	C	7[j]	5		72	10.8	
			I + GM	34[j]	8	NA	71	8.9	NA
				$p = 0.005$	NS		NS	$p = 0.0005$	
104	300	VICE[g]	C	51	5	NA	77	12	18
			C + GM	53	5	NA	78		
			I	55	5	NA	91	15	33
			I + GM	56	5	NA	88		
				NS	NS	NS	NS	$p = 0.014$	*S*
105	233	EVI[h]	C	5[j]	5	0.87	59	9.4	5
			I + GM	7[j]	4	0.73	76	8.7	6
			I + AB	3[j]	3	0.61	70	8.7	6
				NS	NS	NS	0.04	NS	NS
106	244	CDE[i]	C	24	3	0.99	79	12.5	15
			I + G	34	6	1.70	84	12	18
				NS	NS	S	NS	NS	NS

ABBREVIATIONS: C, control arm; AB, arm with antibiotic prophylaxis; I, dose-intensified arm; FN, febrile neutropenia; NA, not available; DI, relative dose intensity; RR, response rate; MST, median survival time; 2YS 2-yr survival; G, arm with granulocyte CSF; GM, arm with granulocyte-macrophage CSF.

[a] CE/ID, cisplatin 50 mg/m² on d 1 and etoposide 75 mg/m² on d 1–2 alternating weekly with ifosfamide 2 g/m² and doxorubicin 25 mg/m² on d 1; G-CSF 5 μg/kg/d when no chemotherapy.

[b] VICE, carboplatin 300 mg/m² and ifosfamide 5 g/m² on d 1, etoposide 120 mg/m² on d 1–2, vincristine 1 mg on d 15; G-CSF 5 μg/kg/d from d 4 to 48 h before next cycle.

[c] CODE, cisplatin 25 mg/m² weekly and vincristine 1 mg/m² on wk 1, 2, 4, 6 and doxorubicin 40 mg/m² + etoposide 80 mg/m² on wk 1, 3, 5, 7; G-CSF 50 μg/m² on days when no chemotherapy.

[d] CE/COD, 3-weekly cisplatin 80 mg/m² on d 1 and etoposide 100 mg/m² on d 1–3 alternating with cyclophosphamide 800 mg/m² and doxorubicin 50 mg/m² and vincristine 1.4 mg/m² on d 1.

[e] CDE, cyclophosphamide 1g/m² and doxorubicin 40 mg/m² on d 1, etoposide iv 120 mg/m² on d 2–3 and etoposide po 240 mg/m² d 4–14 either 3-weekly (standard) or 2-weekly (intensified) with G-CSF.

[f] CDE-C (standard), cyclophosphamide 1.2 g/m² and doxorubicin 40 mg/m² and etoposide 225 mg/m² and cisplatin 100 mg/m²; CDE-C (intensified), cyclophosphamide 1.8 g/m² and doxorubicin 60 mg/m² and etoposide 330 mg/m² and cisplatin 120 mg/m²; GM-CSF 5 μg/kg/d for 10 d.

[g] VICE, vincristine 0.5 mg/m² on d 15, ifosfamide 5 g/m² and carboplatin 300 mg/m² and etoposide 120 mg/m² on d 1–2 every 4 (standard) or 3 (intensified) wk; GM-CSF 250 μg/m²/d for 14 d.

[h] EVI, epirubicin 60 mg/m² and vindesine 3 mg/m² and ifosfamide 5 g/m² on d 1 every 3 weeks (standard) or every 2 wk (intensified); GM-CSF 5 μg/kg d 3–13; or cotrimoxazole d 3 until end of cycle.

[i] CDE, (standard) cyclophosphamide 1 g/m² and doxorubicin 45 mg/m² on d 1, etoposide 100 mg/m² on d 1–3 every 3 wk; (intensified) cyclophosphamide 1.25 g/m² and doxorubicin 55 mg/m² on d 1, etoposide 125 mg/m² on d 1–3 every 2 wk with G-CSF 5 μg/kg/d on d 4–13.

[j] In this study expressed as grade 3 + 4 infections.

Sixty-three patients with extensive disease SCLC were treated with weekly chemotherapy with cisplatin, oncovin, doxorubicin, and etoposide (CODE) with or without rHuG-CSF during 9 wk in a small randomized trial in Japanese patients *(100)*. Dose intensity was the primary endpoint. The trial demonstrated a significantly higher delivered dose intensity in the rHuG-CSF-supported weekly CODE regimen. This result also significantly prolonged median and 2-yr survival rates. In a larger randomized trial, 227 Japanese patients with extensive SCLC were given weekly CODE with rHuG-CSF or standard 3-weekly cisplatin and etoposide alternating with cyclophosphamide, oncovin, and doxorubicin *(101)*. This study could not confirm the previous results, and the received dose intensity in the weekly cohort was lower than in the standard cohort, with no significant differences in median survival or 2-yr survival rates. Patients who received the weekly CODE regimen with rHuG-CSF support had a significant higher incidence of thrombocytopenia and neutropenic fever.

Standard CDE chemotherapy given every 3 wk was compared with accelerated CDE every 2 wk with support of rHuG-CSF in a large randomized trial in 403 patients with SCLC (mainly limited disease) *(102)*. The rHuG-CSF support in the accelerated cohort significantly increased the dose intensity by 32%, but this did not result in a difference in response rate or median survival compared with the standard cohort. Nevertheless, it led to a better survival rate in the intensified cohort, which started at approx 1 yr after treatment and was not associated with worsening of QOL.

The administration of rHuGM-CSF to dose-escalate chemotherapy in patients with SCLC has been studied in three randomized trials. In one of these, a 4-weekly standard-dose cyclophosphamide, doxorubicin, etoposide, and cisplatin (CDE-C) was compared with a 4-weekly high-dose CDE-C with rHuGM-CSF support in patients with extensive SCLC *(103)*. It was concluded that rHuGM-CSF did not allow the delivery of a higher cumulative dose of the four-drug regimen, owing to significantly greater hematologic toxicity (grade 4 neutropenia and thrombocytopenia). Treatment outcome was significantly affected, with a median survival of 8.9 mo in the intensive cohort vs 10.8 mo in the standard cohort ($p = 0.0005$).

Three hundred patients were studied in a trial with a 2 × 2 factorial design with randomization between a slightly modified VICE schedule every 3 wk (intensified) or every 4 wk (standard), and between rHuGM-CSF or placebo *(104)*. FN and dose intensification were the primary endpoints. The intensified-treatment cohort received a 26% higher dose intensity than the standard cohort, with a nonsignificant trend for greater dose intensity for those who received rHuGM-CSF. Nevertheless, the incidence of FN, blood culture-confirmed sepsis, and toxic mortality were not significantly affected by chemotherapy schedule or rHuGM-CSF use. No significant difference in response rate was seen among the four treatment groups. Median survival and 2-yr survival rate were significantly increased in the intensified cohorts compared with the standard cohorts, but not in the rHuGM-CSF group vs the placebo group. The authors concluded that there is a potential survival benefit from dose intensification but that rHuGM-CSF, compared with placebo, did not reduce the incidence of hematologic complications and had no significant impact on either response or survival.

In a three-armed, randomized study with survival as primary endpoint, a 3-weekly chemotherapy course with epirubicin, vindesine, and ifosfamide (EVI) was compared with accelerated 2-weekly EVI chemotherapy supported with rHuGM-CSF or oral antibiotics *(105)*. The administration of EVI chemotherapy could be accelerated with rHuGM-

CSF support. The response was significantly higher in the rhuGM-CSF cohort compared with the control cohort ($p = 0.04$), but the study failed to demonstrate a survival benefit. In contrast to the findings of Steward et al. *(104),* it was impossible to accelerate chemotherapy without rHuGM-CSF support. Hematologic toxicity, consisting mainly of severe thrombocytopenia and nonsevere infections, was increased in the rHuGM-CSF cohort.

Only one randomized phase 3 trial examined the effect of dose intensification based on increasing both the dose density and dose size *(106).* The combined effect of increased dose (by 25%) and increased dose density (by 33%) led to a 70% increase in dose intensity. No statistically significant difference was seen in response rate, median survival time, or 2-yr survival rate. Hematologic and nonhematologic toxicity was increased: grade 4 leukopenia occurred significantly more in the intensified group (79% vs 50%), despite the use of rHuG-CSF, and the incidence of grade 3–4 thrombocytopenia and anemia was significantly higher ($p = 0.001$). A 70% dose increase of CDE chemotherapy thus did not lead to improved outcome in patients with SCLC.

2.1.3. Primary Use of CSF in High-Dose Chemotherapy for SCLC With Stem Cell Support

Approaches used to increase cytotoxic dose intensity can be performed not only with support of CSF, but also with sequential infusion of hematopoietic progenitors in whole blood or autologous bone marrow transplantation. Classic high-dose chemotherapy with support of autologous bone marrow transplantation has been abandoned because of excessive toxicity and conflicting results. A randomized phase 2 trial demonstrated that chemotherapy with ifosfamide, carboplatin, and etoposide can be given at a significant higher dose intensity when it is supported by rHuG-CSF injections and hematopoietic progenitor cell infusion *(107).* No significant difference was seen between the treatment arms in time to progression or overall survival. A sufficiently powered, randomized, phase 3 trial, with survival as primary endpoint, is needed to answer this question.

2.2. Nonsmall-Cell Lung Cancer

The use of CSFs in induction chemotherapy for stage IIIA NSCLC has been restricted to reduction of the risk of neutropenia-related infections to avoid dose reductions or dose omissions. No randomized data to evaluate this approach are available. Some randomized trials focused on the role of high-dose or dose-intensive, cisplatin-based chemotherapy in stage IV NSCLC (Table 7). A very small phase 2 double-blind, placebo-controlled study compared chemotherapy with mitomycin C, vindesine, and cisplatin (MVP) with MVP + rHuGM-CSF *(108).* rHuGM-CSF significantly reduced the duration of grade 3 neutropenia, but no statistically significant difference was seen in response rate or survival. In a large three-arm study, patients were randomly assigned to either a 3-weekly regimen of cisplatin and etoposide, cisplatin and paclitaxel, or cisplatin and paclitaxel + rHuG-CSF *(109).* No differences in response or survival were found between the three cohorts. In another randomized phase 3 trial with MVP, it was observed that rHuGM-CSF reduced the incidence of grade 4 neutropenia, which allowed a 29% increase of the delivered dose intensity, but without changes in the incidence of FN, response rate, or survival *(110).* One Japanese study compared MVP administered every 4 wk or every 3 wk with rHuG-CSF support *(111).* Dose-intensive chemotherapy did not improve median survival compared with standard chemotherapy in patients with stage III

Table 7
Randomized Studies on the Primary Use of White Blood Cell Colony-Stimulating Factors in Chemotherapy for Advanced Nonsmall-Cell Lung Cancer

Ref.	*No.*	*Chemo*	*RR (%)*	*MST (mo)*
108	45	C[a]	26	10
		GM	45	10
			NS	NS
109	571	C[b]	26	9.6
		I + G	31	10.1
			NS	NS
110	123	C[c]	32	7.2
		I + GM	27	9.0
			NS	NS
111	100	C[d]	44	6
		I + G	52	11
			NS	$p = 0.032$

ABBREVIATIONS: C, control; I, dose-intensified arm; MST, median survival time; RR, response rate; MST, median survival time; G, arm with granulocyte CSF; GM, arm with granulocyte-macrophage CSF.

[a] C, cisplatin 100 mg/m^2 and mitomycin 8 mg/m^2 on d 1 + vindesine 3 mg/m^2 on d 1 and 8; GM-CSF 125 μg/m^2 from d 2–16.

[b] C, cisplatin 75 mg/m^2 on d 1 + etoposide 100 mg/m^2 d 1–3 vs cisplatin 75 mg/m^2 on d 2 + paclitaxel 135 mg/m^2 on d 1 (standard) vs cisplatin 75 mg/m^2 on d 2 + paclitaxel 250 mg/m^2 on d 1 + G-CSF 5 μg/kg (intensified).

[c] C, cisplatin 35 mg/m^2 and etoposide 200 mg/m^2 on d 1–3 every 4 wk (standard) vs every 3 wk (intensified); GM-CSF 5 μg/kg from d 4–13.

[d] C, cisplatin 80 mg/m^2 and mitomycin C 8 mg/m^2 on d 1 + vindesine 3 mg/m^2 on d 1 and 8 every 3 wk (intensified) or every 4 wk (standard); G-CSF 2 μg/kg.

NSCLC. In contrast, in patients with stage IV disease, a significant improvement in median survival time was noted. No major toxicity was observed, and hematologic toxicity was acceptable. The low number of patients in the subgroup analysis precludes any meaningful conclusions.

No randomized studies on the use of CSFs in chemotherapy have been reported with new drugs such as gemcitabine, docetaxel, or vinorelbine.

2.3. Recommendations for the Use of White Blood Cell CSFs

2.3.1. Primary Administration

Prospective randomized trials showed that the primary administration of rHuG-CSF in standard-dose chemotherapy for SCLC reduces the severity and duration of neutropenia, leading to a lower incidence of FN (approx 50% lower). This result allows an increase in the number of courses of chemotherapy given on time. Treatment outcome was not the primary endpoint in these studies, but observed response and survival rates were similar in both cohorts of these trials. Because of cost constraints, guidelines recommend reserving primary administration of CSF for patients with an expected incidence rate of FN of at least 40% *(112)*. Thus, for most standard chemotherapy regimens for patients with lung cancer, primary administration of CSF is not recommended. Guidelines, however, recognize that there are some clinical situations in which the use of CSF might be appropriate, as in the case of patients at high risk for postobstructive pneumonia, with extensive prior chemotherapy and/or irradiation, with a history of recurrent FN while receiving earlier chemotherapy, or with decreased immune function. The recommended dose is 5 μg/kg per day for rHuG-CSF (filgrastim) and 250 $\mu g/m^2$ per day for rHuGM-CSF (sargramostim), to be started between 24 and 72 h after chemotherapy until the occurrence of a neutrophil count of $10 \times 10^9/L$. CSFs should be avoided in patients receiving concomitant chemoradiation.

Trials of the primary use of CSF for dose intensification of chemotherapy for SCLC have produced conflicting outcome results. Some studies, particularly those involving patients with mainly extensive disease SCLC, have shown no positive effect on survival. Other studies, mainly involving patients with limited disease SCLC, showed a significant but modest survival benefit in patients randomized to receive the higher dose intensity chemotherapy. In these studies, the incidence of severe neutropenic infections was not reduced. Based on these data, there is currently insufficient evidence to recommend the supportive use of CSFs to increase cytotoxic dose intensity of SCLC chemotherapy in daily practice outside clinical trials.

No proof of benefit exists for the use of CSFs in patients with advanced NSCLC in terms of response rate and survival, and toxicity may even be increased. Outside randomized clinical trials, standard use of CSFs is not recommended for the treatment of patients with NSCLC.

2.3.2. Secondary Prophylaxis With CSFs

Although some limited evidence exists that CSFs can decrease the probability of FN in subsequent cycles of chemotherapy after occurrence in a previous cycle, this type of prophylaxis cannot be recommended *(112)*. The secondary use is rather intuitive and guided by clinical situations. In the absence of clinical data in lung cancer pointing at a clear relationship between maintaining chemotherapy dose intensity and survival, clinicians should consider chemotherapy dose reduction after neutropenic fever or prolonged neutropenia.

2.3.3. Therapeutic Use of CSFs

CSFs are not recommended for routine use in nonfebrile neutropenia *(112)*. In case of FN, >60% of practicing oncologists prescribe CSFs to their patients *(113)*. The available data do not support this practice as an adjunct to antibiotic therapy for most patients. This practice will decrease the duration of grade 4 neutropenia, but its clinical benefit remains unproven. Guidelines, however, recognize that in some clinical instances of FN, the therapeutic use of CSFs might be appropriate. Examples are patients with profound ($<0.1 \times 10^9/L$) neutropenia, high-risk infections such as (postobstructive) pneumonia or sepsis, and advanced age.

REFERENCES

1. Hollen PJ, Gralla RJ, Kris MG, Eberly SW, Cox C. Normative data and trends in quality of life from the Lung Cancer Symptom Scale (LCSS). *Support Care Cancer* 1999; 7:140–148.
2. Curt GA. Impact of fatigue on quality of life in oncology patients. *Semin Hematol* 2000; 37:14–17.

3. Caro JJ, Salas M, Ward A, Goss G. Anemia as an independent prognostic factor for survival in patients with cancer: a systemic, quantitative review. *Cancer* 2001; 91:2214–2221.
4. Watine J. Blood hemoglobin as an independent prognostic factor in surgically resected stages I and II non-small cell patients with lung cancer. *Ann Thorac Surg* 2002; 73:2034–2035.
5. Estrin JT, Schocket L, Kregenow R, Henry DH. A retrospective review of blood transfusions in cancer patients with anemia. *Oncologist* 1999; 4:318–324.
6. Scagliotti GV, Novello S. Role of erythropoietin in the treatment of lung cancer associated anaemia. *Lung Cancer* 2001; 34(suppl 4):91S–94S.
7. Miller CB, Jones RJ, Piantadosi S, Abeloff MD, Spivak JL. Decreased erythropoietin response in patients with the anemia of cancer. *N Engl J Med* 1990; 322:1689–1692.
8. Wood PA, Hrushesky WJ. Cisplatin-associated anemia: an erythropoietin deficiency syndrome. *J Clin Invest* 1995; 95:1650–1659.
9. Dowlati A, R'Zik S, Fillet G, Beguin Y. Anaemia of lung cancer is due to impaired erythroid marrow response to erythropoietin stimulation as well as relative inadequacy of erythropoietin production. *Br J Haematol* 1997; 97:297–299.
10. Moldawer LL, Marano MA, Wei H, et al. Cachectin/tumor necrosis factor-alpha alters red blood cell kinetics and induces anemia in vivo. *FASEB J* 1989; 3:1637–1643.
11. Soria JC, Le Chevalier T. Is cisplatin still the best platinum compound in non-small cell lung cancer? *Ann Oncol* 2002; 13:1515–1517.
12. Pujol JL, Carestia L, Daures JP. Is there a case for cisplatin in the treatment of small cell lung cancer? A meta-analysis of randomized trials of a cisplatin-containing regimen versus a regimen without this alkylating agent. *Br J Cancer* 2000; 83:8–15.
13. Koury MJ, Bondurant MC. Control of red cell production: the roles of programmed cell death (apoptosis) and erythropoietin. *Transfusion* 1990; 30:673–674.
14. Marino P, Preatoni A, Cantoni A. Randomized trials of radiotherapy alone versus combined chemotherapy and radiotherapy in stages IIIa and IIIb non-small cell lung cancer. A meta-analysis. *Cancer* 1995; 76:593–601.
15. De Ruysscher D, Vansteenkiste J. Chest radiotherapy in limited stage small cell lung cancer: facts, questions, prospects. *Radiother Oncol* 2000; 55:1–9.
16. Barrett-Lee PJ, Bailey NP, O'Brien ME, Wager E. Large-scale UK audit of blood transfusion requirements and anaemia in patients receiving cytotoxic chemotherapy. *Br J Cancer* 2000; 82:93–97.
17. Del Mastro L, Gennari A, Donati S. Chemotherapy of non-small cell lung cancer: role of erythropoietin in the management of anemia. *Ann Oncol* 1999; 10(suppl 5):91S–94S.
18. Groopman JE, Itri LM. Chemotherapy-induced anemia in adults: incidence and treatment. *J Natl Cancer Inst* 1999; 91:1616–1634.
19. Tas F, Eralp Y, Basaran M, et al. Anemia in oncology practice: relation to diseases and their therapies. *Am J Clin Oncol* 2002; 25:371–379.
20. Okamoto H, Saijo N, Shinkai T, et al. Chemotherapy-induced anemia in patients with primary lung cancer. *Ann Oncol* 1992; 3:819–824.
21. Cardenal F, Lopez Cabrerizo MP, Anton A, et al. Randomized phase III study of gemcitabine-cisplatin versus etoposide-cisplatin in the treatment of locally advanced or metastatic non-small cell lung cancer. *J Clin Oncol* 1999; 17:12–18.
22. Manegold C, Bergman B, Chemaissani A, et al. Single-agent gemcitabine versus cisplatin-etoposide: early results of a randomised phase II study in locally advanced or metastatic non-small cell lung cancer. *Ann Oncol* 1997; 8:525–529.
23. Perng RP, Chen YM, Ming Liu J, et al. Gemcitabine versus the combination of cisplatin and etoposide in patients with inoperable non-small-cell lung cancer in a phase II randomized study. *J Clin Oncol* 1997; 15:2097–2102.
24. Crino L, Clerici M, Figoli F, et al. Chemotherapy of advanced non-small-cell lung cancer: a comparison of three active regimens. A randomized trial of the Italian Oncology Group for Clinical Research. *Ann Oncol* 1995; 6:347–353.
25. Vansteenkiste JF, Vandebroek JE, Nackaerts KL, et al. Clinical benefit response in advanced non-small cell lung cancer. A multicenter prospective randomized phase III study of single agent gemcitabine versus cisplatin-vindesine. *Ann Oncol* 2001; 12:1221–1230.
26. Rapp E, Pater JL, Willan A, et al. Chemotherapy can prolong survival in patients with advanced non-small cell lung cancer. Report of a Canadian multicenter randomized trial. *J Clin Oncol* 1988; 6:633–641.

27. Vansteenkiste J, Vandebroek J, Marien S, et al. Combination chemotherapy with vindesine-ifosfamide-cisplatin (VIP) in locally advanced unresectable stage III and in stage IV non-small cell lung cancer: A phase II trial. *Lung Cancer* 1995; 13:285–293.
28. Crino L, Scagliotti GV, Ricci S, et al. Gemcitabine and cisplatin versus mitomycin, ifosfamide, and cisplatin in advanced non-small-cell lung cancer: a randomized phase III study of the Italian Lung Cancer Project. *J Clin Oncol* 1999; 17:3522–3530.
29. Gebbia V, Galetta D, Riccardi F, et al. Vinorelbine plus cisplatin versus cisplatin plus vindesine and mitomycin C in stage IIIB-IV non-small cell lung carcinoma: a prospective randomized study. *Lung Cancer* 2002; 37:179–187.
30. Roszkowski K, Pluzanska A, Krzakowski M, et al. A multicenter, randomized, phase III study of docetaxel plus best supportive care versus best supportive care in chemotherapy-naive patients with metastatic or non-resectable localized non-small cell lung cancer (NSCLC). *Lung Cancer* 2000; 27:145–157.
31. Ranson M, Davidson N, Nicolson M, et al. Randomized trial of paclitaxel plus supportive care versus supportive care for patients with advanced non-small cell lung cancer. *J Natl Cancer Inst* 2000; 92:1074–1080.
32. Frasci G, Lorusso V, Panza N, et al. Gemcitabine plus vinorelbine versus vinorelbine alone in elderly patients with advanced non-small cell lung cancer. *J Clin Oncol* 2000; 18:2529–2536.
33. Elderly Lung Cancer Vinorelbine Italian Study Group. Effects of vinorelbine on quality of life and survival of elderly patients with advanced non-small cell lung cancer. *J Natl Cancer Inst* 1999; 91:66–72.
34. Jassem J, Ramlau R, Karnicka-Mlodkowska H, et al. A multicenter randomized phase II study of oral vs intravenous vinorelbine in advanced non-small cell patients with lung cancer. *Ann Oncol* 2001; 12:1375–1381.
35. Comella P, Frasci G, Panza N, et al. Randomized trial comparing cisplatin, gemcitabine, and vinorelbine with either cisplatin and gemcitabine or cisplatin and vinorelbine in advanced non-small cell lung cancer: interim analysis of a phase III trial of the Southern Italy Cooperative Oncology Group. *J Clin Oncol* 2000; 18:1451–1457.
36. Rinaldi M, Crino L, Scagliotti GV, et al. A three-week schedule of gemcitabine-cisplatin in advanced non-small cell lung cancer with two different cisplatin dose levels: a phase II randomized trial. *Ann Oncol* 2000; 11:1295–1300.
37. Schiller JH, Harrington D, Belani CP, et al. Comparison of four chemotherapy regimens for advanced non-small cell lung cancer. *N Engl J Med* 2002; 346:92–98.
38. Scagliotti GV, De Marinis F, Rinaldi M, et al. Phase III randomized trial comparing three platinum-based doublets in advanced non-small cell lung cancer. *J Clin Oncol* 2002; 20:4285–4291.
39. Georgoulias V, Papadakis E, Alexopoulos A, et al. Platinum-based and non-platinum-based chemotherapy in advanced non-small cell lung cancer: a randomised multicentre trial. *Lancet* 2001; 357:1478–1484.
40. Rodriguez J, Pawel J, Pluzanska A, et al. A multicenter, randomized phase III study of docetaxel + cisplatin (DC) and docetaxel + carboplatin (DCB) vs vinorelbine + cisplatin in chemonaive patients with advanced and metastatic non-small cell lung cancer. *Proc Am Soc Clin Oncol* 2001; 20:314A (abstract).
41. Rosell R, Gatzemeier U, Betticher DC, et al. Phase III randomised trial comparing paclitaxel/carboplatin with paclitaxel/cisplatin in patients with advanced non-small cell lung cancer: a cooperative multinational trial. *Ann Oncol* 2002; 13:1539–1549.
42. Kelly K, Crowley J, Bunn PA, et al. Randomized phase III trial of paclitaxel plus carboplatin versus vinorelbine plus cisplatin in the treatment of patients with advanced non-small cell lung cancer: a Southwest Oncology Group trial. *J Clin Oncol* 2001; 19:3210–3218.
43. Wozniak AJ, Crowley JJ, Balcerzak SP, et al. Randomized trial comparing cisplatin with cisplatin plus vinorelbine in the treatment of advanced non-small cell lung cancer: a Southwest Oncology Group study. *J Clin Oncol* 1998; 16:2459–2465.
44. Chen YM, Perng RP, Lee YC, et al. Paclitaxel plus carboplatin, compared with paclitaxel plus gemcitabine, shows similar efficacy while more cost-effective: a randomized phase II study of combination chemotherapy against inoperable non-small cell lung cancer previously untreated. *Ann Oncol* 2002; 13:108–115.
45. Kosmidis P, Mylonakis N, Nicolaides C, et al. Paclitaxel plus carboplatin versus gemcitabine plus paclitaxel in advanced non-small cell lung cancer: a phase III randomized trial. *J Clin Oncol* 2002; 20:3578–3585.

46. Grigorescu AC, Draghici IN, Nitipir C, Gutulescu N, Corlan E. Gemcitabine (GEM) and carboplatin (CBDCA) versus cisplatin (CDDP) and vinblastine (VLB) in advanced non-small cell lung cancer (NSCLC) stages III and IV: a phase III randomised trial. *Lung Cancer* 2002; 37:9–14.
47. Sederholm C. Gemcitabine versus gemcitabine/carboplatin in advanced non-small cell lung cancer: preliminary findings in a phase III trial of the Swedish Lung Cancer Study Group. *Semin Oncol* 2002; 29:50–54.
48. Abels R, Larholt K, Nelson R. Risk of transfusion in small cell patients with lung cancer receiving chemotherapy. *Blood* 1994; 84:664A (abstract)
49. Ray-Coquard I, Le Cesne A, Rubio MT, et al. Risk model for severe anemia requiring red blood cell transfusion after cytotoxic conventional chemotherapy regimens. The Elypse 1 Study Group. *J Clin Oncol* 1999; 17:2840–2846.
50. Pivot X, Guardiola E, Etienne M, et al. An analysis of potential factors allowing an individual prediction of cisplatin-induced anaemia. *Eur J Cancer* 2000; 36:852–857.
51. Non-Small Cell Lung Cancer Collaborative Group. Chemotherapy in non-small cell lung cancer: a meta-analysis using updated data on individual patients from 52 randomised clinical trials. *BMJ* 1995; 311:899–909.
52. Breathnach OS, Freidlin B, Conley B, et al. Twenty-two years of phase III trials for patients with advanced non-small cell lung cancer: sobering results. *J Clin Oncol* 2001; 19:1734–1742.
53. Numico G, Russi E, Merlano M. Best supportive care in non-small cell lung cancer: is there a role for radiotherapy and chemotherapy? *Lung Cancer* 2001; 32:213–226.
54. Ludwig H, Fritz E. Anemia in cancer patients. *Semin Oncol* 1998; 25:2–6.
55. Sarna L. Effectiveness of structured nursing assessment of symptom distress in advanced lung cancer. *Oncol Nurs Forum* 1998; 25:1041–1048.
56. Curt GA, Breitbart W, Cella D, et al. Impact of cancer-related fatigue on the lives of patients: new findings from the Fatigue Coalition. *Oncologist* 2000; 5:353–360.
57. Stone P, Richards M, A'Hern R, Hardy J. A study to investigate the prevalence, severity and correlates of fatigue among patients with cancer in comparison with a control group of volunteers without cancer. *Ann Oncol* 2000; 11:561–567.
58. Cella D. The Functional Assessment of Cancer Therapy-Anemia (FACT-An) Scale: a new tool for the assessment of outcomes in cancer anemia and fatigue. *Semin Hematol* 1997; 34:13–19.
59. Vogelzang NJ, Breitbart W, Cella D, et al. Patient, caregiver, and oncologist perceptions of cancer-related fatigue: results of a tripart assessment survey. The Fatigue Coalition. *Semin Hematol* 1997; 34:4–12.
60. Cella D. Factors influencing quality of life in cancer patients: anemia and fatigue. *Semin Oncol* 1998; 25:43–46.
61. Littlewood TJ, Bajetta E, Nortier JW, Vercammen E, Rapoport B. Effects of epoetin alfa on hematologic parameters and quality of life in cancer patients receiving nonplatinum chemotherapy: results of a randomized, double-blind, placebo-controlled trial. *J Clin Oncol* 2001; 19:2865–2874.
62. Glaspy J, Bukowski R, Steinberg D, Taylor C, Tchekmedyian S, Vadhan Raj S. Impact of therapy with epoetin alfa on clinical outcomes in patients with nonmyeloid malignancies during cancer chemotherapy in community oncology practice. Procrit Study Group. *J Clin Oncol* 1997; 15:1218–1234.
63. Demetri GD, Kris M, Wade J, Degos L, Cella D. Quality-of-life benefit in chemotherapy patients treated with epoetin alfa is independent of disease response or tumor type: results from a prospective community oncology study. Procrit Study Group. *J Clin Oncol* 1998; 16:3412–3425.
64. Case DC, Bukowski RM, Carey RW, et al. Recombinant human erythropoietin therapy for anemic cancer patients on combination chemotherapy. *J Natl Cancer Inst* 1993; 85:801–806.
65. Ludwig H, Sundal E, Pecherstorfer M, et al. Recombinant human erythropoietin for the correction of cancer associated anemia with and without concomitant cytotoxic chemotherapy. *Cancer* 1995; 76:2319–2329.
66. Crawford J, Cella D, Cleeland CS, et al. Relationship between changes in hemoglobin level and quality of life during chemotherapy in anemic cancer patients receiving epoetin alfa therapy. *Cancer* 2002; 95:888–895.
67. Albain KS, Crowley JJ, LeBlanc M, Livingston RB. Survival determinants in extensive-stage non-small cell lung cancer: the Southwest Oncology Group experience. *J Clin Oncol* 1991; 9:1618–1626.
68. Brizel DM, Dodge RK, Clough RW, Dewhirst MW. Oxygenation of head and neck cancer: changes during radiotherapy and impact on treatment outcome. *Radiother Oncol* 1999; 53:113–117.
69. Fein DA, Lee WR, Hanlon AL, et al. Pretreatment hemoglobin level influences local control and survival of T1–T2 squamous cell carcinomas of the glottic larynx. *J Clin Oncol* 1995; 13:2077–2083.

70. Grogan M, Thomas GM, Melamed I, et al. The importance of hemoglobin levels during radiotherapy for carcinoma of the cervix. *Cancer* 1999; 86:1528–1536.
71. Walker RH. Special report: transfusion risks. *Am J Clin Pathol* 1987; 88:374–378.
72. Goodnough LT, Brecher ME, Kanter MH, AuBuchon JP. Transfusion medicine. First of two parts—blood transfusion. *N Engl J Med* 1999; 340:438–447.
73. Piantadosi S, Moores DW, McKneally MF. The adverse effect of perioperative blood transfusion in lung cancer. *Chest* 1994; 106:382S–384S.
74. Dresner SM, Lamb PJ, Shenfine J, Hayes N, Griffin SM. Prognostic significance of peri-operative blood transfusion following radical resection for oesophageal carcinoma. *Eur J Surg Oncol* 2000; 26:492–497.
75. Edna TH, Bjerkeset T. Perioperative blood transfusions reduce long-term survival following surgery for colorectal cancer. *Dis Colon Rectum* 1998; 41:451–459.
76. Platanias LC, Miller CB, Mick R, et al. Treatment of chemotherapy-induced anemia with recombinant human erythropoietin in cancer patients. *J Clin Oncol* 1991; 9:2021–2026.
77. Cascinu S, Fedeli A, Del Ferro E, Luzi Fedeli S, Catalano G. Recombinant human erythropoietin treatment in cisplatin-associated anemia: a randomized, double-blind trial with placebo. *J Clin Oncol* 1994; 12:1058–1062.
78. Oberhoff C, Neri B, Amadori D, et al. Recombinant human erythropoietin in the treatment of chemotherapy-induced anemia and prevention of transfusion requirement associated with solid tumors: a randomized, controlled study. *Ann Oncol* 1998; 9:255–260.
79. Seidenfeld J, Piper M, Flamm C, et al. Epoetin treatment of anemia associated with cancer therapy: a systematic review and meta-analysis of controlled clinical trials. *J Natl Cancer Inst* 2001; 93:1204–1214.
80. Thatcher N, De Campos ES, Bell DR, et al. Epoetin alpha prevents anaemia and reduces transfusion requirements in patients undergoing primarily platinum-based chemotherapy for small cell lung cancer. *Br J Cancer* 1999; 80:396–402.
81. Kunikane H, Watanabe K, Fukuoka M, et al. Double-blind randomized control trial of the effect of recombinant human erythropoietin on chemotherapy-induced anemia in patients with non-small cell lung cancer. *Int J Clin Oncol* 2002; 6:296–301.
82. Egrie JC, Dwyer E, Browne JK, Hitz A, Lykos MA. Darbepoetin alfa has a longer circulating half-life and greater in vivo potency recombinant human erythropoietin. *Exp Hematol* 2003; 31:290–299.
83. Egrie JC, Grant JR, Gillies DK, Aoki KH, Strickland TW. The role of carbohydrate on the biological activity of erythropoietin. *Glycoconj J* 1993; 10:263.
84. Macdougall IC, Gray SJ, Elston O, et al. Pharmacokinetics of novel erythropoiesis stimulating protein compared with epoetin alfa in dialysis patients. *J Am Soc Nephrol* 1999; 10:2392–2395.
85. Heatherington AC, Schuller J, Mercer AJ. Pharmacokinetics of novel erythropoiesis stimulating pro tein (NESP) in cancer patients: preliminary report. *Br J Cancer* 2001; 84(suppl 1):11–16.
86. Kotasek D, Steger G, Faught W, et al. (Aranesp 980291 Study Group) Darbepoetin alfa administered every 3 weeks alleviates anaemia in patients with solid tumours receiving chemotherapy; results of a double-blind, placebo-controlled, randomised study. *Eur J Cancer* 2003; 39:2026–2034.
87. Glaspy JA, Jadeja JS, Justice G, et al. Darbepoetin alfa given every 1 or 2 weeks alleviates anaemia associated with cancer chemotherapy. *Br J Cancer* 2002; 87:268–276.
88. Vansteenkiste J, Pirker R, Massuti B, et al. Double-blind, placebo-controlled, randomised phase III trial of darbepoetin alfa in patients with lung cancer receiving chemotherapy. *J Natl Cancer Inst* 2002; 94:1211–1220.
89. Hedenus M, Hansen S, Taylor K, et al. Randomized, dose-finding study of darbepoetin alfa in anaemic patients with lymphoproliferative malignancies. *Br J Haematol* 2002; 119:79–86.
90. Rizzo JD, Lichtin AE, Woolf SH, et al. Use of epoetin in patients with cancer: evidence-based clinical practice guidelines of the American Society of Clinical Oncology and the American Society of Hematology. *J Clin Oncol* 2002; 20:4083–4107.
91. American Society of Clinical Oncology (ASCO). Recommendations for the use of hematopoietic colony-stimulating factors: evidence-based, clinical practice guidelines. *J Clin Oncol* 1994; 12:2471–2508.
92. Crawford J, Ozer H, Stoller R, et al. Reduction by granulocyte colony-stimulating factor of fever and neutropenia induced by chemotherapy in patients with small-cell lung cancer. *N Engl J Med* 1991; 325:164–170.
93. Trillet-Lenoir V, Green J, Manegold C, et al. Recombinant granulocyte colony stimulating factor reduces the infectious complications of cytotoxic chemotherapy. *Eur J Cancer* 1993; 29A:319–324.

94. Gatzemeier U, Kleisbauer JP, Drings P, et al. Lenograstim as support for ACE chemotherapy of small cell lung cancer: a phase III, multicenter, randomized study. *Am J Clin Oncol* 2000; 23:393–400.
95. Hamm J, Schiller JH, Cuffie C, et al. Dose-ranging study of recombinant human granulocyte-macrophage colony-stimulating factor in small cell lung carcinoma. *J Clin Oncol* 1994; 12:2667–2676.
96. Bunn PA, Crowley J, Kelly K, et al. Chemoradiotherapy with or without granulocyte-macrophage colony-stimulating factor in the treatment of limited-stage small cell lung cancer: a prospective phase III randomized study of the Southwest Oncology Group. *J Clin Oncol* 1995; 13:1632–1641.
97. Arriagada R, Le Chevalier T, Pignon JP, et al. Initial chemotherapeutic doses and survival in patients with limited small-cell lung cancer. *N Engl J Med* 1993; 329:1848–1852.
98. Miles D, Fogarty O, Ash C, Rudd R, et al. Received dose intensity: a randomized trial of weekly chemotherapy with and without granulocyte colony stimulating factor in small cell lung cancer. *J Clin Oncol* 1994; 12:77–82.
99. Woll PJ, Hodgetts J, Lomax L, Bildet F, Cour Chabernaud V, Thatcher N. Can cytotoxic dose-intensity be increased by using granulocyte colony-stimulating factor? A randomized controlled trial of lenograstim in small-cell lung cancer. *J Clin Oncol* 1995; 13:652–659.
100. Fukuoka M, Masuda N, Negoro S, et al. CODE chemotherapy with and without granulocyte colony-stimulating factor in small cell lung cancer. *Br J Cancer* 1997; 75:306–309.
101. Furuse K, Fukuoka M, Nishiwaki Y, et al. Phase III study of intensive weekly chemotherapy with recombinant human granulocyte colony-stimulating factor versus standard chemotherapy in extensive-disease small cell lung cancer. The Japan Clinical Oncology Group. *J Clin Oncol* 1998; 16:2126–2132.
102. Thatcher N, Girling DJ, Hopwood P, Sambrook RJ, Qian W, Stephens RJ. Improving survival without reducing quality of life in small cell patients with lung cancer by increasing the dose-intensity of chemotherapy with granulocyte colony-stimulating factor support: results of a British Medical Research Council multicenter randomized trial. *J Clin Oncol* 2000; 18:395–404.
103. Pujol JL, Douillard JY, Riviere A, et al. Dose-intensity of a four-drug chemotherapy regimen with or without recombinant human granulocyte-macrophage colony-stimulating factor in extensive-stage small-cell lung cancer: a multicenter randomized phase III study. *J Clin Oncol* 1997; 15:2082–2089.
104. Steward WP, von Pawel J, Gatzemeier U, et al. Effects of granulocyte-macrophage colony-stimulating factor and dose intensification of V-ICE chemotherapy in small-cell lung cancer: a prospective randomized study of 300 patients. *J Clin Oncol* 1998; 16:642–650.
105. Sculier JP, Paesmans M, Lecomte J, et al. A three-arm phase III randomised trial assessing, in patients with extensive-disease small cell lung cancer, accelerated chemotherapy with support of haematological growth factor or oral antibiotics. *Br J Cancer* 2001; 85:1444–1451.
106. Ardizzoni A, Tjan-Heijnen VC, Postmus PE, et al. Standard versus intensified chemotherapy with granulocyte colony-stimulating factor support in small cell lung cancer: a prospective European Organization for Research and Treatment of Cancer Lung Cancer Group phase III trial 08923. *J Clin Oncol* 2002; 20:3947–3955.
107. Woll PJ, Thatcher N, Lomax L, et al. Use of hematopoietic progenitors in whole blood to support dose-dense chemotherapy: a randomized phase II trial in small cell patients with lung cancer. *J Clin Oncol* 2001; 19:712–719.
108. Eguchi K, Kabe J, Kudo S, et al. Efficacy of recombinant human granulocyte-macrophage colony-stimulating factor for chemotherapy-induced leukopenia in patients with non-small cell lung cancer. *Cancer Chemother Pharmacol* 1994; 34:37–43.
109. Bonomi P, Kim K, Kusler J, Johnson D. Cisplatin/etoposide vs paclitaxel/cisplatin/G-CSF vs paclitaxel/cisplatin in non-small-cell lung cancer. *Oncology* 1997; 11:9–10.
110. Font A, Moyano AJ, Puerto JM, et al. Increasing dose intensity of cisplatin-etoposide in advanced non-small cell lung carcinoma: a phase III randomized trial of the Spanish Lung Cancer Group. *Cancer* 1999; 85:855–863.
111. Masutani M, Tsujino I, Fujie T, et al. Moderate dose-intensive chemotherapy for patients with non-small cell lung cancer: randomized trial, can it improve survival of patients with good performance status? *Oncol Rep* 1999; 6:1045–1050.
112. Ozer H, Armitage JO, Bennett CL, et al. 2000 update of recommendations for the use of hematopoietic colony-stimulating factors: evidence-based, clinical practice guidelines. American Society of Clinical Oncology Growth Factors Expert Panel. *J Clin Oncol* 2000; 18:3558–3585.
113. Bennett CL, Smith TJ, Weeks JC, et al. Use of hematopoietic colony-stimulating factors: the American Society of Clinical Oncology survey. *J Clin Oncol* 1996; 14:2511–2520.

14 Role of Hematopoietic Growth Factors As Adjuncts to the Treatment of Hodgkin's and Non-Hodgkin's Lymphomas

Marcie R. Tomblyn, MD
and Jane N. Winter, MD

CONTENTS

1. INTRODUCTION

Lymphomas are malignancies of lymphoid cells categorized as either Hodgkin's disease (HD) or non-Hodgkin's lymphomas (NHL). Disease presentations are similar with infiltrations of malignant lymphocytes in lymph nodes or extranodal tissues with or without the presence of constitutional symptoms. Overall, the prognosis for HD is better, with an overall survival rate of >80% at 5 yr *(1)*. NHL is a more complex entity, with many histologies ranging from indolent to highly aggressive in behavior. It occurs in greater frequency in elderly patients with a median age of onset of 50 yr of age *(2)*. In contrast, HD has a bimodal distribution with a peak incidence in the third decade and a second smaller peak in the sixth decade *(1)*. In both HD and NHL, initial treatment consists of chemotherapy, radiation, or both depending on extent of disease. Despite improvements in therapy, however, a significant proportion of patients will progress, relapse, and die from their disease.

Myelosuppression remains a significant complication of combination chemotherapy and is a cause for morbidity and mortality, especially in older patients. The use of

From: *Cancer Drug Discovery and Development*
Hematopoietic Growth Factors in Oncology: Basic Science and Clinical Therapeutics
Edited by: G. Morstyn, M. A. Foote, and G. J. Lieschke © Humana Press Inc., Totowa, NJ

Table 1
Phase 2 Studies Suggesting Improved Relative Dose Intensity in Older Patients With Aggressive NHL

Study Ref.	*No.*	*Median age (range; yr)*	*Treatment*	*Relative dose intensity of anthracycline (%)*	*Complete response rates (%)*	*Overall survival (%)*
13	20	71 (66–80)	CHOP + G-CSF[a]	97.3	60	66 (2 yr)
7	42	74 (70–79)	CHOP + G-CSF[b]	91	87.5	69 (2.5 yr)
4	26	67 (61–84)	CHOP + GM-CSF[c]	93	62	50 (2.5 yr)

[a] Cyclophosphamide 750 mg/m^2 d 1, doxorubicin 50 mg/m^2 d 1, vincristine 1.4 mg/m^2 d 1, prednisone 100 mg d 1–5 repeat every 21 d; recombinant human granulocyte colony-stimulating factor (rHuG-CSF) 5 μg/kg starting d 3 until absolute neutrophil count > 10 × 10^9/L.

[b] Cyclophosphamide 750 mg/m^2 d 1, doxorubicin 50 mg/m^2 d 1, vincristine 1.4 mg/m^2 d 1, prednisone 100 mg d 1–5 repeat every 21 d; rHuG-CSF 2 μg/kg if white blood cell count < 2 × 10^9/L until white blood cell count > 10 × 10^9/L.

[c] Cyclophosphamide 750 mg/m^2 d 1, doxorubicin 50 mg/m^2 d 1, vincristine 1.4 mg/m^2 d 1, prednisone 100 mg d 1–5 repeat every 21 d; rHuGM-CSF 5 μg/kg d 4–13.

hematopoietic growth factors (HGFs) improves the tolerability of standard-dose, increased intensity, or high-dose chemotherapy with benefits in both disease control and overall survival *(3–8)*. HGFs facilitate the collection of peripheral blood progenitor cells (PBPCs) for purposes of autologous and allogeneic hematopoietic stem cell transplantation. Additionally, recombinant human (rHu) HGFs, specifically granulocyte-macrophage colony-stimulating factor (rHuGM-CSF), have been shown to augment the immunogenicity of lymphoma-specific vaccines *(9,10)*.

2. THERAPY IN THE OLDER PATIENT

Age > 60 yr is the single most powerful predictor of shortened overall survival in patients with aggressive NHL *(11)*. Possible reasons for decreased survival in this patient population may be related to the presence of comorbid illness, altered pharmacokinetics resulting in greater treatment-related toxicities, or a more aggressive tumor biology *(5)*. Alternatively, it is possible that physicians, concerned about the potential for toxicity, treat older patients with less intensive chemotherapy and make significant dose reductions, resulting in inferior response rates *(6,12)*. In a retrospective analysis, Kwak and colleagues *(12)* showed that the actual relative dose intensity (RDI) of chemotherapy, specifically doxorubicin, was an important prognostic factor for survival in diffuse large-cell lymphoma. Hence, dose reductions might compromise the outcome of potentially curative therapy. Whereas myelosuppression with its associated risk of infection remains a significant cause of treatment-related morbidity, the addition of HGFs in the older patient may reduce complication rates while allowing for maintenance of planned dose intensity.

Although the results of several small phase 2 studies suggest that the addition of HGFs improves the RDI of administered therapy, resulting in an improvement in response and survival (Table 1), this hypothesis has not been validated in three randomized trials *(4,7,13–16)*. The Nordic Lymphoma Study Group randomized 458 patients over the age of 60 yr with aggressive NHL to receive either cyclophosphamide, doxorubicin, vincristine, and prednisone (CHOP) ± rHu granulocyte colony-stimulating factor (rHuG-CSF) or cyclophosphamide, mitoxantrone, vincristine, and prednisone (CNOP) ± rHuG-CSF in a bifactorial design *(14)*. Decreased rates of neutropenia and infection were seen with the addition of HGFs, but there were no significant effects on rates of complete remission or overall survival. The median actual RDI for the anthracycline was the same whether or not the patient received rHuG-CSF.

The Dutch-Belgian Hemato-Oncology Cooperative Group had similar findings in their study of 303 patients 65 yr of age or older treated with CHOP ± rHuG-CSF *(15)*. In yet another phase 3 trial, Zinzani and colleagues *(16)* evaluated 149 patients 60 yr or older with untreated aggressive NHL. Patients were randomly assigned to receive cyclophosphamide, mitoxantrone, vincristine, etoposide, bleomycin, and prednisone ± rHuG-CSF (5 μg/kg/d) for 5 d. A significant decrease was noted in the number of episodes of neutropenia and infection without a difference in overall response, complete response, and survival. A trend toward a higher RDI was noted in patients receiving rHuG-CSF, but the difference was not statistically significant. Together, these studies show that although there is a decline in myelosuppression-related toxicity with the addition of HGF in patients 60 yr or greater, there is no effect on response rates or overall survival.

The addition of HGFs to standard CHOP chemotherapy has been shown to result in fewer episodes of febrile neutropenia (FN) and a decreased risk of hospitalization with shorter lengths of stay (LOS) *(17,18)*. A retrospective review of patients with NHL treated at a single institution found a potential cost savings through a reduction in neutropenic complications as well as an improvement in administered dose intensity of chemotherapy *(17)*. When specifically studying patients aged 65 yr or greater, Chrischilles and colleagues *(18)* showed that those treated with HGFs were hospitalized for FN an average of 1.2 d less than those not receiving HGF. Consequently, despite the lack of impact on response and overall survival, possibly in part reflecting the presence of comorbid illnesses or alterations in tumor biology, there is a benefit to HGF administration in terms of decreased frequency of neutropenic complications and hospitalizations. Therefore, in accordance with the American Society of Clinical Oncology (ASCO) guidelines, it is appropriate to treat the older patient with lymphoma and a good performance status with conventional-dose chemotherapy supplemented with HGFs to reduce the risk of complications *(19)*.

3. INCREASED DOSE INTENSITY WITHOUT HEMATOPOIETIC STEM CELL SUPPORT

Lymphomas are dose-responsive malignancies *(12)*. For this reason, many studies have evaluated increased doses of chemotherapy in younger patients, using HGF support. Methods to escalate chemotherapy have been used either through increased dosage or more frequent administration, i.e., dose intensity or dose density *(20–28)*. The results of these investigations have been mixed. Two large phase 2 cooperative group studies have analyzed dose intensity in patients with NHL *(20,22)*.

The Cancer and Leukemia Group B (CALGB) conducted dose-escalation pilot studies in patients with aggressive NHL to determine the maximum tolerated dose (MTD) for the CHOPE regimen (chemotherapy with cyclophosphamide, doxorubicin, vincristine, prednisone, and etoposide) with and without the addition of rHuG-CSF *(20)*. Dosing for doxorubicin, vincristine, and prednisone was according to the CHOP regimen

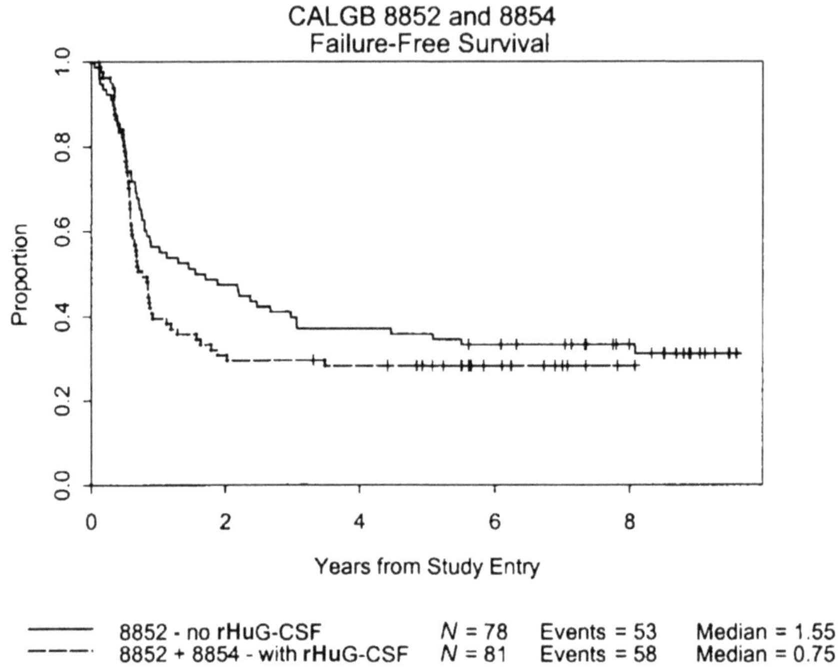

Fig. 1. Failure-free survival for 81 eligible patients who were treated on Cancer and Leukemia Group B (CALGB) Study 8854 or Study 8852 with dose-escalated cyclophosphamide, doxorubicin, vincristine, prednisone, and etoposide (CHOPE) plus recombinant human granulocyte colony-stimulating factor (rHuG-CSF) compared with 78 eligible patients who were treated with CHOPE without rHuG-CSF. (From ref. *20.* © 2001 American Cancer Society. Reprinted with permission of Wiley-Liss, Inc., a subsidiary of John Wiley and Sons, Inc.)

(50 mg/m^2 d 1, 1.4 mg/m^2 [maximum dose of 2 mg] d 1, and 100 mg/d for 5 d, respectively). Without rHuG-CSF supplementation, cyclophosphamide and etoposide could only be escalated to 1000 mg/m^2 on d 1 and 100 mg/m^2 for 3 d, correspondingly. The addition of 200 μg/m^2 of rHuG-CSF administered on d 5–19 of each cycle allowed for maximum doses of 1500 mg/m^2 of cyclophosphamide and 160 mg/m^2 of etoposide. Eighty-one patients were ultimately treated with dose-escalated CHOPE and rHuG-CSF. Despite the increased dosing, the overall response rate and complete response rate of 88 and 43%, respectively, did not differ from the overall response and complete response rates for those patients treated with lower doses without rHuG-CSF. No significant difference was seen in failure-free survival and overall survival (Fig. 1). Although this study was not designed to be a comparative one, the authors concluded that since the response and survival data did not appear significantly better than standard-dose CHOP, there was no reason to pursue a phase 3 study.

In a second phase 2 study evaluating dose intensity, the Eastern Cooperative Oncology Group (ECOG) studied a dose-intensive regimen of 200% ProMACE-CytaBOM (cyclophosphamide [1300 mg/m^2 d 1], doxorubicin [50 mg/m^2 d 1], etoposide [240 mg/m^2 d 1], prednisone [60 mg/m^2 d 1–14], cytarabine [600 mg/m^2 d 8], bleomycin [5 mg/m^2 d 8], vincristine [1.4 mg/m^2 d 8], methotrexate [120 mg/m^2 d 8], and leucovorin) with the addition of HGFs *(22).* Seventy-four patients with stage II bulky, stage III, or stage IV aggressive NHL were evaluated. They reported an overall response rate of 92% with a complete response rate of 69%. The median survival had not been reached at the time of publication. Despite HGF support, hematologic toxicity was significant, including 49% grade 4 thrombocytopenia, 83% grade 4 neutropenia, and 97% grade 4 leukopenia. Although there were marked cytopenias, only 9% of patients had documented infection, and no toxic deaths were observed. This study showed the feasibility of significant dose escalation with the addition of HGF as well as durable responses using this multidrug, dose-intensive regimen for the treatment of aggressive NHL.

To evaluate dose density (treatment frequency), the German High-Grade Non-Hodgkin's Lymphoma Study Group conducted a phase 3 randomized study in younger patients comparing standard dose CHOP every 21 d, CHOP + etoposide 100 mg/m^2 d 1–3 every 21 d, and both regimens in biweekly dosing with rHuG-CSF support starting on d 4 of the 14-d treatments *(26)*. They concluded that there was no significant improvement associated with biweekly chemotherapy but that the complete response rate and time to treatment failure were improved with the addition of etoposide. This finding is in contrast to their data in patients >60 yr, in which there was an improvement in complete response rates with biweekly therapy, especially in patients with increased lactic dehydrogenase *(29)*. Dan and colleagues *(21)* also evaluated the dose-dense treatment regimen of CHOP every 14 d with rHuG-CSF support and found the regimen to be feasible in patients with aggressive NHL. The 96 previously untreated patients had an overall response rate of 100% with a complete response rate of approx 74%. No data on duration of remission were reported, but the 5-yr survival rate was 59%. The data from these dose-dense studies remain controversial but demonstrate the feasibility of shortening the duration of chemotherapy cycles with HGF supplementation. The overall benefit remains to be determined with further randomized studies.

Similar studies addressing the role of HGF support have been evaluated in patients with HD *(27,28,30,31)*. Pfreundschuh and colleagues *(31)* from the German Hodgkin's Lymphoma Study Group escalated doses of etoposide in the Dexa-BEAM regimen (chemotherapy with dexamethasone, carmustine, melphalan, cytarabine, and etoposide) to compare the MTD of etoposide with rHuGM-CSF vs placebo in patients with relapsed or refractory HD. Their data showed both an increased RDI and a substantial overall increase in etoposide dose without a difference in treatment efficacy. The German Hodgkin's Lymphoma Group also published data demonstrating the benefits of the dose-escalated BEACOPP (chemotherapy with bleomycin, etoposide, Adriamycin, cyclophosphamide, vincristine, procarbazine, and prednisone) regimen in patients with advanced-stage HD *(28)*. They showed that with the increase in doses of cyclophosphamide, etoposide, and doxorubicin by 190, 200, and 140%, respectively, the complete response rate was 93%. This regimen was then evaluated in a phase 3 randomized study compared with both COPP/ABVD (cyclophosphamide, vincristine, procarbazine, prednisone, doxorubicin, bleomycin, vinblastine, and dacarbazine) and standard-dose BEACOPP *(27)*. There was a significant improvement in freedom from treatment failure and a trend toward improvement in overall survival for the dose-escalated BEACOPP. These data support the feasibility of dose escalation and are suggestive of clinical benefit in the treatment of HD.

Alternatively, an Italian study used rHuGM-CSF before chemotherapy in a cohort of newly diagnosed HD patients to determine whether there was a myeloprotective effect that would prevent delays in treatment with the MOPP/ABVD (chemotherapy with mechlorethamine, vincristine, procarbazine, prednisone, doxorubicin, bleomycin, vinblastine, and dacarbazine) regimen *(32)*. This randomized, placebo-controlled study enrolled 56 patients with primarily stage III and IV HD who received rHuGM-CSF (5 μg/kg/d) or placebo on d –7 to –4 before chemotherapy with the primary endpoint being adherence to planned drug delivery. No statistical difference was noted between the two groups in dose intensity, but there did appear to be a trend in favor of the rHuGM-CSF group for maintaining dose schedule and delivery, for shortening the duration of neutropenia, and for a higher neutrophil nadir.

Taken together, these studies indicate that dose escalation either as increased intensity or increased density with the support of HGF is feasible. Unfortunately, there does not appear to be a significant benefit compared with standard-dose therapies in terms of response and survival, with the exception of the single randomized, dose-escalated BEACOPP study from the German Hodgkin's Lymphoma Group *(27)*. However, prospective randomized trials for NHL are lacking.

4. USE IN HEMATOPOIETIC STEM CELL TRANSPLANTATION

The PARMA trial clearly showed that high-dose chemotherapy and autologous hematopoietic stem cell transplantation is the optimal treatment for patients with relapsed chemotherapy-sensitive NHL *(33)*. PBPCs collected with HGFs have now supplanted the use of bone marrow progenitors for use in autologous rescue after high-dose chemotherapy *(34)*. Optimal use of HGFs in the mobilization of patients with lymphoma continues to be determined *(35–39)*. Separate studies by Watts and colleagues *(38)* and Pavone and colleagues *(39)* found that lymphoma-specific salvage chemotherapy (ESHAP [etoposide, solumedrol, cytarabine, and cisplatin] or DHAP [cisplatin, cytarabine, and dexamethasone]) followed by rHuG-CSF resulted in PBPC collections similar to those achieved with high-dose cyclophosphamide and rHuG-CSF. When rHuG-CSF and rHuGM-CSF have been compared, there has been no difference in the quality of the harvests, although patients receiving rHuG-CSF for mobilization after cyclophosphamide had a shorter interval to harvest but a relative delay in platelet recovery *(35,36)*. Interestingly, a randomized trial in patients with lymphoma at the New England Medical Center showed that rHuG-CSF alone is adequate for mobilization, eliminating the need for high-dose cyclophosphamide *(37)*. Patients who received only rHuG-CSF collected a lower total number of $CD34^+$ cells/kg, but this did not translate into a significantly longer time to engraftment. Clearly, the optimal role of HGFs in the mobilization of lymphoma patients remains undefined.

The use of HGFs in the post-transplant setting has been studied. Three randomized studies have shown benefit for the addition of rHuG-CSF after high-dose chemotherapy and autologous PBPC transplant *(40–42)*. Linch et al. *(41)* reported that the use of rHuG-CSF beginning on d +1 resulted in a significantly shorter duration of neutropenia with shorter hospitalizations than controls. Lee and colleagues *(40)* found similar results and concluded that health care costs were reduced by approx 22% in patients receiving rHuG-CSF support post transplant. These cost savings were not seen in a similar study from Spain, although the relatively shorter time to engraftment associated with rHuG-CSF was confirmed *(42)*. HGFs have been shown to shorten the duration of neutropenia in the setting of allogeneic stem cell transplant without affecting rates of acute graft-vs-host-disease (GvHD), 100-d transplant-related mortality, or disease-free survival *(43–45)*. The use of HGFs after autologous and allogeneic hematopoietic stem cell transplant clearly shortens the duration of neutropenia, but whether or not this translates into financial savings remains controversial.

5. IMMUNE THERAPY

Direct targeting of tumor cells with naked antibody (Ab) or immunoconjugate remains an attractive approach to the treatment of malignant disease. In the treatment of NHL, this approach has proven benefit in the use of the monoclonal antibody (MAb) rituximab and the immunoconjugate Zevalin® (^{90}Yttrium ibritumomab tiuxetan), both of which target the CD20 molecule present on B lymphocytes. Methods to augment the patient's own immune responses are also under investigation *(9,46–49)*.

Preclinical data suggest that one approach to stimulating the host immune response to the malignant clone is through the use of HGFs *(46,50)*. rHuGM-CSF has been shown to enhance the neutrophil functions of phagocytosis and chemotaxis, to increase the cytotoxicity and cytokine production of monocytes, and to boost the quantity and function of antigen-presenting cells *(46)*. This finding is important given that monocytes have been shown to have defective phagocytic activity in patients with NHL *(50)*. Additionally, both rHuG-CSF and rHuGM-CSF have been shown to augment antibody-dependent cellular cytotoxicity (ADCC), a mechanism of action of rituximab and other MAbs *(49,51,52)*.

Another approach to generating a host immune response to the malignant lymphoma is through the administration of tumor-specific vaccines. The malignant cells in NHL display antigenic determinants, or idiotypes, which are tumor specific and serve as targets for the immune system *(47,48)*. Several studies have shown clinical benefit with production of antitumor immunologic responses consisting of both humoral and cytotoxic T-cell responses *(9,47,48,53,54)*. Bendandi and colleagues *(9)* demonstrated that the immunization of patients using a follicular lymphoma idiotype-specific vaccine supplemented with rHuGM-CSF resulted in molecular complete response in 8/11 patients who before immunization were positive for t(14;18). Furthermore, 19/20 immunized patients developed tumor-specific cytotoxic T-cell responses. They hypothesized that the addition of rHuGM-CSF to the vaccine results in recruitment of antigen-presenting cells and subsequent stimulation of a T-cell response. It has been previously suggested that the T-cell response is the basis for disease control with idiotype vaccines both in murine studies and early clinical trials and that this response is augmented by the addition of rHuGM-CSF *(54,55)*. The use of immune modulation in the treatment of lymphoma is under continued investigation. The supplementation of these mechanisms with HGF needs to be studied further.

6. CONCLUSIONS

Both HD and NHL are chemosensitive diseases for which there is clear evidence of a dose-response curve *(12)*. Consequently, the use of HGFs in the treatment of lymphoma is common practice. In general, both rHuG-CSF and rHuGM-CSF have been shown to improve a patient's tolerance to chemotherapy by decreasing the frequency of hospitalization, shortening the duration of neutropenia, and allowing for maintenance of dose intensity and timing *(17,18,21,31)*. Furthermore, the treatment of older patients with conventional-dose chemotherapy is feasible with HGF supplementation

(13,14,16). Hematopoietic stem cell transplant is a well-recognized therapeutic option for patients with high-risk relapsed lymphoma. The success of this form of treatment has been greatly facilitated by the use of HGFs. The use of HGFs for vaccine therapies and as a potential adjunct to other biologic therapies seems promising but remains to be more fully investigated in clinical trials.

REFERENCES

1. Yahalom J, Straus D. Hodgkin's disease. In: Pazdur R, Coia LR, Hoskins WJ, Wagman LD, eds., *Cancer Management: A Multidisciplinary Approach.* Melville, NY: PRR. 2002:603–622.
2. Molina A, Al-Kadhimi Z, Nicolaou N. Non-Hodgkin's lymphoma. In: Pazdur R, Coia LR, Hoskins WJ, Wagman LD, eds., *Cancer Management: A Multidisciplinary Approach.* Melville, NY: PRR. 2002:623–666.
3. Donnelly G, Glassman J, Long C, et al. Granulocyte-colony stimulating factor (G-CSF) may improve disease outcome in elderly patients with diffuse large cell lymphoma (DLCL) treated with CHOP chemotherapy. *Leuk Lymphoma* 2000; 39:67–75.
4. Gomez H, Mas L, Casanova L, et al. Elderly patients with aggressive non-Hodgkin's lymphoma treated with CHOP chemotherapy plus granulocyte-macrophage colony-stimulating factor: identification of two age subgroups with differing hematologic toxicity. *J Clin Oncol* 1998; 16:2352–2358.
5. Kouroukis C, Meyer R. Treatment strategies in elderly patients with aggressive histology lymphoma. *Ann Hematol* 2001; 80:B86–B88.
6. Kouroukis C, Browman GP, Esmail R, et al. Chemotherapy for older patients with newly diagnosed, advanced-stage, aggressive-histology non-Hodgkin's lymphoma: a systematic review. *Ann Intern Med* 2002; 136:144–152.
7. Niitsu N, Iijima K. Full-dose CHOP chemotherapy combined with granulocyte colony-stimulating factor for aggressive non-Hodgkin's lymphoma in elderly patients: a prospective study. *Ann Hematol* 2001; 80:602–606.
8. Peters F, Fickers MMF, Erdkamp FLG, et al. The effect of optimal treatment on elderly patients with aggressive non-Hodgkin's lymphoma: more patients treated with unaffected response rates. *Ann Hematol* 2001; 80:406–410.
9. Bendandi M, Gocke CD, Kobrin CB, et al. Complete molecular remissions induced by patient-specific vaccination plus granulocyte-monocyte colony-stimulating factor against lymphoma. *Nature* 1999; 5:1171–1177.
10. Borrello I, Sotomayor EM, Cooke S, et al. A universal granulocyte-macrophage colony-stimulating factor-producing bystander cell line for use in the formulation of autologous tumor cell-based vaccines. *Hum Gene Ther* 1999; 10:1983–1991.
11. The International Non-Hodgkin's Lymphoma Prognostic Factors Project. A predictive model for aggressive non-Hodgkin's lymphoma. *N Engl J Med* 1993; 329:987–994.
12. Kwak L, Halpern J, Olshen RA, et al. Prognostic significance of actual dose intensity in diffuse large-cell lymphoma: results of a tree-structured survival analysis. *J Clin Oncol* 1990; 8:963–977.
13. Jacobson J, Grossbard M, Shulman LN, et al. CHOP chemotherapy with preemptive granulocyte colony-stimulating factor in elderly patients with aggressive non-Hodgkin's lymphoma: a dose-intensity analysis. *Clin Lymphoma* 2000; 1:211–217.
14. Bjorkholm M, Osby E, Hagberg H, et al. Randomized trial of r-metHu granulocyte colony-stimulating Factor (G-CSF) as adjunct to CHOP or CNOP treatment of elderly patients with aggressive non-Hodgkin's lymphoma. *Blood* 1999; 94:599a (abstract 2665).
15. Doorduijn J, van der Holt B, van der Hem KG, et al. Randomized trial of granulocyte-colony stimulating factor (G-CSF) added to CHOP in elderly patients with aggressive non-Hodgkin's lymphoma (NHL). *Blood* 2000; 96:133a (abstract 575).
16. Zinzani P, Pavone E, Storti S, et al. Randomized trial with or without granulocyte colony-stimulating factor as adjunct to induction VNCOP-B treatment of elderly high-grade non-Hodgkin's lymphoma. *Blood* 1997; 89:3974–3979.
17. Bobey N, Woodman R. Neutropenic complications in advanced-stage non-Hodgkin's lymphoma: implications for the use of prophylactic recombinant human granulocyte-colony stimulating factor (G-CSF). *Clin Invest Med* 1998; 21:63–70.

18. Chrischilles E, Delgado DJ, Stolshek BS, et al. Impact of age and colony-stimulating factor use on hospital length of stay for febrile neutropenia in CHOP-treated non-Hodgkin's lymphoma. *Cancer Control* 2002; 9:203–211.
19. Ozer H, Armitage JO, Bennett C, et al. 2000 Update of Recommendations for the Use of Hematopoietic Colony-Stimulating Factors. www.asco.org, 2003.
20. Bartlett N, Petroni GR, Parker BA, et al. Dose-escalated cyclophosphamide, doxorubicin, vincristine, prednisone, and etoposide (CHOPE) chemotherapy for patients with diffuse lymphoma. *Cancer* 2001; 92:207–217.
21. Dan K, Ogura M, Oyama A, et al. Long-term follow-up in aggressive non-Hodgkin's lymphoma (NHL) patients treated with rHuG-CSF (lenograstim) combined biweekly CHOP chemotherapy. *Blood* 2001; 98:1452a.
22. Gordon L, Young M, Weller E, et al. A phase II trial of 200% ProMACE-CytaBOM in patients with previously untreated aggressive lymphoma: analysis of response, toxicity, and dose intensity. *Blood* 1999; 94:3307–3314.
23. Itoh K, Ohtsu T, Wakita H, et al. Dose-escalation study of CHOP with or without prophylactic G-CSF in aggressive non-Hodgkin's lymphoma. *Ann Oncol* 2000; 11:1241–1247.
24. Koc H, Arslan O, Gurman G, et al. Use of high-dose chemotherapy plus granulocyte colony-stimulating factor for the salvage of refractory or resistant-relapse lymphoma patients without stem cell support. *Acta Haematol* 1997; 98:136–139.
25. Nikkuni K, Aoki S, Tsukada N, et al. A phase II multicenter clinical trial of high-dose bi-weekly THP-COP with G-CSF support (HDBW-TCOP (G)) for non-Hodgkin's lymphoma. *Blood* 2001; 98:571a.
26. Pfreundschuh M, Trumper L, Kloess M, et al. CHOEP (CHOP + etoposide): the new standard regimen for younger patients with low risk (low LDH) aggressive non-Hodgkin's lymphoma (NHL). *Blood* 2001; 98(abstr 3026):725a.
27. Diehl V, Franklin J, Paulus U, et al. BEACOPP chemotherapy with dose escalation in advanced Hodgkin's disease: final analysis of the German Hodgkin Lymphoma Study Group HD9 Randomized Trial. *Blood* 2001; 98:769a (abstract 3202).
28. Tesch H, Diehl V, Lathan B, et al. Moderate dose escalation for advanced stage Hodgkin's disease using the bleomycin, etoposide, Adriamycin, cyclophosphamide, vincristine, procarbazine, and prednisone scheme and adjuvant radiotherapy: a study of the German Hodgkin's Lymphoma Study Group. *Blood* 1998; 92:4560–4567.
29. Pfreundschuh M, Trumper L, Kloess M, et al. 2-Weekly CHOP (CHOP-4): the new standard regimen for patients with aggressive non-Hodgkin's lymphoma (NHL) > 60 years of age. *Blood* 2001; 98:725a (abstract 3027).
30. Aviles A, Garcia EL, Cuadra I, et al. High dose chemotherapy with G-CSF in refractory Hodgkin's disease. *Leuk Lymphoma* 1999; 361:139–145.
31. Pfreundschuh M, Hasenclever D, Loeffler M, et al. Dose escalation of cytotoxic drugs using haematopoietic growth factors: a randomized trial to determine the magnitude of increase provided by GM-CSF. *Ann Oncol* 2001; 12:471–477.
32. Aglietta M, Montemurro F, Fagioli F, et al. Short term treatment with *Escheria coli* recombinant human granulocyte-macrophage-colony stimulating factor prior to chemotherapy for Hodgkin disease. *Cancer* 2000; 88:454–460.
33. Philip T, Guglielmi C, Hagenbeek A, et al. Autologous bone marrow transplantation as compared with salvage chemotherapy in relapses of chemotherapy-sensitive non-Hodgkin's lymphoma. *N Engl J Med* 1995; 333:1540–1545.
34. Schmitz N, Linch DC, Dreger P, et al. Randomised trial of filgrastim-mobilised peripheral blood progenitor cell transplantation versus autologous bone-marrow transplantation in lymphoma patients. *Lancet* 1996; 347:353–357.
35. Ballestero A, Ferrando F, Garuti A, et al. Comparative effects of three cytokine regimens after high-dose cyclophosphamide: granulocyte colony-stimulating factor, granulocyte-macrophage colony-stimulating factor (GM-CSF) and sequential interleukin-3 and GM-CSF. *J Clin Oncol* 1999; 17:1296–1303.
36. Gazitt Y, Callander N, Freytes CO, et al. Peripheral blood stem cell mobilization with cyclophosphamide in combination with G-CSF, GM-CSF, or sequential GM-CSF/G-CSF in non-Hodgkin's lymphoma patients: a randomized prospective study. *J Hematother Stem Cell Res* 2000; 9:737–748.
37. Narayanasami U, Kanteti R, Morelli J, et al. Randomized trial of filgrastim versus chemotherapy and filgrastim mobilization of hematopoietic progenitor cells for rescue in autologous transplantation. *Blood* 2001; 98:2059–2064.

38. Pavone V, Gaudio F, Guarini A, et al. Mobilization of peripheral blood stem cells with high-dose cyclophosphamide or the DHAP regimen plus G-CSF in non-Hodgkin's lymphoma. *Bone Marrow Transplant* 2002; 29:285–290.
39. Watts M, Ings SJ, Leverett D, et al. ESHAP and G-CSF is a superior blood stem cell mobilizing regimen compared to cyclophosphamide 1.5 g/m^2 and G-CSF for pre-treated lymphoma patients: a matched pairs analysis of 78 patients. *Br J Cancer* 2000; 82:278–282.
40. Lee S, Radford JA, Dobson L, et al. Recombinant human granulocyte colony-stimulating factor (filgrastim) following high-dose chemotherapy and peripheral blood progenitor cell rescue in high-grade non-Hodgkin's lymphoma: clinical benefits at no extra cost. *Br J Cancer* 1998; 77:1294–1299.
41. Linch D, Milligan DW, Winfield DA, et al. G-CSF after peripheral blood stem cell transplantation in lymphoma patients significantly accelerated neutrophil recovery and shortened time in hospital: results of a randomized BNLI trial. *Br J Hematol* 1997; 99:933–938.
42. Ojeda E, Garcia-Bustos J, Aguado MJ, et al. A prospective randomized trial of granulocyte colony-stimulating factor therapy after autologous blood stem cell transplantation in adults. *Bone Marrow Transplant* 1999; 24:601–607.
43. Bishop M, Tarantolo S, Geller R, et al. A randomized, double blind trial of filgrastim (granulocyte colony-stimulating factor) versus placebo following allogeneic blood stem cell transplantation. *Blood* 2000; 96:80–85.
44. Ozcan M, Ustun C, Akcaglayan E, et al. Recombinant human granulocyte colony-stimulating factor (rh-G-CSF) may accelerate hematopoietic recovery after HLA-identical sibling allogeneic peripheral blood stem cell transplantation. *Bone Marrow Transplant* 2001; 27:499–505.
45. Przepiorka D, Smith TL, Folloder J, et al. Controlled trial of filgrastim for acceleration of neutrophil recovery after allogeneic blood stem cell transplantation from human leukocyte antigen-matched related donors. *Blood* 2001; 97:3405–3410.
46. Mellstedt H, Fagerberg J, Frodin JE, et al. Augmentation of the immune response with granulocyte-macrophage colony-stimulating factor and other hematopoietic growth factors. *Curr Opin Hematol* 1999; 6:169–175.
47. Hsu F, Caspar CB, Czerwinski D, et al. Tumor-specific idiotype vaccines in the treatment of patients with B-cell lymphoma—long-term results of a clinical trial. *Blood* 1997; 89:3129–3135.
48. Caspar C, Levy S, Levy R. Idiotype vaccines for non-Hodgkin's lymphoma induce polyclonal immune responses that cover mutated tumor idiotypes: comparison of different vaccine formulations. *Blood* 1997; 90:3699–3706.
49. Masucci G, Wersall P, Ragnhammar P, et al. Granulocyte-monocyte-colony-stimulating factor augments the cytotoxic capacity of lymphocytes and monocytes in antibody-dependent cellular cytotoxicity. *Cancer Immunol Immunother* 1989; 29:288–292.
50. Burgaleta C, Villalba S, Gonzalez N. Defective activity of monocytes from patients with non-Hodgkin lymphoma: the modulatory effect of granulocyte-macrophage-colony stimulating factor. *Cancer* 1999; 86:2133–2137.
51. Ragnhammar P. Anti-tumoral effect of GM-CSF with or without cytokines and monoclonal antibodies in solid tumors. *Med Oncol* 1996; 13:167–176.
52. Stockmeyer B, Elsasser D, Dechant M, et al. Mechanisms of G-CSF- or GM-CSF-stimulated tumor cell killing by Fc receptor-directed bispecific antibodies. *J Immunol Methods* 2001; 248:103–111.
53. Kwak L, Campbell MJ, Czerwinski DK, et al. Induction of immune responses in patients with B-cell lymphoma against the surface-immunoglobulin idiotype expressed by their tumors. *N Engl J Med* 1992; 327:1209–1215.
54. Nelson E, Li X, Hsu FJ, et al. Tumor-specific, cytotoxic T-lymphocyte response after idiotype vaccination for B-cell, non-Hodgkin's lymphoma. *Blood* 1996; 88:580–589.
55. Kwak L, Young HA, Pennington RW, Weeks SD. Vaccination with syngeneic, lymphoma-derived immunoglobulin idiotype combined with granulocyte/macrophage colony-stimulating factor primes mice for a protective T-cell response. *Proc Natl Acad Sci USA* 1996; 93:10972–10977.

15 Use of Granulocyte Growth Factors in Breast Cancer

Eric D. Mininberg, MD
and Frankie Ann Holmes, MD, FACP

CONTENTS

1. INTRODUCTION

In 1976 Bonadonna and colleagues *(1)* revolutionized the treatment of breast cancer when they reported the positive effect of adjuvant cytototoxic chemotherapy in women with node-positive breast cancer. Women with node-positive breast malignancies who had undergone mastectomy with axillary dissection were randomized to observation or 12 cycles of chemotherapy with cyclophosphamide (C), methotrexate (M) and 5-fluorouracil (F). The initial analysis indicated that 24% of the patients in the observation cohort experienced treatment failure, whereas only 5.3% of the patients in the chemotherapy cohort developed disease recurrence. Besides hair loss and amenorrhea, the most common toxicities were thrombocytopenia (platelet count < 130×10^9/L) in 71% and leukopenia (white blood cell count < 4×10^9/L) in 71%. Patients in the treat-

From: *Cancer Drug Discovery and Development*
Hematopoietic Growth Factors in Oncology: Basic Science and Clinical Therapeutics
Edited by: G. Morstyn, M. A. Foote, and G. J. Lieschke © Humana Press Inc., Totowa, NJ

Table 1
Relation of Dose Level of Adjuvant Chemotherapy to 5-Year Relapse-Free Survival (RFS)

Dose level (% of planned dose)	*Total group (% 5-yr RFS)*
≥85	78 (77)
65–84	222 (56)
<65	149 (48)
Total with adjuvant therapy	449 (61)
Controls (no chemotherapy)	179 (45)

ment group had no increased rate of infection. The authors concluded that cytotoxic chemotherapy could be delivered safely with manageable toxicity and that it appeared to have an early impact on disease recurrence *(1)*.

In a retrospective review of this same group of patients 5 yr later, the investigators made a startling discovery: the amount of chemotherapy that a patient received had an effect on outcome, a dose-response effect. Patients who received ≥85% of the planned dose of chemotherapy had a 5-yr relapse-free survival of 77% vs 45% for patients who received no adjuvant therapy (Table 1). Interestingly, patients who received ≤65% of the planned dose had relapse-free and overall survival rates similar to the patients who received no adjuvant therapy *(2)*. After 20 yr of follow-up, the improvement in disease-free and overall survival for women treated with adjuvant CMF chemotherapy has persisted *(3)*. From these data, the concept of dose intensity was born: to have the optimal effect, cytotoxic chemotherapy needs to be given at the right dose over the right time period.

2. DOSE INTENSITY

2.1. Dose Intensity in Breast Cancer: Preclinical and Retrospective Clinical Data

Preclinical in vivo and in vitro data suggest that increasing the dose of chemotherapy increases tumor cell kill, but with significant myelosuppression *(4)*. Hryniuk and Bush *(5)*, in a literature review of regimens for metastatic breast cancer, calculated the dose of CMF chemotherapy given over a unit of time and concluded that a relationship was apparent with dose intensity and response rate in the setting of metastatic breast cancer. For the adjuvant setting, Hryniuk and Levine *(6)* evaluated chemotherapy trials for women with stage II breast cancer treated with CMF-like regimens. In this retrospective study, the authors concluded in both univariate and multivariate analyses that dose intensity was a significant predictor of relapse-free survival *(6)*. These initial observations of dose intensity, although suggestive, were retrospective.

2.2. Prospective Dose-Intensity Trials for Breast Cancer

Tannock et al. *(7)* evaluated the dose-intensity concept in a prospective setting for patients with metastatic breast cancer. Patients were randomly assigned to receive two dose levels of CMF chemotherapy every 3 wk: standard (cyclophosphamide 600 mg/mL, methotrexate 40 mg/mL, 5-fluorouracil 600 mg/mL) and low dose (cyclophosphamide 300 mg/mL, methotrexate 20 mg/mL, 5-fluorouracil 300 mg/mL). Response rates were higher for the standard-dose cohort (30% vs 11%, $p = 0.3$), but there was no statistical difference in overall survival (15.6 mo vs 12.8 mo, $p = 0.12$). Although the rates of toxicity (vomiting, alopecia, myelosuppression, and conjunctivitis) were higher in the standard-dose cohort, patients in the standard-dose cohort had an improved quality of life. Based on the increased response rate, trend to improved survival, and overall improvement in quality of life, the authors concluded that the rate of disease palliation was improved with higher dose therapy.

At the M.D. Anderson Cancer Center, Hortobagyi and colleagues *(8)* evaluated the impact of higher dose anthracycline therapy in metastatic breast cancer. Patients were randomly assigned to receive either standard 5-fluorouracil (F), doxorubicin (A), and cyclophosphamide (C) or 260% higher FAC. The median response durations and overall survival rates were not significantly different. Furthermore, hematologic, infection-related, and gastrointestinal complications were increased in the high-dose FAC group *(8)*. The studies by Tannock et al. *(7)* and Hortobagyi et al. *(8)* seemed to indicate that a threshold dose existed for the treatment of breast cancer, but a large confirmatory trial was needed.

2.3. Threshold Dose in the Treatment of Breast Cancer

The Cancer and Leukemia Group B (CALGB) did a randomized trial evaluating different doses and dose intensities of adjuvant chemotherapy in patients with node-positive breast cancer: 1572 patients were randomized to receive CAF at three dose levels: low-dose (5-flurouracil 300 mg/mL, doxorubicin 30 mg/mL, cyclophosphamide 300 mg/mL), moderate dose (5-fluorouracil 400 mg/mL, doxorubicin 40 mg/mL, cyclophosphamide 400 mg/mL), and high dose (5-fluorouracil 600 mg/mL, doxorubicin 60 mg/mL, cyclophosphamide 600 mg/mL). Women treated in the moderate- and high-dose-intensity groups had significantly longer disease-free and overall survival than those in the low-dose group. Survival was not different between the moderate- and high-dose groups *(9)*. This study validated the idea of a threshold dose in the treatment of breast cancer.

3. DOSE ESCALATION

Several studies have been conducted to assess the benefit, if any, to escalating the dose of chemotherapy beyond the threshold level. The National Surgical Adjuvant Breast and Bowel Project explored dose escalation of cyclophosphamide in two trials, B-22 and B-25 *(10,11)*. Both studies evaluated dose intensification and escalation of cyclophosphamide in women with node-positive breast cancer. Disease-free and overall survival were not significantly different in either trial between patients who received the standard dose and patients who received the escalated dose of chemotherapy. Furthermore, in the B-25 trial, the degree of toxicity correlated positively with dose escalation, and the incidence of acute myeloid leukemia (AML) was disturbingly high.

A similar trial of adjuvant cyclophosphamide 600 mg/m^2 with doxorubicin escalation from the standard 60 mg/m^2 to 25% and 50% higher doses (75 and 90 mg/m^2), respectively failed to show any benefit for the higher doses of doxorubicin *(12)*.

4. IDENTIFYING THE CAUSES OF CHEMOTHERAPY DELAYS OR DOSE REDUCTIONS FOR CHEMOTHERAPY IN BREAST CANCER

Adjuvant chemotherapy for breast cancer has a patient benefit when delivered with a specific dose intensity at a threshold dose beyond which only increased toxicity is gained. Therefore, to maintain dose intensity, clinicians must identify the most common toxicities that cause treatment delays and develop strategies to avoid or eliminate them.

4.1. Common Toxicities

Link and colleagues *(13)* evaluated the chemotherapy use of 13 managed-care, academic, and community practices for the treatment of breast cancer. The aim of the study was to determine the most common regimens used and the incidence of complications. The primary chemotherapy combinations were CMF and doxorubicin-cyclophosphamide (AC) regimens. Thirty percent of patients had dose intensities of <85%, and 27.6% had dose adjustments secondary to neutropenia. The authors concluded that neutropenia was the primary reason that chemotherapy could not be delivered at the optimal dose intensity.

4.2. Myelosuppression/Neutropenia

Antineoplastic agents for the treatment of breast cancer cause myelosuppression and subsequent neutropenia that may cause fever and infection. An early study by Bodey et al. *(14)* at the M.D. Anderson Cancer Center in patients with acute leukemia found that when the absolute neutrophil count (ANC) was between 0.5 and 1.0×10^9/L, the risk of infection was 10%, but when the ANC decreased to $<0.1 \times 10^9$/L, the risk increased to 42%.

4.3. Neutropenia in the Treatment of Breast Cancer

Rahmann et al. *(15)* evaluated the incidence of febrile neutropenia ([FN) body temperature ≥37.2°C and ANC $\leq 1 \times 10^9$/L) in patients with metastatic breast cancer who received systemic chemotherapy. Twenty-three percent of patients developed FN; the incidence of fever did not increase until the ANC was $<0.5 \times 10^9$/L. The risk of infection was not increased until the ANC was $<0.25 \times 10^9$/L; FN occurred in patients with a poor performance status or during the first course of chemotherapy (Fig. 1). The development of FN requires the administration of either combination antibiotics or single agent β-lactam therapy *(16)*. Patients who receive myeolsuppressive therapy are at significant risk for infection and fever that require antibiotic treatment and may delay subsequent courses of chemotherapy.

5. GRANULOCYTE COLONY-STIMULATING FACTOR AND GRANULOCYTE-MACROPHAGE COLONY-STIMULATING FACTOR FOR CHEMOTHERAPY-INDUCED MYELOSUPPRESSION

Granulocyte colony-stimulating factor (G-CSF) and granulocyte-macrophage colony-stimulating factor (GM-CSF) are endogenous glycoproteins that participate in the differentiation and proliferation of granulocytes, monocyte-macrophages, and other cells for hematopoeisis *(17)*. Myelosuppresion is the major toxicity of chemotherapy for solid organ tumors, and prolonged myelosuppression and neutropenia lead to a reduction in chemotherapy dose intensity. Therefore, with the discovery, cloning, and production of recombinant human forms of G-CSF and GM-CSF (rHuG-CSF and

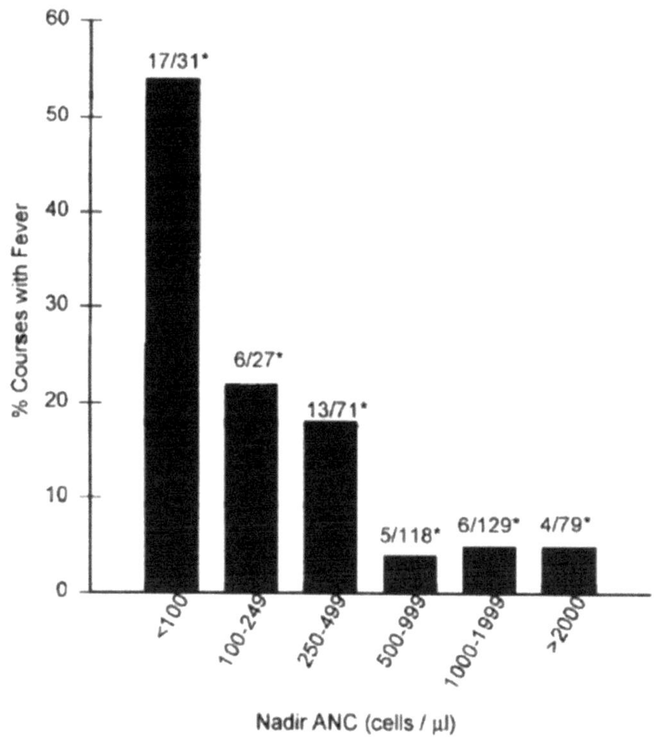

Fig. 1. The relationship between absolute neutrophil count (ANC) and neutropenic fever after salvage chemotherapy is shown for patients with metastatic breast carcinoma. When the ANC decreases to a level below the threshold of 500/µL, the incidence of neutropenic fever increases in a linear trend ($p < 0.01$). *, Number of courses with fever/number of courses with nadir ANC in the same range.

rHuGM-CSF), patients could receive cytotoxic chemotherapy with white blood cell growth factors to counteract the subsequent myelosuppression.

Several studies were performed to evaluate the effect of filgrastim (an rHuG-CSF) and rHuGM-CSF on neutropenia and overall disease outcome in patients receiving chemotherapy for solid tumors. Gabrilove et al. *(18)* performed a study evaluating filgrastim in patients with transitional cell carcinoma of the urothelium. Twenty-seven patients who were receiving MVAC (methotrexate, vinblastine, doxorubicin, and cisplatin) chemotherapy were given filgrastim 60 µg/kg on one of three schedules: before, after, or before and after chemotherapy. Treatment given before chemotherapy increased ANC. Treatment after chemotherapy decreased both the number of days the ANC was $<1.0 \times 10^9$/L and the number of days antibiotics were given compared with fiilgrastim use before chemotherapy. Furthermore, patients who received filgrastim after chemotherapy were able to receive the next course of chemotherapy on the planned day of treatment.

Crawford et al. *(19)* did a randomized, double-blind, placebo-controlled trial in patients with small-cell lung cancer (SCLC) to evaluate the incidence of fever and neutropenia in patients treated with chemotherapy. Two-hundred eleven patients receiving chemotherapy with cyclophosphamide, doxorubicin, and etoposide (CAE) were randomly assigned to placebo or filgrastim on d 4–17 of a 21-d cycle. Patients who received filgrastim experienced a significant reduction in the incidence of fever and neutropenia, duration of grade IV neutropenia defined as ANC < 0.5×10^9/L, days of treatment with intravenous (iv) antibiotics, and culture-confirmed infection. Both studies showed a significant reduction in the incidence of neutropenia in patients receiving chemotherapy who also received filgrastim after chemotherapy and an apparent inferiority, in the first study, of filgrastim administered before chemotherapy. When filgrastim was given prophylactically, patients had less toxicity from myelosuppression and were able to maintain the planned treatment schedule; however, not all patients in these studies developed significant neutropenia and therefore would not require growth factor support.

6. RISK FACTORS FOR FEBRILE NEUTROPENIA

To identify patients who are at highest risk for FN and who may benefit from prophylactic filgrastim, Silber and colleagues *(20)* reviewed a series of patients with breast cancer who had received standard-dose adjuvant chemotherapy. From this series, the authors constructed a predictive model based on three events: ANC < 0.25×10^9/L, occurrence of dose reduction ≤ 15%, and treatment delay ≤ 7 d. Ninety-five patients (development model) were used to develop the model, and 80 patients (conditional model) from the same practice were used as controls to validate it. The charts of patients receiving adjuvant chemotherapy regimens including 5-fluorouracil, doxorubicin, cyclophosphamide, and methotrexate were reviewed to determine the ANC and nadir after the first course of chemotherapy. The degree of neutropenia with the first cycle of chemotherapy was predictive of the occurrence of one of the aforementioned three events in future chemotherapy courses. If the ANC nadir was < 1×10^9/L, the chance for an event was 50%, whereas if the ANC nadir was >1×10^9/L, the chance decreased to 10%.

Rivera et al. *(21)* validated the results of Silber et al. *(20)* in a prospective, nonrandomized trial. Patients were assigned to two risk categories, high-risk and low-risk, based on first-course nadir ANC. High risk was defined as a nadir ANC < 0.5×10^9/L. Low risk was a nadir above that. Patients with a high-risk nadir for course 1 received filgrastim for all subsequent cycles beginning 24 h after the completion of chemotherapy until an ANC ≥ 10×10^9/L. Patients with a low-risk nadir received filgrastim only if they experienced FN. These patients were matched to historical controls. Patients who received filgrastim had improved dose intensity: 4.7% vs 20.1% received ≥85% of planned-dose-on-time chemotherapy. Using these models, patients at high risk for significant neutropenia can be identified and pre-emptively treated with filgrastim to maintain appropriate dose intensity.

7. FILGRASTIM IN THE TREATMENT OF BREAST CANCER

Although filgrastim was known to have an effect on hematopoetic cell lines, it was not clear whether it stimulated nonhematopoetic cells or tumor cells. Several studies were done to elucidate the effect, if any, on human breast cancer cells. Emerman and Eaves *(22)* evaluated human breast epithelial cells from normal and malignant tissues and evaluated the effects of eight cytokines: G-CSF, GM-CSF, Steel factor, interleukin (IL)-2, IL-3, IL-6, transforming growth factor-β (TGF-β), and macrophage inflammatory protein 1-α. The authors found no effect of the cytokines on the growth of normal or malignant breast epithelial cells. Filgrastim appears to be safe in the treatment of breast cancer, but when in the course of chemotherapy is the best time for it to be given?

7.1. Administration of Filgrastim

deWit and colleagues *(23)* determined the optimal time to give filgrastim (before or after chemotherapy) and the protective effect on hematopoietic progenitor cells. From the earlier studies by Gabrilove et al. *(18)* and Crawford et al. *(19)*, it appeared that the most efficacious time for administration of filgrastim was after chemotherapy until ANC recovery. deWit et al. *(23)* randomly assigned 36 patients with locally advanced or metastatic breast cancer who were receiving chemotherapy with doxorubicin 75 mg/mL and cyclophosphamide 1000 mg/mL to receive one of two schedules: filgrastim 5 μg/kg twice a day (bid) for 5 d up until 48 h before chemotherapy or filgrastim 5 μg/kg every day (qd) for 7 d starting 24 h after chemotherapy. No apparent difference was seen in incidence or duration of neutropenia between the two groups. Grade 3–4 thrombocytopenia increased, 54% vs 6%, in the prechemotherapy group. The authors concluded that the preferred schedule for administration of filgrastim is after chemotherapy.

The optimal dose and duration of filgrastim for breast cancer therapy has been extrapolated from studies of other solid tumors as well as breast cancer. The most common schedule is to initiate filgrastim 5 μg/kg daily subcutaneously (sc) 24 h after chemotherapy and to continue until the ANC is 5–10 × 10^9/L *(24)*. The question remains of how filgrastim impacts the delivery and dose intensity of chemotherapy in patients with breast cancer.

7.2. Filgrastim to Maintain Dose Intensity in the Treatment of Breast Cancer

In an initial study by Bronchud et al. *(25)* in patients with advanced breast and ovarian cancer, escalating doses of doxorubicin were followed by infusions of filgrastim given at 14-d intervals for three courses. Administration of filgrastim allowed for an appropriate restoration of neutrophil count at all dose levels. By maintaining neutrophil count, therapy could be continued and dose intensity increased.

7.3. Adjuvant Therapy

As shown by Bonadonna *(1)* and others, administration of adjuvant chemotherapy at >85% of planned dose results in improved outcomes. De Graaf et al. *(26)* assessed the effect of filgrastim in 123 premenopausal, node-positive women receiving standard adjuvant CMF chemotherapy (cyclophosphamide 100 mg/mL orally on d 1–14, methotrexate 40 mg/mL iv on d 1 and 8, and 5-fluorouracil 600 mg/mL iv on d 1 and 8 every 28 d) by evaluating weekly blood counts. Patients whose ANCs were either <3 × 10^9/L on d 1 or <2 × 10^9/L on d 8 were given filgrastim 300 μg sc for 5 d, and treatment was delayed for 1 wk. Filgrastim was continued prophylactically with each subsequent cycle for 10 d from d 15–24. The patients were then divided into three groups: patients without neutropenia, patients with neutropenia treated with filgrastim, and a control group who developed neutropenia but did not receive filgrastim. Although no statistically significant difference was seen in the total dose of chemotherapy received by each group, the difference in dose intensity of the filgrastim-treated group vs the control group was significant: 74% vs 45% ($p < 0.05$) (Table 2). In a smaller pilot study of 19 women who were receiving adjuvant chemotherapy

Table 2
Dose Intensity in Patients Who Received CMF Alone Vs CMF With Filgrastim[a]

Dose intensity (% projected)	*No cytopenias (n = 51)*	*Filgrastim (n = 50)*	*Controls (n = 22)*	*p value*
≥85	46 (90)	37 (74)	10 (45)	<0.05
65–84	3 (6)	9 (13)	10 (45)	<0.05
<65	2 (4)	4 (8)	2 (10)	NS

[a] Data are numbers of patients, with percents in parentheses. Data from ref. *26*.

for breast cancer and who developed FN or a nadir ANC of $<0.5 \times 10^9$/L, patients treated with filgrastim had less chemotherapy delays *(27)*. Thus, in the adjuvant setting, use of prophylactic filgrastim does improve dose intensity for standard therapy.

7.4. Treatment of Metastatic Disease

In the metastatic setting, excluding high-dose chemotherapy, filgrastim has been used prophylactically in highly potent but investigational toxic combination chemotherapy regimens to maintain dose intensity and prevent FN. Doxorubicin 60 mg/m^2 and docetaxel 75 mg/mL administered every 21 d caused objective responses in >70% of patients but resulted in grade 4 neutropenia (ANC $< 0.5 \times 10^9$/L) in 90% of patients and a 38% incidence of FN *(28)*. In similar studies in which prophylactic filgrastim was given, the incidence of grades 3 (ANC $< 1.0 \times 10^9$/L) and 4 neutropenia remained high (74%), but the incidence of FN decreased to 6% *(29)*. At this time, current recommendations do not support the routine use of primary prophylactic rHuG-CSF except in a clinical trial setting or when administered in a regimen in which the probability of FN is >40% *(30)*.

7.5. Cost of Filgrastim

Although the use of filgrastim in the treatment of breast cancer may improve dose intensity in the adjuvant setting and aid in the use of combinations of potent chemotherapeutic agents in the metastatic setting, it is a costly treatment. Several cost analyses have been developed to assess the cost effectiveness of prophylactic filgrastim.

Glaspy et al. *(31)* evaluated 68 patients with SCLC receiving CAE chemotherapy randomly assigned to receive filgrastim or placebo 24 h after chemotherapy until the ANC was $\leq 10 \times 10^9$/L. Patients who received filgrastim had fewer hospitalizations; if they were hospitalized, they had shorter durations of stay and less utilization of resources. The authors concluded that cost savings occurred with the use of filgrastim in patient settings in which the risk of FN was high.

Silber et al. *(32)* used their risk assessment model of first-course nadir ANC and hemoglobin concentration to assess the cost effectiveness of filgrastim in the adjuvant treatment of breast cancer. All patients received their first course of therapy without filgrastim. Patients who were determined to exceed a threshold value that was predetermined based on first-cycle ANC and hemoglobin concentration received filgrastim for subsequent courses of chemotherapy. Although the authors felt that the cost estimates were insensitive to hospitalization costs, if the neediest 50% of patients were treated with filgrastim, a cost-effectiveness ratio of US $34,297 per life-year saved was estimated, on a par for the treatment of other medical conditions.

8. PEGFILGRASTIM IN BREAST CANCER

8.1. Dose-Finding Trial

Johnson et al. *(33)* demonstrated the clinical activity of pegfilgrastim and confirmed the unique biologic behavior of this self-regulating molecule in patients with lung cancer. It was in breast cancer, however, that further development of pegfilgrastim occurred.

Doxorubicin and docetaxel are, arguably, the most effective antineoplastic drugs currently available for breast cancer. The combination of doxorubicin 60 mg/m^2 administered by bolus iv followed by docetaxel 75 mg/m^2 iv over 1 h repeated every 21 d produced a response rate of nearly 70% in patients with metastatic breast cancer with limited prior therapy *(28)*. However, grade 4 myelosuppression occurred in 70% of patients, lasting a median of 5 d (range: 1–13 d), and the incidence of FN was 38%.

Based on the American Society of Clinical Oncology (ASCO) clinical practice guidelines for the use of hematopoeitic growth factors, an incidence of FN $\geq$ 40% was an indication for primary prophylaxis with granulocyte growth factors *(30)*. A once-per-cycle granulocyte growth factor would allow patients the potential benefits of this regimen without the consequences of such a high rate of FN and without the need for daily injections of filgrastim. Thus, this regimen was chosen for the evaluation of pegfilgrastim.

8.2. Dose-Finding Trial Design: Patients and Methods

Eligible patients included those with high-risk stage II (as defined by the investigator, this usually included any or all of these features: four or more positive nodes, HER-2/*neu* overexpressed or amplified, high-grade, high-proliferative rate, stage III, and stage IV disease patients who had received no or one regimen for metastatic disease independent of any adjuvant therapy if the total cumulative dose of doxorubicin did not exceed 240 mg/m^2. Exclusion criteria included progression on a taxane, prior bone marrow or stem cell transplant, radiation within 4 wk of treatment, or a history of any other malignancy. Thus, a patient with stage IV disease may have received one regimen as adjuvant therapy and one regimen for metastatic disease.

In all the studies, both those preceding the pivotal trials as well as the pivotal trials, the regimen of Misset et al. *(28)* was administered for a total of four courses.

On d 2, approx 24 h after chemotherapy, all patients received one of two injections. The first was filgrastim 5 μg/kg daily for 14 d or until the ANC was $\geq 10 \times 10^9$/L after the expected nadir (usually d 7) or whichever came first. The second was pegfilgrastim that was administered according to the scheme in Table 3. To maintain the blind, patients randomized to the pegfilgrastim cohorts received daily placebo injections of the vehicle for filgrastim for the same duration as above, namely, for 14 d or until ANC was $\geq 10 \times 10^9$/L after the expected nadir.

Johnson et al. *(33)* suggested that the optimal dose of pegfilgrastim was 100 μg/kg, so this dose was used in the first randomized trial compared with standard filgrastim. To define the threshold dose of pegfilgrastim, a second randomized trial used pegfilgrastim at 60 μg/kg compared with standard filgrastim. Finally, the threshold dose of pegfilgras-

Table 3
Patient Treatment Comparison Groups in the Dose-Finding Trial

	Treatment	
Group	*Filgrastim*	*Pegfilgrastim*
1	5 μg/kg	100 μg/kg
2	5 μg/kg	60 μg/kg
3	60 μg/kg	30 μg/kg
4	60 μg/kg	100 μg/kg

tim was further explored in two open-label studies comparing pegfilgrastim 30 μg/kg with 60 μg/kg and then 60 μg/kg with 100 μg/kg.

All patients had baseline laboratory studies for serum chemistries, complete blood count with differential and platelets (CBC). During the first course, CBCs were collected daily until ANC recovery and then three times a week. During courses 2–4, CBCs were collected three times weekly until ANC recovery.

Baseline studies for serum antibodies (immunoglobulins G and M) were done and repeated at the end of study. Serum chemistries and uric acid were measured before each course.

Serum samples were collected on d 2 before study drug, then at 1, 2, and 4 h after injection of study drug, and then concurrently with CBCs in courses 1 and 3.

8.3. Trial Objectives

These series of trials were designed to compare the safety, efficacy, and pharmacokinetics of standard filgrastim administered daily with pegfilgrastim administered once per cycle. The primary endpoint was the duration of grade 4 neutropenia (days of severe neutropenia [DSN]), defined as days the ANC was $<0.5 \times 10^9$/L during the first course of chemotherapy. The secondary endpoints were DSN in courses 2–4; the granulocyte profile; and the time to ANC recovery defined as granulocytes $\geq 2.0 \times 10^9$/L. Another objective was to evaluate the rates of FN in each group. The study was not powered for this endpoint, which was collected to evaluate trends.

8.4. Results

In all, 154 women were randomized to each of the four parts of this study (Table 3), 129 to the pegfilgrastim groups and 25 to the filgrastim group. Of these, 152 patients received at least one dose of the study medication; 150 patients were treated per protocol and were eligible for efficacy endpoints. To allow for greater statistical precision, the data from each of the same pegfilgrastim dose groups in the blinded and open-label groups were pooled.

The study evolved as each completed trial suggested a new dose-related question. Additionally, patients were not stratified by any criteria, so patient characteristics are similar within broad ranges, as shown in Table 4.

The efficacy endpoints for course 1 are shown in Table 5. These results define the optimal dose of pegfilgrastim compared with standard filgrastim. As expected, the incidence of grade 4 neutropenia was >70% and the severity correlated inversely with

Table 4
Distribution of Patients by Study Drug Assignment

		Pegfilgrastim		
Parameter	*Filgrastim 5 μg/kg*	*100 μg/kg*	*60 μg/kg*	*30 μg/kg*
No. of patients	25	46	60	19
White (%)	80	76	73	95
Stage II/III (%)	24/36	38/40	42/34	32/47
Stage IV (%)	40	23	24	21

Table 5
Efficacy Endpoints for Filgrastim Vs Pegfilgrastim by Dose Level of Pegfilgrastim

		Pegfilgrastim		
Parameter	*Filgrastim 5 μg/kg*	*100 μg/kg*	*60 μg/kg*	*30 μg/kg*
No. of patients	25	46	60	19
Grade 4 ANC (% pts.)	76	74	90	95
Mean days (SD) grade 4 ANC	1.6 (1.3)	1.3 (1.1)	2 (1.2)	2.7 (1.3)
95% CI for difference in mean DSN between filgrastim and pegfilgrastim	—	–0.81–0.31	–0.21–0.94	0.35–1.93
% Pts. with grade 4 ANC lasting:				
0–2 d	88	87	67	37
≥3 d	12	13	33	63
Time to ANC recovery (d)	9.5	9.4	10.3	11.0
95% CI for difference between filgrastim and pegfilgrastim	—	–0.81–0.93	0.06–1.66	0.2–3.34
FN				
Course 1 (no. of pts [%])	1 (4)	3 (7)	5 (8)	4 (21)
Any course (no. of pts [%])	2 (12)	5 (11)	7 (12)	—

ABBREVIATIONS: ANC, absolute neutropenia count; FN, febrile neutropenia; DSN, days of severe neutropenia when ANC < 0.5×10^9/L; SD, standard deviation.

Date from ref. *34*.

the dose of pegfilgrastim. The primary endpoint, DSN in course 1, favored pegfilgrastim 100 μg over the lower doses. The 95% confidence interval (CI) was calculated for the difference in the mean duration of DSN between each pegfilgrastim group and filgrastim. If the difference is 0 d, the ranges for the 95% CI should overlap 0. The lowest pegfilgrastim dose of 30 μg/kg was inferior, with ranges overlapping 1, suggesting at least a 1-d difference in the DSN.

Two complementary findings of the study included the fact that not only did more patients receiving the lower doses of pegfilgrastim have ≥3 d of neutropenia compared with patients receiving filgrastim or pegfilgrastim 100 μg/kg, but that the time course of ANC recovery was longer. Pegfilgrastim 100 μg/kg and filgrastim 5 μg/kg resulted in a shorter, shallower nadir (Fig. 2). One other clinical observation, which was consistently

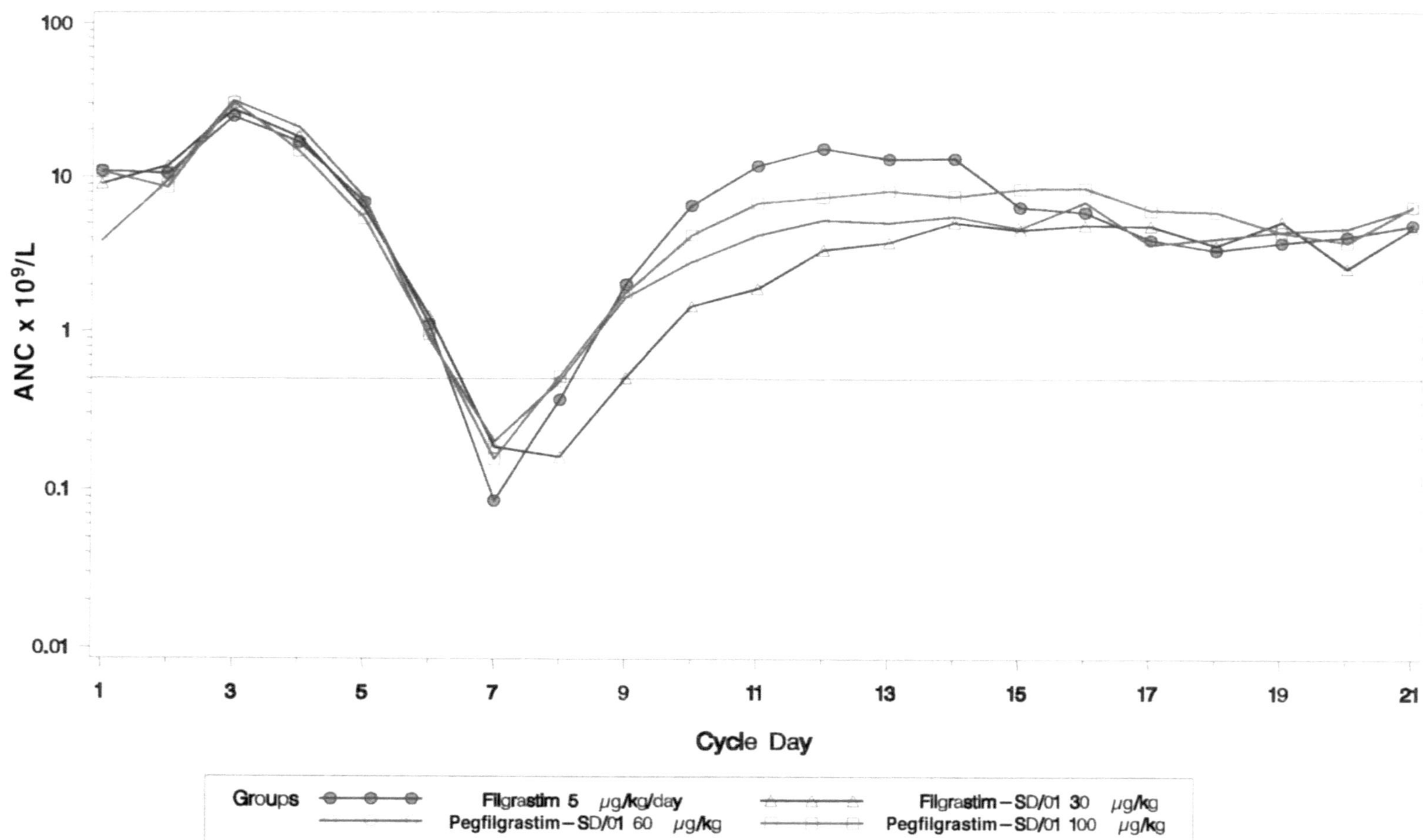

Fig. 2. Median absolute neutrophil count (ANC) by dose of pegfilgrastim and filgrastim. Darker circles, filgrastim 5 μg/kg/day; lighter circles, pegfilgrastim 60 μg/kg; triangles, pegfilgrastim 30 μg/kg; squares, pegfilgrastim 100 μg/kg.

seen in subsequent studies, was that the ANC was less likely to overshoot recovery on d 9–14 with pegfilgrastim than with filgrastim.

The functional result of more prolonged neutropenia is shown in Table 5—a higher incidence of FN. Although the numbers of patients who received the lowest dose of pegfilgrastim are small and the study was not powered for a formal analysis of these data, a trend emerged—a higher percentage of patients experienced FN in course 1. For this reason, these patients received pegfilgrastim at 60 μg/kg for subsequent courses.

No clinical or laboratory findings were observed with pegfilgrastim that had not been observed with filgrastim, nor was the severity or duration of those findings different from what was seen with filgrastim. Bone pain was expected and occurred in 36% and 35%, respectively, for filgrastim and pegfilgrastim. The incidence of bone pain was dose related at 45, 34, and 16%, respectively, for the 100-, 60-, and 30-μg/kg doses of pegfilgrastim.

Transient increase of laboratory variables associated with granulocyte proliferation included alkaline phosphatase, lactose dehydrogenase, and uric acid. No neutralizing antibodies to pegfilgrastim were seen, and all patients had normal recovery of granulocytes after each course of treatment.

This study confirmed and amplified the results of Johnson et al. *(33)*, which showed that pegfilgrastim elimination was inversely related both to the number of circulating granulocytes and to the dose of pegfilgrastim between 30 and 100 μg/kg. At higher doses, pegfilgrastim clearance was reduced, consistent with a saturation effect. A temporal effect on clearance was observed. When courses 1 and 3 were compared, the clearances in course 3 were increased relative to course 1. Based on the known mechanism of clearance, namely, binding to the neutrophil receptor for G-CSF, it is thought that this finding can be explained by the increased myeloid mass, that is, the pool of neutrophils and their precursors.

Clearance of filgrastim was consistent with a previous report with a plasma half-life of 3–4 h *(35)*. Serum values decreased rapidly after administration. A median of 11 injections of filgrastim was required to produce the same clinical effect on granulocyte recovery as a single injection of pegfilgrastim.

8.5. Phase 3 Trials: Weight-Based and Fixed Doses

Formal phase 3 trials to confirm and extend the observations of the phase 2 trials included comparison of pegfilgrastim at the recommended dose, 100 μg/kg, but also a fixed-dose schedule of 6 mg.

The rationale for development of a fixed-dose schedule was threefold. First, mathematical modeling studies based on pharmacokinetic and pharmacodynamic data suggested that a fixed dose would be effective regardless of body weight *(36)*. Second, a retrospective analysis of the actual total administered dose of pegfilgrastim in the dose-finding trial was done to evaluate ANC recovery regardless of weight (Fig. 3). The patients could be divided into three groups based on the total administered dose: 3–4.99, 5–6.99, and 7–8.99 mg. The group receiving 5–6.99 mg pegfilgrastim appeared to be most comparable to filgrastim. Finally, a fixed dose is not only more convenient but also limits the possibility of drug dosing errors.

Thus, two phase 3 trials were done concurrently. Holmes et al. *(37)* continued to evaluate the weight-based dose trial, and Green et al. *(38)* tested the fixed-dose schedule.

The conduct and design of these two trials were identical to those of the dose-finding trial *(34)*, but all patients in both trials were randomly assigned, medication assignment was double-blinded, and stratification criteria were used.

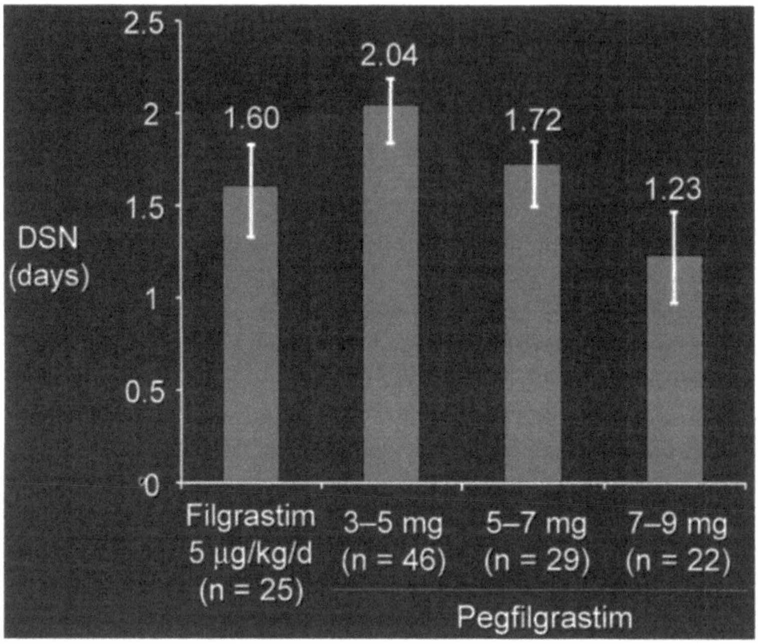

Fig. 3. Rational for pegfilgrastim 6-mg fixed dose. Bar graph showing mean duration of severe neutropenia (absolute neutrophil count [ANC] < 0.5×10^9/L). DSN, days of severe neutropenia. Bars represent standard deviation. Values at top of each bar are mean. (Data on file, Amgen.)

To maintain the blind, all patients assigned to the pegfilgrastim cohort received a daily placebo injection of filgrastim vehicle that was continued with the same guidelines as filgrastim, that is, until the granulocyte recovery (i.e., ANC recovery to $\geq 10 \times 10^9$/L after the expected neutrophil nadir, generally d 7, or for up to 14 d, whichever came first).

Patients were randomized 1:1 in both studies using a stratified permuted-block randomization schedule. Two stratification criteria were common to both trials, namely, previous chemotherapy and center. The weight-based trial was conducted primarily in the United States; the fixed-dose trial included a consortium comprised of physicians from Australia, Canada, the United Kingdom, Spain, Italy, Germany, and The Netherlands. A third stratification criteria, the patient's weight, was required in the fixed-dose trial.

In the weight-based trial, pegfilgrastim 100 µg/kg was given as a sc injection on d 2; in the fixed-dose trial, pegfilgrastim 6 mg was given as a sc injection on d 2.

The weight-based trial included 62 centers enrolling 310 patients, 154 randomized to pegfilgrastim 100 µg/kg and 156 randomized to filgrastim 5 µg/kg daily. In the modified intent-to-treat analysis, 147 and 149 patients, respectively, received pegfilgrastim and filgrastim. The fixed-dose trial included 34 centers enrolling 157 patients, 80 randomly assigned to pegfilgrastim and 77 to filgrastim. In the efficacy analysis of the primary endpoint, 152 patients (97% of the total) were included, of whom 77 received pegfilgrastim 6 mg and 75 received filgrastim 5 µg/kg daily. Patient characteristics by study are shown in Table 6.

Table 6
Patient Characteristics in the Weight-Based and Fixed-Dose Trials

	Weight-based		*Fixed-dose*	
Parameter	*Filgrastim 5 µg/kg/d*	*Pegfilgrastim 100 µg/kg d 2*	*Filgrastim 5 µg/kg/d*	*Pegfilgrastim 6 mg sc d 2*
No. of patients	147	149	75	77
Age (med. yr)	51.9	50.9	52.8	52.1
White (%)	80	75	97	97
Prior chemotherapy	12	9	28	29
Prior radiation therapy	10	9	21	30
Baseline weight (kg)	—	—	72.8	73.5
Range	—	—	49–132	46–125
Stage II/III (%)	49/26	56/25	31/27	25/27
Stage IV (%)	25	19	43	48

The populations were broadly similar with the following differences. The weight-based group included additional ethnic groups (blacks, Hispanics, Asians), and more patients were treated with adjuvant or neoadjuvant chemotherapy compared with the fixed-dose group. Granulocyte response by weight was not analyzed in the weight-based groups.

The results in both studies were remarkably similar (Table 7). Most patients experienced grade 4 neutropenia. The primary endpoints, DSN for pegfilgrastim and filgrastim, respectively, were 1.8 and 1.7 in the weight-based study and 1.6 and 1.8 in the fixed-dose study. The differences between the means were only in hours: 0.03 d and 0.23 d for the weight-based and fixed-dose studies, respectively. The 95% CI for these differences included zero, thus confirming the noninferiority of pegfilgrastim to filgrastim in each of these regimens.

The mean duration of DSN was consistent across treatments throughout the four courses; as in the earlier trials, a mean of 11 daily injections of filgrastim was required compared with a single injection of pegfilgrastim regardless of schedule, and ANC recovery consistently occurred on d 9.

The functional measure of adequate neutrophil reserves, the incidence of FN, showed two results: the rates were always highest in course 1, and the rates were consistently lower in the pegfilgrastim-treated patients.

As a corollary to the higher incidence of FN in course 1 compared with other courses, the granulocyte counts for the weight-based study are listed by course number in Table 8. The nadir granulocyte counts are substantially lower in course 1 compared with subsequent courses. As noted by Bodey et al. *(14)* and Rahman et al. *(15),* the lower the granulocyte counts, the higher the incidence of neutropenic fever. Thus, predictably, in this study as the nadir neutrophil counts for courses 2–4 were higher than in course 1, there was a correspondingly lower rate of FN in these subsequent courses.

This observation of higher granulocyte nadirs in subsequent courses was not a consequence of significant withdrawal of patients or dose reduction. In the weight-based study, >90% of doses were delivered on time, and 90% of patients had an average

Table 7
Efficacy Endpoints of Phase III Trials of Pegfilgrastim Vs Filgrastim

	Weight-based		*Fixed dose*	
Parameters	*Filgrastim daily*	*Pegfilgrastim 100 μg/kg d 2*	*Filgrastim daily*	*Pegfilgrastim 6 mg d 2*
No. of patients	147	149	75	77
Grade 4 ANC course 1 (% pts.)	79	77	83	84
Mean days (SD) grade 4 ANC	1.8 (1.4)	1.7 (1.5)	1.6 (1.1)	1.8 (1.4)
Difference between mean days (pegfilgrastim – filgrastim)	0.03 d		0.23 d	
95% CI for difference in mean DSN between filgrastim and pegfilgrastim	–0.36–0.30 d		–0.15–0.63	
Mean duration of DSN (d) by course				
2	1.1	0.7	0.9	1.1
3	1.2	0.6	0.9	1.1
4	1.3	0.9	1.0	1.0
Time to ANC recovery (d)	9.7	9.3	9.0	9.0
Mean no. of filgrastim injections	11		11	
FN				
Course 1 (no. of pts. [%])	18 (12)	11 (7)	11 (15)	7 (9)
Any course (no. of pts. [%])	27 (18)	14 (9)*	15 (20)	10 (13)

ABBREVIATIONS: ANC, absolute neutrophil count; SD, standard deviation; CI, confidence interval; FN, febrile neutropenia; DSN, days of severe neutropenia when ANC < 0.5×10^9/L.

* $p = 0.029$ (95% CI 16.8, –1.1).

Table 8
Nadir Granulocyte Counts by Course Number in the Weight-Based Trial

Course	*Filgrastim 5 μg/kg d*	*Pegfilgrastim 100 μg/kg d 2*
1	0.181	0.186
2	0.490	0.578
3	0.398	0.609
4	0.396	0.504

received dose intensity of ≥85% *(37,39)*. Granulocyte nadir counts were always higher for the pegfilgrastim group.

The mechanism of these two effects, i.e., a lower incidence of FN and a higher granulocyte nadir in subsequent cycles, may be explained by a study of Allen et al. *(40)*. They treated granulocytes obtained from 12 patients before and after treatment with filgrastim and pegfilgrastim to determine: the time required to double circulating granulocyte counts, the half-life of the stimulated granulocytes, and the levels of granulocyte myeloperoxidase, an enzyme essential for granulocyte killing. Eight patients received standard filgrastim 5 μg/kg daily for 10 d, and four patients received pegfilgrastim 60 μg/kg once. The time to double the granulocyte count was 7 d in the filgrastim-treated

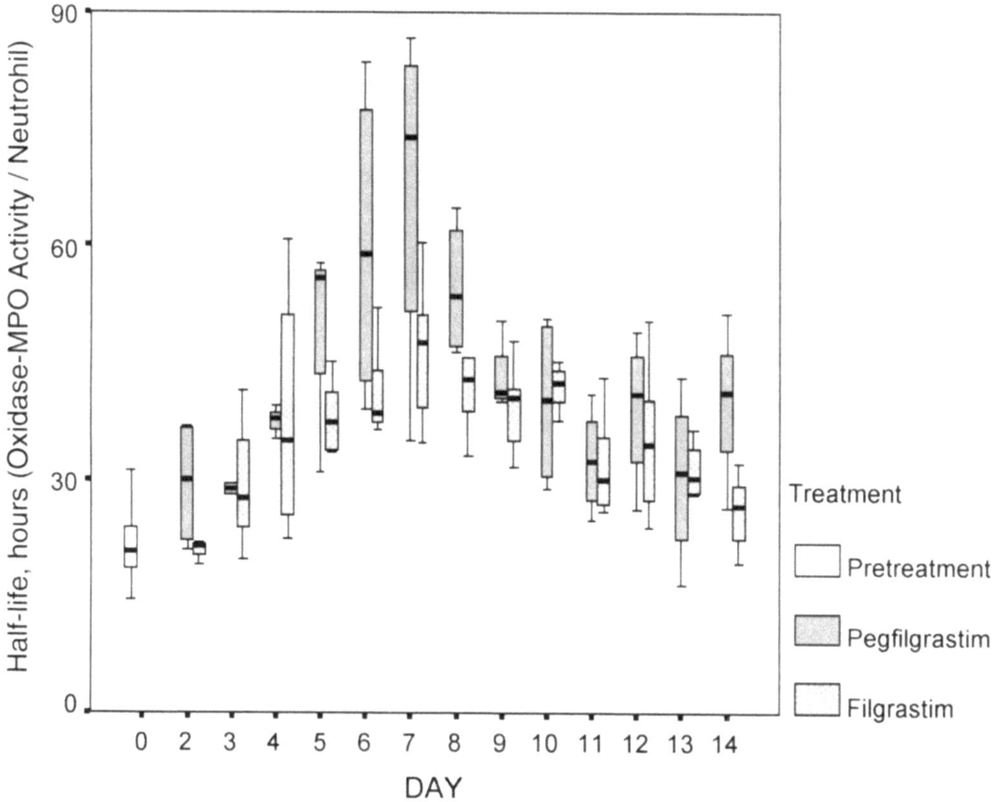

Fig. 4. Half-life, hours (oxidase-myeloperoxidase [MPO] activity/neutrophil) vs day of treatment with either filgrastim or pegfilgrastim. (Courtesy of Robert C. Allen, MD, PhD.)

patients compared with 5 d in the pegfilgrastim-treated patients. The half-lives of the filgrastim- and pegfilgrastim-stimulated granulocytes were, respectively, two- and threefold longer than control granulocytes. Finally, the intragranulocyte concentrations of myeloperoxidase increased more rapidly, peaked higher, and persisted longer in the pegfilgrastim-stimulated granulocytes compared with the filgrastim-stimulated granulocytes (Fig. 4). In sum, both filgrastim and pegfilgrastim produce granulocytes that are superior in function and half-life compared with unstimulated granulocytes; pegfilgrastim-stimulated granulocytes are similarly superior to filgrastim-stimulated granulocytes. These data explain the observed clinical differences in the pivotal trials.

The effect of weight was carefully analyzed by quartile of weight and showed no significant difference (Fig. 5). As in the weight-based study, dose reductions or delays were minimal, and 90% of the patients received chemotherapy as planned *(38)*.

The safety profiles of these two studies were not different compared with the results of the dose-finding trial *(34)*. Bone pain was the most frequent adverse event.

8.6. Pooled Analyses

Because the efficacy endpoints of the two pivotal trials were similar, Shogan et al. *(41)* pooled these data to evaluate the efficacy of pegfilgrastim in patients 65 yr or older

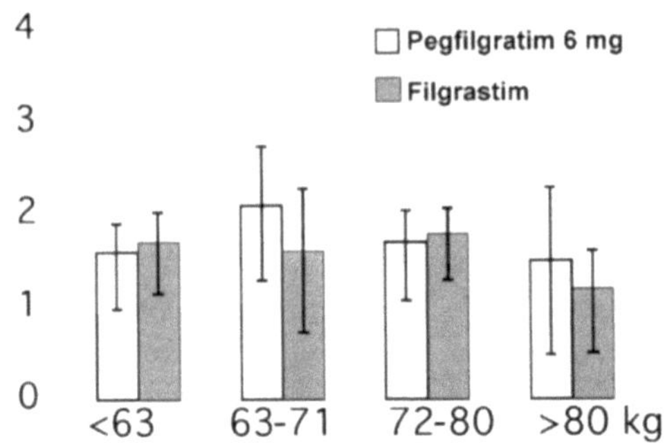

Fig. 5. Days of ANC < 500 by weight quartile, cycle 1. Darker bars, pegfilgrastim 6 mg; lighter bars, filgrastim.

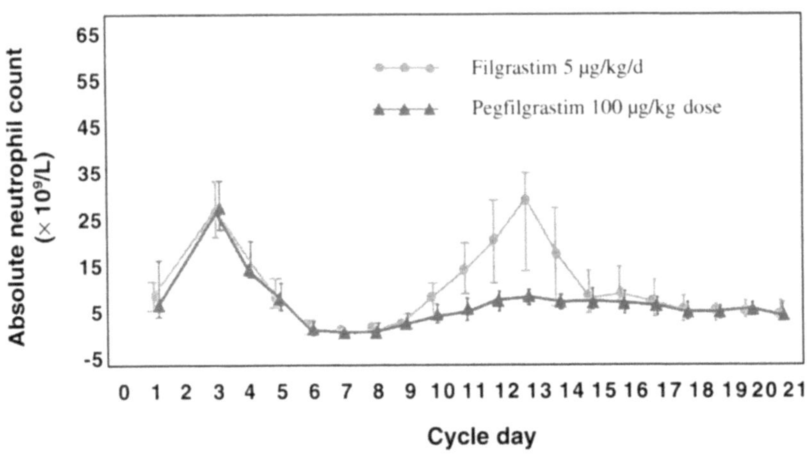

Fig. 6. Pegfilgrastim and filgrastim provide comparable neutrophil recovery: median absolute neutrophil count. (Adapted from ref. *36*.)

using the same endpoints: DSN, rates of FN, antibiotic use, and hospitalization. In the combined trials, 59 patients were aged 65 yr or older, representing 13% of the total population of 456 patients. The distribution of the elderly patients by cohort was 14% (32/225) receiving filgrastim and 12% (27/227) receiving pegfilgrastim.

No difference in the DSN, rates of FN, antibiotic use, or hospitalization by age was seen when the younger and older patients were compared. The pooled data showed a significant decrease in the rates of FN for the pegfilgrastim group regardless of age (Fig. 6).

Shogan et al. *(41)* used these data to evaluate other subgroups at risk for prolonged neutropenia and its complications, namely, patients with prior chemotherapy, prior radiation therapy, a poorer performance status, and advanced (stage IV) vs early disease. In every subgroup, pegfilgrastim was more effective than filgrastim in reducing the incidence of FN (Fig. 7).

Analysis of bone pain using pooled data was attempted by Kubista et al. *(42)*. Bone pain was different between the two studies. The incidence of bone pain was significantly

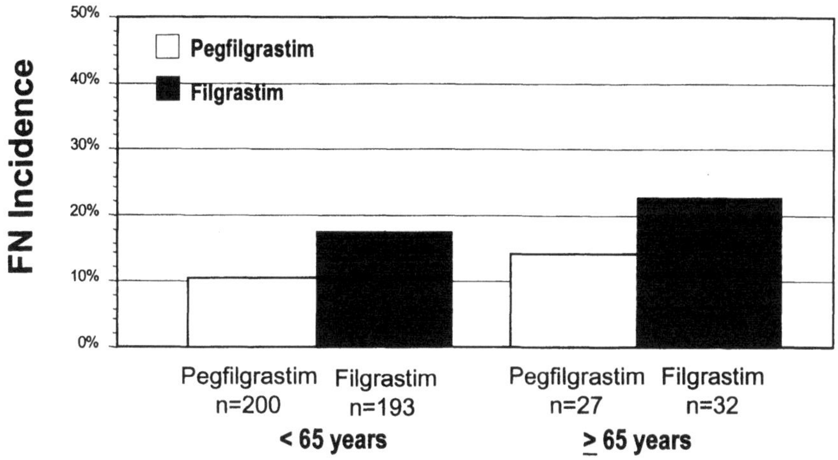

Fig. 7. Incidence of febrile neutrophenia. Open bars, pegfilgrastim; closed bars, filgrastim.

higher in the fixed-dose study compared with the weight-based study ($p = 0.044$), so data could not be pooled. Analyses were performed within each study. In both studies, these analyses showed that bone pain was more severe in the first course compared with later courses ($p < 0.001$), with both filgrastim and pegfilgrastim. Most patients, 60–70%, did not experience bone pain and a few, 5–10%, experienced it in all four courses.

The onset of bone pain tended to be earlier in patients treated with pegfilgrastim compared with filgrastim, but duration or severity was not increased compared with filgrastim. The incidence of bone pain was evaluated by body weight in the fixed-dose study. The numbers of patients in the quartiles were so small that only the extremes were evaluated. Of the 79 patients who received pegfilgrastim, 12 (15%) weighed <60 kg, 60 (76%) weighed between 60 and 100 kg, and 7 (9%) weighed >100 kg. The incidences of bone pain in these groups were 33, 38, and 29%, respectively. The numbers are too small for conclusions, but no obvious trend for more pain in the lighter patients was seen compared with heavier patients.

9. EMERGING ROLES FOR GROWTH FACTORS IN BREAST CANCER THERAPY

9.1. Concurrent Use With Chemotherapy

In 1994, Livingston et al. *(43)* began a series of studies exploring the concept of dose density, namely, multifractioned doses of chemotherapy given at shorter intervals than standard regimens. To prevent dose-limiting myelosuppression, they began intermittent and then continuous neutrophil support with daily filgrastim. In the first study, vinorelbine 35 mg/m^2 was given weekly with continuous filgrastim 5 mg/kg to 40 patients previously treated with anthracyclines and resistant to paclitaxel. They observed that continuous filgrastim allowed a nearly twofold increase in the delivered dose intensity, from 46 to 73%, compared with similar historical series without filgrastim. The increase in delivered dose intensity was suggested as the basis for the observed 25% objective response rate.

This concept of concurrent filgrastim with weekly vinorelbine on d 8 and 15 of each 21-d cycle was extended in trials using concurrent paclitaxel by 96-h infusion *(44)* or docetaxel *(45)*. Both were small trials in patients with resistant disease and produced response rates of 50 and 59%, respectively, with median response duration of 6 mo and median time to progress of 11.7 mo, respectively. No unexpected hematologic events occurred, but these were patients with advanced disease and limited life expectancy.

Use of continuous filgrastim with an alkylating agent, cyclophosphamide 60 mg/m^2/d, continously with doxorubicin 24 mg/m^2/wk was tested preoperatively in 122 patients with locally advanced breast cancer *(46)*. Filgrastim was omitted on the day doxorubicin was administered but was continued on all other days. This regimen produced a 24% pathologic complete response with an additional 22% clinical complete response with only microscopic disease. No untoward hematologic toxicity occurred.

These results were the basis for a second study in 52 high-risk, adjuvant patients treated between October 1992 and June 1997 *(47)*. The initial 30 patients received doxorubicin 20 mg/m^2/wk with 5-flurouracil 300 mg/m^2/wk with oral cyclophosphamide 60 mg/m^2 daily continuously for 24 wk. In the final 22 patients, 5-flurouracil was deleted so doxorubicin could be increased to 26 mg/m^2/wk, and the entire course shortened to 20 weeks. In both groups, filgrastim 5 mg/kg was given as a continuous sc infusion except on the days of chemotherapy. At a median follow-up of 65 mo, the 5-yr actuarial disease-free survival for the combined regimens was 85%, with a projected 86% 5-yr overall survival.

Acute hematologic toxicity included 36.5% grade 3–4 neutropenia, but only 6% (three patients) required admission for FN. Bone pain that was "pulsatile" occurred frequently and required dose reduction of filgrastim in 17%.

One patient died of AML characteristic of anthracyline-related topoisomerase II toxicity: early onset (10 mo after the start of treatment) and with the 11q23 translocation *(48)*. The authors reported, however, that their entire experience with this regimen comprises 185 patients, and only this one patient progressed to leukemia, for an incidence rate of 0.5%, very similar to other reported regimens *(49)*. Moreover, they note that continuous filgrastim is unlikely to enhance leukemogenesis for three reasons: filgrastim does not act at the level of the stem cell, but rather on the neutrophil precursors, filgrastim does not stimulate leukemic blasts, and filgrastim is effective treatment for aplastic anemia.

The dataset for the use of continuous filgrastim with chemotherapy is limited, but these observations do warrant further evaluation, especially with the convenience of pegfilgrastim. These studies would require a redefinition of the concept of a "course" and evaluation of optimal dosing for pegfilgrastim.

This trial, however, still begs the issue about which clinicians and patients routinely ask now that once-per-cycle pegfilgrastim has become available: is it safe (and effective) to administer pegfilgrastim on the same day as intravenous chemotherapy drugs that target DNA, such as doxorubicin or cyclophosphamide? Livingston's group has extensive experience with vinorelbine, an agent that effects microtubules but not DNA directly, and leukemogenesis was not apparent *(43–45)*. However, most of these patients had advanced disease, with limited survival to allow long-term effects to emerge. Although erythropoeitic growth factors are routinely administered on the same day as chemotherapy without apparent loss of efficacy or injury to erythroid precursors, the authors did not administer filgrastim on the same day as doxorubicin.

Doxorubicin's mechanism of action includes DNA intercalation and inhibition of topoisomerase II, the latter of which is postulated as leukemogenic *(48)*. The dose of doxorubicin in the regimens used by Livingston's group was low, only 50–30% of the usual dose, and was administered every week. Although the other DNA-active agent, the alkylator cyclophosphamide, was given concurrently with filgrastim, it was administered orally at only about 10% of the usual intravenous dose. Trials are being designed to answer this question. Many clinicians under the duress of their patient's financial stress and travel logistics have already begun this practice of administering pegfilgrastim on the same day as chemotherapy. Medicare will only pay for pegfilgrastim if it is administered in a physician's office. How does a patient being treated on a Friday or a frail patient with limited transportation resources who lives distant from her doctor's office return for her injection of pegfilgrastim on the day after chemotherapy? These issues demand immediate answers to ensure the safety of our patients for whom we wish, first, to do no harm.

9.2. Dose-Dense Schedules

A related question is the issue of the safety of more frequent, i.e., < every-3-wk administration of pegfilgrastim. The original trial by Johnson et al. *(33)* pretreated patients 15 d before chemotherapy to allow comparison of pegfilgrastim pharmacokinetics in patients whose neutrophil counts were normal and low. No apparent effect on subsequent granulocyte recovery was seen in the subsequent chemotherapy courses.

At the San Antonio Breast Cancer Symposium in December of 2002, the breast cancer community was pleased with the results of CALGB 9741/Intergroup Trial 9741 that evaluated the concept of dose density in the adjuvant setting using the conventional chemotherapy regimen AC-paclitaxel consisting of doxorubicin 60 mg/m^2 with cyclophosphamide 600 mg/m^2 for four courses followed by paclitaxel 175 mg/m^2 for four courses *(50)*. The trial compared the standard 3-wk interval with a compressed, "dose-dense" 2-wk interval given with filgrastim support beginning on d 2 until d 13. The dose-dense cohort showed superior disease-free and overall survival. Additionally, during the limited four courses of therapy, filgrastim support prevented any increase in FN or hospitalizations.

Whether the increased efficacy is a consequence of dose density based on the concepts so well described by Norton and Simon *(51,52)* that can be applied universally to all regimens or whether it is specific to this regimen, particularly the paclitaxel, is unclear. It is obvious that pegfilgrastim administered once on d 2 would make this regimen even more patient-friendly. The initial study of Johnson et al. *(33)* and subsequent studies with Hodgkin's *(53)* and non-Hodgkin's *(54)* lymphoma have suggested that every-14-d administration is safe. The next hurdle will be the economics. A single injection of pegfilgrastim costs the patient $2242 (January 2003) compared with 12 daily injections of filgrastim 300 mg, which costs the patient $1803. Will Medicare and other payors fund this?

9.3. Insufficient Granulocyte Recovery After Pegfilgrastim

Another issue with which clinicians grapple is the patient who returns on d 21 (or d 15) for her next course of chemotherapy but whose granulocyte count has still not recovered despite receiving pegfilgrastim on d 2 after her previous treatment. Although the usual practice has been to delay treatment a few days to a week, this may not be an optimal solution, depending on the severity of the patient's underlying illness, i.e., is this a potentially curative treatment in an adjuvant or neoadjuvant setting or is the patient experiencing rapid disease progression and is she in need of rapid tumor regression to prevent rapid clinical decline. The same logistic and financial issues cited earlier also apply.

Data may help clinicians and patients. The first is, again, the study by Johnson et al. *(33)* that looked at optimal dosing of pegfilgrastim. As with all drugs, there is a dose-response curve. The highest dose tested in the original weight-based studies was 300 mg/kg. This produced a higher granulocyte response than lower doses. This dose was not chosen for subsequent development, however, because it was clearly superior to filgrastim administered at the 5 mg/kg dose, and the objective was to develop pegfilgrastim for use in the same clinical situations with which clinicians had experience and filgrastim was known to be effective. For patients whose bone marrow reserve has been depleted by prior chemotherapy or radiation therapy, however, higher doses may be needed.

This dosing is analogous to our current practice with erythropoietin and darbopoeitin alfa. If patients fail to achieve either a normal hemoglobin concentration or a 2-g increase after four-weekly erythropoietin injections or two-fortnightly darbopoeitin alfa injections, the dose is escalated. In clinical practice, when patients who have received filgrastim on d 2 return and d 21 granulocyte counts are $<1 \times 10^9$/L, we usually increase the granulocyte count by one or two injections of filgrastim 5 mg/kg. For patients on Medicare, however, this may be a problem, as some regional Medicare carriers will not pay for treatment with two similar growth factors.

A second piece of data to help clinicians and patients comes from the dose-dense CALGB 9741 trial *(50)*. To allow retreatment at 14-d intervals and with the assurance that patients randomized to the dose-dense cohort were to receive filgrastim on d 2, the lower limit for retreatment was relaxed to 1×10^9/L. In this short treatment regimen using only eight courses of therapy, cumulative myelosuppression did not occur and hematologic profiles remained normal after completion of treatment.

Thus, from a practical standpoint, it is clear that "standard, one-size-fits all" doses may sometimes be inadequate for patients with inadequate bone marrow reserve. Additional granulocyte growth factor support, either with a higher dose of pegfilgrastim or with additional filgrastim, may be needed. The weight-based studies with pegfilgrastim herein reported were reviewed by the FDA and provide justification for this approach in specific situations. Because of the uncertainty of reimbursement, especially with certain regional Medicare carriers and payors, this approach should not be undertaken without prior discussion with the patient.

9.4. Models to Predict Patients at Risk for Neutropenia and Patients Who Will Benefit From Prophylactic Pegfilgrastim

Appropriate stewardship of limited health care resources compels us to target therapies to prevent costly over utilization. The work of Silber et al. *(32)* was a good beginning. Development of more precise methods to target only those patients at risk for the complications of neutropenia is urgently needed. The cost of hospitalization for an episode of FN may more than offset the cost of prophylactic filgrastim or pegfilgrastim, however.

The issues are complicated by competing priorities that often ignore hidden costs. Clinicians and patients want the safest and easiest treatment, whereas payors are only concerned with cost. A cheaper drug is more cost-effective even if it requires more frequent injections and risks patient compliance. How do payors account for the hidden costs such as days missed from work or transportation costs to medical facilities for patients or their caregivers, in addition to the disruption of lives already tormented by cancer?

Progress has been made. Lyman et al. (this volume) have continued to refine cost estimates by accounting for both the direct costs, which continue to escalate, and these indirect costs. ASCO will be updating practice guidelines for the use of granulocyte growth factors based on these economic analyses and the use of potentially curative dose-dense regimens, as discussed above. Finally, by defining the ultimate risk prediction model from DNA by identification of gene expression profiles—the underlying mystery of cancer itself—we hope to define those patients who will not require granulocyte support for these toxic treatments *(55,56)*.

REFERENCES

1. Bonadonna G, Brusamolino E, Valagussa P, et al. Combination chemotherapy as an adjuvant treatment in operable breast cancer. *N Engl J Med* 1976; 294:405–410.
2. Bonadonna G, Valagussa P. Dose-response effect of adjuvant chemotherapy in breast cancer. *N Engl J Med* 1981; 304:10–15.
3. Bonadonna G, Valagussa P, Moliterni A, et al. Adjuvant cyclophosphamide, methotrexate and fluorouracil in node-positive breast cancer. The results of 20 years of follow up. *N Engl J Med* 1995; 332:901–906.
4. Armstrong DK, Davidson NE. Dose intensity for breast cancer. *Oncology* 2001; 15:701–718.
5. Hryniuk W, Bush H. The importance of dose intensity in chemotherapy of metastatic breast cancer. *J Clin Oncol* 1984; 2:1281–1288.
6. Hryniuk W, Levine MN. Analysis of dose intensity for adjuvant chemotherapy trials in stage II breast cancer. *J Clin Oncol* 1986; 4:1162–1170.
7. Tannock IF, Boyd NF, DeBoer G, et al. A randomized trial of two dose levels of cyclophosphamide, methotrexate and fluorouracil chemotherapy for patients with metastatic breast cancer. *J Clin Oncol* 1988; 6:1377–1387.
8. Hortobagyi GN, Bodey GP, Buzdar AU, et al. Evaluation of high dose versus standard FAC chemotherapy for advanced breast cancer in protected environment units: a prospective randomized study. *J Clin Oncol* 1987; 5:354–364.
9. Wood WC, Budman DR, Korzun AH, et al. Dose and dose intensity of adjuvant chemotherapy for stage II, node-positive breast carcinoma. *N Engl J Med* 1994; 330:1253–1259.
10. Fisher B, Anderson S, Wickerham DL, et al. Increased intensification and total dose of cyclophosphamide in a doxorubicin-cyclophosphamide regimen for the treatment of primary breast cancer: findings from National Surgical Adjuvant Breast and Bowel Project B-22. *J Clin Oncol* 1997; 15:1858–1869.
11. Fisher B, Anderson S, DeCillis A, et al. Further evaluation of intensified and increased total dose of cyclophosphamide for the treatment of primary breast cancer: findings from National Surgical Adjuvant Breast and Bowel Project B-25. *J Clin Oncol* 1999; 17:3374–3388.
12. Henderson IC, Berry DA, Demetri GD, et al. 2003 Improved outcomes from adding sequential Paclitaxel but not from escalating Doxorubicin dose in an adjuvant chemotherapy regimen for patients with node-positive primary breast cancer. *J Clin Oncol*. 2003; 21;963–964.
13. Link B, Budd GT, Scott S, et al. Delivering adjuvant chemotherapy to women with early-stage breast carcinoma. *Cancer* 2001; 92:1354–1367.
14. Bodey GP, Buckley M, Sathe YS, et al. Quantitative relationship between circulating leucocytes and infection in patients with acute leukemia. *Ann Intern Med* 1966; 64:328–340.
15. Rahman Z, Esparza-Guerra L, Yap HY, et al. Chemotherapy-induced neutropenia and fever in patients with metastatic breast carcinoma receiving salvage chemotherapy. *Cancer* 1997; 79:1150–1157.
16. Pizzo PA, Hathorn JW, Hiemenz J, et al. A randomized trial comparing ceftazidime alone with combination antibiotic therapy in cancer patients with fever and neutropenia. *N Engl J Med* 1986; 315:552–558.

17. Metcalf D. The colony stimulating factors. *Cancer* 1990; 65:2185–2195.
18. Gabrilove JL, Jakubowski A, Scher H, et al. Effect of granulocyte colony-stimulating factor on neutropenia and associated morbidity due to chemotherapy for transitional-cell carcinoma of the urothelium. *N Engl J Med* 1988; 318:1414–1422.
19. Crawford J, Ozer H, Stoller R, et al. Reduction by granulocyte colony-stimulating factor of fever and neutropenia induced by chemotherapy in patients with small-cell lung cancer. *N Engl J Med* 1991; 325:164–170.
20. Silber JH, Fridman M, DiPaola RS, et al. First-cycle blood counts and subsequent neutropenia, dose reduction or delay in early-stage breast cancer therapy. *J Clin Oncol* 1998; 16:2392–2400.
21. Rivera E, Erder HM, Fridman M, et al. Delivering full planned dose on time chemotherapy while lowering the incidence of febrile neutropenia hospitalizations: initial results from a prospective study providing filgrastim support to high risk breast cancer patients. *Breast Cancer Res Treat* 2001; 69:209.
22. Emerman JT, Eaves CJ. Lack of effect of hematopoietic growth factors on human breast epithelial cell growth in serum-free primary culture. *Bone Marrow Transplant* 1994; 13:285–291.
23. deWit R, Verweij J, Bontenbal M, et al. Adverse effect on bone marrow protection of prechemotherapy granulocyte colony-stimulating factor support. *J Natl Cancer Inst* 1996; 88:1393–1398.
24. Lieschke GL, Burgess AW. Granulocyte colony-stimulating factor and granulocyte-macrophage colony stimulating factor. *N Engl J Med* 1992; 327:99–106.
25. Bronchud MH, Howell A, Crowther D, et al. The use of granulocyte colony-stimulating factor to increase the intensity of treatment with doxorubicin in patients with advanced breast and ovarian cancer. *Br J Cancer* 1989; 60:121–125.
26. de Graaf H, Pax HB, Bong SB, et al. Dose intensity of standard adjuvant CMF with granulocyte colony stimulating factor for premenopausal patients with node-positive breast cancer. *Oncology* 1996; 53:289–294.
27. Webster J, Kuderer, Lyman GH. Use of G-CSF to sustain dose intensity in breast cancer patients receiving adjuvant chemotherapy: a pilot study. *Cancer Control* 1996; 3:519–522.
28. Misset JL, Dieras V, Gruia G, et al. Dose-finding study of docetaxel and doxorubicin in first-line treatment of patients with metastatic breast cancer. *Ann Oncol* 1999; 10:553–560.
29. Sparano JA, Hu P, Rao RM, et al. Phase II trial of doxorubicin and paclitaxel plus granulocyte colony-stimulating factor in metastatic breast cancer: an Eastern Cooperative Oncology Group study. *J Clin Oncol* 1999; 17:3828–3834.
30. Ozer H, Armitage JO, Bennett CL, et al. 2000 Update of recommendations for the use of hematopoietic colony-stimulating factors: evidence-based, clinical practice guidelines. *J Clin Oncol* 2000; 18:3558–3585.
31. Glaspy JA, Bleecker G, Crawford J, Stoller, Strauss M. The impact of therapy with filgrastim (recombinant granulocyte colony stimulating factor) on the health care costs associated with cancer. *Eur J Cancer* 1993; 29A(suppl 7):S23–30.
32. Silber JH, Fridman M, Shpilsky A, et al. Modeling the cost-effectiveness of granulocyte colony-stimulating factor use in early-stage breast cancer. *J Clin Oncol* 1998; 16:2435–2444.
33. Johnson E, Crawford J, Blackwell S, et al. Randomized, dose-escalation study of SD/01 compared with daily filgrastim in patients receiving chemotherapy. *J Clin Oncol* 2000; 18:2522–2528.
34. Holmes FA, Jones, SE, O Shaughnessy J, et al. Comparable efficacy and safety profiles of once-per-cycle pegfilgrastim and daily injection filgrastim in chemotherapy-induced neutropenia: a multicenter dose-finding study in women with breast cancer. *Ann Oncol* 2002; 13:903–909.
35. Morstyn G, Campbell L, Souza LM, et al. Effects of granulocyte colony stimulating factor on neutropenia induced by cytotoxic chemotherapy. *Lancet* 1988; 1:667–672.
36. Yang BB, Lum PK, Renwick J, et al. Pharmacokinetic rationale for a fixed-dose regimen of a sustained duration form of filgrastim in cancer patients. *Blood* 2000; 96:157b (abstr. 4384).
37. Holmes FA, O Shaughnessy JA, Vukelja S, et al. Blinded, randomized, multicenterstudy to evaluate single administration pegfilgrastim once per cycle versus daily filgrastim as an adjunct to chemotherapy in patients with high-risk stage II or stage III/IV breast cancer. *J Clin Oncol* 2002; 20:727–731.
38. Green MD, Koelbl H, Baselga J, et al. A randomized double-blind multicenter phase III study of fixed-dose single-administration pegfilgrastim versus daily filgrastim in patients receiving myelosuppresive chemotherapy. *Ann Oncol* 2003; 14:29–35.
39. Siena S, Piccart MJ, Holmes FA, et al. A single dose of pegfilgrastim per chemotherapy cycle allows most patients to receive and average dose intensity (ARDI) ≥ 85% (Abstr 535). *Breast Cancer Res Treat* 2002; 76(suppl 1): S135 (http://www.abstracts-on-line.com/abstracts/BCS/aol.asp).

40. Allen RC. Ex vivo half-life of neutrophils from healthy human subjects pre and post treatment with daily filgrastim or single-dose pegfilgrastim. *Blood* 2002; 100:243a (abstract 918).
41. Shogan JE, Koelbl H, Holmes FA, et al. A single dose of pegfilgrastim reduces the incidence of febrile neutropenia in various risk strata compared with daily filgrastim following myelosuppresseive chemotherapy. *Breast Cancer Res Treat* 2002; 76(suppl 1):S135 (abstract 536; http://www.abstracts-on-line.com/abstracts/BCS/aol.asp).
42. Kubista E, Glaspy J, Holmes FA, Green MD, Hackett J, Neumann T. (Pegfilgrastim Study Group) Bone pain associated with once-per-cycle pegfilgrastim is similar to daily filgrastim in patients with breast cancer. *Clin Breast Cancer* 2003; 3:391–398.
43. Livingston RB, Ellis GK, Gralow JR, et al. Dose-intensive vinorelbine with concurrent granulocyte colony-stimulating factor support in paclitaxel-refractory metatastatic breast cancer. *J Clin Oncol* 1997; 15:1395–1400.
44. Ellis GK, Gralow JR, Pierce I, et al. Infusional paclitaxel and weekly vinorelbine chemotherapy with concurrent filgrastim for metastatic breast cancer: high complete response rate in a phase I–II study of doxorubicin-treated patients. *J Clin Oncol* 1999; 17:1407–1412.
45. Gralow JR, Ellis GK, Williams MA, et al. Docetaxel + vinorelbine with concurrent G-CSF support: a phase II study in stage IV breast cancer. *Proc Am Soc Clin Oncol* 2000; 19:106a (abstract 410).
46. Ellis GK, Green J, Livingston RB, et al. Neoadjuvant doxorubicin, cyclophosphamide and G-CSF (AC + G) for locally advanced breast cancer (LABC), a Southwest Oncology Group phase II study. *Proc Am Soc Clin Oncol* 2000; 19:85a (abstract 326).
47. Ellis GK, Livingston RB, Gralow JR, et al. Dose-dense anthracycline-based chemotherapy for node positive breast cancer. *J Clin Oncol* 2002; 20:3637–2643.
48. Arriagada R, Gutierrez J. Anthracyclines: is more better and/or more dangerous? *Ann Oncol* 2003 14:663–665.
49. Bernard-Marty C, Mano M, Paesmans M, et al. Second malignancies following adjuvant chemotherapy: 6-year results from a Belgian randomized study comparing cyclophosphamide, methotrexate and 5-fluorouracil (CMF) with an anthracycline-based regimen in adjuvant treatment of node-positive breast cancer patients. *Ann Oncol* 2003; 14:693–698.
50. Citron M, Berry D, Cirrincione C, et al. Randomized trial of dose-dense versus conventionally scheduled and sequential versus concurrent combination chemotherapy as postoperative adjuvant treatment of node-positive primary breast cancer: First report of Intergroup Trial C9741/Cancer and Leukemia Group B Trial 9741. *J Clin Oncol* 2003; 21 (April 1 electronic version; http://www.jco.org).
51. Norton L, Simon R, Brereton HD, et al. Predicting the course of gompertzian growth. *Nature* 1976; 264:542–545.
52. Norton L. The Norton-Simon hypothesis revisited. *Cancer Treat Rep* 1986; 70:163–169.
53. Younes A, Fayad L, Pro B, et al. Safety and efficacy of prophylactic pegfilgrastim in patients with Hodgkin disease receiving ABVD chemotherapy. *Blood* 2002; 100:171b (abstract 4179).
54. Moore TD, Patel Tarel Segal M, et al. A single pegfilgrastim dose per cycle supports dose-dense (Q14 day) CHOP-R in patients with NHL. *Blood* 2002; 100:571a (abstract 2245).
55. Perou CM, Serlie T, Eisen MB, et al. Molecular portraits of human breast tumors. *Nature* 2000; 406; 747–752.
56. van't Veer IJ, Dai H, Vijver MJ, et al. Gene expression profiling predicts clinical outcomes of breast cancer. *Nature* 2002; 415:530–535.

16 Role of Cytokines in the Management of Chronic Lymphocytic Leukemia

Carol Ann Long, PhD

CONTENTS

1. INTRODUCTION

1.1. Chronic Lymphocytic Leukemia

Chronic lymphocytic leukemia (CLL) is the most common form of leukemia in adults in Western countries. The annual incidence estimate from the American Cancer Society is for approx 7000 new cases in the United States in 2003. (This number suggests an apparent decline in incidence, but it may reflect an increased ability to distinguish CLL from other chronic lymphoid leukemias *[1]*.) CLL tends to be a disease of the elderly; the median age at diagnosis is 62 yr, and only 15% of patients present at an age younger than 50 yr *(2)*.

1.2. Diagnosis

The diagnosis of CLL is most often made incidentally when lymphocytosis is observed in routine blood tests. CLL cells express pan-B antigens (HLA class II, CD19 and CD20) and activation antigens (CD5, CD23, CD25, and CD71), but not terminal differentiation antigens expressed by plasma cells *(3)*. CLL cells have a restricted repertoire of VH1 genes (distinct from that of normal B cells) *(4)*. The two major features that distinguish CLL cells from normal B cells are the expression of CD5 (a T-cell antigen) and the low expression of surface immunoglobulin. These features have been used to diagnose B-cell CLL differentially from other chronic lymphoproliferative diseases:

From: *Cancer Drug Discovery and Development*
Hematopoietic Growth Factors in Oncology: Basic Science and Clinical Therapeutics
Edited by: G. Morstyn, M. Foote, and G. J. Lieschke © Humana Press Inc., Totowa, NJ

prolymphocytic leukemia (PLL), hairy cell leukemia (HCL), non-Hodgkin's lymphomas (NHL) in a leukemic phase, and plasma cell leukemia.

Most patients with CLL are asymptomatic at presentation, and physical examination is normal in 20–30% of patients. Lymphadenopathy or hepatosplenomegaly or both is noted in 40–50% of patients. As the disease progresses, generalized adenopathy and splenomegaly become common features of the disease.

1.3. Clinical Features

Clinical features of the disease include infections, autoimmunity, anemia, pure red cell aplasia, an aggressive transformation, and/or secondary malignancies.

1.3.1. Infections

Infections are the major cause of death in patients with CLL. The basis for the increased susceptibility to infection is multifactorial and relates to both the disease and its treatment. Hypogammaglobulinemia is common, as is defective activation of the complement system and defects in cell-mediated immunity and phagocytosis. Before treatment, the most common pathogens are those that require opsonization for bacterial killing. After treatment, the number of infections with Gram-negative organisms and opportunistic pathogens (especially after treatment with nucleoside analogs) increases *(5,6)*. Infections are the ultimate cause of death in 60–85% of patients with CLL *(7)*.

High-dose, intravenous immunoglobulins have been evaluated for the ability to prevent infections in CLL. Prophylactic use of intravenous immunoglobulins failed to reduce the total number of major infections or incidence of infection, and no improvement in overall survival was reported for patients receiving prophylactic, high-dose, intravenous immunoglobulins *(8)*. Prophylactic antimicrobial regimens are not routinely recommended because the broad spectrum of potential pathogens would require multiple, potentially toxic drugs. Therefore, prophylactic uses of antimicrobial agents or high-dose intravenous immunoglobulins have been restricted to patients with documented, repeated bacterial infections.

1.3.2. Aggressive Transformation

Aggressive transformation of CLL has been reported in 10–15% of patients. The most common transformation (5%) is Richter's syndrome. Transformation is not clearly related to either the nature or extent of primary therapy. Evolution into PLL, acute lymphocytic leukemia (ALL), plasma cell leukemia, multiple myeloma, and Hodgkin's disease (HD) have been reported.

1.3.3. Autoimmunity

Up to 20% of patients may have a positive Coombs' antiglobulin test, although clinical hemolysis occurs in only 50% of these patients. The frequency of immune thrombocytopenia is approx 2%. Autoimmune anemia, or thrombocytopenia, generally responds to a short course of therapy with corticosteroids. In patients unresponsive to corticosteroids, high doses of intravenous immunoglobulin have been used. Splenectomy is an option if systemic approaches fail *(9–11)*.

1.3.4. Anemia and Pure Red Cell Aplasia

Anemia in CLL (defined as hemoglobin [Hb] concentration < 10 g/dL) is frequently observed at presentation (reported incidence of 9–29%) and becomes both more frequent

Table 1
Staging Systems for Chronic Lymphocytic Leukemia

Stage	Simplified three-stage system	Clinical features	Median survival (yr)
Modified Rai staging system			
		Lymphocytosis in blood and marrow only	>10
	Intermediate risk	Lymphocytosis + lymphadenopathy	7
		Splenomegaly ± hepatomegaly	
		Lymphocytosis + anemia	1.5–4
		Thrombocytopenia	
Binet staging system			
A		Less than three areas of clinical lymphadenopathy; no anemia or thrombocytopenia	12
B		Three or more involved node areas; no anemia or thrombocytopenia	7
C		Hb > 10 g/dL and/or platelets < 100×10^9/L	2–4

and more pronounced with disease progression *(12–14)*. Anemia in CLL may be caused by autoimmune hemolysis, extensive bone marrow infiltration, hypersplenism, deficiency of hematopoietic cofactors, blood loss, and/or the anemia of chronic disease (ACD). ACD is characterized by the release of cytokines such as interleukin (IL)-1α and -1β, tumor necrosis factor (TNF)-α, transforming growth factor (TGF)-β, and IL-6, which inhibit endogenous erythropoietin (EPO) production, diminish the responsiveness of erythroid progenitors to EPO, and impair iron utilization *(15–19)*.

Pure red cell aplasia is an uncommon complication characterized by severe anemia without a reticulocyte response or bone marrow normoblast, in the absence of neutropenia or thrombocytopenia. Chemotherapy that effects a clinical response increases the hematocrit in most treated patients. Corticosteroids and cyclosporin may induce responses *(20)*.

1.3.5. Secondary Malignancies

Secondary malignancies occur with increased frequency in patients with CLL and have been attributed both to the immune defects associated with CLL and to iatrogenic consequences of treatment.

1.4. Staging

Patients with CLL exhibit a highly variable course, probably reflecting the underlying molecular heterogenicity of the disease *(21)*. Two staging systems are available and are widely accepted: the Rai classification (commonly used in the United States), and the Binet system (commonly used in Europe). In both systems, increasing incidence and severity of anemia is associated with disease progression (Table 1). Clinical stage is the strongest predictor of outcome, but significant clinical heterogeneity exists within stages of both systems. The Rai system initially identified five stages but has been simplified into a three-stage system. Both systems are cited in the literature.

1.5. Therapy

The current recommendation for patients with early-stage CLL is that treatment should not be initiated without specific indications (i.e., symptomatic progression or a rapid lymphocyte doubling time). This recommendation is based on data demonstrating that currently available therapies do not cure patients with CLL, yet may be associated with significant toxicities *(22)*.

For patients with advanced disease, the most active classes of chemotherapy drugs are alkylating agents (chlorambucil and cyclophosphamide), nucleoside analogs (fludarabine, cladribine, and pentostatin), and monoclonal antibodies (MAbs; alemtuzamab). Myelosuppression is a frequent and often dose-limiting consequence of therapy with these agents.

1.5.1. First-Line Therapy

Fludarabine is the preferred initial treatment for most patients with CLL *(23–25)*. Because of toxicities associated with fludarabine, chlorambucil-based regimens are a first-line treatment option for frail elderly patients, patients with reduced performance status, or those with active infections.

1.5.2. Second-Line Therapies

Fludarabine is the standard agent for second-line therapy of patients who received front-line alkylators. Alemtuzumab has clinical activity in patients refractory to fludarabine and/or alkylating agents *(26)*.

1.5.3. Stem Cell Transplantation

Autologous stem cell transplants are under investigation in CLL. Such transplants usually involve positive and/or negative purging procedures to address the significant amount of leukemic cell contamination in the stem cell source. Data about allogeneic marrow or stem cell transplant are limited in CLL. Given the advanced age at diagnosis (>60 yr) and the fact that currently available therapies rarely eradicate detectable disease, patients with CLL are a high risk for transplantation. Both traditional and submyeloablative allogenic transplants are investigational at this time.

2. TRIALS WITH ERYTHROPOIETIC PROTEINS

2.1. Endogenous Erythropoietin Concentrations

Beguin et al. *(19)* conducted a study of serum EPO concentrations in 47 patients with CLL to determine whether decreased amounts of EPO were a factor in the development of anemia. Hb concentration, hematocrit (Hct), and serum transferrin receptor (sTfR) concentrations were compared with those found in a cohort of 31 normal individuals. Log-transformed EPO and sTfR values were used in statistical analyses. In this study, only 3/47 patients had depressed erythropoiesis because of inadequate EPO stimulation. When the CLL cohort was compared with the normal individual cohort, serum EPO concentration (135.2 ± 3103 vs 14.1 ± 2.8 μm/mL) and sTfR levels (12,380 ± 11,120 vs 5000 ± 1050 ng/mL) were significantly higher in patients with CLL compared with control patients. Serum EPO concentrations were appropriate for the degree

Table 2
Relative Erythropoietin Deficiency Definitions[a]

Hb concentration (g/dL)	*Serum Erythropoietin (U/L)*
>9 and <10	≤100
>8 and ≤9	≤180
≤8	≤300

[a] Serum erythropoietin concentrations were measured at least 7 d after the last transfusion or chemotherapy *(28).*

of anemia observed for patients with active or inactive CLL, early- or late-stage CLL, and in treated vs untreated CLL *(19),* suggesting that the cause of anemia in CLL is more likely to be related to marrow involvement by malignant cells, increased hemolysis, and/or splenic sequestration than to inadequate EPO production.

"Normal" regression equations based on data from 65 normal reference subjects were used to evaluate the relationship between the Hct and EPO or sTfR concentrations and to derive predicted log EPO and log sTfR values for each Hct. Observed-to-predicted values (O/P) were calculated with 95% confidence levels for O/P EPO (0.80–1.20) and O/P sTfR (0.91–1.09). For patients with CLL, Hb concentration was substituted for the Hct value when calculating the regression equations and O/P ratios for individual CLL patients, since the Hct value may be inappropriately large when large numbers of lymphocytes are present. The slope of the regression equation did not differ between the normal reference subjects and the CLL patients ($R + -0.75$, $p < 0.000001$). O/P EPO and O/P sTfR were not different between normal reference subjects and CLL patient cohorts. Inadequate EPO production was reported for three patients with CLL patients (two with active infections), but inappropriately high EPO concentrations were reported for eight patients.

Two randomized pilot studies in patients with hematologic malignancies and anemia evaluated pretreatment factors associated with response to recombinant human erythropoietin (rHuEPO) therapy *(27,28).* In both studies, patients with CLL were included, and analyses reported no differences among patient populations (multiple myeloma, NHL, and CLL). The larger study evaluated different cut points for the O/P ratio of serum EPO, and in a Cox univariate regression analysis of factors associated with time to response, an O/P ratio of serum EPO < 0.9 was statistically significant ($p < 0.01$) *(28).* A cumulative response rate of 89% (Kaplan-Meier method) was found in rHuEPO-treated patients with O/P < 0.6, and nonresponse was predicted by an O/P ratio ≥ 1.2. To translate the information into more clinically accessible data, analyses were conducted using uncorrected serum EPO values. The cumulative response was 76% among patients with values < 50 U/L, whereas in patients with values ≥ 400 U/L, the response rate was only 9%.

A prospective randomized trial required that anemic patients with CLL have low endogenous EPO concentrations at study entry *(29).* Data from this study suggest that 75% of patients with CLL have a relative serum EPO deficiency at baseline. The definitions for relative serum EPO deficiency used in the study are presented in Table 2. Criteria to identify patients who might benefit from rHuEPO therapy have been developed, but their utility in clinical practice is limited (Table 3).

Table 3
Prediction of Response to Exogenous Erythropoietin

Parameter of response	*Predictive factor*	*Comments*
Blunted endogenous EPO response to anemia	Baseline O/P ratio < 0.9	Low predictive accuracy
First signs of therapeutic response	After 2 wk of therapy: reticulocyte counts > 40,000 μL	In patients without chemotherapy
	After 4 weeks of therapy: reticulocyte count > 40,000 μL and ↑ Hb > 1 g/dL	In patients with concomitant chemotherapy
After 2 wk of therapy:		
Combination of endogenous EPO and first signs of therapeutic response	Baseline EPO < 100 mU/mL and ↑ Hb > 0.5 g/dL	Predictive accuracy = 100%
	Baseline EPO < 100 mU/mL and ↑ sTfR > 25%	Predictive accuracy = 96%
	Baseline O/P ratio < 0.9 and ↑ Hb 0.3 g/dL	Predictive accuracy = 88%

ABBREVIATIONS: EPO, erythropoietin; O/P, observed/predicted; sTfR, soluble transferring receptor.
Data from ref. *66*.

2.2. Clinical Trials With Erythropoietic Proteins

Trials conducted with rHuEPO and darbepoetin alfa have shown that exogenous rHuEPO and darbepoetin alfa can reduce transfusion requirements or increse in Hct in patients with CLL. Only one of the trials *(29)* required a low baseline EPO value as part of the entrance criteria (Table 4).

2.2.1. RANDOMIZED TRIALS

Rose et al. *(30)* conducted a randomized, double-blind, placebo-controlled trial of epoetin alfa in 221 anemic patients with CLL. Patients had advanced disease (Rai stage intermediate) with Hct < 32%, and were randomized to receive epoetin alfa 150 U/kg three times/wk sc ($n = 141$) or placebo ($n = 80$) for up to 12 wk. Hct values were measured at baseline and weekly while on study. Quality of life (QOL) (as measured by a self-administered questionnaire addressing energy, physical/social/cognitive role function, and mental health) was assessed at baseline and after 6 and 12 wk of treatment. Treatment groups were balanced for baseline demographics. (Baseline Hct was 27.4% in the treated group vs 27.8% in the control group.) The mean final Hct increased by 5.7 percentage points in the epoetin alfa-treated group and 1.5 percentage points in the placebo group ($p < 0.0001$). Approximately 50% of the epoetin alfa group had a Hct change ≥ 6 points over baseline value, unrelated to transfusion, compared with 15% of the control group ($p < 0.0001$). Overall, approx 30% of the epoetin alfa group and 5% of the placebo group achieved Hct > 38, unrelated to transfusion ($p < 0.0001$). Group differences favoring the epoetin alfa patients were found for the energy scores on the QOL questionnaire ($p < 0.05$). Patients who achieved an Hct ≥ 38% had significant improvements in all aspects of the QOL questionnaire ($p < 0.01$ to $p <$

Table 4
Erythropoietin Activity in Randomized Trials in Anemic, Chronic Lymphocytic Leukemia Patients

Ref.	*Erythropoietin*	*CLL patients (no.)*	*Entry criteria*	*Definition of response*	*Erythropoietin*	*Placebo*	p *value*
30	Epoetin alfa (150 U/kg 3× wk for 12 wks)	*n* = 221 (141 treated, 80 control)	Hct < 32%	Increase in Hct > 6 points from baseline	~ 50%	15%	<0.0001
				Increase in Hct ≥38%	~ 30%	5%	<0.0001
29	Epoetin beta (150 U/kg 3× wk for 16 wk, dose escalation permitted after wk 4)	*n* = 125	Hb < 10 g/dL and "low" serum EPO	Increase in Hb ≥ 2 g/dL from baseline	63%	26%	<0.0001
				Improvement in FACT QOL scale at 16 wk	14.8 ± 28	8.7 ± 28.9	<0.05
31	Darbepoetin alfa (1, 2.25 or 4.5 U/kg 1× wk for 12 wk)	*n* = 11 evaluable (2 placebo, 2, 1, and 6 at the 1, 2.25 and 4.5 U/kg/wk doses)	Hb < 11 g/dL	Increase in Hb ≥ 2 g/dL from baseline	1 U/kg (1/2 N/A) 2.25 U/kg d 1 4.5 U/kg Dose response: 1 U/kg (1/2 N/A) 2.25 U/kg (0/1) 4.5 U/kg (3/6)	Response: 0/2	N/A
32	Epoetin alpha (150 U/kg 3× wk for 12 wk, then 12 wk of open-label drug—dose escalation permitted after wk 12)	*n* = 9 (6 epoetin alfa, 3 placebo)	Hct < 32%	Complete response = Hct ≥ 38%	6/6 responses (wk 12)	0/3 responses wk 12	N/A
				Partial response = Hct > 6 pts from baseline	8/9 responses (wk 24)		

ABBREVIATIONS: Hb, hemoglobin; N/A, not applicable; Hct, hematocrit; FACT, Functional Assessment of Cancer Therapy; QOL, quality of life.

* See Table 2 for definition of "low" serum EPO used.

0.0004). In addition, the need for transfusions was significantly reduced in the epoetin alfa group.

The results of this study have been confirmed in several other randomized trials (Table 4). Österberg et al. *(29)* conducted a double-blind, randomized, placebo-controlled trial of epoetin beta in 343 transfusion-dependent patients with hematologic malignancies (Hb concentration < 10 g/dL) with low serum EPO concentrations. The study was stratified for patients with NHL (n = 106), CLL (n = 126), or multiple myeloma (n = 117). CLL patients were randomized to receive 150 U/kg of epoetin beta sc three times week or placebo for 16 wk. The epoetin beta dose was increased to 300 U/kg three times/wk if no signs of response were observed after 4 wk. Patients were prescreened for low serum EPO concentrations (relative EPO deficiency; *see* Table 2 for definitions). Hb concentrations were measured at baseline and throughout the study. QOL assessments were done at baseline and at wk 4, 8, 12, and 16 using the Functional Assessment of Cancer Therapy-Anemia (FACT-An) questionnaire. The primary endpoint of the study was transfusion-free survival during wk 5 to 16.

The cumulative Hb response rate (defined as a 2-g/dL increase in Hb concentration from baseline) in patients receiving epoetin beta was statistically significantly higher than among placebo patients (63% vs 26%, $p < 0.0001$). Patients receiving epoetin beta in the trial had statistically significant risk reductions of approx 40% in both transfusion-free survival and severe anemia-free survival ($p = 0.02$ and 0.03, respectively). For all patients in the study, a statistically significant increase in FACT-An scores was observed among epoetin beta patients relative to placebo patients at wk 12 and 16 ($p < 0.05$). Regression analysis of the epoetin beta patients evaluating the week-16 Hb concentration and the change in FACT-An over the course of the study demonstrated a statistically significant correlation on the basis of log-linear relationships regression ($r = 0.3167$, $p = 0.001$), but the between-patient variability was considerable.

Hedenus et al. *(31)* conducted a randomized, double-blind, placebo-controlled dose-finding study of darbepoetin alfa in 66 anemic patients with lymphoproliferative malignancies. Anemia was defined as Hb concentration ≤ 11 g/dL. Twelve patients with CLL were randomized within the study: two placebo, two to 1.0 U/kg/wk, one to 225 U/kg/wk, and seven to 4.5 U/kg/wk. No dose increases were allowed during the study. Eleven patients were evaluable for efficacy. Darbepoetin alfa or placebo was administered once a week sc for 12 wk. Hb response was defined as a 2-g/dL increase from the baseline value, and concentrations were measured weekly during the study. For all patients in the study, the proportion of patients achieving an Hb response increased with the darbepoetin alfa dose (from 45% in the 1-U/kg/wk cohort to 62% in the 4.5-U/kg/wk cohort) and was significantly higher for the darbepoetin alfa patients than for placebo patients ($p < 0.01$). Hb responses were observed among CLL patients at a frequency that did not differ from other tumor types by covariate analysis.

Pangalis et al. *(32)* conducted a randomized, closed-label trial of 12 wk of epoetin alfa (n = 6) or placebo (n = 3) in anemic CLL patients (defined as Hct < 32%). Patients were then enrolled in an open-label phase of the study for 12 additional weeks during which all patients received epoetin alfa. During the closed phase, epoetin alfa was administered at 150 U/kg three times/wk. During the open-label phase, increments of 50 U/kg were allowed to a maximum of 300 U/kg if response was slow or unsatisfactory. Complete responses (Hct ≥ 38%) were achieved in 5/9 patients, and partial responses (increase of ≥6 points from baseline) in 3/9 patients. Dose escalation was required in 2/7 responding patients. Patients who received placebo during the closed-label phase of the study showed no evidence of improvement.

2.2.2. Clinical Utilization Issues

Siakantaris et al. *(33)* evaluated the necessity of maintenance therapy in patients who achieved a response to epoetin alfa. The study enrolled 33 patients with chronic lymphoproliferative disorders, among whom were 22 patients with B-CLL. Patients were anemic at entry (Hct < 32%) and were treated with 150 U/kg epoetin alfa three times/wk sc for 12 wk. After 6 wk, escalation of the epoetin alfa doses was permitted in 50-U/kg increments (to a maximum of 300 U/kg three times/wk) for unsatisfactory responses. Unsatisfactory response was defined as an Hct increase from baseline ≤ 2 points. The overall response was determined at wk 12. At that time, 50% of the responding patients received maintenance therapy with epoetin alfa 150 U/kg/wk sc, and the remaining responding patients were discontinued.

At wk 12, 11/22 CLL patients had a complete response (i.e., Hct ≥ 38%), and 6 achieved a partial response (i.e., >6 point increase in Hct from baseline). All responding patients who received maintenance therapy continued to respond (8/8), whereas responding patients who discontinued epoetin alfa relapsed at a median of 2 mo (9/9). The median follow-up time of the maintenance phase was 12 mo. Thus, continued maintenance therapy appears to be necessary to maintain responses to rHuEPO therapy in patients with CLL.

In both the Rai and Binet staging systems, severe anemia (Hb concentration < 11 g/dL and Hct < 33% in Rai, and Hb concentration < 10 g/dL in Binet) is associated with poor prognosis and is part of the definition of an advanced-stage patient. The National Cancer Institute (NCI) guidelines for management of CLL state that B-CLL patients with Hb concentration < 10 g/dL are candidates for chemotherapy *(22)*. Studies have reported that the response to rHuEPO in CLL patients results in the "downstaging" of patients *(32,33)*. Pangalis et al. *(34)* conducted a study to evaluate the clinical impact of the downstaging of CLL patients by improvement of disease-related anemia. The primary endpoint was whether increasing the Hct in patients could postpone the need for cytotoxic therapy and prolong survival.

For this study, 32 consecutive patients with B-CLL diagnosed with Rai stage III (intermediate) or IV (advanced) were eligible to enroll into an epoetin alfa treatment protocol if anemia developed (anemia was defined as Hct < 32% on two occasions 2 wk apart). Of the 32 patients, 11 were anemic at diagnosis, and 14 developed anemia during follow-up (median: 53.5 mo), for a total of 25 study patients with disease-related anemia. Of the 25 patients, 15 had no prior or concurrent chemotherapy, 9 had received prior chemotherapy but had been discontinued for at least 3 mo, and 1 received chlorambucil during the study.

Treatment involved an induction phase with epoetin alfa 150 U/kg three times/wk sc, for a maximum period of 12 wk. If response was slow after 4 wk (Hct increase < 6 points from baseline), the dose was increased in 50-U/kg increments to a maximum of 300 U/kg three times/wk. After the induction period, all responding patients were converted to maintenance therapy with 150 U/kg epoetin alfa sc weekly. After 12 wk of sustained responses on the maintenance schedule, the dosing interval was increased from 7 to 10 d.

The primary endpoint of the study was time to cytotoxic chemotherapy. Blood counts were evaluated every 2 wk during induction and every 4 wk thereafter. In cases of disease progression, cytotoxic therapy was initiated. Complete Hct responses (Hct ≥ 38%) were observed in 18/25 patients. Partial Hct responses (>6-point increase from baseline) were observed in 2 additional patients, for an overall response rate of 80% (20/25). Eighteen/20 responding patients had sustained responses at a median of >30.8 mo. The remaining two patients died of infection while still responding to epoetin alfa. Dose escalation of epoetin alfa to 300 U/kg occurred in seven nonresponding patients, two of whom went on to achieve a complete response.

After induction, responding patients were restaged using Rai criteria. This resulted in the downstaging of 19/20 responding patients from Rai stage III to Rai stage 0 (n = 6), stage I (n = 9), or stage II (n = 4). In the one patient in whom "downstaging" did not occur, anemia was corrected but thrombocytopenia persisted. Disease progression was observed in 4/20 responding patients, triggering initiation of cytotoxic chemotherapy. In addition, one patient developed autoimmune hemolysis, requiring corticosteroids. The 15 remaining patients (11/13 previously untreated and 4/7 previously treated) remained free of antileukemic therapy at a median of 31+ mo. Neither the median time to leukemic therapy nor the median overall survival had been reached at the time of publication. The probability of response to epoetin alfa was decreased in patients with CLL who had increased pretreatment serum EPO concentrations, and among patients with lymphadenopathy and splenomegaly. The probability of response was independent of the extent or pattern of bone marrow infiltration.

As the authors of the study noted, the clinical trial did not prove that exogenous EPO exerts an effect on the biologic course of B-CLL, but it does raise the issue of whether anemia is a suitable criteria for B-CLL staging.

Exogenous EPO have been well tolerated and safe in all clinical trials reported to date in CLL *(27–34)*. Most adverse events were attributed to the underlying malignancies or antitumor therapy and were reported with equal frequency for the erythropoietic and placebo cohorts. Transient skin reaction at the injection sites were the most common rHuEPO-related toxicity.

Two consensus papers were published in 2002 with specific recommendations for the management of disease-related anemia (i.e., multiple myeloma and CLL) with exogenous EPO. These reviews contain critical and extensive analyses of the existing literature and have specific recommendations with regard to patient management *(35,36)*.

3. TRIALS WITH GRANULOCYTE COLONY-STIMULATING AND GRANULOCYTE-MACROPHAGE COLONY-STIMULATING FACTORS

Both recombinant human granulocyte colony-stimulating factor (rHuG-CSF) and granulocyte-macrophage colony-stimulating factor (rHuGM-CSF) have been evaluated for their potential to manage neutropenia in patients with CLL.

3.1. Granulocyte Colony-Stimulating Factor

CLL patients treated with fludarabine have been reported to have a significant incidence of severe infections (i.e., sepsis or pneumonia), especially in patients with advanced-stage disease or those who were pretreated *(37)*. The incidence of severe infections ranged from 12% in previously untreated early-stage patients to 54% in previously treated advanced-stage patients. Grade 3 and 4 neutropenia were frequently reported and resulted in delays in therapy for approx 50% of the patients treated with fludarabine.

Table 5
Comparison of Therapy Delays Between Filgrastim-Treated and Historical Control Patients

Course days	*% of patients*		p Value
	Fludarabine + filgrastim	*Historical control*	
>35	20	50	0.005
>42	12	29	0.03
>49	12	23	0.23

Data from ref. *38*.

In a phase 2 trial, 25 patients with CLL were enrolled in a study of fludarabine 30 mg/m^2 iv for 30 min each day for 5 d, repeated every 4 wk. In addition, rHuG-CSF (filgrastim) was administered at 5 μg/kg/d sc starting on d 6 and continuing until an absolute granulocyte count (AGC) of 10 × 10^9/L. Prophylactic antibiotics were not administered. Data from these 25 patients with CLL were compared with data from an historical control group of 145 CLL patients (previously treated Rai stage III and IV) who received single-agent fludarabine or fludarabine and oral prednisone at a dose of 30 mg/m^2 daily for 5 d per month. Response rates and overall toxic effects were similar among the historical control group patients except for an increase in *Listeria monocytogenes* sepsis and/or *Pneumocystis carinii* pneumonia that occurred only in patients given the combination therapy *(37)*.

No difference was seen in the response rate or in the median time to disease progression between the treatment group and the historical control group *(38)*. A statistically significantly difference with less grade 3 and 4 neutropenia was seen in the treatment groups compared with historical controls for all cycles of therapy (nadir < 1.0 × 10^9/L, 45% vs 79%, p = 0.002; nadir < 0.5 × 10^9/L, 15% vs 63%, p = 0.000) as well as for each individual cycle of therapy. The incidence of prolonged delays in treatment was decreased (Table 5).

The incidence of pneumonia was significantly decreased among treated patients compared with historical controls (8% vs 37%, p = 0.004). Comparison of courses in historical control patients during which pneumonia did or did not develop showed that the only significant factor was neutropenia. Pneumonia occurred in 16% of courses in which AGC was <0.5 × 10^9/L vs 8% of courses for which AGC was >0.5 × 10^9/L (p = 0.009) *(38)*. The incidence of sepsis did not differ between treated and historical control patients in this relatively small trial. Filgrastim therapy was reported to be safe and well tolerated.

3.2. Granulocyte-Macrophage Colony-Stimulating Factor

Two pilot trials have reported on the use of rHuGM-CSF (molgramostim) in patients with CLL *(39,40)*. In one trial, seven patients with CLL were eligible to receive rHuGM-CSF 5 μg/kg/d sc for 28 d if they demonstrated chronic neutropenia ("absolute" neutropenia of <1.5 × 10^9/L, or "relative" neutropenia of 1.5–3.3 × 10^9/L and a history of recurrent bacterial infections). Three patients had "absolute" neutropenia, and four had "relative" neutropenia at baseline. Of the seven patients, five completed 28 d of rHuGM-CSF. Two patients discontinued the study (d 14 and d 25) owing to rHuGM-CSF-related toxicities. All patients had a statistically significant increase in peripheral neutrophils ($p = 0.022$) and eosinophils ($p = 0.034$) at end of study *(39)*.

In a study evaluating the long-term impact of rHuGM-CSF management of patients with CLL, 8 neutropenic CLL patients with a history of recurrent bacterial infections were administered 5 μg/kg/d of rHuGM-CSF sc for a maximum of 3 mo *(40)*. Doses of rHuGM-CSF were adjusted according to the neutrophil count and drug-related adverse effects. Of the eight patients enrolled on the trial, four received rHuGM-CSF for 3 mo. The remaining four patients discontinued treatment after 2, 4, 5, and 7 wk of therapy owing to rHuGM-CSF-related toxicity. (Three had progressive thrombocytopenia, and one had painful local skin reactions.) A statistically significant increase in the median neutrophil and eosinophil counts was reported ($p = 0.01$), as was a statistically significant decrease in the platelet counts ($p = 0.05$). Interestingly, in two patients the size of peripheral lymph nodes decreased by approx 50% while they were receiving rHuGM-CSF therapy. Side effects with rHuGM-CSF treatment were common and included fatigue (6/7), edema (5/7), injection-site reactions (3/7), and transient bone pain (2/7). Of note, five of the patients on the trial received concomitant low-dose chemotherapy with the rHuGM-CSF treatment, owing to active disease at baseline (daily low-dose chlorambucil or cyclophosphamide with or without prednisone). All five patients increased their neutrophil counts while receiving rHuGM-CSF, suggesting that myelotoxicity was not enhanced. In conclusion, although rHuGM-CSF increased neutrophil counts in these patients with CLL, its chronic administration was complicated by adverse effects (fatigue, edema, thrombocytopenia, and local skin reactions). The study size precluded an evaluation of the impact of rHuGM-CSF on the incidence of infection *(40)*.

A pilot study evaluating rHuGM-CSF (sargramostim) in 11 neutropenic patients with lymphoproliferative disorders included 4 patients with CLL *(41)*. rHuGM-CSF was administered by continuous iv infusion for 2 wk on with 2 wk off. Three of the patients with CLL were started at 120 μg/m^2/d and one at 60 μg/m^2/d. For all four patients, increases in neutrophils, monocytes, and eosinophils were observed. Side effects of therapy were generally mild to moderate and well tolerated. Common side effects included fever, chills, myalgia, bone pain, and gastrointestinal disturbances. Again, owing to the limited size of the study, conclusions regarding the impact on infection rates were not possible *(41)*.

3.3. Clinical Experience With Granulocyte-Stimulating Factors in Patients With CLL Receiving Myelosuppresive Therapies

3.3.1. Outpatient Therapies

Support with filgrastim has been used to increase the ability of patients with CLL to tolerate myelosuppressive chemotherapies in trials using primary prophylaxis rHuG-CSF (*see* Table 6 for selected trials).

Alternatively, rHuG-CSF has been used as secondary prophylaxis to maintain planned dose and schedule in patients who have experienced severe and/or prolonged neutropenia (*see* Table 7 for selected trials using secondary prophylaxis rHuG-CSF.)

3.3.2. High-Dose Chemotherapy With Stem Cell Support

B-cell CLL is not curable with conventional therapy. New treatment modalities with curative potential that are being investigated include autologous transplantation (usually with a purging procedure) and reduced-intensity allogeneic transplant.

Table 6
Selected Trials: Primary Prophylactic rHuG-CSF Support of Chemotherapy

Ref.	*Chemotherapy*	*Disease/ condition (no.)*	*Objective response rate to chemotherapy (%)*
67	Fludarabine; cyclophosphamide	Elderly refractory CLL patients (17)	100 (47 CR, 53 PR)
68	Cyclophosphamide; mesna; vincristine; daunoxome; dexamethasone	Richter's syndrome patients (29)	41 (38 CR, 3 PR)
69	Fludarabine; cyclophosphamide	Previously untreated (37)	63.9 (41.7 CR, 22.2 PR)
70	Fludarabine; cyclophosphamide	Previously untreated (17)	100 (47 CR, 53 PR)

ABBREVIATIONS: CR, complete response; PR, partial response.

Table 7
Selected Trials: Secondary Prophylaxis With rHuG-CSF in CLL Chemotherapy Trials

Ref.	*Chemotherapy*	*Patients (no.)*
71	Fludarabine; ara-C; novantrone; dexamethasone	Previously treated (31)
72	Cladribine; cyclophosphamide	Previously untreated (82)
73	Alemtuzamab	Previously treated (18)
74	Alemtuzamab	Previously untreated (41)

Autologous transplant in CLL has several concerns; autografts are usually contaminated with significant numbers of leukemic cells, CLL is a disease of the elderly, that often leads to morbidity and mortality after the transplantation of purged stem cells, and relapses occur frequently, suggesting that reduction of the leukemic burden may be insufficient. The use of rHuG-CSF has allowed investigators to address some of these concerns: the use of rHuG-CSF-mobilized peripheral blood progenitor cells (PBPCs) rather than bone marrow as a source of stem cells has been reported to increase the number of CD34 cells collected significantly and to shorten the duration of post-transplant aplasia resulting from ex vivo-purged autografts *(42,43)*. Furthermore, identification of high-risk patients (high leukocyte count, diffuse bone marrow infiltration, short lymphocyte doubling time, and unfavorable genetics or advanced stage) has, especially in younger patients, facilitated identification of patients for whom an indolent disease course is unlikely and for whom potentially curative therapies are required *(44)*.

Preliminary reports have suggested that myeloablative radiochemotherapy with stem cell support may have curative potential in CLL *(45,46)*. Several trials have used rHuG-CSF for mobilization of PBPCs and for post-transplant support of granulocytopoiesis *(47,48)*. Filgrastim was administered at a dose of 10 μg/kg/d sc through the last day of leukapheresis for stem cell mobilization. Despite the advanced disease of the patients, adequate PBPC harvests were obtained after one (n = 15) or two (n = 5) leukapheresis procedures in all patients *(48)*. (An adequate harvest was defined as >2 × 10^9 $CD34^+$/kg). PBPCs were doubly selected: a positive $CD34^+$ selection followed by a negative anti-CD19/20/23/37 selection. Infusion of the double-purged PBPCs (median $CD34^+$ count: 4.6 × 10^9/kg) was well tolerated and was supported by daily filgrastim (5 μg/kg/d) to accelerate neutrophil recovery. Prompt engraftment of neutrophils (medium: 9 d) and platelets (medium: 10 d) was seen in 19/20 patients. One patient had delayed platelet recovery owing to development of grade 3 veno-occlusive disease. Engraftment was durable, as evidenced by a normal platelet counts 3 mo post transplant in most patients *(48)*. With a median follow-up of 20 mo, 17 patients were in complete clinical remission. One patient died of a pulmonary embolism, one patient had a clinical relapse at 7 mo after transplant, and one patient had an increase in CLL cells in the peripheral blood without meeting criteria for relapse. Continued follow-up is necessary to assess the clinical significance of this approach.

Allogenic transplants for CLL present a different set of concerns than autologous transplants: graft contamination is not an issue, but graft-versus-host disease (GvHD) is. The advanced median age of CLL patients puts them at significant risk for GvHD-mediated morbidity and mortality (ranging from 20 to 40%) *(49)*. The graft-versus-leukemia effect (GvL) is the antileukemic activity of the donor origin immune cells. The ability of allogenic stem cell grafts to eliminate leukemia has been thought to relate both to the intensity of the conditioning regimen and to the number and functional activity of the donor immune cells. However, infused donor lymphocytes in the absence of additional chemotherapy are capable of reinducing complete remission in patients with CLL who have relapsed after allogenic transplantation *(50,51)*. This GVL effect may require several weeks to months after donor lymphocyte infusion to become evident. Persistent engraftment of the allogenic effector cells is presumed to be necessary for GvL effects to occur.

Allogenic stem cell transplant is an effective therapeutic intervention for a select subset of patients with CLL *(52–54)*. The toxicity of high-dose radiochemotherapy conditioning regimens has limited the utility of allogenic transplants in CLL to young patients (<45 yr of age) without comorbid disease. As a result, only a small number of patients with CLL have been eligible for this potentially curative therapy. Reduced intensity conditioning regimens that emphasize GvL as the primary therapeutic approach have been studied in several hematologic malignancies in an attempt to extend the benefits of potentially curative therapy to a wider population. Donor leukocyte infusions have been administered as needed to augment GvL in such patients. Potentially, this clinical strategy may allow older patients and patients with comorbidities to benefit from the effects of GVL *(55)*. Fludarabine is the cornerstone for reduced-intensity conditioning regimens for CLL. This agent is an effective agent in CLL for several reasons *(56)*: it induces lymphocytopenia, it is highly immunosuppressive *(57)*, and it has a mild nonhematologic toxicity.

Two clinical studies have reported on the use of reduced intensity conditioning regimens with allogenic stem cell support *(58,59)*. Khouri et al. *(58)* reported on 15 patients of whom 6 had CLL. Cyclophosphamide (300 mg/m^2 iv on d –5, –4, and –3) and fludarabine (30 mg/m^2 iv on d –5, –4, and –3) were administered as the conditioning regimen. Patients received PBPCs from filgrastim-stimulated (6 μg/kg every 12 h for 4–5 d) HLA-identical donors on day 0. Filgrastim was administered (5 μg/kg daily) from d 0 until recovery of granulocytes to >1 × 10^6/dL. All patients had prompt hematopoietic recovery. Three of the six patients had evidence of donor engraftment, as indicated by marrow studies. Among the three patients who had donor stem cell engraftment, two achieved a complete response and one a partial response. Among the three patients with CLL who did not engraft donor lymphocytes, one had a partial response, one had no response, and one had progressive disease *(58)*.

Perez-Simon et al. *(59)* reported on a series of 34 patients (including 3 with CLL) treated with reduced-intensity conditioning regimen and allogenic transplantation who, because of age, relapse from a prior transplant, or comorbid disease, were considered to be at high risk for a standard allogenic transplant. Patients with CLL received a conditioning regimen that consisted of fludarabine (30 mg/m^2 iv on d –8, –7, –6, –5, and –4) and melphalan (70 mg/m^2 iv on d –3 and –2). Filgrastim-stimulated PBPCs from HLA-matched related donors were infused on d 0. Among the three patients with CLL, two had a complete response and one had a partial response. Acute GvHD was not observed, but one patient had chronic GvHD. The "transplant lite" approach was well tolerated and remains under investigation.

3.3. Clinical Utilization Issues

3.3.1. Safety

Both filgrastim and rHuGM-CSF have been safe and well tolerated in patients with hematologic toxicities. Medullary bone pain, reported in up to 24% of patients, was the only consistently observed adverse reaction attributed to filgrastim therapy. Mild-to-moderate spontaneously reversible increases in uric acid, lactate dehydrogenase, and alkaline phosphatase have been reported in filgrastim-treated patients (27–58% of patients) *(38,65–72)*.

Additional adverse events have been reported with clinical use of the rHuGM-CSF. Sargramostim has been associated with a low incidence of fluid retention (4%), dyspnea secondary to sequestration of granulocytes in the pulmonary circulation, and/or occasional transient supraventricular arrhythmia in addition to medullary bone pain *(39–41,60)*.

3.3.2. Clinical Recommendations

The American Society of Clinical Oncology issued updated guidelines on the recommendations for the use of hematopoietic colony-stimulating factors in 2002. These guidelines contain critical reviews of the existing data and specific recommendations regarding patient management *(61)* (*see* Chap. 10 for more information).

4. COLONY-STIMULATING FACTOR THERAPY FOR ADVANCED UNRESPONSIVE CHRONIC LYMPHOCYTIC LEUKEMIA

Patients with advanced unresponsive B-cell CLL have limited therapeutic options. Patients have often been treated intensively and have limited marrow reserve, resulting in anemia, thrombocytopenia, neutropenia, and recurrent infections. Russo et al. *(62)* conducted a pilot trial in four refractory patients with B-CLL who were managed with a cytokine combination regimen consisting of rHuGM-CSF (2.5 µg/kg/d sc on d 1–14 during induction, and 2.5 µg/kg/d on alternate days during maintenance) and rHuEPO (150 U/kg/d on d 1–14 during induction and 150 U/kg/d on alternate days during maintenance).

Table 8
Response to Previous Therapies of Advanced B-CLL Patients Entered Onto Combination Cytokine Therapy

Patient no.	*First line*	*Response (NCI)/duration*	*Second line*	*Response (NCI)/duration*	*Third line*	*Response (NCI)/duration*
1	CLB/PDN	PR/32 mo	CHOP	PR/15 mo	FAMP	PR/23 mo
2	CLB/PDN	PR/48 mo	CHOP-like	PR/20 mo	FAMP	PR/11 mo
3	CLB/PDN	PR/39 mo	COP	PR/33 mo	FAMP	PR/ND
4	CLB/PDN	PR/45 mo	FAMP	PR/ND	—	—

ABBREVIATIONS: CLB, chlorambucil; PDN, prednisone; FAMP, fludarabine; CHOP, cyclophosphamide + doxorubicin partial response; ND, not determined; PR, partial response; NCI, National Cancer Institute.

Data from ref. *62*.

The rationale for managing patients with advanced refractory B-CLL with combination cytokine therapy includes the following factors:

- Heavily pretreated B-CLL patients were not eligible to receive cytotoxic antileukemic agents because of compromised marrow reserve.
- In vivo and in vitro evidence suggests that cytokines may influence the pathophysiology (especially dysregulated apoptosis and/or cell cycle pathways) in B-CLL lymphocytes *(63)*.
- rHuGM-CSF supports granulocytopoiesis *(38–41)* and may have antileukemic activity in B-CLL *(40)*.
- rHuEPO is highly effective at correcting disease-related anemia in B-CLL *(29–32)* and may have antineoplastic activity *(64,65)*.

The four patients with B-CLL reported in this pilot study had advanced diseases (Binet stage C, Rai high risk) and were heavily pretreated with alkylating agent and nucleoside analog-based regimens (Table 8). At time of entry onto the study all patients had anemia, thrombocytopenia, neutropenia, and lymphocytosis in the bone marrow (Table 9). Systemic symptoms were present in all patients, as were lymphadenopathy and splenomegaly (Table 10).

All patients responded positively to treatment with combination cytokine therapy. Improvements in anemia and neutropenia were observed: 3/4 patients increased their Hb concentrations to >11 g/dL; neutrophils increased to $>1.5 \times 10^9$/L. This translated into a decrease in the number of infections as well as a decrease in the number of transfusions per patient (Table 11). More surprisingly, patients also demonstrated objective tumor responses. All four patients achieved a partial response (Table 11). At the time of publication, three of the patients maintained their partial response (at 4+, 11+, and 12+ mo), and one patient progressed after 10 mo. Lymphadenopathy and splenomegaly decreases of >50% were observed. Leukemic bone marrow infiltrates decreased in all patients. Based on these preliminary data, continued study of combined cytokine therapy in advanced stage B-CLL seems warranted.

5. SUMMARY

B-CLL is at present an incurable disease. The natural progression of the disease involves increasingly frequent recurrent infections as well as increasingly severe anemia.

Table 9
Laboratory Hematologic Values Before Initiating the rHuGM-CSF Plus rHuEPO Schedule

	Before initiation					*One month after initiation*				
	Peripheral blood cells					*Peripheral blood cells*				
Patient no.	*PBL × 10^9/L*	*Hb g/dL*	*PMN × 10^9/L*	*PLT × 10^9/L*	*Bone marrow (% of lymphs.)*	*PBL × 10^9/L*	*Hb g/dL*	*PMN × 10^9/L*	*PLT × 10^9/L*	*Bone marrow (% of lymphs.)*
1	187	7.0	1.2	9	96	>50% decrease	>11	>1.5	>50% increase	80
2	109	7.1	0.8	87	90	>50% decrease	>11	>1.5	>100	72
3	59	8.0	0.9	32	73	>50% decrease	>11	>1.5	>50% increase	60
4	27	6.4	0.3	40	82	>50% decrease	25% increase	>1.5	Stable	78

ABBREVIATIONS: PBL, peripheral blood lymphocytes; Hb, hemoglobin; PMN, polymorphonuclear cells; PLT, platelets.

Table 10
Characteristics of CLL Patients Before and After Initiating rHuGM-CSF Plus rHuEPO Therapy

			Physical examination before initiation				Physical examination 1 mo after initiation				
Patient no.	*ECOG*	*Stage (Binet/Rai)*	*Liver*	*Spleen*	*Node*	*Systemic systems*	*ECOG*	*Liver*	*Spleen*	*Node*	*Systemic symptoms*
1	2	C/high risk	Normal	Palpable (3 cm)	Axillae (2 cm)	Yes	1	Stable	Stable	>50% decrease	Absent
2	2	C/high risk	Palpable (3 cm)	Palpable (10 cm)	Neck, axillae groins (4 cm)	Yes	1	Stable	>50% decrease	50% decrease	Absent
3	2	C/high risk	Normal	Palpable (7 cm)	Neck, axillae groins (3 cm)	Yes	1	Stable	>50% decrease	>50% decrease	Absent
4	2	C/high risk	Palpable (3 cm)	Palpable (6 cm)	Neck, axillae groins (4 cm)	Yes	1	Stable	>50% decrease	Stable	Absent

ABBREVIATIONS: ECOG, Eastern Cooperative Oncology Group.

Table 11
Transfusion Requirement and Infections in Advanced B-Cell Chronic Lymphocytic Leukemia (B-CLL) Patients Managed With rHuGM-CSF and rHuEPO

	Type and duration of response			*1 year before cytokine administration*		*During cytokine therapy (range: 4–13 mo; median: 11)*	
Patient no.	*NCI*	*IW-CLL*	*Duration (mo)*	*Transfusions (units of packed red cells/mo)*	*No. of infections (per mo)*	*Transfusions (units of packed red cells/mo)*	*No. of infections (per mo)*
1	PR	PR	10	1.2	2.4	0.1	0.1
2	PR	PR	12+	0.9	1.3	0.1	0.1
3	PR	PR	11+	0.5	1.7	0.0	0.4
4	PR	PR	4+	0.8	1.6	0.5	0.3

ABBREVIATIONS: PR, partial response; NCI, National Cancer Institute; IW, International Working Party.

Currently available cytotoxic therapies contribute to the risk of anemia and of recurrent infections owing to iatrogenic myelosuppression. Available recombinant human cytokines are safe and well tolerated. They can ameliorate the anemia and recurrent infections in patients with CLL and thereby result in improved patient reported outcomes and increased compliance with the intended therapeutic regimens.

rHuEPO and darbepoetin alfa have been shown to reverse anemia and maintain normal Hb concentrations and Hct in patients receiving myelosuppressive chemotherapy. The potential clinical benefits of "downstaging" patients with CLL through exogenous EPO support warrant further investigation. rHuG-CSF has been shown to decrease the risk of pneumonia, to facilitate recovery from chemotherapy-induced neutropenia, and to support delivery of the planned dose and schedule of therapeutic regimens in patients with CLL. rHuG-CSF has also facilitated the investigation of autologous and allogeneic stem cell transplants as potentially curative therapy for CLL. Finally, early pilot data suggest that combination cytokine therapy may have a role to play in the palliative management of patients with advanced unresponsive B-CLL.

It is hoped that increased understanding of the molecular basis and biologically distinct subsets of CLL will lead to more effective and impactful therapeutic interventions in future. At present, recombinant exogenous cytokines are available to address the anemia and neutropenia that are characteristic symptoms of the disease and to support the delivery of available therapeutic interventions.

REFERENCES

1. American Cancer Society Cancer Facts and Figures 2002;5.
2. Ries LAG, Miller BA, Hankey BF, et al. *Surveillance Epidemiology End Results (SEER) Cancer Statistics Review 1973–1991: Tables and Graphics.* Report no: NIH-94-2789. Bethesda, MD: National Cancer Institute. 1994.
3. Freedman AS, Nadler LM. Immunologic markers in B cell chronic lymphocytic leukemia. In: Cheson BD, ed., *Chronic Lymphocytic Leukemia: Scientific Advances and Clinical Developments,* 2nd ed. Dekker, New York, NY, 2001.
4. Johnson TA, Rassenti LZ, Kipps TJ. Ig VH1 genes expressed in B cell chronic lymphocytic leukemia exhibit distinctive molecular features. *J Immunol* 1997; 158:235–246.

5. Manison YA. The infectious complication of chronic lymphocytic leukemia. *Semin Oncol* 1998; 25:98–106.
6. Heath ME, Cheson BD. Defective complement activation in chronic lymphocytic leukemia. *Am J Hematol* 1985; 19:63–73.
7. Bunch C, Chapel H, Gale RP. Infection complications in CLL. In: Polliack A, Cotouskey D, eds., *Chronic Lymphocytic Leukemia.* London: Harwood Academic. 1988:248–262.
8. Cooperative Group for the Study of Immunoglobulins in Chronic Lymphocytic Leukemia. Intravenous immunoglobulin for the prevention of infection in chronic lymphocytic leukemia. A randomized, controlled clinical trial. *N Engl J Med* 1988; 319:902–907.
9. Kalil N, Cheson BD. Management of chronic lymphocytic leukemia. *Drugs Aging* 2000; 16:9–27.
10. Duhrsen U, Augener W, Zwingers T, et al. Spectrum and frequency of auto immune derangements in lymphoproliferative disorders: analysis of 637 cases and comparison with myeloproliferative diseases. *Br J Haematol* 1987; 67:235–239.
11. Ritch PS, Anderson T. Reversal of autoimmune hemolytic anemia associated with chronic lymphocytic leukemia following high dose immunoglobulin. *Cancer* 1987; 60:2637–2640.
12. Binet J, Auquier A, Dighiero G, et al. A new prognostic classification of chronic lymphocytic leukemia derived from a multivariate survival analysis. *Cancer* 1981; 48:198–206.
13. Rozman C, Montserrat E, Rodriguez-Fernandez JM, et al. Bone marrow histologic pattern—the best single prognostic parameter in chronic lymphocytic leukemia: a multivariate survival analysis of 329 cases. *Blood* 1984; 64:642–648.
14. Pangalis GA, Angelopoulou MK, Vassilakopoulos TP, et al. B-chronic lymphocytic leukemia, small lymphocyte lymphoma and lymphocytic leukemia, lymphoplasmacytic lymphoma including Waldenström's macroglobulinemia: a clinical, morphologic and biologic spectrum of similar disorders. *Semin Hematol* 1999; 36:104–114.
15. Means RT, Krantz SB. Progress in understanding the parthogenesis of the anemia of chronic disease. *Blood* 1992; 80:1639–1642.
16. Sears DA. Anemia of chronic disease. *Med Clin North Am* 1992; 76:567–579.
17. Faquin WC, Schneider TJ, Goldberg MA. Effect of inflammatory cytokines on hypoxia-induced erythropoietin production. *Blood* 1994; 79:1987–1994.
18. Hulkkonen J, Vilpo J, et al. Interleukin/B, interleukin-1 receptor antagonist and interleukin 6 plasma levels and cytokine gene polymorphisms in chronic lymphocytic leukemia: cancellation with prognostic parameters. *Haematologica* 2000; 85:600–606.
19. Beguin Y, Lampertz S, Bron D, et al. Serum erythropoiesis in chronic lymphocytic leukemia. *Br J Haematol* 1996; 93:154–156.
20. Chikkappa G, Pasquale D, Zarrabi MH, et al. Cyclosporine and prednisone therapy for pure red cell aplasia in patients with chronic lymphocytic leukemia. *Am J Hematol* 1992; 41:5–12.
21. Kohlman A, Schoh C, Dugas M, et al. Gene expression profiles of distinct cytogenetic CCL subtypes. *Blood* 2002:100:168a (abstract 169).
22. Cheson BD, Bennet JM, Grever M, et al. National Cancer Institute Working Group guideline for chronic lymphocytic leukemia: revised guidelines for diagnosis and treatment. *Blood* 1996:87:4990–4997.
23. French Cooperative Group on CLL, Johnson S, Smith AG, et al. Randomized trial of fludarabine versus cyclophosphamide, doxorubicin and prednisone for treatment of advanced stage chronic lymphocytic leukemia. *Lancet* 1996; 347:1432–1437.
24. Rai KR, Peterson B, Elias L, et al. A randomized comparison of fludarabine and chlorambucil for patients with previously untreated chronic lymphocytic leukemia. A CALGB, SWOG, CT C/NC1-C and ECOG Intergroup Study. *Blood* 1996; 88:141a (abstract 552).
25. Leporrier S, Chevret B, Cazin B, et al. Randomized comparison of fludarabine CAO and CHOP in 695 previously untreated stage B and C chronic lymphocytic leukemia (CLL): early stopping of the CAP accrual. *Blood* 1997; 90:5290a (abstract 2357).
26. Bowen AL, Zomas A, Emmett E, et al. Subcutaneous CAMPATH-^{1}H in fludarabine resistant/relapsed chronic lymphocytic and B-prolymphocytic leukemia. *Br J Haematol* 1997; 96:617–619.
27. Cazzola M, Messinger D, Battistel V, et al. Recombinant human erythropoietin in the anemia associated with multiple myeloma or non-Hodgkin's lymphoma: dose finding and identification of predictors of response. *Blood* 1995; 86:4446–4453.
28. Österborg A, Boogaerts MA, Cimino R, et al. Recombinant human erythropoietin in transfusion-dependent anemia patients with multiple myeloma and non-Hodgkin's lymphoma: a randomized

multicenter study—The European Study Group of Erythropoietin (Epoetin Beta) Treatment in Multiple Myeloma and Non-Hodgkin's Lymphoma. *Blood* 1996; 87:2675–2682.
29. Österborg A, Brandberg Y, Molostova V, et al. Randomized, double blind, placebo controlled trial of recombinant human erythropoietin, epoetin beta, in hematologic malignancies. *J Clin Oncol* 2002; 20:2486–2494.
30. Rose E, Rai K, Revicki D, et al. Clinical and health status assessments in anemia chronic lymphocytic leukemia (CLL) patients treated with epoetin alfa (EPO). *Blood* 1994; 8:256 (abstract 2091).
31. Hedenus M, Hansen S, Taylor K, et al. Randomized dose finding study of darbepoetin alfa in anemic patients with lymphoproliferative malignancies. *Br J Haematol* 2002; 119:79–86.
32. Pangalis GA, Poziopoulos C, Angelopoulou M, et al. Effective treatment of disease-related anemia in B-chronic lymphocytic leukemia patients with recombinant human erythropoietin. *Br J Haematol* 1995; 89:627–629.
33. Siakantaris M, Angelopoulou M, Vassilakopoulos TP, et al. Correction of disease-related anemia of B-chronic lymphoproliferative disorders by recombinant human erythropoietin: maintenance is necessary to sustain response. *Leuk Lymphoma* 2000; 40:141–147.
34. Pangalis GA, Siakantaris MP, Angelopoulou MK, et al. Downstaging Rai stage III B-chronic lymphocytic leukemia patients with the administration of recombinant human erythropoietin. *Haematologica* 2002; 87:500–506.
35. Rizzo JD, Lichtin AE, Woolf SH, et al. Use of epoetin in patients with cancer: evidence based clinical practice guidelines of the American Society of Clinical Oncology and the American Society of Hematology. *J Clin Oncol* 2002; 20:4083–4107.
36. Ludwig H, Rai K, Blade J, et al. Management of disease-related anemia in patients with multiple myeloma or chronic lymphocytic leukemia: epoetin treatment recommendations. *Hematol J* 2002; 3:121–130.
37. O'Brien S, Kantarjian H, Beran M, et al. Results of fludarabine and prednisone therapy in 264 patients with chronic lymphocytic leukemia with multivariate analysis derived prognostic model for response to treatment. *Blood* 1993; 82:1695–1700.
38. O'Brien S, Kantarjian H, Beran M, et al. Fludarabine and granulocyte colony stimulating factor (G-CSF) in patients with chronic lymphocytic leukemia. *Leukemia* 1997; 11:1631–1635.
39. DeNully Brown P, Hansen M. GMCSF treatment in patients with B-chronic lymphocytic leukemia. *Leuk Lymphoma* 1999; 32:365–368.
40. Itala M, Pelliniemi T-T, Remes K, et al. Long term treatment with GM-CSF in patients with chronic lymphocytic leukemia and recurrent neutropenia infections. *Leuk Lymphoma* 1998; 32:165–174.
41. Vadhan-Raj S, Velasquez W, Butler J, et al. Stimulation of myelopoiesis in chronic lymphocytic leukemia and other lymphoproliferatived isorders by recombinant human granulocyte macrophage colony stimulating factor. *Am J Hematol* 1990; 33:189–197.
42. Dreger P, Neuhoff N, Suttorp M, et al. Rapid engraftment of peripheral blood progenitor cell grafts purged with B cell specific monoclonal antibodies and immunogenic beads. *Bone Marrow Transplant* 1995; 16:627–629.
43. Schmitz N, Linch DC, Dregen P, et al. Randomized trial of filgrastim mobilized peripheral blood progenitor cell transplantation versus autologous bone marrow transplantation in lymphoma patients. *Lancet* 1996; 347:353–357.
44. Rozman C, Montserat E. Chronic lymphocytic leukemia. *N Engl J Med* 1995; 333:1052–1057.
45. Khouri I, Keating M, Vriesendorp H, et al. Autologous and allogeneic bone marrow transplantation for chronic lymphocytic leukemia: preliminary results. *J Clin Oncol* 1994; 12:748–758.
46. Provan D, Bartlett-Pandite L, Zwicky C. Eradication of polymesase chain reaction-detectable chronic lymphocytic leukemia cells is associated with improved outcome after bone marrow transplantation. *Blood* 1996; 88:2228–2235.
47. Dreger P, von Neuhoff N, Kase R, et al. Early stem cell transplantation for chronic lymphocytic leukemia: a chance for cure? *Br J Cancer* 1998; 77:2291–2297.
48. Dreger P, Viehmann K, von Neuhoff, et al. A prospective study of positive/negative ex vivo B-cell depletion in patients with chronic lymphocytic leukemia. *Exp Hematol* 2000; 28:1187–1196.
49. Perez-Simon JA, Caballero D, Diez-Campelo M, et al. Chimerism and minimal residual disease monitoring after reduced intensity conditioning (RIC) allogeneic transplantation. *Leukemia* 2002; 16:1423–1431.
50. Kolb H, Schaltenberg A, Goldman J, et al. Graft versus leukemia effect of donor lymphocyte transfusions in marrow grafted patients. *Blood* 1985; 86:2041–2050.

51. Rondon G, Biralt S, Huh Y, et al. Graft versus leukemia effect after allogeneic bone marrow transplantation for chronic lymphocytic leukemia. *Bone Marrow Transplant* 1996; 18:669–672.
52. Khouri IF, Keating MJ, Vriesendorp HM, et al. Autologous and allogeneic bone marrow transplantation for chronic lymphocytic leukemia: preliminary results. *J Clin Oncol* 1994; 12:748–758.
53. Michallet M, Archimbaud E, Bandini G, et al. HLA-identical sibling bone marrow transplantation in chronic lymphocytic leukemia: 17 cases. Report from the EBMTG. *Bone Marrow Transplant* 1991; 7:275–279.
54. Rabinowe SN, Soiffer RJ, Gribben JG, et al. Autologous and allogeneic bone marrow transplantation for poor prognosis patients with B-cell chronic lymphocytic leukemia. *Blood* 1993; 82:1366–1376.
55. Giralt S, Estey E, Albitar M, et al. Engraftment of allogeneic hematopoietic progenitor cells with purine analog containing chemotherapy: harnessing graft versus leukemia without myeloablative therapy. *Blood* 1997; 89:4531–4536.
56. Keating MJ, Kantarjian H, Talpaz M, et al. Fludarabine: a new agent with major activity against chronic lymphocytic leukemia. *Blood* 1989; 74:19–25.
57. O'Brien S, Kantarjian H, Berane M, et al. Results of fludarabine and prednisone therapy in 264 patients with chronic lymphocytic leukemia with multivariate analysis-derived prognostic model for response to treatment. *Blood* 1993; 82:1695–1700.
58. Khouri IF, Keating MJ, Korbling M, et al. Transplant-lite: induction of graft versus malignancy using fludarabine-based nonablative chemotherapy and allogeneic blood progenitor cell transplantation as treatment for lymphoid malignancies. *J Clin Oncol* 1998; 16:2817–2824.
59. Perez-Simon JA, Caballero Diez-Compelo, et al. Chimerism and minimal residual disease monitoring after reduced intensity conditioning (RIC) allogeneic transplantation. *Leukemia* 2002; 16:1423–1431.
60. Physician's Desk Reference 2002.
61. Ozer H, Armitage JO, Bennett CL, et al. 2000 Update of recommendations for the use of hematopoietic colony-stimulating factors: evidence-based, clinical practice guidelines. *J Clin Oncol* 2000; 18:3558–3585.
62. Russo F, Guadagni R, Mattera G, et al. Combination of granulocyte-macrophage colony stimulating factor (GM-CSF) and erythropoietin (EPO) for the treatment of advanced non-responsive chronic lymphocytic leukemia. *Eur J Haematol* 1999; 63:325–331.
63. Kipps TJ. Signal transduction pathways and mechanisms of apoptosis in CLL-B lymphocytes: their role in CLL pathogenesis. *Hematol Cell Ther* 1997; 39:S17–S27.
64. Wu H, Klingmuller N, Besmer P, et al. Interaction of the erythropoietin and stem cell factor receptors. *Nature* 1995; 377:242–246.
65. Zhang MY, Harhaj EW, Bell L, et al. Bcl-3 expression and nuclear translocation are induced by proliferating human erythroid precursors. *Blood* 1998; 92:1225–1234.
66. Ludwig H. Anemia of hematologic malignancies: what are the treatment options? *Semin Oncol* 2002; 29:45–54.
67. Maretta G, et al. Low dose fludarabine and cyclophosphamide in elderly patients with B cell chronic lymphocytic leukemia refractory to conventional therapy. *Haematologica* 2000; 85:1268–1270.
68. Dabaja B, O'Brien S, Kantarjian H, et al. Franctionated cyclophosphamide, vincristine, liposomal daunobrubin (Daunoxome) and dexamethasone (Hyper CVXD) regimen in Richter's syndrome. *Leuk Lymphoma* 2001; 42:329–337.
69. Flinn I, Jemiai Y, Bennet J, et al. Fludarabine and cyclophosphamide achieves high complete response rate in patients with primarily untreated chronic lymphocytic leukemia ECOG 1997. *Blood* 2001; 98:633a.
70. Flinn I, Byrd JC, Morrison C, et al. Fludarabine and cyclophosphamide with filgrastim support in patients with previously untreated indolent lymphoid malignancies. *Blood* 2000; 96:71–75.
71. Mauro F, Foa R, Meloni G, et al. Fludarabine, ara-C, novantrone and dexamethasone (FAND) in previously treated chronic lymphocytic leukemia patients. *Haematologica* 2002; 87:926–933.
72. Robak T, Blonski J, Kaznicki M, et al. Cladribine combined with cyclophosphamide is highly effective in the treatment of chronic lymphocytic leukemia. *Hematol J* 2002; 3:244–250.
73. McCune S, Gockerman J, Moore L, et al. Alemtuzamab in relapsed or refractory chronic lymphocytic leukemia and prolymphocytic leukemia. *Leuk Lymphoma* 2002; 43:1007–1011.
74. Lundin J, Kimby E. Bjorkholm M, et al. Phase III trial of subcutaneous anti CD-52 monoclonal antibody alemtuzamab (Campath I-H) as first line treatment for patients with B-cell chronic lymphocytic leukemia (B-CLL). *Blood* 2002; 100:768–773.

17 Hematopoietic Growth Factor Therapy for Myelodysplastic Syndromes and Aplastic Anemia

Jason Gotlib, MD, MS *and*
Peter L. Greenberg, MD

CONTENTS

1. INTRODUCTION

Myelodysplastic syndromes (MDS) and idiopathic aplastic anemia (AA) are acquired bone marrow failure states. In AA, cytopenias are primarily caused by immune-mediated destruction of stem cells and concomitant severe compromise of hematopoiesis. In low-risk MDS, excessive intramedullary apoptosis of hematopoietic progenitors and ineffective hematopoiesis often account for the paradox of hypercellular marrows in the setting of chronic refractory cytopenias. Evolution to acute myeloid leukemia (AML) occurs in a proportion of patients with MDS and is frequently associated with reversion of marrow myeloid precursors to a leukemic phenotype. The development of recombinant cytokines has facilitated in vitro and in vivo analysis of the proliferative and differentiation defects involved in MDS and AA

From: *Cancer Drug Discovery and Development*
Hematopoietic Growth Factors in Oncology: Basic Science and Clinical Therapeutics
Edited by: G. Morstyn, M. A. Foote, and G. J. Lieschke © Humana Press Inc., Totowa, NJ

hematopoiesis. Cytokine therapy with recombinant human erythropoietin (rHuEPO) has resulted in clinically important erythroid responses in 20% of patients with MDS, which increases to 40% with addition of granulocyte colony-stimulating factor (rHuG-CSF). Identification of factors that predict response to these hematopoietic growth factors (HGFs) permits tailoring of these treatments to appropriate subsets of MDS patients. The rationale for using HGFs in AA has been to increase the pool of residual stem cells and to stimulate maturation of pre-existing progenitors in an attempt to ameliorate cytopenias; however, their prophylactic use as single agents has not been recommended. Instead, they have primarily been used as adjuncts to immunosuppressive therapy in the setting of clinical trials or in patients refractory to other therapies. Use of rHuG-CSF in AA has caused close scrutiny of the question as to whether the cytokine contributes to the increased risk of late clonal hematologic malignancies observed in a proportion of patients with AA.

2. MYELODYSPLASTIC SYNDROMES

2.1. MDS and In Vitro Hematopoiesis

In vitro culture systems have proved useful for analyzing the proliferative and differentiation effects of various HGFs on the hematopoietic stem/progenitor cell compartments. Such in vitro assays are particularly relevant to the study of MDS in which defective differentiation leads to ineffective hematopoiesis *(1)*. The colony-forming capacities of pluripotent hematopoietic stem cells (granulocyte, erythroid, macrophage, and megakaryocyte colony-forming units [CFU-GEMM]) and their progeny, committed progenitor cells (granulocyte-macrophage colony-forming units [CFU-GM], erythroid burst-forming units [BFU-E], erythroid colony-forming units [CFU-E], and megakaryocyte colony-forming units [CFU-Mk]) are low or absent in most MDS (and AML) patients *(1–5)*.

Two principal hematopoietic regulatory derangements found in MDS are diminished production and decreased responsiveness to HGFs *(1)*. Marrow cells and peripheral blood T cells from patients with MDS produce decreased amounts of GM-CSF, interleukin (IL)-3, monocyte colony-stimulating factor (M-CSF), and IL-6 *(6)*. Levels of monocyte-derived G-CSFs are decreased in patients with MDS and the elderly *(7)*. In clonogenic cultures, CFU-GM stimulated with rHuG-CSF and rHuGM-CSF were subnormal in most MDS patients *(8)*. In MDS, rHuGM-CSF and rHIL-3 generally have greater myeloid proliferative effects in vitro than rHuG-CSF, whereas rHuG-CSF has more potent differentiative effects. These findings are particularly evident in patients with refractory anemia with excess blasts/refractory anemia with excess blasts in transformation (RAEB/RAEB-T) patients and in those with normal cytogenetics *(8)*.

In vitro, MDS erythroid progenitor cells show suboptimal responses to rHuEPO *(9,10)*. Analysis of the relationship between endogenous EPO in MDS and patients' erythroid progenitors indicates that the anemia in MDS was not attributable to an abnormality in the capacity of EPO to induce generation of CFU-E, but was influenced by the size of the BFU-E population, whose severe deficiency resulted in insufficient influx of EPO-responsive cells *(10)*. These findings suggested that treatment of MDS with rHuEPO alone would have limited clinical benefit because the initial growth requirements and generation of BFU-E from more primitive cells were not solely regulated by this hormone. These in vitro predictions have been borne out in therapeutic clinical trials in which rHuEPO has shown modest efficacy in improving anemia. rHuG-CSF synergistically augments the in vitro EPO responsiveness of BFU-E in normal and MDS marrow *(10)*, and in clinical trials of the hormone combination, improved hemoglobin (Hb) responses were observed, particularly in patients with refractory anemia with ringed sideroblasts (RARS). Investigations using serum-free media and purified $CD34^+$ cells with recombinant HGFs have shown decreased responsiveness of MDS hematopoietic progenitors to rHuG-CSF and rHuEPO *(11)*. The mechanisms underlying the altered responsiveness of MDS precursors to cytokines is unclear. G-CSF and IL-3 binding in MDS have not exhibited significantly different receptor numbers or affinity for the receptors *(12)*. Postreceptor signaling pathway abnormalities after EPO binding have been noted in precursors from some patients with MDS *(13)*. These in vitro observations have served as a platform for clinical trial testing of various HGFs in MDS, including rHuEPO, rHuG-CSF *(see* Table 1*)*, as well as rHuGM-CSF, rHuILs, and recombinant thrombopoietic substances.

2.2. rHuEPO

Concentrations of endogenous EPO in patients with MDS may be suboptimally increased for the degree of their anemia. The rationale of rHuEPO therapy is to provide pharmacologic doses of the cytokine to increase serum EPO concentrations and to enhance the proliferation and maturation of marrow erythroid precursors. The clinical objective is to increase Hb concentrations and to reduce the risks associated with transfusion therapy, including infection, red cell alloimmunization, and secondary hemochromatosis. Although various criteria have been used to define response to rHuEPO therapy, and the proportion of low- and high-risk FAB (French-American-British) subtypes differs in each study, the cumulative response rate of numerous published small trials is approx 20% *(14–26)*. The Italian Cooperative Study Group has performed the only double-blind, placebo-controlled, randomized study of rHuEPO in MDS to date *(27)*. Patients with <10% marrow blasts received either placebo or rHuEPO 150 U/kg/d for 8 wk. A statistically significant Hb response was observed in the rHuEPO group, but benefit was limited to the refractory anemia (RA) subtype, and patients with either no prior transfusion requirements or basal endogenous EPO < 200 U/L. Other nonrandomized studies have cited serum EPO < 100 U/L, female sex, or normal karyotype as predictors of response to rHuEPO *(24,28)*. A recent study found that baseline serum EPO concentration predicted survival *(29)*. Patients with serum EPO > 50 U/L experienced a median survival of 17 mo compared with 65 mo in patients with serum EPO < 50 U/L.

Using red blood cell transfusion independence as the minimal criteria for response, one meta-analysis of 115 patients from 10 trials *(30)* and a second meta-analysis of 205 patients from 17 published reports *(31)* reported response rates of 23.5% and 16%, respectively. In the latter analysis, patients with RARS showed a significantly lower response rate (7.5%) than all other patients (21%). Other factors favoring response were the absence of transfusion need (44% vs. 10%) and serum EPO concentration ≤ 200 U/L. Patients without a transfusion requirement and MDS patients other than RARS showed a response rate > 50% irrespective of the serum EPO concentration. No dose-response relationship and no correlation between maximal dose and time to

Table 1
Clinical Trials of rHuEPO ± rHuG-CSF in MDS[a]

Dose	*No. of patients*	*Responses (%)*[b]	*Ref.*
rHuEPO alone			
350 U/kg/wk	16	13%	*15*
450–900 U/kg/wk	20	50%	*16*
900 U/kg/wk or 50,000 U/wk	12	8%	*18*
18,000–72,000 U/wk	14	29%	*19*
800 U/kg/wk	23	30%	*20*
210–1680 U/kg/wk	10	20%	*21*
225–750 U/kg/wk	13	38%	*22*
150 U/kg 3 ×/wk	27	26%	*28*
300–1200 U/kg/wk	20	35%	*23*
450–900 U/kg/wk	100	28%	*24*
450–900 U/kg/wk	12	58%	*25*
450–900 U/kg/wk	41	32%	*26*
1050 U/kg/wk	38	37%	*27*
150 U/kg 3×/wk	281	45%	*33*
150–200 U/kg 3×/wk	68	33%	*29*
Various doses and schedules[c]	110	24%	*30*
Various doses and schedules[c]	205	16%	*31*
rHuG-CSF and rHuEPO			
G-CSF 1 μg/kg/d EPO 150–300 U/kg/d	24	42%	*43*
G-CSF 0.3–3.0 μg/kg/d EPO 60–120 U/kg/d	21	38%	*44*
G-CSF 1 μg/kg/d EPO 150–300 U/kg/d	44	48%	*45*
G-CSF 0.3–3.0 μg/kg/d EPO 60–300 U/kg/d	98	36%	*46*
G-CSF 30–150 μg/d EPO 5000–10,000 U/d	47	38%	*47*
G-CSF 1 μg/kg 3×/wk EPO 300 U/kg 3×/wk	14	50%	*49*
G-CSF 1.5 μg/kg/d EPO 200–400 U/kg 3×/wk	25,28[d]	61%, 80%	*50*
G-CSF 75–300 μg/d EPO 10,000 U 5×/wk	53	42%	*48*

ABBREVIATIONS: rHuEPO, recombinant human erythropoietin; rHuG-CSF, recombinant human granulocyte colony-stimulating factor; MDS, myelodysplastic syndromes.

[a] Clinical trials enrolling 10 or more patients are shown.

[b] Response criteria differ between studies.

[c] Metaanalysis.

[d] Twenty-five patients evaluated in 12-wk follow-up with 61% response rate; 28 evaluated in 36-wk follow-up with 80% response rate.

response was seen. The optimal dose was generally in the range of 450–1000 U/kg/wk. The limited clinical efficacy of rHuEPO in these trials partly reflects the suboptimal responsiveness of myelodysplastic BFU-E to rHuEPO in vitro *(9,10)*.

Durability of rHuEPO response has been studied in two trials. In a small study of 18 primarily low-risk MDS patients treated with rHuEPO 10,000 U three times weekly, three patients were still responding at 30, 41, and 56 mo *(32)*. Two of these patients were maintained on a lower rHuEPO dose, and one was still responding 48 mo after rHuEPO had been discontinued. In seven patients, anemia recurred with tapering of the initial rHuEPO dose, and a second course of rHuEPO resulted in responses in 5 of 6 retreated patients. The remaining eight patients died during or soon after the initial treatment period, three from transformation to AML. At the time of follow-up, five patients maintained Hb responses with a median duration of 36+ mo.

A phase 2 study of 281 patients evaluated whether response rates to rHuEPO increase with prolonged administration *(33)*. Using a dose of 150 U/kg three times weekly, the overall erythroid response rate was 18.1% at 12 wk and increased to 45.1% at 26 wk. The median duration of response was 68 wk. Significant predictors of response included serum EPO < 150 U/L, good cytogenetic risk group by International Prognostic Scoring System (IPSS) criteria, and RA compared with RARS and RAEB FAB subtypes.

2.3. rHuEPO Plus Other Agents

In recent phase 2 trials, amifostine added to rHUEPO ± rHuGSF has generally not resulted in clinically significant erythroid responses or improvements in other blood lineages *(34–37)*. Sustained but limited multilineage responses (11%) were noted with all-*trans* retinoic acid plus EPO in low- and intermediate-risk MDS patients. Further study is warranted to evaluate this combination *(38)*.

2.4. rHuG-CSF

In a 6–8-wk dose-escalation phase 1–2 trial of subcutaneous (sc) rHuG-CSF at doses of 0.1–3.0 μg/kg/d *(39)*, 16/18 patients had an increase in the absolute neutrophil count (ANC) from 5- to 40-fold. Cessation of treatment resulted in return of counts to baseline values over a 2–4-wk period. Bone marrow myeloid maturation improved in 16/18 patients. No other significant lineage responses were noted. Eleven patients from this initial cohort were subsequently enrolled in a long-term maintenance trial of rHuG-CSF *(40)*. Ten patients responded with persistent improvements in neutrophil counts for up to 16 mo. In a retrospective analysis, there was a significant reduction in bacterial infection risk during periods with an ANC > 1.5 × 10^9/L with rHuG-CSF therapy compared with periods with an ANC < 1.5 × 10^9/L. Enhancement of in vitro neutrophil function (phagocytosis and chemotaxis) persisted during the maintenance phase. Of 10 anemic patients, 2 nontransfusion patients had >20% improvement in the Hb concentration, and another 2 patients had decreases in their transfusion requirements. Cytogenetic abnormalities, when present, persisted after rHuG-CSF treatment, indicating differentiation of the abnormal clone. Three patients progressed to AML after 3–16 mo of treatment. Chronic rHuG-CSF administration was well tolerated without clinically significant toxicities.

A phase 3 multi-institutional randomized trial of 102 patients with high-risk MDS determined the impact of rHuG-CSF on the natural history of the disease *(41)*. Fifty patients with RAEB or RAEB-T were treated with sc rHuG-CSF 1–5 μg/kg/d, and 52 patients received only supportive care. rHuG-CSF was well tolerated, with a low incidence of minor side effects. The rate and time to progression to AML was similar in RAEB and RAEB-T patients in both groups of the study. The survival of RAEB-T patients was comparable in both groups; however, the median survival of RAEB patients was significantly shorter in patients receiving rHuG-CSF (10.4 vs. 21.4 mo), owing to a higher rate of disease-related nonleukemic deaths, primarily from bleeding. A retrospective analysis found that RAEB patients receiving rHuG-CSF had a median survival time comparable to previously reported RAEB survival data in the literature; in contrast, RAEB patients in the supportive care group had prolonged survival. An increased proportion of RAEB patients receiving rHuG-CSF (29% vs. 14%) were in the high prognostic risk category, using a scoring system that stratified MDS patients according to the percentage of bone marrow blasts, platelets, and age. Decreased survival was only observed in this subgroup of poor-risk RAEB patients receiving rHuG-CSF. The survival differences in RAEB patients may therefore be attributed to either the increased number of high-risk patients in the rHuG-CSF-treated group or the unusually long survival of high-risk patients receiving only supportive measures. rHuG-CSF was not shown to alter the rate of infections in these patients.

2.5. rHuG-CSF and rHuEPO

Synergy between the HGFs rHuEPO and rHuG-CSF has been shown in vitro for the production of both normal and MDS marrow BFU-E numbers *(42)*. rHuG-CSF enhances the development of early precursors into EPO-responsive hematopoietic progenitors *(42)*. Two phase 2 studies confirmed improved in vivo erythroid responses to combined rHuEPO and rHuG-CSF treatment compared with either agent alone *(43,44)*. These trials initially used rHuG-CSF at doses of 1 μg/kg (0.3–3 μg/kg) sc daily to normalize or double the neutrophil count. rHuEPO 100 U/kg/d was administered sc and dose-escalated to 150–300 U/kg/d every 4 wk, or maintained at 120 U/kg/d in the other study, while continuing rHuG-CSF. Ten (42%) of 24 patients in one study *(43)* and 8 (38%) of 21 patients in the second study *(44)* had substantial erythroid responses, characterized by increased Hb values and decreased transfusion requirements. Nearly all patients had improvements in neutrophil counts. Responders had lower endogenous serum EPO (<200–500 U/L), less advanced pancytopenia, and less pretreatment red cell transfusion needs. Responses were seen in all FAB subtypes, the best rate (60%) being observed in RARS patients, who respond poorly to rHuEPO alone. A subsequent study of maintenance rHuG-CSF treatment showed that approx 50% of the patients lost their response upon rHuG-CSF withdrawal and regained it when rHuG-CSF was resumed *(45)*.

In a multi-institutional Scandinavian-American trial of 98 MDS patients treated with rHuG-CSF and rHuEPO, a similar erythroid response rate of 36% was observed *(46)*. Multivariate analysis showed that baseline serum EPO and initial transfusion needs predicted responses to combination therapy. Using pretreatment serum EPO as a ternary variable (<100, 100–500, or >500 U/L) and red cell transfusion requirement as a binary variable (<2 or ≥2 units per month), a scoring system was devised as a means of predicting erythroid response (Table 2). Patients were divided into three groups: a group with a high probability of erythroid responses (74%), an intermediate group

Table 2
Model for Predicting Erythroid Responses to rHuG-CSF and rHuEPO in Patients With Myelodysplastic Syndromes

	Score[a]					
Variable	*–3*	*–2*	*–1*	*0*	*+1*	*+2*
Serum EPO (U/L)	>500				100–500	<100
RBC transfusions (U/mo)		≥2				<2

	Response group	
Predictive score	*Type*	*% Responders (no. of patients)*
>+1	High	74 (22/29)
±1	Intermediate	23 (7/31)
<–1	Low	7 (3/34)

ABBREVIATIONS: rHuG-CSF, recombinant human granulocyte colony-stimulating factor; EPO, erythropoietin; RBC, red blood cell.

[a] Multivariate logistic regression analysis; weighted logistic coefficients. From Hellstrom-Linberg et al. *(46)*, with permission from Blackwell Science, Ltd.

(23%), and a group with poor responses to treatment (7%). A subsequent randomized phase 2 study verified the results of the Scandinavian-American trial and established a durable median response time of 24 mo *(47)*. Response rates were identical in two treatment groups primed with either rHuG-CSF (4 wk) or rHuEPO (8 wk), indicating that initial treatment with rHuG-CSF was not necessary.

The Scandinavian MDS Group has provided further data validating the Scandinavian-American model defining subgroups of patient with good, intermediate, and poor erythroid responses to the combination of rHuG-CSF and rHuEPO. This study also indicated improved quality of life for responding patients *(48)*. The Scandinavian-American score was useful in predicting erythroid responses in a Spanish multicenter study of 32 patients with RA or RARS and serum EPO at study entry of ≤250 U/L *(49)*. A 50% erythroid response rate was observed among the subset of 14 patients treated with rHuG-CSF 1 μg/kg in addition to rHuEPO 300 U/kg three times weekly. In a phase 2 German study, Mantovani and colleagues *(50)* assessed a prolonged schedule of combined rHuEPO and rHuG-CSF treatment. After 12 wk of treatment, the erythroid response rate was 61% and increased to 80% after 36 wk. After 1 and 2 yr of ongoing combined cytokine treatment, 50% of the initial responders showed continuing responses.

2.6. GM-rHuCSF

Despite the use of different schedules and routes of administration, numerous phase 1–2 studies have shown that rHuGM-CSF produces dose-dependent increases in neutrophil counts in most patients with MDS *(51–62)*. A European Organization for Research and Treatment of Cancer (EORTC) randomized multicenter study evaluated the effects of up to 2-mo rHuGM-CSF treatment in MDS patients with <10% bone marrow blasts *(63)*. Approximately two-thirds of patients responded at dose levels of 108 or 216 µg sc daily. The small number of patients and limited duration of treatment precluded determination of the effects of rHuGM-CSF therapy on disease progression and infection frequency. Another multicenter study randomized MDS patients to rHuGM-CSF 3 µg/kg sc daily for 3 mo vs. observation *(64)*. After 3 mo of therapy, patients could cross over from the observation to the rHuGM-CSF cohort if infections were documented. A marked increase in neutrophils and fewer infections were observed in the rHuGM-CSF group. rHuGM-CSF was not associated with an increased rate of conversion to leukemia. Survival benefit could not be assessed because of the study's crossover design. These multicenter trials of rHuGM-CSF have generally shown no clinically significant erythroid responses, and many thrombocytopenic patients developed lower platelet counts during treatment, necessitating more platelet transfusions *(63,64)*. In addition, a significant proportion of patients discontinued treatment with rHuGM-CSF because of side effects, including pulmonary infiltrates, flu-like syndromes, hyperleukocytosis, and bone pain *(63–65)*.

2.7. *rHuGM-CSF and rHuEPO*

Similar to trials of rHuG-CSF and rHuEPO, investigators have assessed the clinical efficacy of combined rHuGM-CSF and rHuEPO treatment in patients with MDS. In small phase 2 trials of concurrent or sequential rHuEPO and rHuGM-CSF treatment, increases in Hb concentrations or decreased transfusion requirements occurred in 23–46% of patients *(66–69)*. A 12-wk randomized, placebo-controlled trial of rHuGM-CSF (0.3–5.0 µg/kg/d) and rHuEPO therapy (150 U/kg three times weekly) stratified 66 MDS patients to endogenous EPO <500 or >500 U/L *(70)*. Combined rHuGM-CSF and rHuEPO therapy significantly improved neutrophil counts, but platelet counts were unaffected. A trend toward reduced red blood cell transfusion requirements was observed in patients with EPO < 500 U/L, but only 9% of patients in the combined cytokine group achieved an Hb response (≥2 g/dL). In a study of 19 patients, sequential rHuGM-CSF (3 µg/kg) and rHuEPO (60–120 U/kg) were administered weekly for 3 mo *(71)*. Ten of 19 (53%) responded, with 7 patients achieving a good response and 3 patients a partial response. All responding RARS patients continued to have erythroid responses during 3–24 mo of follow-up, whereas one RA and two RAEB patients did not have continuing responses at 2–12 mo. Although these studies of rHuGM-CSF and rHuEPO treatment suggest some clinically important erythroid responses, the combination of rHuG-CSF and rHuEPO is at least as effective and is generally better tolerated because of the greater toxicity associated with rHuGM-CSF.

2.8. *rHuIL-3*

Three phase 1–2 studies have evaluated the effects of short-term treatment with rHuIL-3 in MDS *(72–74)*. These preliminary studies suggested that rHuIL-3 could increase neutrophil counts but not as prominently as rHuGM-CSF or rHuG-CSF. Furthermore, rHuIL-3 transiently improves thrombocytopenia in some patients, but erythropoiesis was rarely stimulated. A longer term study of 3-mo rHuIL-3 therapy elicited improvements in two of five patients with initial platelet counts < 50×10^9/L, without notable changes in the other lineages *(75)*. The issue as to whether combination HGF support with rHuIL-3 and rHuEPO could augment erythroid responses was evaluated in 22 MDS patients *(76)*. The combination increased reticulocyte counts in five patients, but only two patients experienced decreased red cell transfusion requirements. The erythroid response was comparable to that in studies of rHuEPO alone, but rHuIL-3 produced toxicity requiring dose reduction in most patients.

2.9. rHuIL-6

The in vitro stimulatory effect of rHuIL-6 on thrombopoiesis prompted its evaluation in a phase 1 study of 22 low-risk MDS patients with thrombocytopenia *(77)*. Eight (36%) patients experienced a transient increase in platelet counts, but only three were classified as major responders. rHuIL-6 increased the frequency of higher ploidy megakaryocytes without increasing the number of megakaryocyte progenitors, consistent with its known maturation-inducing effect. Nondose-dependent anemia developed in most patients, and no neutrophil responses were documented. Constitutional symptoms and anemia were seen in most patients, precluding all but three patients from receiving maintenance therapy. The marginal activity and significant therapy-related toxicity of rHuIL-6 makes it of limited value as a thrombopoietic agent in MDS.

2.10. rHuIL-11

Because of rHuIL-11-associated toxicity (e.g., peripheral and pulmonary edema) at doses of 50 µg/kg/d, Kurzrock and coworkers *(78)* initiated a study of lower dose rHuIL-11 at 10 µg/kg/d in patients with bone marrow failure. Six (38%) of 16 patients showed clinically significant platelet responses to rHuIL-11. The median increase in peak platelet counts was 95 × 10^9/L above baseline (range increase of 55–130 × 10^9/L above baseline). Responses were seen in 5/11 MDS patients and in one patient with aplastic anemia. Responses lasted for 12, 13, 14, 25, 30, and 30+ wk. Side effects of rHuIL-11 were mild in severity and included peripheral edema, conjunctival injection, and myalgias.

2.11. rHuTPO

In 1994 the ligand of the c-mpl receptor was cloned and found to be thrombopoietin (TPO, c-mpl ligand) *(79–83)*. TPO acts as a lineage-specific HGF by promoting the proliferation and differentiation of megakaryocytes into platelets *(84)*. TPO has also been found to have effects on hematopoietic stem cells, promoting their survival and stimulating their growth in combination with other cytokines such as IL-3 or stem cell factor (SCF) *(85,86)*. Preclinical studies in animals, and several phase 1–2 studies in humans have shown that rHuTPO can reduce the severity and duration of thrombocytopenia after chemotherapy-induced myelosuppression *(87–92)*. There has been great interest in using rHuTPO to improve the thrombocytopenia and multilineage responses in patients with MDS.

Plasma TPO concentrations are inversely correlated to platelet count and bone marrow megakaryocyte mass *(93)*. Plasma TPO concentrations have generally been found to be higher in MDS patients than in normal individuals *(94)*. RA patients had higher plasma TPO concentrations than RAEB/RAEB-T patients, irrespective of similar platelet counts in these groups. The plasma TPO concentration was upregulated and inversely correlated with the platelet count in RA patients, but not in RAEB/RAEB-T or CMML patients *(95,96)*. These findings suggest that the physiologic pathways for TPO production and metabolism are intact in patients with low-risk MDS but may be deranged in the advanced stages of MDS, in which the leukemic clone has progressed. One study found that the number of TPO receptors (c-mpl) was decreased in MDS marrow cells compared with normal cells, a similar finding across all MDS FAB subtypes *(96)*. Reduced numbers of TPO receptors, in addition to thrombocytopenia, may contribute to the increased plasma TPO concentrations found in MDS patients.

In vitro studies have assessed the effects of recombinant TPO on the proliferation and differentiation of MDS and AML bone marrow progenitor cells. In short-term liquid cultures and progenitor assays, recombinant human megakaryocyte growth and development factor (rHuMGDF) stimulated DNA synthesis and potentiated leukemic cluster growth of marrow mononuclear cells in approx 25% of patients with MDS *(97)*. rHuMGDF-induced blast cell proliferation correlated with increased expression of c-mpl. rHuMGDF stimulated CFU-MK growth in 45% of these patients. In another study, rHuTPO increased blast number from cultured marrow cells from high-risk MDS patients, but not lower-risk individuals (RA/RARS) *(98)*. High lactic dehydrogenase values were associated with rHuTPO-induced blast proliferation in high-risk patients. In a study of 7-d suspension cultures, rHuMGDF increased CFU-MK growth in 1/10 AML and 6/16 MDS marrows, and $CD61^+$ (a marker of megakaryocytes) cell numbers were increased in 9/13 AML and 12/15 MDS samples *(99)*. In this series, rHuMGDF did not increase CFU-GM colony or cluster growth. Stimulation of in vitro megakaryopoiesis by rHuMGDF in MDS samples could be augmented by rHuIL-3 and rHuSCF *(100)*. When fetal calf serum and rHuEPO were added to MDS marrow samples, rHuTPO induced MDS CFU-GM and BFU-E cell proliferation in a dose-dependent manner by up to 100% *(101)*. These in vitro effects were comparable to previous results obtained with rHuG-CSF, rHuGM-CSF, and rHuIL-3. rHuTPO also augmented the stimulatory effects of these cytokines on MDS marrow cells. These in vitro studies indicate that rHuTPO can induce differentiation of MDS megakaryocyte precursors; however, the potential for fostering leukemic cell growth also exists, a concern that needs to be carefully scrutinized in future clinical trials of recombinant rHuTPO in MDS.

A phase 1–2 open-label, sequential dose-escalation study evaluated the effects of a 14-d course of intravenous pegylated rHuMGDF in patients with MDS and AA who had average baseline platelet counts $< 30 \times 10^9$/L without transfusion *(102)*. Preliminary data indicated that the drug was well tolerated, but only modest increases in platelet counts were observed in the dose range of 1.25–5.0 μg/kg/d.

3. MECHANISMS OF ACTION OF EPO AND G-CSF

In response to EPO, DNA synthesis, GATA-1 binding activity, and signal transducer and activator of transcription (STAT)5 activation were found to be absent or severely decreased in MDS compared with normal marrow cells *(13)*; however, another study determined that ineffective erythropoiesis was more strongly correlated with stimulation of Fas-mediated proapoptotic pathways than with defective antiapoptotic signaling by the JAK2-STAT5 pathway *(103)*. In some cases, both mechanisms appear to be operative. Apoptosis is associated with increased Fas ligand production during the stage of erythroid differentiation stage, a process that can be inhibited by a chimeric

Fas-Fc protein *(104)*. Using both morphology and fluorescent *in situ* hybridization (FISH) in cytogenetically categorized patients with MDS, rHuEPO treatment in responding patients resulted in a significantly lower proportion of FISH-abnormal erythroid precursors compared with before rHuEPO treatment *(105)*. In addition, patients responding to rHuEPO had a significantly lower percentage of FISH abnormal erythroid precursors compared with unresponsive individuals. The results are consistent with rHuEPO-induced proliferation of residual karyotypically normal erythroid precursors in MDS marrows.

Studies of apoptosis within MDS marrow progenitor cells have begun to unravel the mechanism whereby rHuG-CSF synergistically works with rHuEPO to improve the Hb concentration in patients with MDS. In the RARS subgroup, rHuG-CSF inhibited the increased Fas-induced apoptosis of MDS bone marrow cells *(106)*. rHuG-CSF mediated reductions in caspase-8 and caspase-3-like activity, with concomitant reductions in the amount of late cellular apoptotic changes. Erythroid progenitor cells from patients with MDS also spontaneously released cytochrome c from mitochondria, with subsequent activation of caspase-9, an additional apoptotic pathway that can be inhibited by rHuG-CSF *(107)*. Among low-risk MDS patients studied, this effect was most pronounced in erythroid progenitors from RARS patients.

4. APLASTIC ANEMIA

Aplastic anemia (AA) is an acquired bone marrow stem cell disorder characterized by hypocellular bone marrows and variable degrees of pancytopenia. Morbidity and mortality are related to disease-associated cytopenias and primarily include infection and bleeding. Therapy has principally consisted of either immunosuppressive therapy with antithymocyte or antilymphocyte globulin (ATG/ALG) and cyclosporine as single agents or in combination, or allogeneic bone marrow/stem cell transplantation. Both treatment modalities result in high response rates and prolongation of disease-free survival. HGF therapy has been used to increase neutrophil counts in patients with AA in the setting of severe infections, as an adjunct to immunosuppressive therapy, and as treatment in patients refractory other treatment modalities. The European Bone and Marrow Transplant group (EBMT) has recommended that HGFs not be used as initial treatment for newly diagnosed AA patients for several reasons, including increased risk of human leukocyte antigen (HLA) sensitization and refractoriness to platelet transfusions from random donors; possible exposure and sensitization to minor histocompatibility antigens, thereby increasing the possibility of graft failure after allogeneic bone marrow transplantation; and delay of more appropriate therapy such as immunosuppression or transplant *(108,109)*. Mostly nonrandomized, single-arm trials enrolling small numbers of patients with AA have assessed the efficacy of various recombinant cytokines as single agents, or in combination, including recombinant forms of EPO, G-CSF, GM-CSF, IL-1, IL-3, IL-6, and SCF (Table 3; *73, 74, 134–152*).

4.1. Aplastic Anemia and In Vitro Hematopoiesis

Quantitative deficits in the hematopoetic stem cell compartment are present in AA, exemplified by marked in vitro reductions in long-term culture-initiating cells or the number of hematopoietic progenitors by clonogenic studies (e.g., BFU-E, CFU-M, CFU-GM, CFU-MK) *(110,111)*. Qualitative abnormalities of CD34 cells, such as

Table 3
Clinical Trials of Hematopoietic Growth Factors Used Alone in Patients With Aplastic Anemia

Treatment	*No. of patients*	*Ref.*
rHuGM-CSF	8	*135*
rHuGM-CSF	4	*136*
rHuGM-CSF	10	*134*
rHuGM-CSF	11	*137*
rHuGM-CSF	8	*138*
rHuGM-CSF ± rHuEPO	12	*144*
rHuGM-CSF	37	*139*
rHuG-CSF	14	*140*
rHuG-CSF	5	*141*
rHuG-CSF	27	*142*
rHuG-CSF	10	*143*
rHuG-CSF + rHuEPO	27	*145*
rHuG-CSF + rHuEPO	20	*146*
rHuG-CSF + rHuEPO	110	*147*
rHuIL-1	4	*150*
rHuIL-3	9	*149*
rHuIL-3	8	*73*
rHuIL-3	7	*74*
rHuIL-3	15	*148*
rHuIL-6	11	*151*
rHuG-CSF ± rHuSCF	15	*152*

Abbreviations: GM-CSF, granulocyte-macrophage colony-stimulating factor; G-CSF, granulocyte colony-stimulating factor; EPO, erythropoietin; IL, interleukin; SCF, stem cell factor; rHu, recombinant human.

accelerated apoptosis, also contribute to impairment of stem cell function *(112)*. It has generally been found that stromal layers from patients with AA can support normal hematopoiesis *(113,114)*, but with some in vitro culture systems, abnormal stroma has been seen and may play a role in the pathogenesis of selected AA cases *(115,116)*.

Amounts of various HGFs (e.g., G-CSF, GM-CSF, IL-6, and SCF) secreted from AA marrow stromal layers were normal using different assays *(117–119)*. Except for SCF, which may be low or normal *(120–122)*, serum concentrations of most HGF are increased *(123–127)*. In addition, both serum and marrow amounts of TPO are increased *(93,128–130)*. As has been previously reviewed, local marrow concentrations of cytokines, which mediate paracrine interactions between stem cells and their microenvironment, are probably more important than serum HGF concentrations *(109)*. Addition of single cytokines (e.g., rHuSCF) or combinations of HGF (e.g., rHuIL-3 and rHuGM-CSF) to AA long-term bone marrow cultures have resulted in stimulation of CFU-GM in some cases, but results are variable, and interpretation is confounded by several methodologic issues *(109,131,132)*. However, in vitro experiments have shown that rHuG-CSF can often restore to normal the reduced cloning efficiency of purified AA CD34 cells *(133)*.

4.2. rHuGM-CSF and rHuG-CSF

A study by Vadhan-Raj and colleagues *(134)* established that rHuGM-CSF could stimulate myelopoiesis in AA patients. rHuGM-CSF 60–500 μg/m^2 was administered daily by continuous iv infusion for 2 wk followed by a 2-wk rest period in 10 patients with moderate-to-severe disease severity. White cell counts increased from 1.6- to 10-fold, and neutrophil counts increased by 1.5- to 20-fold, with nine of the patients achieving neutrophil counts > 1.5 × 10^9/L. The median duration of treatment was 16 wk (range: 8–32 wk). With discontinuation of the rHuGM-CSF infusion, neutrophil counts returned to pretreatment values. Bone marrow cellularity increased with treatment, manifested primarily by increased myeloid precursors. Patients with less severe AA had better hematologic responses. Five additional studies with rHuGM-CSF *(135–139),* and four studies of rHuG-CSF *(140–143)* in patients with AA have reached similar conclusions: rHuGM-CSF/rHuG-CSF can increase neutrophil counts in a moderate proportion of patients, but responses are less common among patients with severe AA and poorly preserved myelopoiesis; improvements in white cell counts are usually transient and return to baseline with discontinuation of therapy; and very few patients experience improvement in red cell and platelet counts. In an attempt to decrease the costs and side effects of cytokine therapy, a regimen of "very low-dose" rHuGM-CSF has been studied (5–20 μg/m^2/d), with neutrophil responses observed in 5/12 patients *(144).*

4.3. rHuEPO and rHuG-CSF

As in MDS, rHuEPO can synergize with rHuG-CSF to increase the rate of multilineage responses in patients with AA; however, such responses have generally not been sustained, and rHuEPO ± rHuG-CSF therapy has generally not been considered a useful regimen. In one study, combined rHuG-CSF and rHuEPO therapy elicited erythroid responses in 6/14 (43%) patients with moderate AA after 10 wk, and a delayed response was noted in 3 additional patients *(145).* Erythroid responses were less impressive among individuals with severe AA (3/13, 23%). Durable trilineage responses were observed in 6/27 (22%) patients, but in 5 of these patients, count improvement was not manifest until after 10 wk of therapy. In this study, rHuG-CSF 400 μg/m^2 iv daily and rHuEPO 100 U/kg sc daily were considered to be doses sufficient to increase neutrophil counts and Hb concentrations, respectively. In another trial of 20 patients, rHuG-CSF (50–100 μg/m^2 sc daily) with addition of rHuEPO (2000–8000 U/m^2 three times weekly), started 2 wk after rHuG-CSF initiation, resulted in red cell transfusion independence in 7 (35%) patients with long-term administration, with at least bilineage responses seen in the same proportion of patients *(146).* A multicenter randomized, controlled study compared rHuG-CSF alone with two dosages of rHuEPO (200 U/kg or 400 U/kg three times weekly) in addition to rHuG-CSF *(147).* Erythroid responses in the 400-U/kg rHuEPO group were significantly higher (36.8%) than either the lower dose rHuEPO group (14.6%) or the rHuG-CSF-alone group (12.9%); however, red cell transfusion independence was not observed. Factors predicting response included nonsevere AA, lower serum EPO, higher Hb concentration, reticulocyte count, and level of serum transferrin receptors.

4.4. rHu-Interleukins

IL-3 elicits hematologic responses in a small proportion of AA patients, and they are generally transient in nature. In 15 patients with severe AA, nonsustained increases in white blood cell counts were observed in 7/9 patients and 2/6 patients at dose levels of 1–2 µg/kg/d and 4–16 µg/kg/d, respectively, administered as 21-d continuous iv infusions *(148)*. Responses were not elicited in other blood lineages. In a phase 1–2 study of 21 AA and MDS patients evaluating rHuIL-3 dose levels of 0.5–10 µg/kg/d sc for 21 d, 2 AA patients experienced improvements in red cell transfusion requirements *(74)*. Two additional small trials reported neutrophil and platelet responses in a few patients, but erythroid responses were not observed *(73,149)*. Studies of both rHuIL-1 and rHuIL-6 in patients with refractory severe AA patients have not shown any efficacy *(150,151)*. Nonhematologic side effects produced by rHuIL-6 included fever, headache, arthralgia, tachycardia, and hypertension. Hematologic toxicity included worsening of pre-existing anemia and thrombocytopenia. The study was discontinued early because of the toxicities attributed to rHuIL-6.

4.5. Stem Cell Factor

rHuSCF was evaluated in AA patients with moderate and severe disease who had failed ATG or cyclosporine A therapy *(152)*. When rHuSCF was used alone, 14/17 patients exhibited neutrophil responses, with only one trilineage response observed. Addition of rHuG-CSF to rHuSCF resulted in trilineage responses in 5/15 patients. rHuSCF use has resulted in anaphylactoid reactions including laryngeal edema and bronchospasm. The rate of severe allergic reactions was 8% in this study.

5. HGFs AS ADJUNCTIVE THERAPY TO IMMUNOSUPPRESSION

The rationale for adding rHuG-CSF to trials of ATG/ALG or cyclosporine was to reduce the morbidity and mortality related to infectious complications during the window of neutropenia before patients exhibited hematologic responses to immunosuppressive therapy. The Severe Aplastic Anemia Working Party of the EBMT conducted a pilot study of 40 patients using rHuG-CSF on d 1–90 in addition to treatment with ALG and cyclosporine, as well as a tapering course of methylprednisolone *(153)*. Compared with previous data, the results showed comparatively favorable trilineage response rates (82%) and actuarial survival (92%), as well as a relatively low number of deaths from infection (8%). In a Gruppo Italiano Trapianti di Milolio Osseo/EBMT update of 100 patients using the same treatment regimen, the 5-yr actuarial survival was similar (87%) *(154)*. Patients not achieving a white count of 5×10^9/L exhibited a relatively lower response rate (37%) and a higher mortality rate (42%), indicating a significant effect of neutrophil counts on response. In a more recent phase 3 randomized study of patients with severe AA by the EBMT, there was no significant difference between groups treated with immunosuppression with or without rHuG-CSF with regard to survival, hematologic responses, and incidence of secondary leukemia *(155)*. Therefore, at least some of the relatively high response and survival rates attributed to rHuG-CSF observed in the 1990s may be owing to other factors, including improvements in supportive care, longer term immunosuppressive regimens, and the addition of cyclosporine to ATG/ALG *(109)*.

6. G-CSF THERAPY AND THE RISK OF MDS/AML TRANSFORMATION IN APLASTIC ANEMIA

Three studies have enumerated a 5–15% risk of transformation to MDS/AML in AA patients treated with immunosuppression *(156–158)*. With the initial reports of MDS and AML arising in patients with AA after rHuG-CSF therapy *(159,160)*, studies began to analyze whether the cytokine contributed to this increased risk of clonal evolution. In two Japanese studies of children and adults with AA, factors associated with a higher incidence rate of transformation to MDS or AML included high doses of rHuG-CSF (>10 μg/kg/d) and prolonged use (>1 yr) *(161,162)*. In addition, evolution to MDS or AML in both studies was only noted among patients receiving immunosuppression plus rHuG-CSF and not among patients receiving immunosuppression alone. In the childhood study, a cumulative 47% transformation rate to MDS/AML was observed after 6 yr and was linked to emergence of monosomy 7 in 10/11 cases. Results of the Japan Childhood Aplastic Anemia Study Group, published in 2000, indicated an overall 3% risk of MDS/AML at 4 yr, which was not influenced by rHuG-CSF treatment *(163)*. In the adult trial, the probability of clonal evolution was 8% after 2 yr and 39% after 3 yr. In a more recent Japanese study of adult AA patients with 1-yr follow-up, 16% of patients developed a clonal cytogenetic abnormality, with monosomy 7 being most common *(164)*. Evolution to MDS was noted in 8% of 65 evaluable patients. More recent studies of adult AA patients suggest a lower risk of MDS/AML evolution. For example, in the phase 3 EBMT randomized study of patients with severe AA receiving immunosuppressive therapy with or without rHuG-CSF, there was only one case of secondary leukemia in each group *(155)*. The Italian Aplastic Anaemia Study Group found no increased risk of MDS or leukemia associated with addition of rHuG-CSF to immunosuppressive therapy *(165)*. These findings are consistent with those indicated above in the randomized trial for high-risk MDS patients *(41)*, comparing chronic rHuG-CSF administration to observation only, in which no increased risk of AML evolution occurred in the treatment arm.

7. SUMMARY

To date, clinical trials have provided a reasonable composite picture of the safety and efficacy of HGF in MDS and AA. In AA, future studies should aim to better characterize the additional benefit derived from the use of rHuG-CSF with immunosuppressive therapy and to define further the risk associated with rHuG-CSF and the later development of clonal hematologic disorders. In MDS, quality-of-life and pharmacoeconomic comparisons between rHuEPO therapy and red blood cell transfusions will assist physician and patient decision making regarding individual treatment options and will shape the debate regarding health care resource allocation for these diseases *(166)*.

Novel longer-acting recombinant cytokines such as darbepoetin alfa and pegfilgrastim have shown comparable safety and efficacy in studies of cancer patients with anemia owing to chronic disease or multicycle chemotherapy. Currently, phase 1–2 trials of darbepoetin alfa in MDS are evaluating whether less frequent dosing of this potent erythropoietin can add to the convenience of therapy of these chronic anemias. The recent establishment of consensus response criteria by the International Working Group will permit better interpretation of the results of trials of these cytokines and other agents in MDS *(167)*.

REFERENCES

1. Greenberg PL. Biologic and clinical implications of marrow culture studies in the myelodysplastic syndromes. *Semin Hematol* 1996; 33:163–175.
2. Greenberg PL, Mara B. The preleukemic syndrome: correlation of in vitro parameters of granulopoiesis with clinical features. *Am J Med* 1979; 66:951–958.

3. Chui DH, Clarke BJ. Abnormal erythroid progenitor cells in human preleukemia. *Blood* 1982; 60:362–367.
4. Juvonen E, Partanen S, Knuutila S, Ruute T. Megakaryocyte colony formation by bone marrow progenitors in myelodysplastic syndromes. *Br J Haematol* 1986; 63:331–334.
5. Nagler A, Ginzton N, Negrin RS, Bang D, Donlon T, Greenberg, PL. In vitro differentiative and proliferative effects of human recombinant colony-stimulating factors on marrow hemopoiesis in myelodysplastic syndromes. *Leukemia* 1990; 4:193–202.
6. Schipperus MR, Sonneveld P, Lindemans J, et al. The combined effects of IL-3, GM-CSF, and G-CSF on the in vitro growth of myelodysplastic myeloid progenitor cells. *Leuk Res* 1990; 14:1019–1025.
7. Greenberg PL, Mackichan ML, Negrin R. Production of granulocyte colony-stimulating factor by normal and myelodysplastic syndrome peripheral blood cells. *Blood* 1990; 76:146a (abstract).
8. Nagler A, Binet C, Mackichan ML, et al. Impact of marrow cytogenetics and morphology on in vitro hemopoiesis in the myelodysplastic syndromes: comparison between recombinant human granulocyte colony-stimulating factor and granulocyte-monocyte colony-stimulating factor. *Blood* 1990; 76:1299–1307.
9. Merchav S, Nielsen OJ, Rosenbaum H, et al. In vitro studies of erythropoietin-dependent regulation of erythropoiesis in myelodysplastic syndromes. *Leukemia* 1990; 4:771–774.
10. Greenberg PL, Negrin RS, Ginzton N. G-CSF synergizes with erythropoietin for enhancing erythroid colony-formation in myelodysplastic syndromes. *Blood* 1991; 78:38a (abstract).
11. Sawada K, Sato N, Tarumi T, et al. Proliferation and differentiation of myelodysplastic CD34+ cells in serum-free medium: response to individual colony-stimulating factors. *Br J Haematol* 1993; 83:349–358.
12. Budel LM, Dong F, Lowenberg B, Touw IP. Hematopoietic growth factor receptors: structure variations and alternatives of receptor complex formation in normal hematopoiesis and in hematopoietic disorders. *Leukemia* 1995; 9:553–561.
13. Hoefsloot LH, van Amelsvoort MP, Broeders LC, et al. Erythropoietin-induced activation of STAT5 is impaired in the myelodysplastic syndrome. *Blood* 1997; 89:1690–1700.
14. Oster W, Krumwieh D, Brune T, et al. Evaluation of erythropoietin (EPO) in the treatment of patients with myelodysplastic syndromes (MDS)-preclinical data supporting a rationale for sequential therapy with granulocyte-macrophage colony-stimulating factor (GM-CSF) and EPO. *J Cancer Clin Oncol* 1990; 116:280.
15. Kurzrock R, Talpaz M, Estey E, O'Brien S, Estrov Z, Gutterman JU. Erythropoietin treatment in patients with myelodysplastic syndrome and anemia. *Leukemia* 1991; 5:985–990.
16. Adamson JW, Schuster M, Allen S, Haley NR. Effectiveness of recombinant human erythropoietin therapy in myelodysplastic syndromes. *Acta Haematol* 1992; 87:20–24.
17. Shepherd JD, Currie CJ, Sparling TG, Krystal G, Eaves AC. Erythropoietin therapy of myelodysplastic syndromes. *Blood* 1992; 79:1891–1892.
18. Ganser A, Hoelzer D. Treatment of myelodysplastic syndromes with hematopoietic growth factors. *Hematol Oncol Clin North Am* 1992; 6:633–653.
19. Yoshida Y, Anzai N, Kawabata H, Kohsaka Y, Okuma M. Serial changes in endogenous erythropoietin levels in patients with myelodysplastic syndromes and aplastic anemia undergoing erythropoietin treatment. *Ann Hematol* 1993; 66:175–180.
20. Aloe Spiriti MA, Petti MC, Latagliata R, et al. Is recombinant human erythropoietin treatment in myelodysplastic syndromes worthwhile? *Leuk Lymphoma* 1993; 9:79–83.
21. Mohr B, Herrmann R, Huhn D. Recombinant human erythropoietin in patients with myelodysplastic syndromes and myelofibrosis. *Acta Haematol* 1993; 90:65–70.
22. Ghio R, Balleari E, Ballestrero A, et al. Subcutaneous recombinant human erythropoietin for the treatment of anemia in myelodysplastic syndromes. *Acta Haematol* 1993; 90:58–64.
23. Stone RM, Bernstein SH, Demetri G, et al. Treatment with recombinant human erythropoietin in patients with myelodysplastic syndromes. *Leuk Res* 1994; 18:769–776.
24. Rose EH, Abels RI, Nelson RA, McCullough OM, Lessin L. The use of r-HuEPO in the treatment of anaemia related to myelodysplasia (MDS). *Br J Haematol* 1995; 89:831–837.
25. DiRaimondo F, Longo G, Cacciola E Jr, et al. A good response rate to recombinant erythropoietin alone may be expected in selected myelodysplastic patients. A preliminary clinical study. *Eur J Haematol* 1996; 56:7–11.
26. Stasi R, Brunetti M, Bussa S, et al. Response to recombinant human erythropoietin in patients with myelodysplastic syndromes. *Clin Cancer Res* 1997; 3:733–739.

27. Italian Cooperative Study Group for rHuEpo in Myelodysplastic Syndromes. A randomized double-blind placebo-controlled study with subcutaneous recombinant human erythropoietin in patients with low-risk myelodysplastic syndromes. *Br J Haematol* 1998; 103:1070–1074.
28. Stenke L, Wallvik J, Celsing F, Hast R. Prediction of response to treatment with human recombinant erythropoietin in myelodysplastic syndromes. *Leukemia* 1993; 7:1324–1327.
29. Wallvik J, Stenke L, Bernell P, Nordahl G, Hippe E, Hast R. Serum erythropoietin (EPO) levels correlate with survival and independently predict response to EPO treatment in patients with myelodysplastic syndromes. *Eur J Haematol* 2002; 68:180–185.
30. Rodriguez JN, Dieguez JC, Muniz R, et al. [Human recombinant erythropoietin in the treatment of myelodysplastic syndromes anemia. Meta-analytic study.] *Sangre (Barc)* 1994; 39:435–439 [in Spanish].
31. Hellström-Lindberg E. Efficacy of erythropoietin in the myelodysplastic syndromes: a meta-analysis of 205 patients from 17 studies. *Br J Haematol* 1995; 89:67–71.
32. Hast R, Wallvik J, Folin Abernell P, Stenke L. Long-term follow-up of 18 patients with myelodyplastic syndromes responding to recombinant erythropoietin treatment. *Leuk Res* 2001; 25:13–18.
33. Terpos E, Mougiou A, Kouraklis A, et al. for the Greek MDS Study Group. Prolonged administration of erythropoietin increases erythroid response rate in myelodysplastic syndromes: a phase II trial in 281 patients. *Br J Haematol* 2002; 118:174–180.
34. Tefferi A, Elliott MA, Steensma DP, et al. Amifostine alone and in combination with erythropoietin for the treatment of favorable myelodysplastic syndrome. *Leuk Res* 2001; 25:183–185.
35. Neumeister P, Jaeger G, Eibl M, Sormann S, Zinke W, Linkesch W. Amifostine in combination with erythropoietin and G-CSF promotes multilineage hematopoiesis in patients with myelodysplastic syndrome. *Leuk Lymphoma* 2001; 40:345–349.
36. Tsiara SN, Kapsali HD, Panteli K, Christou L, Bourantas KL. Preliminary results of amifostine administration in combination with recombinant human erythropoietin in patients with myelodysplastic syndromes. *J Exp Clin Cancer Res* 2001; 20:35–38.
37. Grossi A, Musto P, Santini V, et al. Combined therapy with amifostine plus erythropoietin for the treatment of myelodysplastic syndromes. *Haematologica* 2002; 87:322–323.
38. Stasi R, Brunetti M, Terzoli E, Amadori S. Sustained response to recombinant human erythropoietin and intermittent all-trans retinoic acid in patients with myelodysplastic syndromes. *Blood* 2002; 99:1578–1584.
39. Negrin RS, Haeuber DH, Nagler A, et al. Treatment of myelodysplastic syndromes with recombinant human granulocyte colony-stimulating factor. *Ann Intern Med* 1989; 110:976–984.
40. Negrin RS, Haeuber DH, Nagler A, et al. Maintenance treatment of patients with myelodysplastic syndromes using recombinant human granulocyte colony-stimulating factor. *Blood* 1990; 76:36–43.
41. Greenberg P, Taylor K, Larson R, et al. Phase III randomized multicenter trial of recombinant human G-CSF in MDS. *Blood* 1993; 82:196a (abstract).
42. Greenberg PL, Negrin RS, Ginzton N. In vitro-in vivo correlations of erythroid responses to G-CSF plus erythropoietin in myelodysplastic syndromes. *Exp Hematol* 1992; 20:733 (abstract).
43. Negrin RS, Stein R, Doherty K, et al. Treatment of the anemias of MDS using recombinant human granulocyte colony-stimulating factor in combination with erythropoietin. *Blood* 1993; 82:737–743.
44. Hellström-Lindberg E, Birgegard G, Carlsson M, et al. A combination of granulocyte colony-stimulating factor and erythropoietin may synergistically improve the anaemia in patients with myelodysplastic syndromes. *Leuk Lymphoma* 1993; 11:221–228.
45. Negrin RS, Stein R, Doherty K, et al. Maintenance treatment of the anemia of myelodysplastic syndromes with recombinant human granulocyte colony-stimulating factor and erythropoietin: evidence for in vivo synergy. *Blood* 1996; 87:4076–4081.
46. Hellström-Lindberg E, Negrin R, Stein R, et al. Erythroid response to treatment with G-CSF plus erythropoietin for the anaemia of patients with myelodysplastic syndromes: proposal for a predictive model. *Br J Haematol* 1997; 99:344–351.
47. Hellström-Lindberg E, Ahlgren T, Beguin Y, et al. Treatment of anemia in myelodysplastic syndromes with granulocyte colony-stimulating factor plus erythropoietin; results from a randomized phase II study and long-term follow-up of 71 patients. *Blood* 1998; 92:68–75.
48. Hellström-Lindberg E, Gulbrandsen N, Lindberg G, et al. A validated decision model for treating the anaemia of myelodysplastic syndromes with erythropoietin + granulocyte colony-stimulating factor: significant effects on quality of life. *Br J Haematol* 2003; 120:1037–1046.

49. Remacha AF, Arrizabalaga B, Villegas A, et al. Erythropoietin plus granulocyte colony-stimulating factor in the treatment of myelodysplastic syndromes. Identification of a subgroup of responders. *Haematologica* 1999; 84:1058–1064.
50. Mantovani L, Lentini G, Hentschel B, et al. Treatment of anaemia in myelodysplastic syndromes with prolonged administration of recombinant human granulocyte colony-stimulating factor and erythropoietin. *Br J Haematol* 2000; 109:367–375.
51. Vadhan-Raj S, Keating M, LeMaistre A, et al. Effects of recombinant human granulocyte-macrophage colony-stimulating factor in patients with myelodysplastic syndromes. *N Engl J Med* 1987; 317:1545–1552.
52. Antin JH, Weinberg DS, Rosenthal DS. Variable effect of recombinant human granulocyte-macrophage colony-stimulating factor on bone marrow fibrosis in patients with myelodysplasia. *Exp Hematol* 1990; 18:266–270.
53. Ganser A, Volkers B, Greher J, et al. Recombinant human-granulocyte-macrophage colony-stimulating factor in patients with myelodysplastic syndromes a phase I/II trial. *Blood* 1989; 73:31–37.
54. Hermann F, Lindemann A, Klein H, Lubbert M, Schultz G, Mertelsmann R. Effect of recombinant human granulocyte-macrophage colony-stimulating factor in patients with myelodysplastic syndrome with excess blasts. *Leukemia* 1989; 3:335–338.
55. Hoelzer D, Ganser A, Greher J, Volkers B, Walther F. Phase I/II study with GM-CSF in patients with myelodysplastic syndromes. *Behring Inst Mitt* 1988; 83:134–138.
56. Thompson JA, Douglas JL, Kidd P, et al. Subcutaneous granulocyte macrophage colony-stimulating factor in patients with myelodysplastic syndrome: toxicity, pharmacokinetics, and hematological effects. *J Clin Oncol* 1989; 7:629–637.
57. Dunbar CE, Smith D, Kimball J, et al. Sequential treatment with recombinant human growth factors to compare activity of GM-CSF and IL3 in the treatment of primary myelodysplasia. *Blood* 1990; 76:141a (abstract).
58. y EH, Kurzrock R, Talpaz M, et al. Effects of low doses of recombinant human granulocyte-macrophage colony-stimulating factor (GM-CSF) in patients with myelodysplastic syndromes. *Br J Haematol* 1991; 77:291–295.
59. Rosenfeld CS, Sulecki M, Evans C, Shadduck RK. Comparison of intravenous versus subcutaneous recombinant human granulocyte-macrophage colony-stimulating factor in patients with primary myelodysplasia. *Exp Hematol* 1991; 19:273–277.
60. Gradishar WJ, LeBeau MM, O'Laughlin R, Vardiman JW, Larson RA. Clinical and cytogenetic responses to granulocyte-macrophage colony-stimulating factor in therapy-related myelodysplasia. *Blood* 1992; 80:2463–2470.
61. Takahashi M, Yoshida Y, Kaku K, et al. Phase II study of recombinant granulocyte-macrophage colony-stimulating factor in myelodysplastic syndrome and aplastic anemia. *Acta Haematol* 1993; 89:189–194.
62. Rose C, Wattel E, Bastion Y, et al. Treatment with very low-dose GM-CSF in myelodysplastic syndromes with neutropenia. A report on 28 cases. *Leukemia* 1994; 8:1458–1462.
63. Willemze R, Van Der Lely N, Zwierzina H, et al. A randomized phase-I/II multicenter study of recombinant human granulocyte-macrophage colony-stimulating factor (GM-CSF) therapy for patients with myelodysplastic syndromes and a relatively low risk of acute leukemia. *Ann Hematol* 1992; 64:173–180.
64. Schuster MW, Thompson JA, Larson R, et al. Randomized phase II study of recombinant granulocyte macrophage-colony stimulating factor (rGM-CSF) in patients with neutropenia secondary to myelodysplastic syndrome (MDS). *Blood* 1995; 86:338a (abstract).
65. Yoshida Y, Nakahata T, Shibata A, et al. Effects of long-term treatment with recombinant human granulocyte-macrophage colony-stimulating factor in patients with myelodysplastic syndrome. *Leuk Lymphoma* 1995; 18:457–463.
66. Runde V, Aul C, Ebert A, Grabenhorst U, Schneider W. Sequential administration of recombinant human granulocyte-macrophage colony-stimulating factor and human erythropoietin for treatment of myelodysplastic syndromes. *Eur J Haematol* 1995; 54:39–45.
67. Hansen PB, Johnsen HE, Hippe E, Hellstrom-Lindberg E, Ralfkiaer E. ecombinant human granulocyte-macrophage colony-stimulating factor plus recombinant human erythropoietin may improve anemia in selected patients with myelodysplastic syndromes. *Am J Hematol* 1993; 44:229–236.
68. Bernell P, Stenke L, Wallvik J, Hippe E, Hast R. A sequential erythropoietin and GM-CSF schedule offers clinical benefits in the treatment of anemia in myelodysplastic syndromes. *Leuk Res* 1996; 20:693–699.

69. Stasi R, Pagano A, Terzoli E, Amadori S. Recombinant human granulocyte-macrophage colony-stimulating factor plus erythropoietin for the treatment of cytopenias in patients with myelodysplastic syndromes. *Br J Haematol* 1999; 105:141–148.
70. Thompson J, Gilliland G, Prchal J, et al. The use of GM-CSF+ r-HuEPO for the treatment of cytopenias associated with myelodysplastic syndromes. *Blood* 1995; 86:337a (abstract).
71. Economopoulos T, Mellou S, Papageorgiou E, et al. Treatment of anemia in low risk myelodysplastic syndromes with granulocyte-macrophage colony-stimulating factor plus recombinant human erythropoietin. *Leukemia* 1999; 13:1009–1012.
72. Ganser A, Seipelt G, Lindemann A, et al. Effects of recombinant human interleukin-3 in patients with myelodysplastic syndromes. *Blood* 1990; 76:455–462.
73. Kurzrock R, Talpaz M, Estrov Z, Rosenblum MG, Gutterman JU. Phase I study of recombinant human interleukin-3 in patients with bone marrow failure. *J Clin Oncol* 1991; 9:1241–1250.
74. Nimer SD, Paquette RL, Ireland P, Resta D, Young D, Golde DW. A phase I/II study of interleukin-3 in patients with aplastic anemia and myelodysplasia. *Exp Hematol* 1994; 22:875–880.
75. Ganser A, Ottmann OG, Seipelt G, et al. Effect of long-term treatment with recombinant human interleukin-3 in patients with myelodysplastic syndromes. *Leukemia* 1993; 7:696–701.
76. Miller AM, Noyes WE, Taetle R, List AF. Limited erythropoietic response to combined treatment with recombinant human interleukin 3 and erythropoietin in myelodysplastic syndrome. *Leuk Res* 1999; 23:77–83.
77. Gordon MS, Nemunaitis J, Hoffman R, et al. A phase I trial of recombinant human interleukin-6 in patients with myelodysplastic syndromes and thrombocytopenia. *Blood* 1995; 85:3066–3076.
78. Kurzrock R, Cortes J, Thomas DA, Jeha S, Pilat S, Talpaz M. Pilot study of low-dose interleukin-11 in patients with bone marrow failure. *J Clin Oncol* 2001; 19:4165–4172.
79. Lok S, Kaushansky K, Holly RD, et al. Cloning and expression of murine thrombopoietin cDNA and stimulation of platelet production in vivo. *Nature* 1994; 369:565–568.
80. De Sauvage FJ, Hass PE, Spencer SD, et al. Stimulation of megakaryocytopoiesis and thrombopoiesis by the c-mpl ligand. *Nature* 1994; 369:533–538.
81. Kaushansky K, Lok S, Holly RD, et al. Promotion of megakaryocyte progenitor expansion and differentiation by the c-mpl ligand thrombopoietin. *Nature* 1994; 369:568–571.
82. Wendling F, Maraskovsky E, Debili N, et al. cMpl ligand is a humoral regulator of megakaryocytopoieisis. *Nature* 1994; 369:571–574.
83. Bartley TD, Bogenberger J, Hunt P, et al. Identification and cloning of a megakaryocyte and development factor that is a ligand for the cytokine receptor mpl. *Cell* 1994; 77:1117–1124.
84. Debili N, Wendling F, Katz A, et al. The Mpl-ligand or thrombopoietin of megakaryocyte growth and differentiative factor has both direct proliferative and differentiative activities on human megakaryocyte progenitors. *Blood* 1995; 86:2516–2525.
85. Sitnicka E, Lin N, Priestley GV, et al. The effect of thrombopoietin on the proliferation and differentiation of murine hematopoietic stem cells. *Blood* 1996; 87:4998–5005.
86. Katayama N, Itoh R, Kato T, et al. Role for C-MPL and its ligand thrombopoietin in early hematopoiesis. *Leuk Lymphoma* 1997; 28:51–56.
87. Molineaux G, Hartley C, McElroy P, McCrea C, McNiece IK. Megakaryocyte growth and development factor accelerates platelet recovery in peripheral blood progenitor cell transplant recipients. *Blood* 1996; 88:366–376.
88. Farese AM, Hunt P, Grab LB, MacVittie TJ. Combined administration of recombinant human megakaryocyte growth and development factor and granulocyte colony-stimulating factor enhances multilineage hematopoietic reconstitution in non-human primates after radiation-induced marrow aplasia. *J Clin Invest* 1996; 97:2145–2151.
89. Basser RL, Rasko JE, Clarke K, et al. Thrombopoietic effects of pegylated recombinant human megakaryocyte growth and development factor (PEG-rHuMGDF) in patients with advanced cancer. *Lancet* 1996; 348:1279–1281.
90. Vadhan-Raj S, Murray LJ, Bueso-Ramos C, et al. Stimulation of megakaryocyte and platelet production by a single dose of recombinant human thrombopoietin in patients with cancer. *Ann Intern Med* 1997; 126:673–681.
91. Basser RL, Rasko JE, Clarke K, et al. Randomized, blinded, placebo-controlled phase I trial of pegylated recombinant human megakaryocyte growth and development factor with filgrastim after dose-intensive chemotherapy in patients with advanced cancer. *Blood* 1997; 89:3118–3128.
92. Fanucchi M, Glaspy J, Crawford J, et al. Effects of polyethylene glycol-conjugated recombinant human megakaryocyte growth and development factor on platelet counts after chemotherapy for lung cancer. *N Engl J Med* 1997; 336:404–409.

93. Emmons RV, Reid DM, Cohen RL, et al. Human thrombopoietin levels are high when thrombocytopenia is due to megakaryocyte deficiency and low when due to increased platelet destruction. *Blood* 1996; 87:4068–4071.
94. Wang W, Matsuo T, Yoshida S, et al. Colony-forming unit-megakaryocyte (CFR-meg) numbers and serum thrombopoietin concentrations in thrombocytopenic disorders: an inverse correlation in myelodysplastic syndromes. *Leukemia* 2000; 14:1751–1756.
95. Zwierzina H, Rollinger-Holzinger I, Nuessler V, Herold M, Meng YG. Endogenous serum thrombopoietin concentrations in patients with myelodysplastic syndromes. *Leukemia* 1998; 12:59–64.
96. Tamura H, Ogata K, Luo S, et al. Plasma thrombopoietin (TPO levels) and expression of TPO receptor on platelets in patients with myelodysplastic syndromes. *Br J Haematol* 1998; 103:778–784.
97. Fontenay-Roupie M, Dupont JM, Picard F, et al. Analysis of megakaryocyte growth and development factor (thrombopoietin) effects on blast cell and megakaryocyte growth in myelodysplasia. *Leuk Res* 1998; 22:527–535.
98. Luo SS, Ogata K, Yokose N, Kato T, Dan K. Effect of thrombopoietin on proliferation of blasts from patients with myelodysplastic syndromes. *Stem Cells* 2000; 18:112–119.
99. Adams JA, Liu Yin JA, Brereton ML, Briggs M, Burgess R, Hyde K. The in vitro effect of pegylated recombinant human megakaryocyte growth and development factor (PEG rHuMGDF) on megakarypoiesis in normal subjects and patients with myelodysplasia and acute myeloid leukemia. *Br J Haematol* 1997; 99:139–146.
100. Liu Yin JA, Adams JA, Brereton ML, Hann A, Harrison BD, Briggs M. Megakaryopoiesis in vitro in myelodysplastic syndromes and acute myeloid leukemia: effect of pegylated recombinant human megakaryocyte growth and development factor in combination with other growth factors. *Br J Haematol* 2000; 108:743–746.
101. Ferrajoli A, Talpaz M, Kurzrock R, et al. Thrombopoietin stimulates myelodysplastic syndrome granulocyte-macrophage and erythroid progenitor proliferation. *Leuk Lymphoma* 1998; 30:279–292.
102. Komatsu N, Okamoto T, Yoshida T, et al. Pegylated recombinant human megakaryocyte growth and development factor (PEG-rHuMGDF) increased platelet counts (PLT) in patients (pts) with aplastic anemia (AA) and myelodysplastic syndrome (MDS). *Blood* 2000; 96:296a (abstract).
103. Fontenay-Roupie M, Bouscary D, Guesnu M, et al. Ineffective erythropoiesis in myelodysplastic syndromes: correlation with Fas expression but not with lack of erythropoietin receptor signal transduction. *Br J Haematol* 1999; 106:464–473.
104. Claessens YE, Bouscary D, Dupont JM, et al. In vitro proliferation and differentiation of erythroid progenitors from patients with myelodysplastic syndromes: evidence for Fas-dependent apoptosis. *Blood* 2002; 99:1594–1601.
105. Rigolin GM, Della Porta M, Bigoni R, et al. rHuEPO administration in patients with low-risk myelodysplastic syndromes: evaluation of erythroid precursors response by fluorescence in situ hybridization on May-Grünwald-Giemsa-stained bone marrow samples. *Br J Haematol* 2002; 119:652–659.
106. Schmidt-Mende J, Tehranchi R, Forsblom AM, et al. Granulocyte colony-stimulating factor inhibits Fas-triggered apoptosis in bone marrow cells isolated from patients with refractory anemia with ringed sideroblasts. *Leukemia* 2001; 15:742–751.
107. Tehranchi R, Fadeel B, Forsblom AM, et al. Granulocyte colony-stimulating factor inhibits spontaneous cytochrome c release and mitochondria-dependent apoptosis of myelodysplastic syndrome hematopoietic progenitors. *Blood* 2003; 101:1080–1086.
108. Marsh JCW, Socie G, Schrezenmeier H, et al. Haemopoietic growth factors in aplastic anaemia: a cautionary note. *Lancet* 1994; 344:172–173.
109. Marsh JCW. Hematopoietic growth factors in the pathogenesis and for the treatment of aplastic anemia. *Semin Hematol* 2000; 37:81–90.
110. Brereton ML, Adams JA, Briggs M, et al. The in vitro effect of pegylated recombinant human megakaryocyte growth and development factor (PEGrHuMGDF) on megakaryopoiesis in patients with aplastic anaemia. *Br J Med* 1994; 104:119–126.
111. Marsh JCW, Testa NG. In: Schrezenmeier H, Bacigalupo A, eds., *Aplastic Anaemia*. Cambridge, UK: Cambridge University Press. 1999:2–20.
112. Philpott NJ, Scopes J, Marsh JC, Gordon-Smith EC, Gibson FM. Increased apoptosis in aplastic anemia bone marrow progenitor cells: possible pathophysiological significance. *Exp Hematol* 1995; 23:1642–1648.
113. Marsh JCW, Chang J, Testa NG, Hows JM, Dexter TM. In vitro assessment of marrow stem cell and stromal cell function in aplastic anaemia. *Br J Haematol* 1991; 78:258–267.

114. Novitzky N, Jacobs P. Immunosuppressive therapy in bone marrow aplasia: the stroma functions normally to support hemopoiesis. *Exp Hematol* 1995; 23:1472–1477.
115. Holmberg LA, Seidel K, Leisenring W, Torok-Storb B. Aplastic anemia: analysis of stromal cell function in long term marrow culture. *Blood* 1994; 84:3685–3690.
116. Nissen C, Wodnar-Filipowicz A, Slanicka Krieger M, et al. Persistent growth impairment of bone marrow stroma after antilymphocyte globulin treatment for severe aplastic anaemia and its association with relapse. *Eur J Haematol* 1995; 55:255–261.
117. Hirayama Y, Kohgo Y, Matsunaga T, Ohi S, Sakamaki S, Niitsu Y. Cytokine mRNA expression of bone marrow stromal cells from patients with aplastic anaemia and myelodysplastic syndrome. *Br J Haematol* 1993; 85:676–683.
118. Stark R, Andre C, Thierry D, Cherel M, Galibert F, Gluckman E. The expression of cytokine and cytokine receptor genes in long term bone marrow culture in congenital and acquired marrow hypoplasias. *Br J Haematol* 1993; 83:560–566.
119. Kojima S, Matsuyama T, Kodera Y. Hemopoietic growth factors releases from marrow stromal cells from patients with aplastic anemia. *Blood* 1992; 79:2256–2261.
120. Kojima S, Matsuyama T, Kodera Y. Plasma levels and production of soluble stem cell factor by marrow stromal cells in patients with aplastic anaemia. *Br J Haematol* 1997; 99:440–446.
121. Nimer SD, Leung DHY, Wolin MJ, Golde DW. Serum stem cell factor levels in patients with aplastic anemia. *Int J Hematol* 1994; 60:185–189.
122. Wodnar-Filipowicz A, Yancik S, Moser Y, et al. Levels of soluble stem cell factor in serum of patients with aplastic anemia. *Blood* 1993; 81:3259–3264.
123. Kojima S. Hemopoietic growth factors and marrow stroma in aplastic anemia. *Int J Hematol* 1998; 68:19–28.
124. Schrezenmeier H, Noe G, Raghavachar A, Rich IN, Heimpel H, Kubanek B. Serum erythropoietin and serum transferring receptor levels in aplastic anaemia. *Br J Haematol* 1994; 88:286–294.
125. Kojima S, Matsuyama T, Kodera Y, et al. Measurement of endogenous plasma granulocyte colony stimulating factor in patients with acquired aplastic anemia by a sensitive chemiluminescent assay. *Blood* 1996; 87:1303–1308.
126. Schrezenmeier H, Raghavachar A, Heimpel H. Granulocyte-macrophage colony stimulating factor in the serum of patients with aplastic anemia. *Clin Invest* 1993; 71:102–108.
127. Wodnar-Filipowicz A, Lyman SD, Gratwohl A, Tichelli A, Speck B, Nissen C. Flt-3 ligand level reflects hemopoietic progenitor cell function in aplastic anemia and chemotherapy induced bone marrow aplasia. *Blood* 1996; 88:4493–4499.
128. Hirayama Y, Sakamaki S, Matsunaga T, et al. Concentrations of thrombopoietin in bone marrow in normal subjects, and in patients with idiopathic thrombocytopenic purpura, aplastic anemia and essential thrombocythemia correlates with its mRNA expression of bone marrow stromal cells. *Blood* 1998; 92:46–52.
129. Kojima S, Matsuyama T, Kodera Y, Tahara T, Kato T. Measurement of endogenous plasma thrombopoietin in patients with acquired aplastic anaemia by a sensitive enzyme-linked immunoabsorbent assay. *Br J Haematol* 1997; 97:538–543.
130. Marsh JCW, Gibson FM, Prue RL, et al. Serum thrombopoietin levels in patients with aplastic anaemia. *Br J Haematol* 1996; 95:605–610.
131. Gibson FM, Scopes J, Daly S, et al. In vitro response of normal and aplastic anemia bone marrow to mast cell growth factor and in combination with granulocyte macrophage colony stimulating factor and interleukin-3. *Exp Hematol* 1994; 22:302–312.
132. Wodnar-Filipowicz A, Chlouskaia E, Manz CY, et al. Effect of flt3 ligand on in vitro growth and expansion of colony forming bone marrow cells from patients with aplastic anemia. *Exp Hematol* 1997; 25:573–581.
133. Scopes J, Daly S, Atkinson R, et al. Aplastic anemia: evidence for dysfunctional bone marrow progenitor cells and the corrective effect of granulocyte colony stimulating factor in vitro. *Blood* 1996; 87:3179–3185.
134. Vadhan-Raj S, Buescher S, Broxmeyer HE, et al. Stimulation of myelopoiesis in patients with aplastic anemia by recombinant human granulocyte-macrophage colony-stimulating factor. *N Engl J Med* 1988; 319:1628–1634.
135. Antin JH, Smith BR, Holmes W, Rosenthal DS. Phase I/II study of rhGM-CSF in aplastic anemia and myelodysplastic syndromes. *Blood* 1988; 72:705–713.
136. Nissen C, Tichelli A, Gratwohl A, et al. Failure of rhGM-CSF therapy in aplastic anemia patients with very severe neutropenia. *Blood* 1988; 72:2045–2046.

137. Champlin RE, Nimer SD, Ireland P, Oette DH, Golde DW. Treatment of refractory aplastic anemia with recombinant human granulocyte-macrophage colony stimulating factor. *Blood* 1989; 73:694–699.
138. Guinan EC, Sieff CA, Oette DH, Nathan DG. A phase I/II trial of human granulocyte-macrophage colony stimulating factor for children with aplastic anemia. *Blood* 1990; 76:1077–1082.
139. Takahashi M, Yoshida Y, Kaku K, et al. Phase II study of recombinant human granulocyte-macrophage colony stimulating factor in myelodysplastic syndrome and aplastic anemia. *Acta Haematol* 1993; 89:189–194.
140. Kojima S, Fukuda M, Miyajima Y, Matsuyama T, Horibe K. Treatment of aplastic anemia in children with recombinant human granulocyte-colony stimulating factor. *Blood* 1991; 77:937–941.
141. Sonoda Y, Yashige H, Fujii H, et al. Bilineage response in refractory aplastic anemia patients following long-term administration of recombinant granulocyte-colony stimulating factor. *Eur J Haematol* 1992; 48:41–48.
142. Sonoda Y, Ohno Y, Fujii H, et al. Multilineage response in refractory aplastic anemia patients following long-term administration of filgrastim (recombinant human granulocyte colony stimulating factor). *Stem Cells* 1993; 11:543–554.
143. Kojima S, Matsuyama T. Stimulation of granulopoiesis by high-dose recombinant human granulocyte colony stimulating factor in children with aplastic anemia and very severe neutropenia. *Blood* 1994; 83:1474–1478.
144. Kurzrock R, Talpaz M, Gutterman JU. Very low doses of GM-CSF administered alone or with erythropoietin in aplastic anemia. *Am J Med* 1992; 93:41–48.
145. Imamura M, Kobayashi M, Kobayashi S, et al. Combination therapy with recombinant human granulocyte colony-stimulating factor and erythropoietin in aplastic anemia. *Am J Hematol* 1995; 48:29–33.
146. Yonekura S, Kawada H, Watanabe S, et al. Hematologic response in patients with aplastic anemia after long-term administration of recombinant human granulocyte colony-stimulating factor and erythropoietin. *Clin Ther* 1997; 19:1394–1407.
147. Bessho M, Hirashima K, Asano S, et al. Treatment of anemia of aplastic anemia patients with recombinant human erythropoietin in combination with granulocyte colony-stimulating factor: a multicenter randomized controlled study. Multicenter Study Group. *Eur J Haematol* 1997; 58:265–272.
148. Bargetzi MJ, Gluckman E, Tichelli A, et al. Recombinant human interleukin-3 in refractory severe aplastic anaemia: a phase I/II trial. *Br J Haematol* 1995; 91:306–312.
149. Ganser A, Lindermann A, Seipelt G, et al. Effect of recombinant human interleukin-3 in aplastic anemia. *Blood* 1990; 76:1287–1292.
150. Walsh CE, Liu JM, Anderson SM, Rossio JL, Nienhuis AW, Young NS. A trial of recombinant human interleukin-1 in patients with severe aplastic anaemia. *Br J Haematol* 1992; 80:106–110.
151. Schrezenmeier H, Marsh JCW, Stromeyer P, et al. A phase I/II trial of recombinant human interleukin-6 in patients with aplastic anaemia. *Br J Haematol* 1995; 90:283–292.
152. Kurzrock R, Paquette R, Gratwohl A, et al. Use of stem cell factor (Stemgen, SCF) and filgrastim (G-CSF) in aplastic anemia patients who have failed ATG/ALG therapy. *Blood* 1997; 90:173 (abstract).
153. Bacigalupo A, Broccia G, Corda G, et al. Antilymphocyte globulin, cyclosporin, and granulocyte colony-stimulating factor in patients with acquired severe aplastic anemia (SAA): a pilot study of the EBMT SAA Working Party. *Blood* 1995; 85:1348–1353.
154. Bacigalupo A, Bruno B, Saracco P, et al. Antilymphocyte globulin, cyclosporine, prednisolone, and granulocyte colony-stimulating factor for severe aplastic anemia: an update of the GITMO/EBMT study on 100 patients. European Group for Blood and Marrow Transplantation (EBMT) Working Party on Severe Aplastic Anemia and the Gruppo Italiano Trapianti di Midolio Osseo (GITMO). *Blood* 2000; 95:1931–1934.
155. Gluckman E, Rokicka-Milewska R, Hann I, et al. Results and follow-up of a phase III randomized study of recombinant human-granulocyte stimulating factor as support for immunosuppressive therapy in patients with severe aplastic anaemia. *Br J Haematol* 2002; 119:1075–1082.
156. DePlanque M, Bacigalupo A, Wursch A, et al. Long-term follow-up of severe aplastic anaemia patients treated with antithymocyte globulin. Severe Aplastic Anaemia Working Party of the European Cooperative Group for Bone Marrow Transplantation (EBMT). *Br J Haematol* 1989; 73:121–126.
157. Socie G, Henry AM, Bacigalupo A, et al. Malignant tumours occurring after treatment of aplastic anemia. European Bone Marrow Transplant Severe Aplastic Anemia Working Party. *N Engl J Med* 1993; 329:1152–1157.
158. Tichelli A, Gratwohl A, Wursch A, Nissen C, Speck B. Late haematological complications in severe aplastic anaemia. *Br J Haematol* 1988; 69:413–418.

159. Kojima S, Tsuchida M, Matsuyama T. Myelodysplasia and leukemia after treatment of aplastic anemia with granulocyte colony stimulating factor. *N Engl J Med* 1992; 326:1294–1295.
160. Imashuku S, Hibi S, Kataoka MY, et al. Myelodysplasia and acute myeloid leukaemia in cases of aplastic anaemia and congenital neutropenia following G-CSF administration. *Br J Haematol* 1995; 89:188–191.
161. Ohara A, Kojima S, Hamajima N, et al. Myelodysplasia and acute myeloid leukemia as a late clonal complication in children with acquired aplastic anemia. *Blood* 1997; 90:1009–1013.
162. Kaito K, Kobayashi M, Katayama T, et al. Long-term administration of G-CSF for aplastic anaemia is closely related to the early evolution of monosomy 7 MDS in adults. *Br J Haematol* 1998; 103:297–303.
163. Kojima S, Hibi S, Kosaka Y, et al. Immunosuppressive therapy using antithymocyte globulin, cyclosporine, and danazol with or without human granulocyte colony-stimulating factor in children with acquired aplastic anemia. *Blood* 2000; 2049–2054.
164. Bessho M, Hotta T, Ohyashiki K, et al. Multicenter prospective study of clonal complications in adult aplastic anemia patients following recombinant human granulocyte colony-stimulating factor (lenograstim) administration. *Int J Hematol* 2003; 77:152–158.
165. Locasciulli A, Arcese W, Locatelli F, Di Bona E, Bacigalupo A. Italian Aplastic Anaemia Study Group. *Lancet* 2001; 357:43–44.
166. Bowen DT, Hellstrom-Lindberg E. Best supportive care for the anaemia of myelodysplasia: inclusion of recombinant erythropoietin therapy? *Leuk Res* 2001; 25:19–21.
167. Cheson BD, Bennett JM, Kantarjian H, et al. Report of an international working group to standardize response criteria for myelodysplastic syndromes. *Blood* 2000; 96:3671–3674.

18 Use of Hematopoietic Growth Factors in AIDS-Related Malignancies

MaryAnn Foote, PhD

CONTENTS

1. INTRODUCTION

Malignancies develop in approx 30–40% of patients with human immunodeficiency virus (HIV) infections *(1)*. In 1993, The Centers for Disease Control listed three malignancies as acquired immunodeficiency syndrome (AIDS)-defining conditions, Kaposi's sarcoma; intermediate or high-grade, B-cell non-Hodgkin's lymphoma (NHL); and invasive cervical cancer *(2)*. Other malignancies with an increased incidence in people with HIV infection include angiosarcoma, Hodgkin's disease (HD), multiple myeloma, brain cancer, and seminoma *(3)*. Survival has increased in patients with HIV infection and malignancy owing to better prevention, diagnosis, and treatment of opportunistic infections as well as more effective antiretroviral therapies. Unfortunately, improved survival may result in an increased incidence of malignancies, particularly those not considered AIDS-defining conditions, i.e., Kaposi's sarcoma *(1)*.

Chemotherapy administration to patients with advanced-stage AIDS and a malignancy can decrease tumor size and improve survival *(4)*. Unfortunately, patients with HIV infection often receive less dose-intense chemotherapy regimens to minimize the risk of exacerbating neutropenia, which occurs as a result of multiple interrelated

From: *Cancer Drug Discovery and Development*
Hematopoietic Growth Factors in Oncology: Basic Science and Clinical Therapeutics
Edited by: G. Morstyn, M. A. Foote, and G. J. Lieschke © Humana Press Inc., Totowa, NJ

Table 1
Factors Contributing to Neutropenia in Patients With HIV Infection

Antiretroviral therapies (e.g., zidovudine)
Chemotherapy
Hematopoietic growth factor deficiencies
HIV infection
Apoptosis acceleration
Malignancies
Nutritional deficiencies
Opportunistic infections involving the bone marrow
Prophylactic therapies (e.g., acyclovir, trimethoprim/sulfamethoxazole)

Data from refs. *5* and *6*.

factors (Table 1) *(5,6)*. Administration of hematopoietic growth factors (HGFs) may allow for the administration of more dose-intense chemotherapy regimens and, ultimately, an improvement in clinical outcome. This chapter describes the use of recombinant human granulocyte-colony stimulating factor (rHuG-CSF) and recombinant human granulocyte macrophage-colony stimulating factor (rHuGM-CSF) in patients with HIV infection and malignancy including Kaposi's sarcoma, NHL, invasive cervical cancer, and HD. Both comparative and noncomparative studies are reviewed. Most studies were not randomized and were not specifically designed to evaluate the benefits of HGF administration. Because of differences in patient characteristics and the rapid evolution of AIDS therapies, readers should be careful about comparing findings from different treatment groups within studies and should avoid the temptation to compare findings from different studies.

2. USE OF rHuG-CSF OR rHuGM-CSF IN PATIENTS WITH HIV INFECTION AND MALIGNANCY

The effects of rHuG-CSF and rHuGM-CSF on HIV-infected cells were evaluated in vitro. Exposure to rHuG-CSF in vitro did not increase HIV replication in HIV-infected monocyte, macrophage, and bone marrow stem cells *(7–9)*. Exposure to rHuGM-CSF in vitro had various effects in HIV-infected monocytes, macrophages, brain cells, and bone marrow stem cells. Results from some *(7–14)* but not all *(15–19)* in vitro studies suggest that rHuGM-CSF can increase HIV replication. Interestingly, in some studies, the antiretroviral activity of dideoxynucleoside agents was increased with concurrent rHuGM-CSF exposure *(9,11,14–16)*.

Results from clinical studies evaluating the virologic effect of rHuG-CSF and rHuGM-CSF in patients with HIV infection are similar to those from in vitro studies. A clinical study evaluating rHuG-CSF administration to patients with HIV infection found no evidence of enhanced viral replication *(20)*. A systematic, nonquantitative review of all known rHuGM-CSF studies in patients with HIV infection published in 1998 reported no convincing evidence of enhanced viral replication *(21)*.

Both rHuG-CSF and rHuGM-CSF have been administered to patients with HIV infection conditions other than malignancies including the treatment of HIV-associated neutropenia, the adjunctive treatment of established infections, and mobilization of stem cells for genetic alteration *(22,23)*. The safe and effective treatment of HIV-associated neutropenia with rHuG-CSF and rHuGM-CSF in patients with HIV infection and without malignancy has led to their use in patients with HIV infection and malignancy. It is hoped that rHuG-CSF or rHuGM-CSF use in this patient population will allow for the administration of chemotherapy doses in combination with myelotoxic drugs, such as antiretrovirals and prophylactic therapies. Ultimately, the goal of HGF administration is to improve clinical outcomes and patient quality of life.

3. KAPOSI'S SARCOMA

Kaposi's sarcoma, the most common malignancy in patients with HIV infection, occurs in 20–30% of patients *(24)*. The incidence of Kaposi's sarcoma is 300-fold higher in patients with HIV infection compared with those without HIV infection *(3)*. The adjusted incidence rate for Kaposi's sarcoma decreased from 15.2 per 1000 person-years from 1992 through 1996 to 4.9 per 1000 person-years from 1997 through 1999 in developed countries because of the administration of highly active antiretroviral therapy (HAART) *(25)*.

Current treatment strategies for Kaposi's sarcoma are not curative. Treatment should be individualized based on the extent and rate of tumor growth, tumor-related symptoms, immune system condition, social and cosmetic needs of the patient, and the presence of other HIV-associated illnesses. Treatment options include both local and systemic therapies. Local therapies include surgical excision, laser therapy, cryotherapy, radiotherapy, and intralesion injections. Systemic therapies include HAART, immune-response modifiers, and chemotherapy. HGFs have been used in combination with several systemic therapies including the immune-response modifier interferon-α (IFN-α) and numerous chemotherapy regimens.

3.1. IFN-α

Systemic IFN-α (36–50 MU/m^2/d) produced responses in 18–46% of patients with Kaposi's sarcoma *(1)*; combination IFN-α (1–10 MU/d) and zidovudine produced responses in approx 40–50% of patients with Kaposi's sarcoma *(26,27)*. The major dose-limiting toxicity for combination IFN-α-zidovudine therapy is myelosuppression.

The use of HGF in combination with IFN-α and zidovudine for the treatment of Kaposi's sarcoma was evaluated in two published studies. Daily rHuGM-CSF 5 μg/kg sc as primary prophylaxis in combination with daily zidovudine 1200 mg orally and IFN-α 5, 10, or 20 MU sc was administered in the first study *(28)*. The rHuGM-CSF dose was titrated to maintain a white blood cell count between 1 and 5 × 10^9/L. The second study administered rHuGM-CSF as secondary prophylaxis in combination with daily zidovudine 1200 mg orally and IFN 9 MU sc *(29)*. Patients received daily rHuGM-CSF 125 μg/m^2 sc if the absolute neutrophil count (ANC) was <1 × 10^9/L; rHuGM-CSF dose was titrated to maintain an ANC > 1 × 10^9/L. In both studies, rHuGM-CSF administration increased white blood cell counts. Tumor response rates (41 and 50%) were similar to results from studies not incorporating HGF. Flu-like symptoms were the most commonly reported adverse effects. No consistent changes in immune function or HIV activity were reported.

3.2. Chemotherapy

Systemic chemotherapy treatment of Kaposi's sarcoma is typically reserved for second-line therapy or for patients with widespread, symptomatic disease including

Table 2
Hematopoietic Growth Factors As Primary or Secondary Prophylaxis in Patients With HIV Infection and Kaposi's Sarcoma

Ref.	*Hematopoietic growth factor*	*Antiretroviral*	*Chemotherapy*	*No. of evaluable patients (no. receiving CSF)*	*Response (%)*	
					Overall	*Complete*
Primary prophylaxis						
33	rHuGM-CSF	None	Doxorubicin, bleomycin, vincristine	6 (6)	67	17
34	rHuGM-CSF	Zidovudine	Doxorubicin, bleomycin, vincristine	16 (16)	69	13
35	rHuG-CSF	Didanosine	Doxorubicin, bleomycin, vincristine	25 (25)	58	18
Secondary Prophylaxis						
36	rHuGM-CSF	Unspecified	Doxorubicin, bleomycin, vindesine	27 (13)	70	11
37	rHuG-CSF	Zidovudine, didanosine, or zalcitabine	Liposomal daunorubicin	116 (37)	25	3
			Doxorubicin, bleomycin, vincristine	111 (20)	28	1
38	Unspecified	Unspecified	Paclitaxel	56 (15)	59	2
39	rHuG-CSF	Zidovudine, didanosine, zalcitabine	Doxorubicin, bleomycin, vinblastine, vincristine, dactinomycin, dacarbazine	18 (8)	83	50
40	Unspecified	Unspecified	Paclitaxel	107 (NR)	56	4
41	rHuG-CSF	Nucleoside reverse-transcriptase inhibitors	Paclitaxel	28 (10)	71	10

ABBREVIATIONS: CSF, colony-stimulating factor; rHuG-CSF, recombinant human granulocyte colony-stimulating factor; rHuGM-CSF, recombinant human granulocyte-macrophage colony-stimulating factor; NR, not reported.

visceral disease. Response rates of 10–76% have been reported for single-agent therapies; response rates of 23–88% have been reported for combination therapies *(1,4,30–32)*. Myelosuppression occurs with both single-agent and combination therapies. Current recommendations are to administer single-agent therapy with a liposomal anthracycline or with paclitaxel, a bleomycin-*Vinca* alkaloid combination, or a three-drug doxorubicin combination. Concomitant HAART and an HGF should also be administered.

HGFs have been administered as primary and secondary prophylaxis of infections in published studies designed to evaluate both single-agent and combination therapies for Kaposi's sarcoma (Table 2). The use of rHuG-CSF or rHuGM-CSF administered as primary prophylaxis was the focus in two of the three primary prophylaxis studies *(33,35)*. The use of rHuG-CSF and rHuGM-CSF administered as secondary prophylaxis was the focus in two of the six published secondary prophylaxis studies *(36,39)*.

3.3. Primary Prophylaxis

Gill and co-workers *(33)* determined the maximum tolerated dose of rHuGM-CSF administered in combination with doxorubicin, bleomycin, and vincristine (ABV) given every 14 d. Antiretroviral and myelosuppressive medications were discontinued 2 wk before study entry. Patients received ABV on d 1 and daily rHuGM-CSF 250 or 500 μg/m^2 sc on d 2–12. The overall response rate was 67%, and the complete response rate was 17%. White blood cell counts increased similarly with both rHuGM-CSF doses. Dose-limiting toxicities, such as grade 3 fever, fatigue, and diarrhea, were more common with the 500-μg/m^2 dose. No patient required a change in chemotherapy schedule because of neutropenia. No patient developed a bacterial infection; one patient developed an opportunistic infection (cytomegalovirus retinitis).

Mastroianni and coworkers *(35)* evaluated the use of rHuG-CSF in combination with ABV administered every 14 d. Patients received rHuG-CSF 5 μg/kg before and after ABV administration. Concomitant antiretroviral therapy with didanosine and *Pneumocystis carinii* prophylaxis with trimethoprim sulfamethoxazole was allowed. The overall response rate to ABV was 58%, and the complete response rate was 18%. Median survival was 11 mo. Administration of rHuG-CSF decreased the incidence of hematologic toxicity and morbidity from febrile neutropenia (FN) and increased patient quality of life. Serious bacterial infections occurred in five (20%) and opportunistic infections in three (12%) patients. Adverse effects occurring in >40% of patients included nausea, vomiting, and headache.

3.4. Secondary Prophylaxis

Sloand and coworkers *(39)* evaluated the use of rHuGM-CSF or rHuG-CSF in combination with doxorubicin, bleomycin, vinblastine, vincristine, actinomycin D, and dacarbazine administered every 21 d. Antiretroviral therapy was continued with zidovudine, zalcitabine, or didanosine. Chemotherapy doses were decreased for neutropenia. In addition, patients received compassionate use rHuGM-CSF 5 μg/kg sc daily if the ANC was $<0.5 \times 10^9$/L. After it became commercially available, rHuG-CSF 300 μg was administered sc daily if the ANC was $<1 \times 10^9$/L. HGF support continued until the ANC was $>1.5 \times 10^9$/L. The overall response rate to therapy was 83%, and the complete response rate was 50%. Median survival was 9 mo. A total of eight patients received either rHuGM-CSF (three patients) or rHuG-CSF (five patients). Survival was longer in patients who required less than three compared with those who required three or more decreases in chemotherapy doses for neutropenia. No dosage reductions were necessary in patients who received rHuG-CSF. Serious bacterial infections occurred in three (17%) and opportunistic infections in two (11%) patients. HGF use in these patients with infections was not reported.

Bakker and co-workers *(36)* evaluated the use of rHuGM-CSF in combination with doxorubicin, bleomycin, and vindesine administered every 14 d. Antiretroviral therapy was continued. Patients received daily rHuGM-CSF 5 μg/kg sc on d 2–12 if their ANC was <0.5 × 10^9/L or if their chemotherapy doses had to be consistently reduced. The overall response rate was 70%, and the complete response rate was 11%. Median survival was 30 wk. A total of 13 patients received rHuGM-CSF. In general, white blood cell counts increased to >2 × 10^9/L with rHuGM-CSF administration. Adverse events with rHuGM-CSF were minimal. No bacterial infections were reported; five opportunistic infections occurred, two in patients who received rHuGM-CSF.

4. NON-HODGKIN'S LYMPHOMA

NHL is the second most common malignancy in patients with HIV infection. The incidence of NHL is increased 113-fold and cerebral lymphoma is increased approx 3600-fold in patients with HIV infection compared with those without HIV infection *(3,6)*. The incidence of NHL has decreased since the introduction of HAART; however, the decrease in incidence is less than that seen with Kaposi's sarcoma *(25)*. The adjusted incidence rate for NHL decreased from 6.2 per 1000-person years from 1992 through 1996 to 3.6 per 1000-person years from 1997 through 1999 in developed countries since the introduction of HAART. Analysis by morphologic type or anatomic site showed variations among cerebral lymphoma, immunoblastic lymphoma, and Burkitt's lymphoma. The rate ratio for 1997–1999 vs. 1992–1996 was 0.58 for all NHL, 0.42 for cerebral lymphoma, 0.57 for immunoblastic lymphoma, and 1.18 for Burkitt's lymphoma *(3)*.

The current recommendation for treating all NHL, except cerebral lymphoma, is systemic chemotherapy. The current recommendation for treating cerebral lymphoma is whole brain radiotherapy; adjunctive chemotherapy may increase response rates in young patients with high performance status *(6)*. As of 2003, the optimal chemotherapy regimen for treating NHL has not been identified. Median survival with chemotherapy is ≤12 mo *(1)*. Prognostic factors associated with a poor outcome include age >35 years, intravenous drug abuse, stage III or IV disease, CD4 lymphocyte count < 0.1 × 10^9/L, history of Kaposi's sarcoma or an opportunistic infection, Karnofsky performance score ≤70%, and extranodal disease, particularly of the bone marrow *(6,42)*.

Numerous chemotherapy regimens have been evaluated as first-line therapy for patients with HIV infection and NHL. However, grade 4 leukopenia or neutropenia occurred in 44–79%, and FN and sepsis occurred in 25–50% of patients *(43)*. Administration of half-dose chemotherapy regimens did not decrease the incidence of grade 4 leukopenia or FN *(43)*.

The use of HGF in treating patients with HIV infection and NHL was evaluated in several published comparative, but not necessarily randomized, studies (Table 3). Kaplan and coworkers *(45)* compared administration of cyclophosphamide, doxorubicin, vincristine, and prednisone (CHOP) alone with CHOP and either early rHuGM-CSF administration (d 1–10) or late rHuGM-CSF administration (d 4–13). The dosage of rHuGM-CSF administered was 10–20 μg/kg sc daily. A total of 6 of 9 patients (67%) who received CHOP alone, 3 of 5 patients (60%) who received CHOP and early rHuGM-CSF, and 7 of 10 patients (70%) who received CHOP and late rHuGM-CSF had a complete response; partial responses were not reported. Median survival was 9 mo for patients who received CHOP alone, 8 mo for those who received CHOP plus early rHuGM-CSF, and 11 mo for those who received CHOP plus late rHuGM-CSF. Administration of CHOP and late rHuGM-CSF administration compared with CHOP

Table 3
Hematopoietic Growth Factor in Patients With HIV Infection and Non-Hodgkin's Lymphoma in Comparative Trials[a]

Ref.	Antiretroviral	Chemotherapy	No. of evaluable patients	Response (%) Overall	Response (%) Complete
44	NR	Modified COP-BLAM + rHuGM-CSF	64	85	72
		Modified COP-BLAM	↑	↑	↑
			73	81	62
45	NR	CHOP + early rHuGM-CSF	5	NR	60
		CHOP + late rHuGM-CSF	10	NR	70
		CHOP	9	NR	67
46	Unspecified,	m-BACOD + rHuGM-CSF (all patients)	81	78	52
	no zidovudine	Reduced-dose m-BACOD + rHuGM-CSF (as needed)	94	69	41
47	HAART	CHOP + rHuG-CSF	23	57	48
		Modified CHOP	40	60	30
48	NR	ProMACE-CytaBOM + rHuG-CSF	20	65	40
		ProMACE-CytaBOM	11	82	82
43,49	NR	LNH 84 or CHVmP/VCR-BLM + rHuG-CSF	18	78	69
		LNH 84 or CHVmP/VCR-BLM	19	88	67

ABBREVIATIONS: NR, not reported; LNH84, cyclophosphamide, doxorubicin, vindesine, bleomycin, methylprednisolone, methotrexate; CHVmP/VCR-BLM, cyclophosphamide, doxorubicin, teniposide, vincristine, bleomycin, prednisone; rHuG-CSF, recombinant human granulocyte colony-stimulating factor; CHOP, cyclophosphamide, doxorubicin, vincristine, prednisone; COP-BLAM, cyclophosphamide, vincristine, prednisolone, bleomycin, doxorubicin, procarbazine; rHuGM-CSF, recombinant human granulocyte macrophage colony-stimulating factor; m-BACOD, methotrexate, bleomycin, doxorubicin, cyclophosphamide, vincristine, dexamethasone; ProMACE-CytaBOM, prednisone, doxorubicin, cyclophosphamide, etoposide, cytarabine, bleomycin, vincristine, methotrexate, leucovorin; HAART, highly active antiviral therapy.

[a] Trials were designed to evaluate the effects of hematopoietic growth factor administration.

alone was associated with an increase in ANC, shortened mean duration of neutropenia, decreased number of chemotherapy cycles complicated by neutropenia and fever, decreased number of hospital days for neutropenia and fever, decreased number of chemotherapy dosage reductions, and decreased number of delays in chemotherapy administration. No difference in outcome was reported for patients who received CHOP alone and CHOP plus early rHuGM-CSF. Three opportunistic infections occurred, one in each treatment group. Bacteremia occurred in a few patients, and the incidence was similar between the treatment groups.

Gerhartz and co-workers *(44)* compared administration of cyclophosphamide, vincristine, prednisolone, bleomycin, doxorubicin, and procarbazine (COP-BLAM) plus rHuGM-CSF 400 μg subcutaneously on d 8–14 with COP-BLAM alone. A response occurred in 54 patients (85%) who received COP-BLAM plus rHuGM-CSF and in 59 patients (81%) who received COP-BLAM alone. A complete response occurred in 46 patients (72%) who received COP-BLAM plus rHuGM-CSF and in 45 patients (62%) who received COP-BLAM alone. Mean number of days with fever ($p = 0.04$), number of patients who required antibiotics ($p = 0.02$), mean days of intravenous antibiotics ($p = 0.02$), number of patients hospitalized for infection ($p = 0.02$), and mean number of hospital days for infection ($p = 0.01$) were significantly reduced for patients who received COP-BLAM plus rHuGM-CSF compared with COP-BLAM alone.

Tirelli and Vaccher *(43,49)* administered cyclophosphamide, doxorubicin, vindesine, bleomycin, methylprednisolone, and methotrexate (LNH 84) or cyclophosphamide, doxorubicin, teniposide, vincristine, bleomycin, and prednisone (CHVmP + VB) plus rHuG-CSF 5 µg/kg sc for 13 d beginning 24 h after chemotherapy administration or LNH 84 or CHVmP + VB alone. An overall response occurred in 16 patients (78%) who received either LNH 84 or CHVmP + VB plus rHuG-CSF and 15 patients (88%) who received LNH 84 or CHVmP + VB alone. A complete response occurred in 14 patients (69%) who received either LNH 84 or CHVmP + VB plus rHuG-CSF and 13 patients (67%) who received LNH 84 or CHVmP + VB alone. Median survival was 4 mo in patients who received rHuG-CSF and 10 mo in those who received only chemotherapy ($p = 0.04$). The authors attributed this difference to a lower CD4 count in rHuG-CSF-treated patients. Administration of rHuG-CSF significantly decreased the mean duration of delays between chemotherapy cycles ($p = 0.01$) and the mean hospitalization duration for toxicity ($p = 0.003$). Cost was also decreased with rHuG-CSF administration from US $3232 to US $2282 per chemotherapy cycle (p = not significant). The incidence of opportunistic infections was higher in patients who did not receive rHuG-CSF. The incidence of FN was comparable between the two treatment groups; however, infections in the group not receiving rHuG-CSF were more severe and required more hospitalization days and antibiotic therapy.

Rossi and co-workers *(48)* compared prednisone, doxorubicin, cyclophosphamide, etoposide, cytarabine, bleomycin, vincristine, methotrexate, and leucovorin (ProMACE-CytaBOM) plus rHuG-CSF 300 µg sc on d 9–20 with ProMACE-CytaBOM alone. A response occurred in 13 patients (65%) who received ProMACE-CytaBOM plus rHuG-CSF and in 9 patients (82%) who received chemotherapy alone. A complete response occurred in eight patients (40%) who received ProMACE-CytaBOM plus rHuG-CSF and in nine patients (82%) who received ProMACE-CytaBOM alone. The authors noted that patients who received ProMACE-CytaBOM plus rHuG-CSF had worse prognostic features, more advanced HIV disease, and lower white blood cell counts than patients who received ProMACE-CytaBOM alone. Administration of rHuG-CSF significantly decreased the number of reduced-dose chemotherapy cycles administered ($p < 0.001$) and the number of delayed chemotherapy cycles ($p < 0.001$). Opportunistic infections occurred in three patients (25%) who received ProMACE-CytaBOM alone and in six patients (29%) who received ProMACE-CytaBOM plus rHuG-CSF.

Ratner and co-workers *(47)* compared administration of low-dose CHOP with full-dose CHOP plus rHuG-CSF 300 µg sc daily for patients <70 kg or 480 µg daily for patients >70 kg. All patients received antiretroviral therapy consisting of stavudine, lamivudine, and indinavir. A response occurred in 13 patients (57%) who received full-dose CHOP plus rHuG-CSF and 24 patients (60%) who received low-dose CHOP. A complete response occurred in 11 patients (48%) who received full-dose CHOP plus rHuG-CSF and 12 patients (30%) who received low-dose CHOP. Grade 3 or 4 neutropenia occurred in 13% of patients who received full-dose CHOP plus rHuG-CSF and 25% of patients who received low-dose CHOP. FN developed in one patient who received low-dose CHOP.

Finally, Kaplan and co-workers *(46)* compared low- with standard-dose methotrexate, bleomycin, doxorubicin, cyclophosphamide, vincristine, and dexamethasone (m-BACOD). All patients who received standard-dose m-BACOD received rHuGM-CSF 5 μg/kg sc on d 4–13; only patients who received low-dose m-BACOD and had an ANC $< 1 \times 10^9$/L on d 22 or $<0.5 \times 10^9$/L during the chemotherapy cycle received rHuGM-CSF 5 μg/kg sc. Patients could receive any antiretroviral therapy except zidovudine. A response occurred in 65 patients (69%) who received low-dose m-BACOD and 63 patients (78%) who received standard-dose m-BACOD plus rHuGM-CSF. A complete response occurred in 39 patients (41%) who received low-dose m-BACOD and 42 patients (52%) who received standard-dose m-BACOD plus rHuGM-CSF. Median survival was 8 mo in patients who received low-dose m-BACOD and 7 mo in those who received standard-dose m-BACOD plus rHuGM-CSF. Hospitalization was significantly longer for patients who received standard-dose m-BACOD plus rHuGM-CSF compared with those receiving low-dose m-BACOD ($p = 0.03$). Opportunistic infections occurred in 22 patients (22%) receiving low-dose m-BACOD and in 22 patients (23%) receiving standard-dose m-BACOD plus rHuGM-CSF. Grade 4 neutropenia occurred in 49 patients (50%) who received low-dose m-BACOD and in 65 patients (69%) who received standard-dose m-BACOD plus rHuGM-CSF.

Numerous published studies evaluating various chemotherapy regimens for NHL have included HGF administration; however, these studies were not designed to evaluate the benefit of growth factor administration (Table 4). Overall response rates ranged from 7 to 96%, and complete response rates ranged from 0 to 87%. Grade 3 or 4 neutropenia was reported in 40–79% of patients receiving HGFs as primary prophylaxis.

Two published reports describe the use of rHuG-CSF administration for stem cell mobilization in patients with HIV-associated lymphoma receiving HAART *(64,65)*. Patients received myeloablative chemotherapy with autologous stem cell transplantation. Hematopoietic recovery occurred after stem cell transplantation. Most patients remained in remission for >19 mo.

The optimal treatment for NHL has not been identified. Administration of standard-dose chemotherapy regimens with HGF support has not consistently improved outcomes. Current recommendations are to administer lower doses of aggressive chemotherapy regimens such as m-BACOD, CDE, or CHOP with or without HGFs to patients with poor prognostic factors. Standard chemotherapy doses with HGFs should be administered to patients without poor prognostic factors.

5. CERVICAL CANCER

Invasive cervical cancer is the least common AIDS-defining malignancy. Unlike Kaposi's sarcoma and NHL, the adjusted incidence rate for invasive cervical cancer has not decreased over time. The adjusted incidence rate was 1.1 per 1000 person-years from 1992 through 1996 and 2.1 per 1000 person-years from 1997 through 1999 *(25)*.

Cervical cancer, unlike other AIDS-defining malignancies, is caused by an infection with certain types of human papillomaviruses and can be prevented with early detection and treatment of premalignant conditions. Treatment options for premalignant conditions include loop electrosurgical excision, cryoablation, conization, or laser surgery. Unfortunately, invasive cervical cancer does occur and is a more aggressive disease than that seen in patients without HIV infection *(66)*. Treatment strategies for

Table 4

Hematopoietic Growth Factor As Primary or Secondary Prophylaxis in Patients With HIV Infection and Non-Hodgkin's Lymphoma in Noncomparative Trial[a]

Ref.	*Hematopoietic growth factor*	*Antiretroviral*	*Chemotherapy*	*No. of evaluable patients*	*Response (%)*	
					Overall	*Complete*
50	rHuG-CSF	Lamivudine, zidovudine, indinavir	Cyclophosphamide, vincristine, mitoxantrone, bleomycin	29	72	72
50	rHuG-CSF	Zidovudine, didanosine	Cyclophosphamide, vincristine, epirubicin, bleomycin	60	54	54
51	rHuG-CSF	Unspecified	Dexamethasone, cisplatin, cytarabine	13	7	0
			Etoposide, cisplatin, methlyprednisolone, cytarabine	13	54	31
52	rHuG-CSF	Zidovudine	Doxorubicin, cyclophosphamide, vindesine, bleomycin, prednisolon	32	56	44
53	rHuG-CSF	None	Cyclophosphamide, mitoxantrone, vincristine, prednisone	21	43	19
54	RHuG-CSF	Zidovudine, didanosine	Cyclophosphamide, epirubicin, vincristine, prednisolone	14	57	50
55	RHuG-CSF	NR	Cyclophosphamide, vincristine, bleomycin, etoposide, doxorubicin, prednisone	23	96	87
56	RHuG-CSF	Nucleoside analog	Doxorubicin, cyclophosphamide, vindesine, bleomycin, prednisolone, followed by cyclophosphamide, etoposide, methotrexate	52	85	71
57	rHuG-CSF	Unspecified	Lomustine, etoposide, cyclophosphamide, procarbazine	20	70	30
58	rHuG-CSF	Didanosine	Cyclophosphamide, doxorubicin, etoposide	24	63	58
59	rHuG-CSF	Unspecified	Cyclophosphamide, doxorubicin, etoposide	40	28	10
60	rHuG-CSF	HAART	Rituximab, cyclophosphamide, doxorubicin, etoposide	26	90	86
61	rHuG-CSF	NR	Liposomal daunorubicin	31	39	7
62	rHuGM-CSF	HAART	Cyclophosphamide, doxorubicin, vincristine, prednisone	24	NR	50
	or rHuG-CSF	None	Cyclophosphamide, doxorubicin, vincristine, prednisone	75	NR	36
63	rHuGM-CSF	None	Bleomycin, doxorubicin, cyclophosphamide, vincristine, dexamethasone	16	Not reported	50

Abbreviations: rHuG-CSF, recombinant human granulocyte colony-stimulating factor; rHuGM-CSF, recombinant human granulocyte-macrophage colony-stimulating factor; NR, not reported; HAART, highly active antiretroviral therapy.

[a] Trials were not designed to evaluate the effects of hematopoietic growth factor administration.

Table 5
Hematopoietic Growth Factor As Primary Prophylaxis in Patients With HIV Infection and Hodgkin's Disease

Ref.	*Hematopoietic growth factor*	*Antiretroviral*	*Chemotherapy*	*No. of evaluable patients*	*Response (%)*	
					Overall	*Complete*
68	rHuG-CSF	Zidovudine or didanosine	Epirubicin, bleomycin, vinblastine	35	91	74
69	rHuG-CSF	None	Doxorubicin, bleomycin, vinblastine, dacarbazine	21	62	43
70	rHuG-CSF	HAART	Stanford V	59	89	81

ABBREVIATIONS: HAART, highly active antiretroviral therapy; Stanford V, doxorubicin, vinblastine, meclorethamine, etoposide, vincristine, bleomycin, prednisone; rHuG-CSF, recombinant human granulocyte colony-stimulating factor.

invasive cervical cancer are the same for women with and without HIV infection because women with HIV infection are more likely to die from invasive cervical cancer than from complications of HIV infection *(66)*. Treatment strategies include radical hysterectomy and pelvic lymphadenectomy, radiation, and chemotherapy. Chemotherapy regimens administered include cisplatin alone or in combination with bleomycin and vincristine. HGFs can be administered in combination with myelotoxic chemotherapy regimens to optimize dose intensity and ultimately improve clinical outcome. HGFs should be administered during the expected peak time of myelosuppression based on the administered chemotherapy regimen.

6. HODGKIN'S DISEASE

HD is the most common malignancy not considered an AIDS-defining condition in patients with HIV infection. The risk for developing HD in patients with HIV infection is approx 8.5 times higher than for patients without HIV infection *(1)*. The adjusted incidence rate for HD has remained fairly steady during the 1990s in developed countries. The adjusted incidence rate was 0.5 per 1000 person-years from 1992 through 1996 and 0.4 per 1000 person-years from 1997 through 1999 *(25)*. Unfortunately, patients with HIV infection typically present with advanced-stage HD. The presence of systemic symptoms such as fever, night sweats, and weight loss is common. More than 75% of patients have Ann Arbor stage III or IV disease, and most have unfavorable histologic subtypes.

Current treatment strategies include administration of systemic combination chemotherapy such as mechlorethamine, vincristine, procarbazine, and prednisone (MOPP) or doxorubicin, bleomycin, vinblastine, and dacarbazine (ABVD). Response rates with combination chemotherapy in patients with HIV disease are generally less than those in patients without HIV disease. Several published studies were designed to evaluate the use of rHuG-CSF administered in combination with chemotherapy for HD (Table 5); however, no published studies were designed to evaluate specifically the use of HGF in patients with HIV infection and HD. Response rates with combination chemotherapy and rHuG-CSF range from 62 to 91% *(69–71)*. Grade 3 or 4 neutropenia is common and occurred in 29–78% of patients despite rHuG-CSF administration.

7. OTHER CANCERS

HGF can be administered to patients with HIV disease and other types of cancers to optimize chemotherapy dose intensity and improve clinical outcomes. HGF administration should be based on the myelosuppressive profile of the administered chemotherapy regimen and should be given during the expected peak time of myelosuppression based on the administered chemotherapy regimen. The optimal dose of rHuG-CSF and rHuGM-CSF for patients with HIV infection receiving myelotoxic chemotherapy has not been determined and should be based on patient clinical status, laboratory values, and the administered chemotherapy regimen.

8. CONCLUSIONS

Patients with HIV infection and a malignancy can be safely treated with an HGF. Administration of rHuG-CSF does not increase HIV replication in vitro or in vivo, but administration of rHuGM-CSF has variable effects on HIV replication in vitro and in vivo. HIV replication increased in some, but not all, studies involving rHuGM-CSF; however, administration of rHuGM-CSF in conjunction with an antiretroviral agent does not appear to increase HIV replication. HGF use may allow for administration of higher chemotherapy doses or more myelosuppressive therapy. Studies are needed to determine the ideal dosage of HGF and how they should be combined with chemotherapy. Until those findings are available, dosages of rHuG-CSF or rHuGM-CSF should be based on the myelosuppressive profile of the chemotherapy regimen administered.

ACKNOWLEDGMENTS

Cindy Hamilton, PharmD, and Beth Lesher, PharmD, assisted with the writing of this chapter.

REFERENCES

1. Spina M, Vaccher E, Carbone A, Tirelli U. Neoplastic complications of HIV infection. *Ann Oncol* 1999; 10:1271–1286.
2. 1993 revised classification system for HIV infection and expanded surveillance case definition for AIDS among adolescents and adults. *MMWR Recomm Rep* 1992; 41:1–19.
3. Goedert JJ, Cote TR, Virgo P, et al. Spectrum of AIDS-associated malignant disorders. *Lancet* 1998; 351:1833–1839.
4. Lee FC, Mitsuyasu RT. Chemotherapy of AIDS-related Kaposi's sarcoma. *Hematol Oncol Clin North Am* 1996; 10:1051–1068.
5. Kuritzkes DR. Neutropenia, neutrophil dysfunction, and bacterial infection in patients with human immunodeficiency virus disease: the role of granulocyte colony-stimulating factor. *Clin Infect Dis* 2000; 30:256–260.
6. Mitsuyasu R. Oncological complications of human immunodeficiency virus disease and hematologic consequences of their treatment. *Clin Infect Dis* 1999; 29:35–43.
7. Kitano K, Abboud CN, Ryan DH, Quan SG, Baldwin GC, Golde DW. Macrophage-active colony-stimulating factors enhance human immunodeficiency virus type 1 infection in bone marrow stem cells. *Blood* 1991; 77:1699–1705.
8. Koyanagi Y, O'Brien WA, Zhao JQ, Golde DW, Gasson JC, Chen IS. Cytokines alter production of HIV-1 from primary mononuclear phagocytes. *Science* 1988; 241:1673–1675.

9. Perno CF, Cooney DA, Gao WY, et al. Effects of bone marrow stimulatory cytokines on human immunodeficiency virus replication and the antiviral activity of dideoxynucleosides in cultures of monocyte/macrophages. *Blood* 1992; 80:995–1003.
10. Denis M, Ghadirian E. Interleukin 13 and interleukin 4 protect bronchoalveolar macrophages from productive infection with human immunodeficiency virus type 1. *AIDS Res Hum Retroviruses* 1994; 10:795–802.
11. Kandanearatchi A, Zuckerman M, Smith M, Vyakarnam A, Everall IP. Granulocyte-macrophage colony-stimulating factor enhances viral load in human brain tissue: amelioration with stavudine. *AIDS* 2002; 16:413–420.
12. Novak RM, Holzer TJ, Kennedy MM, Heynen CA, Dawson G. The effect of interleukin 4 (BSF-1) on infection of peripheral blood monocyte-derived macrophages with HIV-1. *AIDS Res Hum Retroviruses* 1990; 6:973–976.
13. Perno CF, Yarchoan R, Cooney DA, et al. Replication of human immunodeficiency virus in monocytes. Granulocyte/macrophage colony-stimulating factor (GM-CSF) potentiates viral production yet enhances the antiviral effect mediated by 3′-azido-2′3′-dideoxythymidine (AZT) and other dideoxynucleoside congeners of thymidine. *J Exp Med* 1989; 169:933–951.
14. Schuitemaker H, Kootstra NA, van Oers MH, van Lambalgen R, Tersmette M, Miedema F. Induction of monocyte proliferation and HIV expression by IL-3 does not interfere with anti-viral activity of zidovudine. *Blood* 1990; 76:1490–1493.
15. Hammer SM, Gillis JM. Synergistic activity of granulocyte-macrophage colony-stimulating factor and 3′-azido-3′-deoxythymidine against human immunodeficiency virus in vitro. *Antimicrob Agents Chemother* 1987; 31:1046–1050.
16. Hammer SM, Gillis JM, Pinkston P, Rose RM. Effect of zidovudine and granulocyte-macrophage colony-stimulating factor on human immunodeficiency virus replication in alveolar macrophages. *Blood* 1990; 75:1215–1219.
17. Kedzierska K, Maerz A, Warby T, et al. Granulocyte-macrophage colony-stimulating factor inhibits HIV-1 replication in monocyte-derived macrophages. *AIDS* 2000; 14:1739–1748.
18. Kornbluth RS, Oh PS, Munis JR, Cleveland PH, Richman DD. Interferons and bacterial lipopolysaccharide protect macrophages from productive infection by human immunodeficiency virus in vitro. *J Exp Med* 1989; 169:1137–1151.
19. Matsuda S, Akagawa K, Honda M, Yokota Y, Takebe Y, Takemori T. Suppression of HIV replication in human monocyte-derived macrophages induced by granulocyte/macrophage colony-stimulating factor. *AIDS Res Hum Retroviruses* 1995; 11:1031–1038.
20. Miles SA, Mitsuyasu RT, Moreno J, et al. Combined therapy with recombinant granulocyte colony-stimulating factor and erythropoietin decreases hematologic toxicity from zidovudine. *Blood* 1991; 77:2109–2117.
21. Ross SD, DiGeorge A, Connelly JE, Whiting GW, McDonnell N. Safety of GM-CSF in patients with AIDS: a review of the literature. *Pharmacotherapy* 1998; 18:1290–1297.
22. Armstrong WS, Kazanjian P. Use of cytokines in human immunodeficiency virus-infected patients: colony-stimulating factors, erythropoietin, and interleukin-2. *Clin Infect Dis* 2001; 32:766–773.
23. Frumkin LR. Role of granulocyte colony-stimulating factor and granulocyte-macrophage colony-stimulating factor in the treatment of patients with HIV infection. *Curr Opin Hematol* 1997; 4:200–206.
24. Hermans P. Kaposi's sarcoma in HIV-infected patients: treatment options. *HIV Med* 2000; 1:137–142.
25. Highly active antiretroviral therapy and incidence of cancer in human immunodeficiency virus-infected adults. *J Natl Cancer Inst* 2000; 92:1823–1830.
26. Fischl MA, Finkelstein DM, He W, Powderly WG, Triozzi PL, Steigbigel RT. A phase II study of recombinant human interferon-alpha 2a and zidovudine in patients with AIDS-related Kaposi's sarcoma. AIDS Clinical Trials Group. *J Acquir Immune Defic Syndr Hum Retrovirol* 1996; 11:379–384.
27. Kovacs JA, Deyton L, Davey R, et al. Combined zidovudine and interferon-alpha therapy in patients with Kaposi sarcoma and the acquired immunodeficiency syndrome (AIDS). *Ann Intern Med* 1989; 111:280–287.
28. Krown SE, Paredes J, Bundow D, Polsky B, Gold JW, Flomenberg N. Interferon-alpha, zidovudine, and granulocyte-macrophage colony-stimulating factor: a phase I AIDS Clinical Trials Group study in patients with Kaposi's sarcoma associated with AIDS. *J Clin Oncol* 1992; 10:1344–1351.
29. Scadden DT, Bering HA, Levine JD, et al. GM-CSF as an alternative to dose modification of the combination zidovudine and interferon-alpha in the treatment of AIDS-associated Kaposi's sarcoma. *Am J Clin Oncol* 1991; 14:S40–44.

30. Davey RT Jr, Davey VJ, Metcalf JA, et al. A phase I/II trial of zidovudine, interferon-alpha, and granulocyte-macrophage colony-stimulating factor in the treatment of human immunodeficiency virus type 1 infection. *J Infect Dis* 1991; 164:43–52.
31. Lee FC, Mitsuyasu R. Use of myeloid hematopoietic growth factors in AIDS-related malignancies. In: Morstyn G, Dexter TM, Foote M, eds., *Filgrastim (r-metHuG-CSF) in Clinical Practice,* 2nd ed. New York: Marcel Dekker. 1998: pp. 323–340.
32. Levine AM, Tulpule A. Clinical aspects and management of AIDS-related Kaposi's sarcoma. *Eur J Cancer* 2001; 37:1288–1295.
33. Gill PS, Bernstein-Singer M, Espina BM, et al. Adriamycin, bleomycin and vincristine chemotherapy with recombinant granulocyte-macrophage colony-stimulating factor in the treatment of AIDS-related Kaposi's sarcoma. *AIDS* 1992; 6:1477–1481.
34. Gill PS, Mitsuyasu RT, Montgomery T, et al. AIDS Clinical Trials Group Study 094: a phase I/II trial of ABV chemotherapy with zidovudine and recombinant human GM-CSF in AIDS-related Kaposi's sarcoma. *Cancer J Sci Am* 1997; 3:278–283.
35. Mastroianni A, Coronado O, Cancellieri C, Manfredi R, Pignatari S, Chiodo F. Pulmonary Kaposi's sarcoma in AIDS patients treated with combined chemotherapy and recombinant human granulocyte colony-stimulating factor. *J Chemother* 1998; 10:405–410.
36. Bakker PJ, Danner SA, ten Napel CH, et al. Treatment of poor prognosis epidemic Kaposi's sarcoma with doxorubicin, bleomycin, vindesine and recombinant human granulocyte-monocyte colony stimulating factor (rhGM-CSF). *Eur J Cancer* 1995; 2:188–192.
37. Gill PS, Wernz J, Scadden DT, et al. Randomized phase III trial of liposomal daunorubicin versus doxorubicin, bleomycin, and vincristine in AIDS-related Kaposi's sarcoma. *J Clin Oncol* 1996; 14:2353–2364.
38. Gill PS, Tulpule A, Espina BM, et al. Paclitaxel is safe and effective in the treatment of advanced AIDS-related Kaposi's sarcoma. *J Clin Oncol* 1999; 17:1876–1883.
39. Sloand E, Kumar PN, Pierce PF. Chemotherapy for patients with pulmonary Kaposi's sarcoma: benefit of filgrastim (G-CSF) in supporting dose administration. *South Med J* 1993; 86:1219–1224.
40. Tulpule A, Groopman J, Saville MW, et al. Multicenter trial of low-dose paclitaxel in patients with advanced AIDS-related Kaposi sarcoma. *Cancer* 2002; 95:147–154.
41. Welles L, Saville MW, Lietzau J, et al. Phase II trial with dose titration of paclitaxel for the therapy of human immunodeficiency virus-associated Kaposi's sarcoma. *J Clin Oncol* 1998; 16:1112–1121.
42. Straus DJ, Huang J, Testa MA, Levine AM, Kaplan LD. Prognostic factors in the treatment of human immunodeficiency virus-associated non-Hodgkin's lymphoma: analysis of AIDS Clinical Trials Group protocol 142—low-dose versus standard-dose m-BACOD plus granulocyte-macrophage colony-stimulating factor. National Institute of Allergy and Infectious Diseases. *J Clin Oncol* 1998; 16:3601–3606.
43. Errante D, Vaccher E, Tirelli U. Are hematopoietic colony-stimulating factors useful in association with chemotherapy in the treatment of HIV-related non-Hodgkin's lymphomas? *Ann Oncol* 1996; 7:233–237.
44. Gerhartz HH, Engelhard M, Brittinger G, et al. Recombinant human granulocyte-macrophage colony-stimulating factor as adjunct to chemotherapy in aggressive non-Hodgkin's lymphomas. *Semin Oncol* 1994; 21:25–28.
45. Kaplan LD, Kahn JO, Crowe S, et al. Clinical and virologic effects of recombinant human granulocyte-macrophage colony-stimulating factor in patients receiving chemotherapy for human immunodeficiency virus-associated non-Hodgkin's lymphoma: results of a randomized trial. *J Clin Oncol* 1991; 9:929–940.
46. Kaplan LD, Straus DJ, Testa MA, et al. Low-dose compared with standard-dose m-BACOD chemotherapy for non-Hodgkin's lymphoma associated with human immunodeficiency virus infection. *N Engl J Med* 1997; 336:1641–1648.
47. Ratner L, Lee J, Tang S, et al. Chemotherapy for human immunodeficiency virus-associated non-Hodgkin's lymphoma in combination with highly active antiretroviral therapy. *J Clin Oncol* 2001; 19:2171–2178.
48. Rossi G, Donisi A, Casari S, et al. Effects of recombinant granulocyte colony-stimulating factor (G-CSF) in patients treated with ProMACE-CytaBOM for HIV-related non-Hodgkin's lymphoma (NHL). *Haematologica* 1998; 83:317–322.
49. Tirelli U, Vaccher E. Economic and clinical evaluation of therapy of HIV-related non-Hodgkin's lymphoma with chemotherapy and granulocyte colony-stimulating factor (G-CSF). *Eur J Cancer* 1994; 30A:1589–1590.
50. Aviles A, Nambo MJ, Halabe J. Treatment of acquired immunodeficiency syndrome-related lymphoma with a standard chemotherapy regimen. *Ann Hematol* 1999; 78:9–12.

51. Bi J, Espina BM, Tulpule A, Boswell W, Levine AM. High-dose cytosine-arabinoside and cisplatin regimens as salvage therapy for refractory or relapsed AIDS-related non-Hodgkin's lymphoma. *J Acquir Immune Defic Syndr* 2001; 28:416–421.
52. Gabarre J, Lepage E, Thyss A, et al. Chemotherapy combined with zidovudine and GM-CSF in human immunodeficiency virus-related non-Hodgkin's lymphoma. *Ann Oncol* 1995; 6:1025–1032.
53. Kersten MJ, Verduyn TJ, Reiss P, Evers LM, de Wolf F, van Oers MH. Treatment of AIDS-related non-Hodgkin's lymphoma with chemotherapy (CNOP) and r-hu-G-CSF: clinical outcome and effect on HIV-1 viral load. *Ann Oncol* 1998; 9:1135–1138.
54. Newell M, Goldstein D, Milliken S, et al. Phase I/II trial of filgrastim (r-metHuG-CSF), CEOP chemotherapy and antiretroviral therapy in HIV-related non-Hodgkin's lymphoma. *Ann Oncol* 1996; 7:1029–1036.
55. Niitsu N, Okamoto M, Kuraishi Y, Nakamura S, Kodama F, Hirano M. CyclOBEAP (cyclophosphamide, vincristine, bleomycin, etoposide, doxorubicin, prednisolone) regimen with granulocyte colony-stimulating factor (G-CSF) for patients with aggressive non-Hodgkin's lymphoma: a pilot study. The Adult Lymphoma Treatment Study Group (ALTSG). *Eur J Haematol* 2000; 65:188–194.
56. Oksenhendler E, Gerard L, Dubreuil ML, et al. Intensive chemotherapy (LNHIV-91 regimen) and G-CSF for HIV associated non-Hodgkin's lymphoma. *Leuk Lymphoma* 2000; 39:87–95.
57. Remick SC, Sedransk N, Haase RF, et al. Oral combination chemotherapy in conjunction with filgrastim (G-CSF) in the treatment of AIDS-related non-Hodgkin's lymphoma: evaluation of the role of G-CSF; quality-of-life analysis and long-term follow-up. *Am J Hematol* 2001; 66:178–188.
58. Sparano JA, Wiernik PH, Hu X, et al. Pilot trial of infusional cyclophosphamide, doxorubicin, and etoposide plus didanosine and filgrastim in patients with human immunodeficiency virus-associated non-Hodgkin's lymphoma. *J Clin Oncol* 1996; 14:3026–3035.
59. Spina M, Vaccher E, Juzbasic S, et al. Human immunodeficiency virus-related non-Hodgkin lymphoma: activity of infusional cyclophosphamide, doxorubicin, and etoposide as second-line chemotherapy in 40 patients. *Cancer* 2001; 92:200–206.
60. Tirelli U, Spina M, Jaeger U, et al. Infusional CDE with rituximab for the treatment of human immunodeficiency virus-associated non-Hodgkin's lymphoma: preliminary results of a phase I/II study. *Recent Results Cancer Res* 2002; 159:149–153.
61. Tulpule A, Rarick MU, Kolitz J, et al. Liposomal daunorubicin in the treatment of relapsed or refractory non-Hodgkin's lymphoma. *Ann Oncol* 2001; 12:457–462.
62. Vaccher E, Spina M, di Gennaro G, et al. Concomitant cyclophosphamide, doxorubicin, vincristine, and prednisone chemotherapy plus highly active antiretroviral therapy in patients with human immunodeficiency virus-related, non-Hodgkin lymphoma. *Cancer* 2001; 91:155–163.
63. Walsh C, Wernz JC, Levine A, et al. Phase I trial of m-BACOD and granulocyte macrophage colony stimulating factor in HIV-associated non-Hodgkin's lymphoma. *J Acquir Immune Defic Syndr* 1993; 6:265–271.
64. Krishnan A, Molina A, Zaia J, et al. Autologous stem cell transplantation for HIV-associated lymphoma. *Blood* 2001; 98:3857–3859.
65. Molina A, Krishnan AY, Nademanee A, et al. High dose therapy and autologous stem cell transplantation for human immunodeficiency virus-associated non-Hodgkin lymphoma in the era of highly active antiretroviral therapy. *Cancer* 2000; 89:680–689.
66. Maiman M, Fruchter RG, Guy L, Cuthill S, Levine P, Serur E. Human immunodeficiency virus infection and invasive cervical carcinoma. *Cancer* 1993; 71:402–406.
67. Maiman M. Management of cervical neoplasia in human immunodeficiency virus-infected women. *J Natl Cancer Inst Monogr* 1998; 23:43–49.
68. Errante D, Gabarre J, Ridolfo AL, et al. Hodgkin's disease in 35 patients with HIV infection: an experience with epirubicin, bleomycin, vinblastine and prednisone chemotherapy in combination with antiretroviral therapy and primary use of G-CSF. *Ann Oncol* 1999; 10:189–195.
69. Levine AM, Li P, Cheung T, et al. Chemotherapy consisting of doxorubicin, bleomycin, vinblastine, and dacarbazine with granulocyte-colony-stimulating factor in HIV-infected patients with newly diagnosed Hodgkin's disease: a prospective, multi-institutional AIDS clinical trials group study (ACTG 149). *J Acquir Immune Defic Syndr* 2000; 24:444–450.
70. Spina M, Gabarre J, Rossi G, et al. Stanford V regimen and concomitant HAART in 59 patients with Hodgkin disease and HIV infection. *Blood* 2002; 100:1984–1988.
71. Evison J, Jost J, Ledergerber B, Jost L, Strasser F, Weber R. HIV-associated non-Hodgkin's lymphoma: highly active antiretroviral therapy improves remission rate of chemotherapy. *AIDS* 1999; 13:732–734.

IV Safety and Economic Implications

19 The Safety of Hematopoietic Growth Factors

Roy E. Smith, MD and Barbara C. Good, PhD

Contents

This manuscript is dedicated to the memory of Helen Louise Smith.

1. INTRODUCTION

Recombinant DNA technology has permitted the production of recombinant hematopoietic growth factors (HGFs) in amounts generous enough to allow both a wide array of cell culture-based laboratory experimentation and rapid introduction into clinical application. The introduction of these proteins into clinical trials has led to the detection of both expected and unexpected adverse events.

This chapter discusses those recombinant HGF that have found their way into the clinical armamentarium: recombinant human interleukin-11 (rHuIL-11, oprelvekin); recombinant human stem cell factor (rHuSCF, ancestim); recombinant human erythropoietin (rHu-EPO, epoetin); recombinant human thrombopoietin (rHuTPO); recombinant human granulocyte-macrophage colony-stimulating factor (rHuGM-CSF; sargramostim and molgramostim); and recombinant human granulocyte colony-stimulating factor (rHuG-CSF; filgrastim, lenograstim, and pegfilgrastim). For each of these, the molecular characteristics and functions, clinical indications, and advantages and disadvantages are briefly addressed, with special emphasis on the adverse events associated with administration.

2. IMMUNE RESPONSE CONSIDERATIONS

The administration of medicinal recombinant proteins raises the potential that the human immune system will recognize these proteins as foreign *(1)*. A number of factors

From: *Cancer Drug Discovery and Development*
Hematopoietic Growth Factors in Oncology: Basic Science and Clinical Therapeutics
Edited by: G. Morstyn, M. A. Foote, and G. J. Lieschke © Humana Press Inc., Totowa, NJ

have been shown to either encourage or discourage immune assault. Oral or intravenous administration illicits weak immune responses, whereas subcutaneous or repeated administration strengthens the response *(2,3)*. The immune response is sometimes exaggerated in patients with autoimmune disease and in patients with cancer or those treated with immunosuppressive therapies *(4)*. The presence of extraneous proteins acquired during the industrial manufacturing may act as immune adjuvants, resulting in a heightened immune reaction *(5)*.

Simple proteins, proteins with tertiary and quarternary structures similar to other "self" proteins, and proteins that are soluble tend to be either nonimmunogenic or less immunogenic than those that are complex, degraded, aggregated, or denatured *(3,6)*. Glycosylation prevents exposure of the protein's molecular backbone to immuno-effectors and reduces the opportunity for the protein to encourage an immune response *(7)*.

An exaggerated or abnormal immune response to the administration of an exogenous protein may have detrimental effects and result in adverse events. Antibodies (Abs) directed against the administered protein may cause the formation of antigen/Ab complexes that can affect that administered protein's pharmacokinetics, increasing clearance and decreasing efficacy. They can also be deposited in the skin or kidneys, leading to damage or malfunction *(1)*. Neutralizing Abs may decrease the protein's expected potency and efficacy. Perhaps one of the most dreaded complications with the administration of HGFs is the occurrence of crossreacting Abs that are directed toward identical or similar endogenous proteins *(8,9)*. Other concerns include the eliciting of either acute or delayed hypersensitivity reactions that may be so severe that they are life-threatening *(7)*.

3. CLINICALLY USED HEMATOPOIETIC GROWTH FACTORS

HGFs are glycosylated proteins that interact with specific receptors to regulate the production and function of hematopoietic cells. Originally detected by their characteristic ability to stimulate the growth and maturation of immature bone marrow-derived hematopoietic target cells, these proteins have been generally labeled as colony-stimulating factors (CSFs). Since the time they were first detected, the number of HGFs identified has increased markedly.

3.1. rHuIL-11

3.1.1. Background

Oprelvekin is a recombinant form of IL-11 produced in *E. coli* by recombinant DNA technology *(10)* and approved by the Food and Drug Administration (FDA) to prevent severe thrombocytopenia and reduce the need for platelet transfusions after myelosuppressive chemotherapy in patients with nonmyeloid cancers. rHuIL-11 increases the size and DNA content of megakaryocytes and stimulates thrombopoiesis, increasing production and release of normally functioning platelets *(10,11)*. Its nonhematologic effects include the modulation of intestinal epithelial growth that leads to increased rates of intestinal healing, enhanced fat deposition, an increase in the synthesis of acute-phase proteins, and osteoclastic maturation *(10–13)*. rHuIL-11 may promote the growth of myeloid and megakaryocytic and plasma cell lines *(14–16)*.

3.1.2. Studies

In a review by Smith *(17)*, the safety and tolerability of rHuIL-11 administered sc at the recommended dose of 50 μg/kg/d was compared with placebo in two phase 2 studies. The dataset included 308 patients, ranging from 8 mo to 75 yr of age, who received up to eight sequential 1–28-d courses of oprelvekin. In this group, aside from complications associated with underlying malignancy or cytotoxic chemotherapy, most adverse events were of mild or moderate severity and were reversible after cessation of the growth factor. The incidence and type of adverse events were similar between patients who received oprelvekin and those who received placebo. Edema, dyspnea, tachycardia, conjunctival injection, palpitations, and pleural effusion occurred more frequently in the oprelvekin-treated patients. Adverse events that occurred in ≥10% of patients and were observed in equal or greater frequency among patients receiving placebo included asthenia, pain, chills, abdominal pain, infection, anorexia, constipation, dyspepsia, ecchymosis, myalgia, bone pain, and alopecia. Patient withdrawal owing to an adverse event (most commonly atrial fibrillation/flutter) was more frequent among those receiving oprelvekin compared with placebo (11% vs 6%). An analysis of data derived from these patients has led to the speculation that oprelvekin treatment, along with age, history of atrial arrythmias or cardiac disease, or alcohol use, are risk factors for the development of these arrythmias. Thrombotic events, the number of red blood cell (RBC) transfusions, and the duration of neutropenia (absolute neutrophil count [ANC] $< 0.5 \times 10^9$/L) were similar in both groups. The incidence of ≥grade 3 adverse events was similar in oprelvekin-treated and placebo-treated patients. Although the incidence of asthenia was similar between these two groups (65% vs 64%, $p = 1.0$), ≥grade 3 was more common in the former (14% vs 3%, $p = 0.03$).

Retrospective analysis of the phase 2 placebo-controlled chemotherapy studies (studies 1 and 2) showed a significantly ($p < 0.01$) lower incidence of bleeding complications—primarily ecchymosis and epitaxis—among patients in the oprelvekin group (28%) compared with those in the placebo group (51%). None of the patients treated with oprelvekin ($n = 69$) developed severe or life-threatening bleeding complications (grade 3 hemorrhage, hemorrhagic cystitis, or vaginal hemorrhage); these occurred only among placebo-treated patients (3/67, 4.5%).

In the two phase 2 placebo-controlled chemotherapy studies, the only biochemical laboratory abnormalities that occurred significantly more frequently with oprelvekin than with placebo were decreases in serum albumin and total protein concentrations. These changes were without clinical consequence, and laboratory values returned to baseline levels after drug discontinuation. Mean decreases in serum albumin of up to 0.6 g/dL (10–15%) were noted in the first phase 2 study.

In the second phase 2 study, the observed mean decreases in serum albumin and total protein concentrations were 22% in the oprelvekin group vs 6% in the placebo group ($p = 0.0006$). The investigators determined that these changes seem to have resulted from the combined effects of oprelvekin-induced increased plasma volume and decreased nutritional intake by the patients because of the gastrointestinal and central toxicity of chemotherapeutic agents.

In a later representative phase 3 trial ($n = 133$), all grades of edema, dyspnea, and dizziness were more frequent among patients who received oprelvekin than among those who received placebo (45% vs 20%; 34% vs 13%; 44; 34% vs 13%; 44% vs 20%, respectively), although the proportion of patients with ≥grade 3 was similar between the two groups (4% vs 2%; 2% vs 4%; 2% vs 0%, respectively). In this trial, metabolic abnormalities led to drug discontinuation in 5% of the oprelvekin-treated patients. Hypokalemia was more frequent in this group (7% vs 4%); the investigators concluded that this difference was probably owing to diuretic use.

The incidence and type of adverse events in the phase 3 chemotherapy study were similar to those seen in the two placebo-controlled phase 2 studies, with the exception of dizziness, which was attributed to concomitant diuretic use *(18)*. As in the phase 2 placebo-controlled trials, most adverse events in the phase 3 trial were mild or moderate in severity (grade 1 or 2) and resolved without sequelae after discontinuation of the study drug. The oprelvekin and placebo groups did not differ significantly in overall incidence of grade 3 and 4 adverse events (36% [oprelvekin] and 38% [placebo]); however, the incidence of grade 3 or 4 chills was reported significantly ($p = 0.04$) more frequently in the placebo group (n = 3, 7%) than in the oprelvekin group (n = 0). In addition, the only episodes of grade 3 or 4 gastrointestinal hemorrhage (two patients) or pulmonary infarct (one patient) occurred in the placebo group.

As in the phase 2 patients, in the phase 3 study, bleeding events contributing to hospitalization occurred in a higher percentage of patients in the placebo group (5/45, 11.1%) than in the oprelvekin group (3/88, 3.4%). These observations reflect the lack of adverse effects of oprelvekin on platelet function or blood coagulation.

Most adverse events associated with oprelvekin (e.g., edema, dyspnea, pleural effusions, and conjunctival injection) are believed to be the result of fluid retention and increased plasma volume *(19)*. Mild, reversible dilutional anemia characterized by moderate decreases in hemoglobin (Hb) concentration (15–19% reductions from baseline) and hematocrit levels (approx 20% reduction from baseline) secondary to plasma volume expansion has occurred during oprelvekin therapy in phase 1 studies in healthy volunteers *(19)* and in nonmyelosuppressed patients with cancer *(20)*. In the latter population, anemia developed within 2–3 d of initiation of oprelvekin therapy and reached a nadir during the second week of administration *(20)*. Hb concentrations returned to baseline levels within 2 wk after the completion of oprelvekin therapy. Although this dilutional anemia occurred in approx 20% of patients who received oprelvekin in phase 1 trials, it was not associated with statistically significant increases in the incidence of clinically significant anemia or with mean requirements for RBC transfusions in those who received oprelvekin compared with those who received placebo *(21,22)*. Across the phase 2 studies, anemia was reported in only 10% of oprelvekin-treated patients, compared with 6% of placebo patients *(17)*. The mean number of RBC units transfused per patient was 1.9 in the oprelvekin group and 1.7 in the placebo group.

3.1.3. Other Hematologic Effects

rHuIL-11 increases fibrinogen and von Willebrand factor levels. Nevertheless, in the placebo-controlled studies with oprelvekin, thrombotic and thromboembolic events occurred infrequently and with similar incidence in oprelvekin and placebo groups.

Thromboembolic sequelae such as stroke have been observed in patients receiving oprelvekin who experienced atrial arrythmias. Since patients with histories of thrombotic events or disseminated intravascular coagulation have been excluded from most clinical protocols, it is difficult to determine whether oprelvekin heightens their risk. Postmarketing surveillance has shown spontaneous reports of thrombotic events in patients receiving oprelvekin *(17)*; however, a causal relationship has not been ascertained.

Cumulative toxicity and bone marrow exhaustion are not a consequence of repetitive treatment with oprelvekin. The frequency and severity of adverse events appear to be stable after prolonged administration. Maintenance of platelet nadirs, neutrophil recovery times, and requirements for RBC transfusion have not been seen to increase during sequential treatments *(22)*.

Oprelvekin is occasionally recognized as a foreign protein. The incidence of Ab reactivity to oprelvekin among subjects who have received more than one dose of oprelvekin is reported to be 1.4–4%. The development of these Abs has not been associated with anaphylactoid reactions or neutralizing properties. Specifically, no unexpectedly prolonged thrombocytopenia has been described.

No significant differences between patients receiving oprelkevin or placebo are reported with respect to median time to neutrophil recovery after chemotherapy, the duration of neutropenia, or the incidence of neutropenic fever (48% vs 42%; $p = 0.5$).

3.1.4. Oprelvekin and Tumor Growth

In placebo-controlled chemotherapy studies, the rate of disease progression was similar between groups treated with oprelvekin or placebo, suggesting that oprelvekin does not interfere with the antitumor effectiveness of cytotoxic therapy and has no inherent tumorigenic effects. Preclinical observations suggest that oprelvekin does not stimulate the growth of cells from human primary solid tumors in vitro *(17)*. Furthermore, retrospective analysis of follow-up data from three randomized studies showed no adverse effects on overall survival or progression-free survival.

3.1.5. Concomitant Administration

Almost all patients treated with oprelvekin have been treated concurrently with rHuG-CSF (filgrastim) without evidence of an adverse pharmacodynamic interaction between these two cytokines.

Oprelvekin has been administered concomitantly with acetaminophen, ondansetron, prochlorperazine, diphenhydramine, dexamethasone, lorazepam, ciprofloxacin, or furosemide in most (≥65%) patients involved in the two phase 2 placebo-controlled chemotherapy studies ($n = 69$), with no evidence of significant drug interactions. At the recommended dose, there does not appear to be any effect of oprelkevin on the liver cytochrome P450 microsomal enzyme system *(17)*.

3.2. *rHuSCF*

3.2.1. Background

SCF, also referred to as Steel locus factor, mast cell growth factor, and c-kit ligand, is a glycoprotein growth factor that modulates the proliferation of hematopoietic progenitor cells and mast cells. The action of SCF is based on its interaction with the tyrosine kinase receptor encoded by the c-*kit* proto-oncogene *(23)*, resulting in the stimulation of mature and immature hematopoietic cells of multiple lineages (myeloid, erythroid, and megakaryocytic progenitors) and the expansion of the stem cell compartment *(24–26)*. SCF alone appears to have a modest effect on its target cell's proliferation and mobilization and has an enhanced influence in the presence of other HGFs *(27,28)*. It was the ability of SCF alone and in combination with other growth factors to induce proliferation, prolong survival, encourage lineage commitment, and stimulate the mobilization of hematopoietic progenitor cells that led to the development of rHuSCF and its further development in nonhuman primate and human clinical trials. rHuSCF is produced by DNA technology and expressed in *E. coli* as a 166-amino acid nonglycosylated protein with methionine included at the N-terminus.

3.2.2. Studies

The adverse event profile associated with r-metHuSCF was first defined in two small phase 1 clinical trials investigating its utility in patients with cancer receiving chemotherapy *(29,30)*. When administered to 17 patients with nonsmall-cell lung cancer in incremental doses of 10, 25, and 50 μg/kg/d before the administration of chemotherapy, a specific pattern of adverse events emerged. At the lowest dose level, adverse events were limited to the injection site. At dose levels > 10 μg/kg/d, adverse events occurred as multisystem systemic reactions. Dose-related mild-to-moderate reactions occurred in all patients at all dose levels and included edema, urticaria, erythema, and pruritus. These reactions, mild to severe, as well as angioedema and dermatographia, occurred at distant cutaneous sites. Cough, throat tightness, sore throat, dyspepsia, and hypotension were transient and did not result in patient withdrawal from the study *(29)*. In another phase 1 trial of identical design, rHuSCF was administered to patients (n = 17) with advanced breast cancer. The adverse event profile was similar to that described above *(30)*.

Larger phase 2 and phase 3 clinical trials investigating the value of combining rHuSCF with rHuG-CSF (filgrastim) for the mobilization of bone marrow progenitor cells have demonstrated adverse event patterns like those seen in the earlier phase 1 trials. In a phase 1–2 trial (n = 38) of rHuSCF plus filgrastim in patients with non-Hodgkin's lymphoma (NHL), >80% of those who received rHuSCF had local injection site reactions, and 12% (three patients) had cough, dyspnea, and chest tightness with distant urticaria that resolved with the continuation of filgrastim *(31)*. In a small randomized apheresis study comparing filgrastim alone with filgrastim plus dose-escalated rHuSCF in patients with breast cancer (n = 62), rHuSCF-related injection site reactions occurred in 89% (n = 39) of patients *(32)*. These local reactions consisted of erythema, urticaria, and pruritus and were of mild-to-moderate severity. All occurred within 24 h of start of therapy and resolved within 96 h of onset. Six patients (14%) developed similar reactions at distant sites; these followed the same time sequence as those seen at the local injection site. Other adverse events that occurred more frequently among patients receiving rHuSCF compared with placebo included mild transient decreases in blood pressure (n = 4), fever (n = 6), and nausea (n = 5). One patient developed angioedema (periorbital, perioral, and tongue edema, hoarseness) with generalized urticaria and pruritus requiring treatment with corticosteroids and H1 antagonists.

A randomized phase 2 trial comparing cyclophosphamide plus filgrastim alone vs the same with filgrastim plus rHuSCF for the mobilization of progenitor cells in patients with breast cancer (n = 215) showed that 88% of patients receiving rHuSCF had drug-related injection site reactions and 4% pruritus, 3% rash, and 3% dyspnea *(33)*. In a similarly designed phase 3 trial for patients with breast cancer (n = 203), rHuSCF-related injection site reactions occurred in 92% of patients, dyspnea in 8%, and pruritus in 6% *(34)*. Another phase 3 trial that compared progenitor cell mobilization with cyclophosphamide plus filgrastim or the same with rHuSCF in patients with multiple myeloma (n = 102) found that injection site erythema and reaction occurred in 44% (n = 24) and 22% (n = 12) of patients receiving rHuSCF. Distant rash and erythema, respectively, were seen in 13% ($n = 7$) and 5% ($n = 3$) of rHuSCF-treated patients and 0% and 2% ($n = 1$) of filgrastim alone-treated patients. Although the number of patients experiencing skeletal pain was small, rHuSCF appeared to increase its frequency compared with placebo (7% vs 2%) *(35)*. This adverse event profile associated with rHuSCF administration, which is consistently demonstrated in multiple clinical trials, appears to be mast cell-related. SCF (mast cell growth factor) has been shown to stimulate cutaneous mast cell proliferation and degranulation *(36,37)*, and the occurrence of injection site and distant erythema, rash, and urticaria as well angioedema strongly supports this finding. Therapeutic evidence of this mast cell effect includes the fact that H1 and H2 receptor blockers favorably influence the severity of rHuSCF-induced cutaneous and systemic reactions.

c-kit or a c-kit variant is found in a variety of normal and neoplastic hematopoietic and nonhematopoietic tissues *(38–50)*. In particular, a mutation of codon 816 (Asp^{816}) has been identified in mast cell leukemia, acute myeloblastic leukemia (AML), and germ cell tumors *(51)* that confers cytokine independence and constitutive activation of signal transducer and activator of transcription 3 (STAT3). The presence of both normal and abnormal c-kit offers an opportunity for therapeutic intervention and the risk that treatment with rHuSCF may accelerate the neoplastic process. The c-kit tyrosine kinase inhibitor (ST1571) has significant activity in patients with chronic myelocytic leukemia and gastrointestinal stromal tumors *(52)*. Likewise, the inhibition of c-kit tyrosine kinase decreases the proliferation of human colorectal and small cell lung cancer cell lines *(52,53)*. Cell lines derived from patients with mastocytosis demonstrate the presence of an activating c-kit mutation that is supersensitive to the presence of SCF, resulting in an increase in the rate of progenitor proliferation and the accumulation of mast cells in an SCF concentration-dependent manner *(54,55)*. The neoplastic process has not been reported to be worsened by exposure to rHuSCF.

No rHuSCF-related neutralizing Abs have been reported in patients who have received either rHuSCF alone or in combination with other HGF.

3.3. rHuEPO

3.3.1. Background

EPO is an endogenous HGF that interacts with EPO receptors present on hematopoietic precursor and nonhematopoietic cells. EPO stimulates the production, maturation, and release of RBCs from the bone marrow storage compartment. Produced primarily by the kidneys in response to hypoxia, EPO acts on the bone marrow hematopoietic progenitor cells (mainly erythroid colony-forming units [CFU-E]) after their commitment to further erythroid development. EPO maintains a proliferation compartment of erythroid progenitor cells, allows for continued maturation of progenitor cells committed to the erythroid cell line, recruits uncommitted progenitor cells into the erythroid progenitor pool, and inhibits the naturally occurring apoptosis of CFU-E.

rHuEPO has been produced by DNA recombinant technology in Chinese hamster ovary (CHO) cells using the gene that codes for human EPO. Epoetin alfa, epoetin beta, and darbepoetin alfa are three erythropoietic proteins available for human use. Epoetin alfa and epoetin beta are 165-amino acid glycoproteins with an amino acid sequence and biologic activity identical to that of endogenous EPO. Darbepoetin alfa differs from epoetin alfa and epoetin beta by the substitution of five amino acids in the primary amino acid sequence by creating two new *N*-linked glycosylation sites using site-directed mutagenesis *(56,57)*. Darbepoetin alfa has five *N*-linked carbohydrate chains compared with both endogenous EPO and epoetin alfa, which have only three *(58)*. The presence of the extra carbohydrate chains results in a biochemically different analog. Compared with epoetin alfa and epoetin beta, darbepoetin alfa has a greater molecular weight and sialic acid content and a negative charge *(58)*. The in vivo biologic activity of both recombinant analogs of endogenous EPO is positively correlated with the number of sialic acid residues present on the molecule *(59)*. In comparison with epoetin alfa, which has 14 sialic acid residues per molecule, darbepoetin alfa has 22 sialic acid residue per molecule *(58)*. As a result of these differences, darbepoetin alfa has a longer half-life, decreased affinity for the erythropoietin receptor, and increased biologic activity compared with epoetin alfa.

3.3.2. Studies

All three clinically available recombinant erythropoietic proteins are well tolerated and share similar adverse event profiles. Sowade et al. *(60)* reviewed the collected unpublished (epoetin beta) and published (epoetin alfa) adverse events in patients registered on randomized trials comparing treatment with either epoetin alfa or epoetin beta with placebo. The adverse event profiles of each rHuEPO differed according to indication and generally reflected the influence of the underlying illness or invasive procedure (renal disease or elective cardiac, general, or orthopedic surgery). With most indications, no relevant differences in the incidences of adverse events were observed between patients treated with rHuEPO or placebo. Only in the rHuEPO therapy of renal disease was an increased incidence of hypertensive events observed in the rHuEPO-treated subjects, a finding not observed among patients treated with other indications. The results of this review generally parallel those reported in the package inserts for epoetin alfa *(61)*. Among 131 patients with cancer who were receiving chemotherapy and were randomly assigned to treatment with either epoetin alfa or placebo, diarrhea (21% vs 7%, $p = 0.041$) and edema (17% vs 1%, $p = 0.0016$) were reported to be more frequent among the epoetin alfa-treated group *(61)*, although the rate of deep vein thrombotic events has been reported to be similar among patients receiving rHuEPO and placebo *(60–62)*. The occurrence of thrombotic events may be related to the rate and amount of increase of red cell mass *(63,64)*. In patients receiving dialysis, the frequency of arteriovenous shunt occlusion and other thrombotic events is higher among patients receiving epoetin alfa than among patients not receiving epoetin alfa (39% vs 29%, $p < 0.001$), and myocardial infarction, vascular ischemic events, and venous thrombosis were higher in patients with target hematocrits maintained at 41–43 compared with those with hematocrits maintained at 30–33 *(61)*. In patients having elective orthopedic surgery, treatment with epoetin alfa is not generally considered to increase the risk of clinically detected thrombotic events, but the incidence of postoperative deep vein thrombosis detected by ultrasonograpy or surveillance venography among patients with pretreatment Hb concentrations > 13 g/dL does appear to be increased among those treated with epoetin alfa compared with those not receiving it (11% vs 6%) *(60,61,65)*.

The adverse event profiles associated with darbepoetin alfa use among patients with chronic renal disease and anemia associated with cancer are similar in frequency and severity to those seen with in patients treated with rHuEPO or placebo *(66)*. Studies comparing the adverse events seen in patients randomly assigned to either epoetin alfa or darbepoetin alfa are few, but all report similar kinds and frequencies of events between the treatment groups and according to underlying illness *(67–70)*.

At this time, rHuEPO-induced IgG human EPO-neutralizing Abs have been reported only in patients with renal disease receiving either epoetin alfa or epoetin beta. These patients presented with severe anemia and were subsequently found to have pure red cell aplasia. Most were also undergoing dialysis at the time of presentation. Casadevall et al. *(9)* carefully characterized the Abs found in 13 such patients. Scatchard analysis showed a linear pattern of EPO binding by the anti-EPO Ab in each patient's serum; this linearity is thought to indicate the presence of a homogeneous population of Abs, the interaction of the anti-EPO Ab with a single epitope on the EPO molecule, or both. Deglycosylation of epoetin resulted in an increase the Ab's affinity for EPO, suggesting that the bulking carbohydrate chains somehow protected epitopes found on the molecules' protein backbone. Among the patients with Abs associated with epoetin alfa use, denaturation of epoetin resulted in a lack of binding to EPO. Thus, the anti-EPO Ab appeared to interact with conformational epitopes only. Serum from the patients who received only epoetin beta contained Abs that bound both native and denatured epoetin, suggesting that these patients' Abs bound to both linear and conformational antigens and that epoetin beta-induced Abs may differ from those induced by epoetin alfa.

The incidence of antibody development in patients receiving darbepoetin alfa has not been adequately determined. Radioimmunoprecipitation assays were performed on sera from 1534 patients with chronic renal failure and 833 patients with cancer treated with darbepoetin alfa in clinical studies. High-titer Abs were not detected in patients with chronic renal failure, but assay sensitivity may have been inadequate to detect lower titers reliably. Abs were detected by radioimmunoprecipitation in sera from three patients with cancer; neutralizing activity, possibly related to Abs, was detected in one of these three patients. The patient had no evidence of pure red cell aplasia *(66)*.

No reports exist for patients with polycythemia vera, hematologic malignancies, or solid cancers who were treated with rHuEPO whose worsening illness could be attributed to the growth factor therapy.

3.4. rHuTPO

3.4.1. Background

In addition to IL-11, other lineage-dominant regulators of megakaryocyte development and platelet production exist. One of these, the ligand for c-Mpl, is produced in the liver, kidney, brains, and testes and has been shown to enhance megakaryocyte development, size, number, and ploidy *(71,72)* and to increase platelet production markedly *(71)*. It is important to point out that thrombopoiesis is controlled by several different cytokines. IL-3, G-CSF, GM-CSF, and SCF modulate megakaryocte progenitors; IL-6 influences maturation in the later stages of megakaryocytic development; and TPO and IL-11 stimulate all phases of megakaryocytopoiesis. In addition, TPO acts in synergy with EPO to stimulate the growth of erythroid progenitor cells *(73)*, and TPO acts in conjunction with IL-3 or SCF to cause the proliferation and prolongation in survival of hematopoietic progenitors. c-Mpl ligand has been successfully isolated, cloned, and produced using recombinant DNA technology. Recombinant c-Mpl-ligand (TPO) is a glycosylated protein that specifically binds to the megakaryocyte c-Mpl receptor or to c-Mpl receptors found in megakaryocytic descendants *(74–76)*.

Two kinds of recombinant thrombopoietins have been introduced into clinical trials. rHuTPO is a full polypeptide chain, whereas polyethylene glycol-recombinant human megakaryocyte growth and development factor (PEG-rHuMGDF) consists of the ligand portion of the molecule that has been chemically modified by the addition of polyethylene glycol to extend its half-life after administration. Both molecules have similar biologic activities and adverse event profiles.

3.4.2. Studies

Thrombopoietins, whether rHuTPO or PEG-rHuMGDF, appear to be well tolerated. Much of the safety data available on this HGF are derived from preclinical trials in animals and from clinical randomized trials comparing patients with various malignancies treated with chemotherapy plus TPO vs patients treated with chemotherapy alone. The therapeutic efficacy and toxicity of TPO have been evaluated in mice, rats, dogs, and nonhuman primates. In all cases, the administration of either form of TPO was without significant complication. Major organ dysfunction (liver, kidney, lung, bone marrow) did not occur. Capillary leak was not evident (by weight gain, respiratory symptoms, or edema), nor were thrombosis, hemorrhage, or acute-phase reaction *(77)*. In a single experiment, the administration of rHuTPO to monkeys after treatment with sublethal doses of irradiation caused a functional iron deficiency *(78)*, implying that TPO has an effect on erythropoiesis and that iron replacement may be indicated.

Clinical trials performed in humans support the findings in the preclinical trials *(79)*. In all trials, in which either rHuTPO or PEG-rHuMGDF were administered to patients planned to receive chemotherapy, a profound stimulation of platelet production was seen. Since the indication and safety of TPO in these trials were tentative, patients with known cardiac, pulmonary, or vascular disease were excluded. In most of the trials, study design limited the administration of TPO to a single course. In these trials, there were no detected significant differences in vital signs and weight loss or frequency of bone pain, organ dysfunction, or thrombosis between patients receiving TPO and those not receiving TPO. In a blinded, randomized, placebo-controlled, two-cycle crossover trial to determine the value of PEG-rHuMGDF for increasing platelet counts and platelet harvest yields in healthy subjects, reported adverse events were related to increasing doses of PEG-rHuMGDF, and the development of thrombocytosis was an infrequent event, with platelet counts achieving peak values ranging from 1.1- to 3.6-fold greater than baseline values *(80)*. The occurrence of anti-TPO antibodies was reported in one patient; however, this low incidence of the development of anti-TPO Abs could be attributed to the brief exposure to therapeutic rHuTPO *(81)*.

Although it is unusual, the development of thrombocytopenia in patients receiving PEG-rHuMGDF has been reported *(8)*. These patients presented with easy bruising, heavy menses, severe thrombocytopenia (6, 9, and 2×10^9/L, respectively), and IgG-neutralizing Abs to both PEG-rHuMGDF and endogenous TPO. More recently, pancytopenia and aplastic anemia-like syndrome have been reported in a patient with cancer who developed an anti-TPO Ab after the subcutaneous administration of PEG-rHuMGDF *(82)*. Although anti-TPO Abs have been reported to occur with exposure to rHuTPO, they were transient and had no neutralizing activity *(81,83)*.

The occurrence of thrombosis has been reported in some clinical trials involving PEG-rHuMGDF. It is important to emphasize, however, that these were trials including patients with underlying malignancies who had been treated with other potential thrombogenic interventions. Both rHuTPO and PEG-rHuTPO increase the sensitivity of platelets to subthreshold levels of platelet agonists *(84,85)*, providing a rationale for the occurrence of rHuTPO- or PEG-rHuTPO-induced proclivity to thrombosis. It is important, however, to point out that the evidence for this is weak. When these growth factors were used to increase platelet counts and harvest yields in healthy subjects, there were no reported thrombotic episodes *(80)*. Likewise, when platelets harvested from subjects stimulated with PEG-rHuMGDF were transfused into patients with various malignancies who were also thrombocytopenic, no thrombotic events were reported *(86)*.

One adverse event that may be related to long-term rHuTPO exposure or may become evident as clinical application expands is the possible development of bone marrow fibrosis; although it has not yet been observed in humans receiving rHuTPO, mice induced to overexpress TPO develop increased megakaryocytopoiesis and marrow fibrosis *(87)*. The TPO receptor c-Mpl is not exclusive to the megakaryocyte and its marrow descendents. The TPO receptor (c-Mpl) has been reported to occur in nonmegakaryocytic hematopoietic cells lines, in nonhematopoietic cells, and in cell lines derived from malignancies, leading to the speculation that treatment with rHuTPO could negatively affect patients by transforming the natural history of diseases such as essential thrombocythemia, polycythemia vera, acute and chronic myeloblastic leukemia, lymphomas, and hepatocellular carcinoma. Furthermore, since c-Mpl has been identified in normal liver endothelial cells, and endothelial cells can be induced to proliferate, it is at least possible that prolonged or repetitive exposure to TPO with or without high-dose chemotherapy may result in increased risk for the development of veno-occlusive disease in some patients *(88,89)*.

3.5. rHuGM-CSF and rHuG-CSF

3.5.1. Background

GM-CSF supports the survival, clonal expansion, and differentiation of hematopoietic progenitor cells. GM-CSF induces partially committed progenitor cells to divide and differentiate in the granulocyte-macrophage pathway through its interaction with specific surface receptors located on the target cells. It also enhances the phagocytic and antibacterial activity of mature granulocytes and macrophages. GM-CSF has a multilineage effect, and in addition to its effects on cells committed to the macrophage-granulocyte pathway, it can also promote, in conjunction with appropriate and target-specific other HGFs, the proliferation and maturation of megakaryocytic and erythroid precursors. rHuGM-CSF (sargramostim) is produced by DNA technology in a yeast *(Saccharomyces cerevisiae)*-expressing system. Sargramostim is a glycoprotein that differs from natural occurring human GM-CSF by a leucine substitution at the 23 position of the amino acid sequence and differences in the carbohydrate content. Another rHuGM-CSF (molgramostim) is produced in an *E. coli*-expressing system and is nongylcosylated. Because it is not clinically available in the United States, it will not be discussed. Information about studies in which other forms of rHuGM-CSF were used is included in the following section.

G-CSF is a lineage-specific glycoprotein produced by monocytes, fibroblasts, and endothelial cells that regulates the production and function of marrow neutrophils by stimulating the proliferation, differentiation, and maturation of neutrophilic precursor and end-cell activation through direct interaction with ligand-specific receptors on the target cells *(90)*. Filgrastim (r-metHuG-CSF) is a nonglycosylated, rHuG-CSF with an N-terminal methionine group produced by DNA technology in *E. coli.* The molecule is identical to that of endogenous G-CSF in every way except for the N-terminal methionine group (which is required for *E. coli* expression) and the nonglycosylation. Another form of rHuG-CSF (lenograstim) is glycosylated and is produced in CHO cells. It is not commercially available in the United States and will not be discussed.

A further modification of filgrastim (pegfilgrastim, PEG-r-metHuG-CSF) is derived by adding a 20-kDa monomethoxypolyethylene glycol molecule to the N-terminal residue. The resulting compound has increased size, molecular weight, and prolonged half-life, allowing for less frequent administration than its parent compound (filgrastim) *(91)*.

Filgrastim and sargramostim are used commonly in normal donors and in patients to mobilize peripheral blood progenitor cells (PBPCs) for harvesting in preparation for bone marrow or stem cell transplantation, in patients with cancer receiving myelosuppressive or myeloablative chemotherapy, and less commonly for the treatment of patients with severe chronic neutropenia (SCN). Pegfilgrastim has been approved in the United States for use in cancer patients receiving chemotherapy to reduce the risk of neutropenic fever, for neutropenia-induced treatment delays, and in cases of chemotherapy dose reduction *(92)*.

3.5.2. Studies

The adverse events reported in subjects receiving either filgrastim or sargramostim are similar. The most frequently reported adverse events attributed to filgrastim are bone pain, injection site reaction, rash, acute neutrophilic dermatoses, allergic reactions, worsening of inflammatory conditions, and splenic enlargement. For sargramostim, they are bone pain, fever, headache, chills or muscle ache, rash or injection site reactions, shortness of breath, and edema or capillary leak *(93)*.

The most common adverse event associated with patients receiving filgrastim relative to placebo-treated patients is bone pain (15–39% vs 0–21%) *(93)*. This dose-related adverse event appears to begin shortly after beginning treatment with filgrastim and may occur again or worsen just before neutrophilic recovery among patients who have previously received myelosuppressive chemotherapy *(93)*. Both filgrastim and sargramostim can cause benign transient increases in serum concentrations of lactic dehydrogenase (LDH), alkaline phosphatase, and uric acid. Although the mechanisms of these increases are poorly understood, they are probably related to increased cell turnover in chemotherapy *(94)*. The administration of sargramostim is associated with heightened activities of several cytokines (such as IL-1, IL-6, tumor necrosis factor-α, and leukotrienes), which may explain some of the asymmetry in that HGF's adverse event profile relative to that of filgrastim. In particular, the presence of fever may confuse the clinician, leading to the conclusion that an active infection may be present when it is not or may result in the fever's being prolonged. There is some evidence that prolonged treatment with molgramostim or filgrastim may cause thrombocytopenia; however, this is evidently not the case for yeast-derived sargramostim *(93)*. One proposed mechanism for the occurrence of rHuGM-CSF-associated thrombocytopenia is the stimulation of Kupffer cells in the liver. Since splenomegaly has been reported to occur with filgrastim treatment, it is not unreasonable to assume a similar mechanism for the thrombocytopenia associated with this agent. Because most patients treated with either filgrastim or sargramostim have either received myelosuppressive chemotherapy or are being prepared for PBPC harvesting, it is impossible to separate the cause of CSF-associated thrombocytopenia from a chemotherapy or leukophoresis effect. Interestingly, 17% of patients with SCN (who were not receiving chemotherapy) had platelet counts $< 100 \times 10^9$/L while being treated with filgrastim *(90)*. Unfortunately, since one-third of these patients also had pretreatment splenomegaly and pretreatment thrombocytopenia, it is difficult to determine whether this occurrence represents a worsening of their underlying illness, activation of liver Kupffer cells, or liver macrophage proliferation. Splenomegaly and splenic rupture have been reported to occur with treatment with either filgrastim or sargramostim, although both adverse advents appear to be more common with the former *(95–100)*.

Venous and arterial thrombosis has been associated with both types of HGFs, with the reported cases being more frequent in patients with cancer receiving intravenous sargramostim (4.2%) than in those receiving filgrastim (4.2% vs 1.2%; $p < 0.01$) *(101–105)*. A review of 13 controlled clinical trials involving 838 cancer patients supported an increased incidence of thrombosis with rHuGM-CSF treatment relative to nontreated control patients (6.6% vs 3.6%, $p < 0.05$). When a pooled meta-analysis was performed on the data from each of these trials, a statistically significant difference in the incidence of thrombosis was noted in rHuGM-CSF-treated patients vs those who did not receive rHuGM-CSF *(106)*. Although the mechanism for these thrombotic episodes is unknown, there is evidence that treatment with rHuGM-CSF results in platelet, endothelial cell, neutrophilic, and surface coagulation activation, which further results in a hypercoagulable state that affects both the right and left side of the circulation *(107,108)*.

Acute dyspnea with or without pulmonary infiltrates, fluid retention, and hypotension has been reported to occur with sargramostim *(109)*. Both sargramostim and filgrastim have been reported to cause a so-called first-dose reaction characterized by dyspnea, rigors, and hypotension, although this adverse event appears to be more commonly associated with the brief intravenous or prolonged subcutaneous administration of rHuGM-CSF than with filgrastim treatment *(110–112)*. This syndrome often disappears with subsequent doses of the CSF and may be in part preventable by primary or secondary prophylaxis with analgesics, antihistamines, and corticosteroids *(113)*. Acute respiratory distress syndrome has also been associated with both drugs and can occur either as a first-dose phenomenon or either immediately before or during neutrophil recovery from myelosuppressive or myeloablative chemotherapy. The risk is heightened for the development of this serious complication when the patient has received chemotherapeutic agents that can damage the lung or has a known previous lung injury or pulmonary infection and experiences a brisk neutrophil recovery from myelosuppression while receiving filgrastim or sargramostim. It is believed that the CSF-activated neutrophils are retained in the lung vasculature and that either the release of other cytokines or highly oxidizing moieties damage the lung's blood vessels and/or parenchyma *(114,115)*. A review of all the reported cases of pulmonary toxicity associated with rHuG-CSF administration found that few of the cases could be attributed to the CSF alone, since most patients also received chemotherapy that could have caused lung damage *(116)*.

Filgrastim and sargramostim may play a permissive role in the pathophysiology of sickle cell crisis, suggested by increased concentrations of GM-CSF in the plasma of a disproportionate number of patients in sickle cell crisis relative to the proportion of noncrisis sickle cell patients *(117)*. In addition, at least one case has been reported of a patient with breast cancer and sickle cell trait treated with myelosuppressive chemotherapy and filgrastim who developed sickle cell crisis and severe multiorgan failure including the lung *(118)*.

An unusual severe, atypical peripheral neuropathy characterized by the presence of severe neuropathic foot pain and marked motor weakness of the lower extremities without an associated weakness of the upper extremities has been described in patients receiving vincristine-containing chemotherapy for NHL *(119)*. Comparing the frequency of this neuropathy in 54 patients receiving either filgrastim or sargramostim or no CSF, there was a strong association between CSF exposure and the occurrence of the neuropathy (39% vs 4%, $p = 0.0024$). It is speculated that the relationship between sargramostim exposure and neuropathy may be caused by a chemotherapy-induced modulation of CSF effect on nerve growth or to an alteration in vincristine clearance.

Neutrophilic dermatosis (Sweet's syndrome) and leukocytoclastic vasculitis have been associated with filgrastim and sargramostim *(120)* in patients with myeloproliferative diseases and various other benign conditions, nonmyeloid cancers, and bullous pyoderma in patients with lung cancer *(121,122)*.

Hyperleukocytosis occurs with treatment with either sargramostim or filgrastim *(90,123)*. Patients with various myeloproliferative disorders and hematologic and nonhematologic malignancies theoretically could be worsened by treatment with either of these CSFs; however, there is little evidence to support this contention *(124)*. The risk of leukemic/myelodysplastic transformation among patients with congenital neutropenia, a heterogeneous group of diseases commonly treated from the time of diagnosis with filgrastim, has been reported to be approx 1.7% each year. No relationship has been shown between this conversion risk and patient age or duration of exposure to filgrastim. Comparison with a nontreated group of similar patients is not possible, since most die of infections before the third year of life *(125)*. A retrospective review of six prospective trials in which patients with breast cancer received standard chemotherapy or intensified or increased chemotherapy with or without filgrastim or sargramostim support indicated that the risk of developing AML/MDS was greater among those who received increased or intensified chemotherapy, in-breast irradiation, and a CSF *(126)*. A prospective analysis of children with acute lymphoblastic leukemia treated with radiation therapy and intense chemotherapy ± filgrastim demonstrated that the subsequent risk of developing AML/MDS was significantly increased among all groups receiving filgrastim *(127)*.

The development of neutralizing Abs has not been reported in patients treated for prolonged periods with filgrastim *(90)*. Neutralizing Abs have been detected in 2.3% of patients receiving sargramostim by both intravenous and subcutaneous routes; however, because of the patients' underlying illnesses, the effect on endogenous GM-CSF and hematopoietic reconstitution could not be ascertained *(123)*.

A retrospective review of the comparative safety of filgrastim and sargramostim as reported from 10 outpatient chemotherapy centers indicated that fever unexplained by infection was more common with sargramostim compared with filgrastim (7% vs 1%, $p < 0.001$), as were fatigue, diarrhea, injection site reactions, other dermatologic disorders, and edema (all $p < 0.05$). Bone pain was more frequent with filgrastim ($p < 0.06$). Patients initially treated with sargramostim more frequently change to filgrastim as an alternative than vice versa ($p < 0.001$) *(128)*.

To date, little published information exists about the adverse event profile associated with pegfilgrastim treatment, which is understandable given the recent approval of pegfilgrastim. Adverse events with this growth factor appear to be similar to those observed with its parent compound (filgrastim) *(129,130)*. Mild-to-moderate bone pain that is easily managed with non-narcotic analgesics is the most frequently observed adverse event, being reported by approx 25% of patients receiving pegfilgrastim *(129,130)*. Joint pain, muscle aches, headache, leukocytosis, thrombocytopenia, and heightened liver test, LDH, and uric acid values have been observed *(129–131)*. Hypersensitivity reactions have not been reported with pegfilgrastim; however, since it (like filgrastim) is derived from *E. coli,* patients who have had hypersensitivity reactions when receiving *E. coli*-derived proteins should not be offered this drug. Other unusual but life-threatening adverse events that have not been observed with pegfilgrastim treatment but have been seen among patients receiving filgrastim have included adult respiratory distress syndrome, splenic rupture, and sickle cell crisis.

4. CONCLUSIONS

Chemotherapy-associated myelosuppression has long been a major limitation to a patient's tolerance of anticancer therapy. The toxicities caused by chemotherapeutic agents have negatively impacted the patient's quality of life and have caused treatment delays that can affect response to treatment or even survival. The use of HGFs alleviated many of these problems but also introduced new toxicities caused by the growth factors themselves. The challenge to the physician lies in the judicious and carefully monitored use of those HGFs that are now clinically available.

REFERENCES

1. Porter S. Human immune response to recombinant human proteins. *J Pharm Sci* 2001; 90:1–11.
2. Schwartz RH, In: Paul WE, ed., *Fundamental Immunology.* Philadelphia: Lippincot-Raven. 1999:701–740.
3. Braun A, Kwee L, Labow MA, et al. Protein aggregates seem to play a key role among the parameters influencing the antigenicity of interferon alpha (IFN-alpha) in normal and transgenic mice. *Pharm Res* 1997; 14:1472–1478.
4. Meager A, Wadhwa M, Bird C, et al. Spontaneously occurring neutralizing antibodies against granulocyte-macrophage colony-stimulating factor in patients with autoimmune disease. *Immunology* 1999; 97:536–532.
5. Wadhwa M, Skog A-LH, Bird C, et al. Immunogenicity of granulocyte-macrophage colony-stimulating factor (GM-CSF) products in patients undergoing combination therapy with GM-CSF. *Clin Cancer Res* 1999; 5:1353–1361.
6. Josic D, Buchacher A, Kannicht C, et al. Degradation products of factor VIII which can lead to increased immunogenicity. *Vox Sang* 1999; 77:90–99.
7. Koren E, Zuckerman LA, Mire-Sluis AR. Immune responses to therapeutic proteins in humans—clinical significance, assessment and prediction. *Curr Pharm Biotechnol* 2002; 3:349–360.
8. Li Y, Yang C, Xia Y, et al. Thrombocytopenia caused by the development of antibodies to thromopoietin. *Blood* 2001; 98:3241–3248.
9. Casadevall N, Nataf J, Viron B, et al. Pure red-cell aplasia and antierythropoietin antibodies in patients treated with recombinant erythropoietin. *N Engl J Med* 2002; 346:469–475.
10. Neumega (oprelvekin) package insert. Cambridge, MA: Genetics Institute. July, 1998.
11. Teramura M, Kobayashi S, Yoshinaga K, et al. Effect of interleukin 11 on normal and pathological thrombopoiesis. *Cancer Chemother Pharmacol* 1996; 38:S99–S102.
12. Du X, Williams DA. Interleukin-11: review of molecular, cell biology, and clinical use. *Blood* 1997; 89:3897–3908.

13. Du X, Williams DA. Interleukin-11: a multifunctional growth factor derived from the hematopoietic microenvironment. *Blood* 1994; 83:2023–2030.
14. Hu JP, Cesano A, Santoli D, et al. Effects of interleukin-11 on proliferation and cell cycle status of myeloid leukemic cells. *Blood* 1993; 81:1586–1592.
15. Kobayashi S, Teramura M, Sugawara I, et al. Interleukin-11 acts as an autocrine growth factor for human megakaryoblastic cell lines. *Blood* 1993; 81:889–893.
16. Zhang XG, Gu JJ, Lu ZY, et al. Ciliary neurotropic factor, interleukin 11, leukemia inhibitory factor, and oncostatin M are growth factors for human myeloma cell lines using the interleukin 6 signal transducer gp130. *J Exp Med* 1994; 179:1337–1342.
17. Smith JW. Tolerability and side-effect profile of rhIL-11. *Oncology (Huntingt)* 2000; 14:41–47.
18. Smith JW, Beach K, Bedrosian CL, et al. Neumega (oprelvekin: rhIL-11) prevents severe chemotherapy-induced thrombocytopenia in abbreviated phase III study. *Blood* 1998; 92:377a (abstract 1555).
19. Ault K, Mitchell J, Knowles C. Recombinant human interleukin eleven (Neumega) rhIL-11 growth factor increases plasma volume and decreases urine sodium excretion in normal human subjects. *Blood* 1994; 84:276a (abstract).
20. Gordon MS, McCaskill-Stevens WJ, Battiato LA, et al. A phase I trial of recombinant human interleukin-11 (Neumega rhIL-11 growth factor) in women with breast cancer receiving chemotherapy. *Blood* 1996; 87:3615–3624.
21. Tepler I, Elias L, Smith JW, et al. A randomized placebo-controlled trial of recombinant human interleukin-11 in cancer patients with severe thrombocytopenia due to chemotherapy. *Blood* 1996; 87:3607–3614.
22. Isaacs C, Robert NJ, Bailey FA, et al. Randomized placebo-controlled study of recombinant human interleukin-11 to prevent chemotherapy-induced thrombocytopenia in patients with breast cancer receiving dose-intensive cyclophosphamide and doxorubicin. *J Clin Oncol* 1997; 15:3368–3377.
23. Williams DE, Eisenman J, Baird A, et al. Identification of a ligand for the c-kit proto-oncogene. *Cell* 1990; 63:167–174.
24. Broxmeyer HE, Cooper S, Lu L, et al. Effect of murine mast cell growth factor (c-kit proto-oncogene ligand) on colony formation by human marrow hematopoietic progenitor cells. *Blood* 1991; 77:2142–2149.
25. McNiece IK, Langley KE, Zsebo KM. Recombinant human stem cell factor synergises with GM-CSF, G-CSF, IL-3 and EPO to stimulate human progenitor cells of the myeloid and erythroid lineages. *Exp Hematol* 1991; 19:226–231.
26. Andrews RG, Bensinger WI, Knitter GH, et al. The ligand for c-kit, stem cell factor, stimulates the circulation of cells that engraft lethally irradiated baboons. *Blood* 1992; 80:2715–2720.
27. Ulich TR, del Castillo JC, McNiece IK, et al. Stem cell factor in combination with granulocyte colony-stimulating factor (CSF) or granulocyte-macrophage CSF synergistically increases granulopoiesis in vivo. *Blood* 1991; 78:1954.
28. Pietsch T, Kyas U, Steffens U, et al. Effects of human stem cell factor (c-kit ligand) on proliferation of myeloid leukemia cells: heterogeneity in response and synergy with other hematopoietic growth factors. *Blood* 1992; 80:1199–1206.
29. Crawford I, Lau D, Erwin R, et al. A phase I trial of recombinant methionyl human stem cell factor (SFC) in patients (PTS) with advanced non-small cell lung carcinoma (NSCLC). *Proc Am Soc Clin Oncol* 1993; 12:135 (abstract 338).
30. Demetri G, Costa J, Hayes D, et al. A phase I trial of recombinant methionyl human stem cell factor (SFC) in patients with advanced breast carcinoma pre- and post-chemotherapy (CHEMO) with cyclophosphamide (C) and doxorubicin (A). *Proc Am Soc Clin Oncol* 1993; 12:142 (abstract 367).
31. Moskowitz CH, Stiff P, Gordon MS, et al. Recombinant methionyl human stem cell factor and filgrastim for peripheral blood progenitor cell mobilization and transplantation in non-Hodgkin's lymphoma patients—results of a phase I/II trial. *Blood* 1997; 89:3136–3147.
32. Basser RL, To LB, Begley CG, et al. Rapid hematopoietic recovery after multicycle high-dose chemotherapy: enhancement of filgrastim-induced progenitor-cell mobilization by recombinant human stem0cell factor. *J Clin Oncol* 1998; 16:1899–1908.
33. Glaspy JA, Shpall EJ, LeMaistre CF, et al. Peripheral blood progenitor cell mobilization using stem cell factor in combination with filgrastim in breast cancer patients. *Blood* 1997; 90:2939–2951.
34. Shpall EJ, Wheeler CA, Turner SA, et al. A randomized phase III study of peripheral blood progenitor cell mobilization with stem cell factor and filgrastim in high-risk breast cancer patients. *Blood* 1999; 93:2491–2501.

35. Facon T, Harousseau J-L, Maloisel F, et al. Stem cell factor in combination with filgrastim after chemotherapy improves peripheral blood progenitor cell yield and reduces apheresis requirements in multiple myeloma patients: a randomized, controlled trial. *Blood* 1999; 94:1218–1225.
36. Costa JJ, Demetri GD, Harrist PJ, et al. Recombinant human stem cell factor (c-kit ligand) promotes human mast cell and melanocyte hyperplasia and functional activation in vivo. *J Exp Med* 1996; 183:2681–2686.
37. Columbo M, Horowitz EM, Botana LM, et al. The human recombinant c-kit receptor ligand, rhSCF, induces mediator release from human cutaneous mast cells and enhances IgE-dependent mediator release from both skin mast cells and peripheral blood basophils. *J Immunol* 1992; 149:599–608.
38. Caceres-Cortes JR, Alvarado-Moreno JA, Waga K, et al. Implication of tyrosine kinase receptor and steel factor in cell density-dependent growth in cervical cancers and leukemias. *Cancer Res* 2001; 61:6281–6289.
39. Tamborini E, Papini D, Messelani A, et al. c-kit and c-kit ligand (SCF) in synovial sarcoma (SS): an mRNA expression analysis in 23 cases. *Br J Cancer* 2001; 85:405–411.
40. Metcalfe DD, Akin C. Mastocytosis: molecular mechanisms and clinical disease heterogeneity. *Leuk Res* 2001; 25:577–582.
41. Bellone G, Carbone A, Sibona N, et al. Aberrant activation of c-kit protects colon carcinoma cells against apoptosis and enhances their invasive potential. *Cancer Res* 2001; 61:2200–2206.
42. Yamamotot T, Umeda T, Nishioka K. Immunohistological distribution of stem cell factor and kit receptor in angiosarcoma. *Acta Derm Venereol* 2000; 80:443–445.
43. Landuzzi L, De Giovanni C, Nicoletti G, et al. The metastatic ability of Ewing's sarcoma cells is modulated by stem cell factor and by its receptor c-kit. *Am J Pathol* 2000; 157:2123–2131.
44. Simak R, Capodieci P, Cohen DW, et al. Expression of c-kit and kit-ligand in benign and mailgnant prostatic tissues. *Histol Histopathol* 2000; 15:365–374.
45. Miettinen M, Majidi M, Lasota J. Pathology and diagnostic criteria of gastrointestinal stromal tumors (GISTs): a review. *Eur J Cancer* 2002; 38:S39–S51.
46. Esposito I, Kleeff J, Bischoff SC, et al. The stem cell factor-c-kit system and mast cells in human pancreatic cancer. *Lab Invest* 2002; 82:1481–1492.
47. Aldinucci D, Poletto D, Nanni P, et al. Hodgkin and Reed-Sternberg cells express functional c-kit receptors and interact with primary fibroblasts from Hodgkin's disease-involved lymph nodes through soluble and membrane-bound stem cell factor. *Br J Haematol* 2002; 118:1055–1064.
48. Wu B, Liu XL, Xuan WL, et al. Detection of stem cell factor mRNA expression in leukemic cells by in situ reverse transcriptase-PCR. *Di Yi Jun Yi Da Xue Xue Bao* 2002; 22:490–492.
49. Akin C, Jaffe ES, Raffeld M, et al. An immunohistochemical study of the bone marrow lesions of systemic mastocytosis: expression of stem cell factor by lesional mast cells. *Am J Clin Pathol* 2002; 118:242–247.
50. Moses AV, Jarvis MA, Raggo C, et al. Kaposi's sarcoma-associated herpesvirus-induced upregulation of the c-kit proto-oncogene, as identified by gene expression profiling, is essential for the transformation of endothelial cells. *J Virol* 2002; 76:8383–8399.
51. Smith MA, Court EL, Smith JG. Stem cell factor: laboratory and clinical aspects. *Blood Rev* 2001; 15:191–197.
52. Attoub S, Rivat C, Rodrigues S, et al. The c-kit tyrosine kinase inhibitor STI571 for colorectal cancer therapy. *Cancer Res* 2002; 62:4879 4883.
53. Krystal GW, Honsawek S, Litz J, et al. The selective tryosine kinase inhibitor ST1571 inhibits small cell lung cancer growth. *Clin Cancer Res* 2000; 6:3319–3326.
54. Dror Y, Leaker M, Caruana G, et al. Mastocytosis cells bearing a c-kit activating point mutation are characterized by hypersensitivity to stem cell factor and increased apoptosis. *Br J Haematol* 2000; 108:729–736.
55. Kambe N, Miyachi Y. A possible mechanism of mast cell proliferation in mastocytosis. *J Dermatol* 2002; 29:1–9.
56. Cases A. Novel erythropoiesis stimulating protein. Antianemic: NESP. *Drugs Fut* 2000; 25:246–248.
57. Macdougall IC. Novel erythropoiesis stimulating protein. *Semin Nephrol* 2000; 20:375–381.
58. Egrie JC, Browne JK. Development and characterization of novel erythropoiesis stimulating protein (NESP). *Br J Cancer* 2001; 84:S3–S10.
59. Egrie JC, Grant JR, Gillies DK, et al. The role of carbohydrate on the biological activity of erythropoietin. *Glycoconjugate J* 1993; 10:263 (abstract).

60. Sowade B, Sowade O, Mocks J, et al. The safety of treatment with recombinant human erythropoietin in clinical use: a review of controlled studies. *Int J Mol Med* 1998; 1:303–314.
61. Procrit (Epoetin alfa) package insert. Raritan, NJ: OrthoBiotech. November, 2002.
62. Vansteenkiste J, Pirker R, Massuti B, et al. Double-blind, placebo-controlled, randomized phase III trial of darbepoetin alfa in lung cancer patients receiving chemotherapy. *J Natl Cancer Inst* 2002; 94:1211–1220.
63. Koenig W, Ernst E. The possible role of hemorheology in atherothrombogenesis. *Atherosclerosis* 1992; 94:93–107.
64. Lowe GD, Forbes CD. Blood rheology and thrombosis. *Clin Haematol* 1981; 10:343–367.
65. de Andrade JR, Frei D, Guilfoyle M. Integrated analysis of thrombotic/vascular event occurrence in epoetin alfa-treated patients undergoing major, elective orthopedic surgery. *Orthopedics* 1999; 22:s113–s118.
66. Aranesp (darbepoetin alfa) package insert. Thousand Oaks, CA: Amgen. September, 2001.
67. Glaspy J, O'Byrne J, Armstrong S, et al. Randomised, active-controlled phase I/II dose escalation study of novel erythropoiesis stimulating protein (NESP) in patients with solid tumours (presented by the NESP Oncology Group) *Ann Oncol* 2000; 11:146 (abstract).
68. Glaspy J, Jadeja JS, Justice G, et al. A dose-finding and safety study of novel erythropoiesis stimulating protein (NESP) for the treatment of anaemia in patients receiving multicycle chemotherapy. *Br J Cancer* 2001; 84(suppl. 1);17–23.
69. Glaspy JA, Jadeja JS, Justice G, et al. Darbepoetin alfa given every 1 or 2 weeks alleviates anaemia associated with cancer chemotherapy. *Br J Cancer* 2002; 87:268–276.
70. Nissenson AR, Swan SK, Lindberg JS, et al. Randomized, controlled trial of darbepoetin alfa for the treatment of anemia in hemodialysis patients. *Am J Kidney Dis* 2002; 40:110–118.
71. de Sauvage F, Hass P, Spencer S, et al. Stimulation of megakaryocytopoiesis and thrombopoiesis by the c-Mpl ligand. *Nature* 1994; 369:533–538.
72. van de Ven C, Fernandez GW, Herbst T, et al. Thrombopoietin (TPO) significantly increases neonatal (NB) rat myelopoiesis and thrombopoiesis: Additive effect of IL-3 and IL-11 with lower doses of TPO (2 μg/kg). *Blood* 1995; 86:910 (abstract).
73. Pavithran K, Doval DC. Thrombopoietin—biology and clinical applications. *Oncol Forum* 2001; 5:20–24.
74. Vigon I, Mornon JP, Cocault L, et al. Molecular cloning and characterization of mpl, the human homolog of the V-mpl oncogene: identification of a member of the hematopoietic growth factor receptor super family. *Proc Natl Acad Sci USA* 1992; 89:5640–5644.
75. Methia N, Louache F, Vainchencker W, et al. Oligodeoxynucleotides antisense to the pronto-oncogene c-mpl specifically inhibit in vitro megakaryocytopoiesis. *Blood* 1993; 82:1395–1401.
76. Debili N, Wendling F, Cosman D, et al. The Mpl receptor is expressed in the mega-karyocytic lineage from late progenitors to platelets. *Blood* 1995; 85:391–401.
77. Kaushansky K. Thrombopoietin. *N Engl J Med* 1998; 339:746–754.
78. Neelis KJ, Qingliang L, Thomas GR, et al. Prevention of thrombocytopenia by thrombopoietin in myelosuppressed rhesus monkeys accompanied by prominent erythropoietic stimulation and iron depletion. *Blood* 1997; 90:58–63.
79. Basser RL, Rasko JE, Clarke K, et al. Thrombopoietic effects of pegylated recombinant human megakaryocyte growth and development factor (PEG-rHuMGDF) in patients with advanced cancer. *Lancet* 1996; 348:1279–1281.
80. Kuter DJ, Goodnough LT, Romo J, et al. Thrombopoietin therapy increases platelet yields in healthy platelet donors. *Blood* 2001; 98:1339–1345.
81. Vadhan-Raj S, Murray LJ, Bueso-Ramos C, et al. Stimulation of megakaryocyte and platelet production by a single dose of recombinant human thrombopoietin in patients with cancer. *Ann Intern Med* 1997; 126:673–681.
82. Basser RL, O'Flaherty E, Green M, et al. Development of pancytopenia with neutralizing antibodies to thrombopoietin after multicycle chemotherapy supported by megakaryocyte growth and development factor. *Blood* 2002; 99:2599–2602.
83. Vadhan-Raj S. Clinical experience with recombinant human thrombopoietin in chemotherapy-induced thrombocytopenia. *Semin Hematol* 2000; 37:28–34.
84. Ezumi Y, Takayama H, Okuma M. Thrombopoietin, c-Mpl ligand, induces tyrosine phosphorylation of Tyk2, JAK2 and STAT3, and enhances agonist-induced aggregation in platelets in vitro. *FEBS Lett* 1995; 374:48–52.

85. Toombs CF, Young CH, Glaspy JA. Megakaryocyte growth and development factor (MGDF) moderately enhances in vitro platelet aggregation. *Thromb Res* 1995; 80:23–33.
86. Goodnough LT, Kuter DJ, McCullough J, et al. Prophylactic platelet transfusions from healthy apheresis platelet donors undergoing treatment with thrombopoietin. *Blood* 2001; 98:1346–1351.
87. Yan XQ, Lacey D, Fletcher F, et al. Chronic exposure to retroviral vector encoded MGDF (mpl-ligand) induces lineage-specific growth and differentiation of megakarocytes in mice. *Blood* 1995; 88:4025–4033.
88. Cardier JE. Effects of megakaryocyte growth and development factor (thrombopoietin) on liver endothelial cells in vitro. *Microvasc Res* 1999; 58:108–113.
89. Cardier JE, Dempsey J. Thrombopoietin and its receptor, c-mpl, are constitutively expressed by mouse liver endothelial cells: evidence of thrombopoietin as a growth factor for liver endothelial cells. *Blood* 1998; 91:923–929.
90. Neupogen (filgrastim) package insert. Thousand Oaks, CA: Amgen. June, 2000.
91. Morstyn G, Foote M, Walker T, et al. Filgrastim (r-metHuG-CSF) in the 21st century:SD/01. *Acta Haematol* 2001; 105:151–155.
92. Neulasta (pegfilgrastim) package insert. Thousand Oaks, CA: Amgen. September, 2002.
93. Wagner LM, Furman WL. Haemopoietic growth factors in paediatric oncology. *Paediatr Drugs* 2001; 3:195–217.
94. Murata M, Harada M, Kato S, et al. Peripheral blood stem cell mobilization and apheresis: analysis of adverse events in 94 normal donors. *Bone Marrow Transplant* 1999; 24:1065–1071.
95. Becker PS, Wagle M, Matous S, et al. Spontaneous splenic rupture following administration of granulocyte colony-stimulating factor (G-CSF): occurrence in an allogeneic donor of peripheral blood stem cells. *Biol Blood Marrow Transplant* 1997; 3:45–49.
96. Boxer LA, Hutchinson R, Emerson S. Recombinant human granulocyte-colony-stimulating factor in the treatment of patients with neutropenia. *Clin Immunol Immunopathol* 1992; 62:s39–s46.
97. Bonilla MA, Dale D, Zeidler C, et al. Long-term safety of treatment with recombinant human granulocyte colony-stimulating factor (r-metHuG-CSF) in patients with severe congenital neutropenias. *Br J Haematol* 1994; 88:723–730.
98. Platzbecker U, Prange-Krex G, Bornhauser M, et al. Spleen enlargement in healthy donors during G-CSF mobilization of PBPCs. *Transfusion* 2001; 41:184–189.
99. Delmer A, Karmochkine M, Cadiou M, et al. Recurrent spleen enlargement during cyclic granulocyte-macrophage colony-stimulating factor therapy for myelodysplastic syndrome. *Am J Hematol* 1990; 34:73–74.
100. Zimmer BM, Berdel WE, Ludwig WD, et al. Fatal spleen rupture during induction chemotherapy with rh GM-CSF priming for acute monocytic leukemia. Clinical case report and in vitro studies. *Leuk Res* 1993; 17:277–283.
101. Tolcher AW, Giusti RM, O Shaughnessy JA, et al. Arterial thrombosis associated with granulocyte-macrophage colony-stimulating factor (GM-CSF) administration in breast cancer patients treated with dose-intensive chemotherapy: a report of two cases. *Cancer Invest* 1995; 13:188–192.
102. O'Reilly SE, Gelmon KA, Onetto N, et al. Phase I trial of recombinant human granulocyte-macrophage colony-stimulating factor derived from yeast in patients with breast cancer receiving cyclophosphamide, doxorubicin, and fluorouracil. *J Clin Oncol* 1993; 11:2411–2416.
103. Conti JA, Scher HI. Acute arterial thrombosis after escalated-dose methotrexate, vinblastine, doxorubicin, and cisplatin chemotherapy with recombinant granulocyte colony-stimulating factor. A possible new recombinant granulocyte colony-stimulating factor toxicity. *Cancer* 1992; 70:2699–2702.
104. Gozdasoglu S, Unal E, Yavuz G, et al. Granulocyte-macrophage colony stimulating factor (rh-GM-CSF) in the treatment of chemotherapy-induced neutropenia. *J Chemother* 1995; 7:467–469.
105. Grem JL, McAtee N, Murphy RF, et al. Phase I and pharmacokinetic study of recombinant human granulocyte-macrophage colony-stimulating factor given in combination with fluorouracil plus calcium leucovorin in metastatic gastrointestinal adenocarcinoma. *J Clin Oncol* 1994; 12:560–568.
106. Barbui T, Finazzi G, Grassi A, et al. Thrombosis in cancer patients treated with hematopoietic growth factors: a meta-analysis. On behalf of the Subcommittee on Haemostasis and Malignancy of the Scientific and Standardization Committee of the ISTH. *Thromb Haemost* 1996; 75:368–371.
107. Canales MA, Arrieta R, Gomez-Rioja R, et al. Induction of a hypercoagulability state and endothelial cell activation by granulocyte colony-stimulating factor in peripheral blood stem cell donors. *J Hematother Stem Cell Res* 2002; 11:675–681.

108. Kawachi Y, Watanabe A, Uchida T, et al. Acute arterial thrombosis die to platelet aggregation in a patient receiving granulocyte colony-stimulating factor. *Br J Haematol* 1996; 94:413–416.
109. Ruef C, Coleman DL. GM-CSF and G-CSF: cytokines in clinical application. *Schweiz Med Wochenschr* 1991; 121:297–412.
110. Stern AC, Jones TC. The side-effect profile of GM-CSF. *Infection* 1992; 20:s124–s127.
111. Lieschke GJ, Cebon J, Morstyn G. Characterization of the clinical effects after the first dose of bacterially synthesized recombinant human granulocyte-macrophage colony-stimulating factor. *Blood* 1989; 74:2634–2643.
112. Cebon J, Lieschke GJ, Bury RW, et al. The dissociation of GM-CSF efficacy from toxicity according to route of administration: a pharmacodynamic study. *Br J Haematol* 1992; 80:144–150.
113. Edmonson JH, Hartmann LC, Long HJ, et al. Granulocyte-macrophage colony-stimulating factor. Preliminary observations on the influences of dose, schedule, and route of administration in patients receiving cyclophosphamide and carboplatin. *Cancer* 1992; 70:2529–2539.
114. Takahashi Y, Kobayashi Y, Chikayama S, et al. Effect of granulocyte/colony-stimulating factor on the onset of the adult respiratory distress syndrome. *Acta Haematol* 1999; 101:124–129.
115. Akasheh M, Eastwood D, Vesole DH. Engraftment syndrome after autologous hematopoietic stem cell transplant supported by granulocyte-colony-stimulating factor (G-CSF) versus granulocyte-macrophage colony-stimulating factor (GM-CSF). *Bone Marrow Transplant* 2003; 31:113–116.
116. Azoulay E, Attalah H, Harf A, et al. Granulocyte colony-stimulating factor or neutrophil-induced pulmonary toxicity: myth or reality? Systematic review of clinical case reports and experimental data. *Chest* 2001; 120:1695–1701.
117. Haider MZ, Raghupathy R, Azizieh F, et al. GM-CSF in sickle cell anemia patients with elevated Hb F. *Acta Haematol* 2000; 102:140–143.
118. Grigg A. Granulocyte colony-stimulating factor-induced sickle cell crisis and multiorgan dysfunction in a patient with compound heterozygous sickle cell/β+ thalassemia. *Blood* 2001; 97:3998–3999.
119. Weintraub M, Adde MA, Venzon DJ, et al. Severe atypical neuropathy associated with administration of hematopoietic colony-stimulating factors and vincristine. *J Clin Oncol* 1996; 14:935–940.
120. Spiekermann K, Roesler J, Emmendoerffer A, et al. Functional features of neutrophils induced by G-CSF and GM-CSF treatment: differential effects and clinical implications. *Leukemia* 1997; 11:466–478.
121. Arbetter KR, Hubbard KW, Markovic SN, et al. Case of granulocyte colony-stimulating factor-induced Sweet's syndrome. *Am J Hematol* 1999; 61:126–129.
122. Ross HJ, Moy LA, Kaplan R, et al. Bullous pyoderma gangrenosum after granulocyte colony-stimulating factor treatment. *Cancer* 1991; 68:441–443.
123. Leukine (sargramostim) package insert. Richmond, CA: Berlex Laboratories. 2003.
124. Brodsky RA, Bedi A, Jones RJ. Are growth factors leukemogenic? *Leukemia* 1996; 10:175–177.
125. Cottle TE, Fier CJ, Donadieu J, et al. Risk and benefit of treatment of severe chronic neutropenia with granulocyte colony-stimulating factor. *Semin Hematol* 2002; 39:134–140.
126. Smith RE, Bryant J, DeCillis A, et al. Acute myeloid leukemia and myelodysplastic syndrome after doxorubicin-cyclophosphamide adjuvant therapy for operable breast cancer: the National Surgical Adjuvant Breast and Bowel Project Experience. *J Clin Oncol* 2003; 21:1195–1204.
127. Relling MV, Boyett JM, Blanco JG, et al. Granulocyte colony-stimulating factor and the risk of secondary myeloid malignancy after etoposide treatment. *Blood* 2003; 15:3862–3867.
128. Milkovich G, Moleski RJ, Reitan JF, et al. Comparative safety of filgrastim versus sargramostim in patients receiving myelosuppressive chemotherapy. *Pharmacotherapy* 2000; 20:1432–1440.
129. Holmes F, O Shaughnessy J, Vukelja S, et al. Blinded, randomized, multicenter study to evaluate single administration pegfilgrastim once per cycle versus daily filgrastim as an adjunct to chemotherapy in patients with high-risk stage II or stage III/IV breast cancer. *J Clin Oncol* 2002; 20:727–731.
130. Green MD, Koelbl H, Baselga J, et al. (International Pegfilgrastim 749 Study Group) A randomized double-blind multicenter phase III study of fixed dose single-administration pegfilgrastim versus daily filgrastim in patients receiving myelosuppressive chemotherapy. *Ann Oncol* 2003; 14:29–35.
131. Johnston E, Crawford J, Blackwell S, et al. Randomized, dose-escalation study of SD/01 compared with daily filgrastim in patients receiving chemotherapy. *J Clin Oncol* 2002; 18:2522–2528.

20 Long-Term Safety of Filgrastim in Chronic Neutropenias

Karl Welte, MD, PhD

CONTENTS

1. INTRODUCTION

Twenty years after the detection of human granulocyte colony-stimulating factor (G-SCF) *(1)* and 10 years since commercial launch of the recombinant human form, filgrastim, millions of patients have been treated to decrease the incidence of infection, as manifested by neutropenia *(2)*. Filgrastim has utility in patients with nonmyeloid malignancies who are receiving myelosuppressive anticancer drugs. These drugs are associated with a significant incidence of severe febrile neutropenia (FN) in the settings of bone marrow transplantation (BMT), severe chronic neutropenia (SCN), and mobilization of peripheral blood progenitor cells (PBPCs). In addition to adverse events reported in these licensed indications, postmarket reports in nonlicensed clinical settings, i.e., human immunodeficiency virus (HIV) infection, myelodysplastic syndromes (MDS), and noncytotoxic drug-induced neutropenia, have been published *(3)*.

In all studies, the safety profile and patient tolerance of filgrastim have been very good, with medullary bone pain (seen in approx 10–20% of the patients treated by the conventional subcutaneous route) as the only clinically significant and relatively frequent side effect. Safety data are available from several clinical settings including

From: *Cancer Drug Discovery and Development*
Hematopoietic Growth Factors in Oncology: Basic Science and Clinical Therapeutics
Edited by: G. Morstyn, M. A. Foote, and G. J. Lieschke © Humana Press Inc., Totowa, NJ

standard-dose chemotherapy, high-dose therapy with or without BMT or PBPC support, and SCN *(2,3)*.

In all studies, overall events attributed to filgrastim were infrequent. Local reactions (pain, swelling, and redness at the injection site) were very rarely reported, and fever and chills were not observed. The laboratory changes (i.e., increases in alkaline phosphatase, leukocyte alkaline phosphatase, and uric acid) were sustained during treatment, but diminished or resolved without clinical sequelae when treatment was stopped. The percentage of reports by indication for filgrastim usage shows that 64% of the adverse events reported were for the adjunct to chemotherapy indication, whereas 9% were for the SCN indication *(3)*. The reporting frequency of adverse events mirrors actual usage in the clinical setting. The body systems most frequently affected were the body as a whole (19%), hematologic (16%), skin (14%), appendages (14%), musculoskeletal (12%), respiratory (9%), cardiovascular (7%), nervous system (6%), metabolic (4%), application sites (4%), gastrointestinal (3%), liver (1.5%), and urinary (1.3%).

The label for filgrastim contains a precaution that safety and efficacy has not been stipulated when filgrastim is administered simultaneously with antimetabolites (e.g., 5-fluorouracil), nitosoureas, or mitocytin C, or with concomitant radiotherapy. This precaution is not unique to filgrastim, however. The label for other myeloid factors, such as the recombinant human granulocyte-macrophage colony-stimulating factors (rHuGM-CSFs) (i.e., sargramostim and molgramostim) contain the same precaution.

Patients with SCN should have spleen size monitored by computed tomography or magnetic resonance imaging, as clinical trial data suggest that this organ tends to increase early in filgrastim treatment and then, for most patients, to decrease toward baseline values.

In normal-donor studies, the side effects of filgrastim reported have been limited to musculoskeletal pain, and normal volunteers given a short course of filgrastim have not shown any evidence of abnormal bone marrow findings *(3)*.

With any drug, the number of patients enrolled in clinical trials is small compared with the number of patients receiving the commercial product. Consequently, very rare events may not be characterized during the clinical trial period. With increased market exposure, new safety issues may emerge, changing or adding to the premarket safety profile since the drug is being observed and tested under a wide range of clinical conditions. Spontaneously reported events are analyzed in detail by drug manufacturers to look for potential indications of important, previously unknown safety factors. Postmarketing safety surveillance is a means of identifying these potential problems; however, in the postmarket setting, the determination of real quantification of rates of suspected reactions is not possible. It is difficult to ascertain objective causality, which is of less importance in the context of raising an early suspicion or signal.

The use of filgrastim in patients with chronic diseases offers an opportunity to study the long-term safety of this HGF. Because rHuGM-CSF and recombinant human stem cell factor (rHuSCF) have not received marketing approval for long-term use, no comparable data are available. A recombinant human thrombopoietic factor, megakaryocyte growth and development factor (rHuMGDF) has been used on a compassionate basis in a patient with idiopathic thrombocytic purpura with no apparent ill effect *(4)*. Given these limitations, selected safety issues were identified from spontaneous reports and the published literature and are discussed below.

2. DERMATOLOGIC EVENTS

Neutrophilic dermatosis, including Sweet's syndrome and pyoderma gangrenosum, are rare events that have been reported in patients receiving chemotherapy with filgrastim support *(3)*. With the increased use of filgrastim, the reporting incidence of these events has not dramatically increased. Neutrophilic dermatosis is approx <1 in 33,000 patients. Sweet's syndrome has been identified as a paraneoplastic syndrome seen in the patient population that typically receives filgrastim. Although filgrastim administration was temporally associated in several of the cases reported, its role in the pathogenesis of this syndrome is uncertain. In these reported cases, it is doubtful that filgrastim induced Sweet's syndrome, as these cases are similar to those reported in the literature in patients who were not receiving filgrastim or any other cytokines, and in a few reported cases other drugs were identified as co-suspect. It has been suggested that the pathogenesis of Sweet's syndrome may be secondary to an inappropriate secretion of one or more endogenous cytokines *(5)*. Whether exogenous administration of filgrastim participates directly or indirectly in the development of Sweet's syndrome remains speculative.

3. RESPIRATORY EVENTS

The possibility that filgrastim, or the rapid increase of white blood cells, might augment bleomycin pulmonary toxicity has been discussed in the literature. Bleomycin is known to cause pulmonary toxicity in approx 10% of patients, lethal pulmonary fibrosis in approx 1–2% of patients, and nonlethal pulmonary fibrosis in 2–3% of patients *(6)*. The incidence of pulmonary toxicity appears to increase when bleomycin is used in combination with other drugs and administered to patients with reduced renal function. The possible augmentation of bleomycin pulmonary toxicity by filgrastim has been addressed by studies in animal models *(7,8)* and by both nonrandomized and randomized clinical trials *(9–11)*. Although anecdotal case reports of pulmonary adverse events have been published, the available evidence from controlled clinical trials argues against an excess morbidity in filgrastim-treated individuals. Determination of a causal relationship between filgrastim and the possible augmentation of bleomycin pulmonary toxicity is complicated in these cases by confounding variables and contributory risk factors. It should be noted that the rHuGM-CSF products have labeled precautions recommending close monitoring in patients with pulmonary disease *(12)*.

4. RHEUMATOLOGIC EVENTS

Since the commercial introduction of filgrastim, the reporting rate of arthritis in patients treated with filgrastim has been <1 in 63,000 patients *(3)*. Most of these reports of arthritis occurred in patients with Felty's syndrome; however, other diagnoses including histories of rheumatoid arthritis, inflammatory joint disease (osteoarthritis and migratory polyarthritis), and Sjögren's syndrome were also represented. In most cases, arthritis developed within the first 10 d of filgrastim administration. Resolution of symptoms occurred in approx 50% of patients after treatment with analgesics and/or nonsteroidal anti-inflammatory agents. In rare cases, steroids were required. Filgrastim was discontinued in approx 75% patients who reported arthritis flares. Symptoms recurred in all patients who were rechallenged, but in a few patients, symptoms abated with treatment during filgrastim therapy. Of interest are several published case reports discussing filgrastim use in patients with Felty's syndrome that did not show an association with exacerbation of arthritis *(13)*.

5. PEDIATRIC STUDIES

Many studies of filgrastim administration after chemotherapy in children with acute leukemias or solid tumors have shown that the incidences of adverse events were similar in patients receiving placebo/no drug or filgrastim. In our own study of patients with high-risk acute lymphoblastic leukemia comparing 121 chemotherapy cycles plus filgrastim and 137 control chemotherapy cycles, only one World Health Organization grade III vasculitis was considered to be attributed to filgrastim *(2)*. This topic is reviewed in Lerhrnbecher and Welte *(14)*.

6. PREGNANCY

When filgrastim was first licensed, little information was available regarding placental transfer of the protein. Since that time, two publications have addressed this issue, and filgrastim was shown to cross the placenta and specifically induce bone marrow and spleen myelopoiesis in the fetus and neonate in a preclinical rat study *(15,16)*.

No well-controlled trials have been done to study the use of filgrastim in human pregnancies; however, the transplacental passage of a measurable amount of filgrastim in women who received a single dose of filgrastim and in whom preterm delivery was imminent was reported *(17)*. Concentrations of G-CSF and neutrophils were measured in maternal blood and umbilical venous cord blood after administration of a single intravenous (iv) 25-μg/kg dose of filgrastim in 11 women in whom preterm delivery was imminent. These measurements were compared with values from 34 control women and 35 cord sera. The transplacental passage of a measurable quantity of filgrastim was noted, especially in those women who received filgrastim at least 30 h before delivery. According to the authors, this amount of filgrastim can have a biologic effect on the fetus.

7. PATIENT SUBGROUPS

7.1. Cancer Patients

Dose-dependent musculoskeletal pain remains the most consistently observed adverse event across all cancer patient populations in multiple settings including adjunct to chemotherapy, PBPC, and BMT. Medullary bone pain was reported in 14% of patients who received filgrastim doses ranging from 0.4 to 12 μg/kg/d and in 27% of patients who received filgrastim doses ranging from 20 to 120 μg/kg/d. Musculoskeletal pain was controlled with non-narcotic analgesia in most patients. The cause of musculoskeletal pain is not known, although it appears to be related to myelopoietic stimulation. Other reported adverse events included thrombocytopenia and anemia consistent with complications of cytotoxic chemotherapy; the potential for receiving full doses of chemotherapy on the prescribed schedule may put the patient at a greater risk of hematologic complications. Other variables including disease, infection, and treatment can also contribute to the frequency, duration, and severity of thrombocytopenia in these patients. It is difficult to determine whether filgrastim treatment contributes to the development of thrombocytopenia in chemotherapy-treated patients. Dose-dependent, predictable, and spontaneously reversible increases in serum alkaline phosphatase, lactic dehydrogenase, and uric acid were reported. No serious clinical sequelae were reported in association with biochemistry abnormalities.

7.2. Severe Chronic Neutropenia Patients

The longest exposure to daily administration of filgrastim has been in patients with SCN. Daily subcutaneous injections of filgrastim for >10 yr in over 1000 patients worldwide, documented in the Severe Chronic Neutropenia International Registry (SCNIR), lead to neither exhaustion of myelopoiesis nor to anti-G-CSF antibody production.

Chronic daily administration of filgrastim to patients with SCN neither exhausts myelopoiesis nor produces anti-G-CSF antibodies, and causes relatively few adverse events; those that do occur are mild and easily managed. The number and duration of reported adverse events related to filgrastim decreases with the duration of treatment. Bone pain is noted early in treatment and tends to decrease in frequency with long-term therapy.

7.2.1. Severe Congenital Neutropenia (Kostmann's Syndrome)

7.2.1.1. Pathophysiology. The underlying genetic defect of this group of disorders, including Kostmann's syndrome, has been only partially identified. The original hypothesis for Kostmann's syndrome included a genetic predisposition resulting in defective production of G-CSF or defective response of the neutrophilic precursors to G-CSF or other HGFs; however, serum from these patients contains normal or increased amounts of G-CSF, and in vitro assays demonstrate a normal biologic activity of the endogenous G-CSF. Myeloid cells from patients with Kostmann's syndrome express slightly increased numbers of G-CSF receptors with a normal binding constant for G-CSF to its receptor.

Kostmann *(18)* originally described a Swedish kindred with congenital neutropenia inherited as an autosomal recessive trait without additional hematologic changes or other congenital abnormalities. With the recent detection of various mutations within the neutrophil elastase gene as the cause of cyclic neutropenia *(19)*, genetic screening for mutations of the neutrophil elastase was started in patients diagnosed with congenital neutropenia *(19–21)*. Despite phenotypical uniformity, characterized by congenital neutropenia and a maturation arrest of myelopoiesis in the bone marrow at the promyelocyte/myelocyte stage, neutrophil elastase mutations were present only in a major subgroup of patients with congenital neutropenia. All mutations identified to date are present in only one allele. Analysis of families with Kostmann's syndrome showed that only one parent carried the mutated elastase gene, suggesting an autosomal dominant inheritance *(19)*.

In patients with Kostmann's syndrome who developed leukemia, acquired G-CSF receptor mutations affecting the cytoplasmic domain were present in most patients tested *(22–25)*, suggestive of an important role of these mutations in the leukemogenesis. None of the G-CSF receptor mutations was detectable from birth, indicating that these mutations are not causative for the neutropenia. A small subgroup of patients develops these mutations during the course of life, most likely caused by genetic instability. G-CSF receptor analyses cannot be used to discriminate between the different diseases causing severe neutropenia, but they might be helpful for screening for risk of leukemia. The time between acquisition of a G-CSF receptor mutation and development of leukemia varies considerably. In a few patients, a G-CSF receptor is only present in the leukemic cells, whereas other patients show single or multiple mutations of the G-CSF receptor gene several years before leukemic transformation *(24)*. Like the elastase mutations, the G-CSF receptor mutations affect only one allele in most patients. No evidence exists that a G-CSF receptor mutation leads to a change in the clinical response to G-CSF treatment irrespective of any increase or decrease in G-CSF dose.

7.2.1.2. Clinical Features. All patients with SCN have absolute neutrophil counts (ANCs) continuously <200 µL, and in many patients peripheral blood neutrophils are completely absent. The estimated frequency of SCN is approx 1–2 cases per million with equal distribution between males and females. If the disease is diagnosed during the first months of life, antineutrophil antibodies should be excluded.

In patients with SCN, severe bacterial infections frequently occur during the first year of life. Postnatal omphalitis may be the first symptom, but later otitis media, pneumonitis, infections of the upper respiratory tract, and abscesses of the skin or liver are also common infections, which often lead to the diagnosis of SCN. Blood cultures are positive for staphylococci or streptococci, but other bacteria, e.g., *Pseudomonas* and *Peptostreptococcus,* and fungi were reported. In addition, rare infections like a clostridial gas gangrene infection may occur in these patients. The outcome of these fulminant infections is often lethal owing to lack of neutrophil defense. Most patients have frequent aphthous stomatitis and gingival hyperplasia, leading to an early loss of permanent teeth.

7.2.1.3. Blood Values. To confirm the diagnosis, repeated differential blood counts are required indicating persistent ANC within a range of $0–0.2 \times 10^9$/L. Blood counts often indicate additional mild anemia and thrombocytosis. Blood monocytes and eosinophils may be increased. Immunoglobulin concentrations for IgG are increased for most patients independent of their infectious status. The specific immunologic competence after vaccination is normal. Blood chemistry is within the normal, age-dependent range for electrolytes, and kidney and liver function values.

7.2.1.4. Bone Marrow. The bone marrow usually shows a maturation arrest of neutrophil precursors at an early stage (promyelocyte/myelocyte level) with few cells of the neutrophilic series beyond the promyelocyte stage. Promyelocytes often reveal morphologic atypical nuclei and vacuolization of the cytoplasma. The number of promyelocytes is slightly increased *(26),* with a median percentage of promyelocytes of 8% before filgrastim treatment. While receiving filgrastim, the percentage of promyelocytes decreases to 3%, whereas myelocyte and neutrophil counts increase. Marrow eosinophilia and monocytosis is common, and monocyte counts may change during treatment. Cellularity is usually normal or slightly decreased. Megakaryocytes are normal in number and morphology. The in vitro growth of granulocyte colonies in granulocyte-macrophage colony-forming unit (CFU-GM) assays is often defective, with a maturation arrest that mimics the disease.

7.2.1.5. Cytogenetic Evaluation and Molecular Testing. Normal bone marrow cytogenetics at diagnosis may change during the course of the disease, with monosomy 7 being the most frequent aberration in approx 50% of abnormal cytogenetic results. Abnormal cytogenetics are often associated with morphologic changes of the bone marrow indicating the onset of myelodysplasia or leukemia (*see* Subheading 7.2.1.8 below).

Studies of the G-CSF receptor gene have shown that mutations occur mainly within a critical region (nucleotide position 2300–2500) of the intracellular part of the receptor *(22,23)*. These are acquired mutations in a subgroup of patients. Individual patients may develop single or multiple mutations within this critical region. Analysis of the G-CSF receptor gene to detect acquired mutations can be performed from blood and bone marrow.

7.2.1.6. Differential Diagnosis. The most common of these rare diseases are cyclic neutropenia, Shwachman-Diamond syndrome, glycogen storage disease type 1b, and autoimmune neutropenia in infancy. A very important differential diagnostic evaluation is testing for neutrophilic antibodies: in children aged 1–3 yr with autoimmune neutropenia, the presence of neutrophil-specific autoantibodies can increase peripheral destruction of neutrophils. Although peripheral blood neutrophil counts may be as low as in SCN patients, these patients usually do not have severe bacterial infections. In the serum of these patients, granulocyte-specific antibodies are detectable by various immunologic tests *(27)*.

7.2.1.7. Treatment. Since 1987, filgrastim has been available for the treatment of SCN. Phase 1–3 studies have demonstrated the efficacy of filgrastim for increasing the number of neutrophils and reducing infections *(28,29)*. In contrast, granulocyte-macrophage colony-stimulating factor (GM-CSF) treatment does not lead to an increase in blood neutrophils, but only blood eosinophils *(30)*.

In 1994, the Severe Chronic Neutropenia Registry (SCNIR) was established to collect data on the clinical course and outcome of these rare disorders. As of December 2000, 383 patients with SCN were enrolled in the SCNIR. Of these 383 patients, >95% responded to filgrastim treatment with an increase in their ANC to 1.0×10^9/L and above (Fig. 1). Most patients with SCN respond to a dose between 3 and 10 μg/kg/d.

After initiation of filgrastim at 5 μg/kg/d, the dose should be increased to 10 μg/kg/d and then by increments of 10 μg/kg at 14-d intervals if the ANC remains $<1.0 \times 10^9$/L. As soon as the ANC can be maintained at 1.0×10^9/L or above, the filgrastim dose does not need to be further increased since the occurrence of bacterial infection is dramatically reduced with an ANC at this level. The filgrastim dose can be reduced if the ANC increases to 5.0×10^9/L or above to maintain the patient at the lowest dose necessary for maintaining a sufficient neutrophil count to avoid and overcome infections. Patients who do not respond to filgrastim are defined as patients failing to respond to filgrastim doses exceeding 120 μg/kg/d. Partial responders can increase their ANC to $0.5–1.0 \times 10^9$/L, but still have bacterial infections. In these patients, the dose of filgrastim cannot be increased because of the large volume and the frequency of injections required. In some of these patients, a combination of filgrastim with rHuSCF increases the ANC; however, because of potential allergic side effects from rHuSCF, this treatment combination was used exclusively during severe infections for hospitalized patients who receive concomitant antihistaminic medication (*see* Chap. 8 for further information). For patients who do not respond to filgrastim treatment alone or in combination with rHuSCF, transplantation of human stem cells (HSCT) is currently the only treatment available *(31,32)*. After successful HSCT, the patients have a normal hematopoiesis and no longer require cytokine treatment.It appears difficult to recommend a transplantation, if patients benefit from filgrastim and do not show any evidence of an impending malignant transformation.The risks associated with a transplant from an HLA-identical sibling may outweigh the risk of leukemic transformation when filgras-

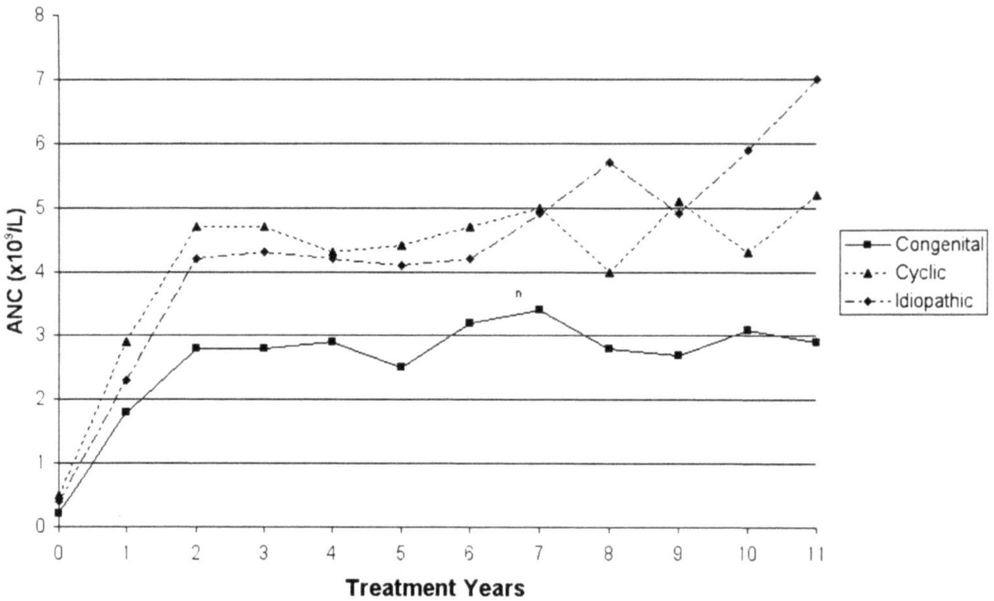

Fig. 1. Mean absolute neutrophil count (ANC) by year of G-CSF treatment. Congenital: n = 323; cyclic: n = 128; idiopathic: n = 204.

tim is continued in responding patients.If the risks of HSCT could be further decreased by new regimens, then HSCT from a matched sibling donor may be an early curative option in the future.

7.2.1.8. Long-Term Safety

7.2.1.8.1. Leukemia Development. Before the availability of cytokine therapy, it was recognized that leukemic transformation occurred in patients with congenital neutropenia *(33,34);* however, in the precytokine era, in 42% of all published cases the patients died in the first 2 yr of life, usually from sepsis or pneumonia. Thus, the true risk of congenital neutropenia patients developing MDS/acute myeloid leukemia (AML) could not be defined. Because filgrastim therapy is available, most of the patients survive well beyond 2 yr of age. Therefore, it is unknown whether prolonged survival unmasks the natural course of the disease with an increased risk of leukemic transformation independent of any treatment; however, the possibility cannot be excluded that filgrastim therapy further increases the basic risk of leukemic transformation.

From the initiation of clinical trials with filgrastim in 1987 through December 2000, 45 patients with SCN who developed MDS/AML were reported to the SCNIR, all of whom had a diagnosis of congenital neutropenia. The overall incidence or crude rate of MDS/AML conversion is 11.7% for SCN patients (45 cases among 383 exposed cases), with an average follow-up of approx 5–6 yr. Two of the 45 patients with congenital neutropenia and secondary MDS/leukemia were diagnosed as having Shwachman-Diamond syndrome. No cases of MDS/AML occurred in the subgroup of patients with cyclic or idiopathic neutropenia.

Conversion to MDS/AML in SCN patients was associated with one or more cellular genetic abnormalities, e.g., monosomy 7, ras mutation, or G-CSF receptor mutation, which may be useful to identify subgroups of patients at high risk *(22,23)*. Marrow cells from 11 patients with SCN who transformed to MDS/AML showed point mutations in the gene for G-CSF receptor, resulting in a truncated C-terminal cytoplasmic region of the receptor that is crucial for maturation signaling.

As illustrated by the cases described herein, the development of MDS/AML is a multistep process characterized by a series of cellular genetic changes indicating a genetic predisposition to malignant transformation. Whether and how filgrastim has an impact on this predisposition remains unclear; unfortunately, no historical controls are available for comparison available. To address further the issue of risk vs benefit of filgrastim in the SCN setting with regard to MDS/AML, all available data were critically reviewed *(35)*. The advisory board of the SCNIR recommends annual marrow cytogenetic testing for patients with congenital neutropenia to identify monosomy 7 or other changes indicating malignant transformation to allow early therapeutic intervention such as BMT.

7.2.1.8.2. Osteoporosis. The initial observation of bone pain and pathologic fractures in a number of our patients led us to investigate bone mineral density in a cohort of 30 patients *(36)*; 15/30 patients (50%) showed evidence of osteopenia/osteoporosis, and in 5 of these 15 patients osteoporosis became a clinical problem with either pathologic fractures or moderate back pain.

Within the SCNIR, bone density measurements have been reported for 121 patients with congenital neutropenia measured by different techniques including quantitative computer tomography, dual-energy X-ray absorptiometry, single-photon absorptiometry, and lumbar X-ray. Sixty-six of the 121 patients (54.4%) had varying degrees of abnormal results; however, these results were not quantified. Most patients did not show clinical symptoms of osteopenia/osteoporosis, such as bone pain or fractures, explaining why diagnostic procedures for bone density evaluation were not reported in >70% of SCNIR patients. The real incidence continues to remain unknown. The pathophysiology of osteopenia/osteoporosis has not been elucidated. Serum chemistry did not reveal a typical pattern in patients with osteopenia/osteoporosis. Furthermore, patients did not receive a higher dose of filgrastim compared with all SCNIR patients.

7.2.1.8.3. Vasculitis. Vasculitis was reported in 3.3% (9/270) of patients with congential neutropenia. Symptoms of vasculitis generally developed simultaneously with an increase in ANC and abated when ANC decreased. Patients with recurrent vasculitis or with renal involvement need to be evaluated for other diseases. Vasculitis may be associated with autoimmune disorders or an underlying malignancy. After a temporary disruption of filgrastim administration, the vasculitis has abated in all patients.

7.2.1.8.4. Splenomegaly. In patients with congenital neutropenia, the incidence of a palpable splenomegaly (2 cm below the costal margin) before treatment with filgrastim was 20.6%. During the first year of filgrastim therapy, the incidence increased to 38.9% and remained approx at this level of occurrence (33.8–47.6%) through 10 yr of therapy. Spleen size appears to increase in relation to time on filgrastim treatment. Additionally, in some individuals, splenomegaly is associated with infections or with transformation to MDS/AML.

7.2.2. Cyclic Neutropenia

7.2.2.1. Pathophysiology. Cyclic neutropenia is another rare disorder characterized by repetitive infectious episodes, fever, and mouth ulcers during regularly recurring phases of severe neutropenia. This disorder was first described by Leale in 1910 *(37)* as recurrent furunculosis in an infant showing an unusual blood picture. Many years later the autosomal dominant inheritance was first recognized by a collection of affected families.

An oscillatory production of precursor cells in the bone marrow causes fluctuations of almost all types of blood cells. In most patients, the disease is autosomal dominantly inherited, but sporadic cases were also identified. Molecular genetic studies showed that different mutations in the gene for neutrophil elastase located on chromosome 19p13.3 are responsible for this disease in both autosomal dominant and sporadic cases *(20,21)*.

7.2.2.2. Clinical Features. The diagnosis of cyclic neutropenia should be considered if a child presents with regularly recurring fever, mouth ulcers, pharyngitis, and lymphadenopathy, or recurrent skin infections. Usually these symptoms are already present in children <1 yr of age. Symptoms may last for >1 wk. Patients with painful deep mouth ulcers are often unable to eat and may present with loss of body weight. Almost all patients with periods of severe neutropenia (ANC $< 0.2 \times 10^9$/L) every 3 wk show at least some symptoms with almost every cycle. The frequency of bacterial infections depends on the length of the neutropenic period and therefore patients with longer neutropenic periods are more susceptible to infections; however, severe bacterial infections like pneumonia and septicemia are usually rare *(38)*. In between the neutropenic phases, patients are without symptoms and have normal physical examinations.

7.2.2.3. Blood Values. Blood cells show a cyclic pattern with a typical cycle length of 21 d *(38,39)*. In clinically obvious cyclic neutropenia, neutrophil counts decrease to $<0.2 \times 10^9$/L. After 3–5 d neutrophils increase and reach counts within the lower normal level.

If cyclic neutropenia is suspected, serial blood counts need to be performed at least three times per week over 6 wk to document the typical cyclic pattern of blood neutrophils. In most patients periodic oscillations of reticulocytes and platelets are detectable as well, and sometimes even eosinophils and lymphocytes cycle.

7.2.2.4. Bone Marrow. In cyclic neutropenia, bone marrow morphology changes during a cycle. Serial bone marrow aspirates have shown an early maturation arrest of myelopoiesis, comparable to that of congenital neutropenia, at the onset of the neutropenic phase. Usually, within 3–5 d myeloid maturation recovers and myelopoiesis up to band neutrophils is present in bone marrow aspirates. Erythroid precursors also show oscillations in the bone marrow. Colony assays from patients with cyclic neutropenia have shown that various types of cells fluctuate at the same periodicity.

7.2.2.5. Treatment. For patients with cyclic neutropenia, the availability of filgrastim changed the clinical course significantly, since there was no effective treatment before *(38,39)*. Clinical trials have shown that daily application of filgrastim (2–5 μg/kg) increased the amplitude of neutrophil oscillations and shortened the duration of the neutropenic phase. With filgrastim, the cycle length changes from 21 to approx 14 d. The significant decrease of infectious episodes is mainly owing to a shortening of the severe neutropenic period. A response to filgrastim could be maintained over >12 yr with daily or alternate-day administration of filgrastim at doses of 5 μg/kg/d or less.

7.2.2.6. Long-Term Safety. For patients with cyclic neutropenia, filgrastim treatment significantly reduced mouth ulcers and febrile and infectious episodes *(38,39)*. A modest increase in spleen size is probably common, but significant splenomegaly was not documented.

During the past 10 yr, leukemic development was not reported in patients with cyclic neutropenia with or without filgrastim treatment. In contrast to congenital neutropenia, cyclic neutropenia seems not to be a preleukemic disorder.

In light of the reported studies and longitudinal data from the SCNIR, we suggest that the use of filgrastim should remain the first-line treatment for most patients with chronic neutropenia and clinically symptomatic patients with cyclic neutropenia.

8. COMPARATIVE SAFETY OF FILGRASTIM VS OTHER HGFS

In a study comparing rates of adverse events with filgrastim vs sargramostim (rHuGM-CSF) when given prophylactically to patients receiving myelosuppressive chemotherapy, 490 patients treated for lung, breast, lymphatic system, or ovarian tumors were analyzed. The frequency and severity of adverse events were assessed. Fever unexplained by infection was more common with sargramostim (7% vs 1%; $p < 0.001$), as were fatigue and diarrhea; however, skeletal pain was more frequent with filgrastim. Overall, adverse events were less frequent with filgrastim than with sargramostim *(40)*.

ACKNOWLEDGMENTS

I thank all my colleagues associated with the Data Collection Centers of the Severe Chronic Neutropenia International Registry at the University of Washington, Seattle, WA, and the Medizinische Hochschule, Hannover, Germany for their continued assistance, and I am also grateful to the many physicians worldwide who faithfully and generously submitted data on their patients.

REFERENCES

1. Welte K, Platzer E, Lu L, et al. Purification and biochemical characterization of human pluripotent hematopoietic colony-stimulating factor. *Proc Natl Acad Sci USA* 1985; 82:1526–1530.
2. Welte K, Gabrilove J, Bronchud MH, Platzer E, Morstyn G. Filgrastim (r-metHuG-CSF): the first 10 years. *Blood* 1996; 88:1907–1929.
3. Patterson KL, Masuda SY, Brown SL. Safety profile of filgrastim (r-metHuG-CSF). In: Morstyn G, Dexter TM, Foote MA, ed., *Filgrastim (r-metHuG-CSF) in Clinical Practice,* 2nd ed. Totowa, NJ: Humana. 1998:583–602.
4. stRice L, Nichol JL, McMillan R, Roskos LK, Bacile-M. Cyclic immune thrombocytopenia responsive to thrombopoietic growth factor therapy. *Am J Hematol* 2001; 68:210–214.
5. Reuss-Borst MA, Muller CA, Waller HD. The possible role of G-CSF in the pathogenesis of Sweet's syndrome. *Leuk Lymphoma* 1994; 15:261–264.
6. Bleomycin at www.dhs.sa.gov/cancare. Accessed 12 May 2003.
7. Adach K, Suzuki M, Sugimoto T, et al. Granulocyte colony-stimulating factor exacerbates the acute lung injury and pulmonary fibrosis induced by intratracheal administration of bleomycin in rats. *Exp Toxicol Pathol* 2002; 53:501–510.
8. Hay J, Shahzeidi S, Laurent G. Mechanisms of bleomycin-induced lung damage. *Arch Toxicol* 191; 65:81–94.
9. Takamizawa A, Koyama S, Sato E, et al. Bleomycin stimulates lung fibroblasts to release neutrophil and monocyte chemotactic activity. *J Immunol* 1999; 162:6200–6208.

10. Saxman SB, Nichols CR, Einhorn LH. Pulmonary toxicity in patients with advanced-stage germ cell tumors receiving bleomycin with and without granulocyte colony stimulating factor. *Chest* 1997; 111:657–660.
11. Lei KI, Leung WT, Johnson PJ. Serious pulmonary complications in patients receiving recombinant granulocyte colony-stimulating factor during BACOP chemotherapy for aggressive non-Hodgkin's lymphoma. *Br J Cancer* 1994; 70:1009–10013.
12. Sargramostim. http:/csi.micromedex.com. Accessed 12 May 2003.
13. Stanworth SJ, Bhavnani N, Chatopadhya C, Miller H, Swinson DR. Treatment of Felty's syndrome with the haemopoietic growth factor granulocyte colony-stimulating factor (G-CSF). *Q J Med* 1998; 91:49–56.
14. Lehrnbecher T, Welte K. Haematopoietic growth factors in children with neutropenia. *Br J Haematol* 2002; 116:28–56.
15. Medlock ES, Kaplan DL, Cecchini M. Ulich TR, delCastillo J, Andresen J. Granulocyte colony-stimulating factor crosses the placenta and stimulates fetal rat granulopoiesis. *Blood* 1993; 81:91–92.
16. Novales JS, Salva AM, Modanlou HD, et al. Maternal administration of granulocyte-stimulating factor improves neonatal rat survival after a lethal group B streptococcal infection. *Blood* 1993; 15:81:923–927.
17. Calhoun DA, Donnelly WH, Du Y, Dame JB, Li Y, Christensen RD. Distribution of granulocyte colony-stimulating factor (G-CSF) and G-CSF-receptor mRNA and protein in the human fetus. *Pediatr Res* 1999; 46:333–338.
18. Kostmann R. Infantile genetic agranulocytosis. *Acta Pediatr Scand* 1956; 45:1–78.
19. Horwitz M, Benson KF, Person RE, et al. Mutations in ELA2, encoding neutrophil elastase, define a 21-day biological clock in cyclic haematopoesis. *Nature Genet* 1999; 23:433–436.
20. Dale DC, Person RE, Bolyard AA, et al. Mutations in the gene encoding neutrophil elastase in congenital and cyclic neutropenia. *Blood* 2000; 96:2317–2322.
21. Germeshausen M, Schulze H, Ballmaier M, et al. Mutations in the gene encoding neutrophil elastase (ELA2) are not sufficient to cause the phenotype of congenital neutropenia. *Br J Haematol* 2001; 115:1–4.
22. Dong F, Russel KB, Tidow N, et al. Mutations in the gene for the granulocyte-colony stimulating factor receptor in patients with acute myeloid leukemia preceded by severe congenital neutropenia. *N Engl J Med* 1995; 333:487–493.
23. Tidow N, Pilz C, Teichmann B, et al. Clinical relevance of point mutations in the cytoplasmatic domain of the granulocyte-colony stimulating factor gene in patients with severe congenital neutropenia. *Blood* 1997; 88:2369–2375.
24. Tschan CA, Pilz C, Zeidler C, et al. Time course of increasing numbers of mutations in the granulocyte colony-stimulating factor receptor gene in a patient with congenital neutropenia who developed leukemia. *Blood* 2001; 97:1882–1884.
25. Bernard T, Gale R, Evans J, et al. Mutations of the granulocyte-colony stimulating factor receptor in patients with severe congenital neutropenia are not required for transformation to acute myeloid leukaemia and may be a bystander phenomenon. *Br J Haematol* 1998; 101:141–149.
26. Welte K, Boxer L. Severe chronic neutropenia: pathophysiology and therapy. *Semin Hematol* 1997; 34:267–278.
27. Bux J, Behrens G, Jaeger G, et al. Diagnosis and clinical course of autoimmune neutropenia in infancy: analysis of 240 cases. *Blood* 1998; 91:181–186.
28. Bonilla M, Dale D, Zeidler C, et al. Long-term safety of treatment with recombinant human granulocyte colony-stimulating factor (r-metHuG-CSF) in patients with severe congential neutropenias. *Br J Hematol* 1994; 88:723–730.
29. Bonilla M, Gillio A, Ruggeiro M, et al. Effects of recombinant human granulocyte colony-stimulating factor on neutropenia in patients with congenital agranulocytosis. *N Engl J Med* 1989; 320:1574–1580.
30. Welte K, Zeidler C, Reiter A, et al. Differential effects of granulocyte-macrophage colony-stimulating factor and granulocyte colony-stimulating factor in children with severe congenital neutropenia. *Blood* 1990; 75:1056–1063 .
31. Zeidler C, Welte K, Barak Y, et al. Stem cell transplantation in patients with severe congenital neutropenia without evidence of leukemia transformation. *Blood* 2000; 95:1195–1198.
32. Rappeport J, Parkman R, Newburger P, et al. Correction of infantile granulocytosis (Kostmann syndrome) by allogeneic bone marrow transplantation. *Am J Med* 1980; 68:605–609.
33. Rosen R, Kang S. Congenital agranulocytosis terminating in acute myelomonocytic leukemia. *J Pediatr* 1979; 94:406–408.

34. Gilman P, Jackson D, Guild H. Congenital agranulocytosis: prolonged survival and terminal acute leukemia. *Blood* 1970; 36:576–585.
35. Freedman MH, Alter BP. Risk of myelodysplastic syndrome and acute myeloid leukemia in congenital neutropenias. *Semin Hematol* 2002; 39:128–133.
36. Yakisan E, Schirg E, Zeidler C, et al. High incidence of significant bone loss in patients with severe congenital neutropenia (Kostmann's syndrome). *J Pediatr* 1997; 131:592–597.
37. Leale M. Recurrent furunculosis in an infant showing an unusual blood picture. *JAMA* 1910; 54:1854–1855.
38. Dale D, Bonilla M, Davis M, et al. A randomized controlled phase III trial of recombinant human granulocyte colony-stimulating factor (G-CSF) for treatment of severe chronic neutropenia. *Blood* 1993; 81:2496–2502.
39. Dale DC, Bolyard AA, Aprikyan A. Cyclic neutropenia. *Semin Hematol* 2002; 39:89–94.
40. Milkovitch G, Moleski RJ, Reitan JF, et al. Comparative safety of filgrastim versus sargramostim in patients receiving myelosuppressive chemotherapy. *Pharmacotherapy* 2000, 20:1432–1440.

21 Economics of Hematopoietic Growth Factors

Gary H. Lyman, MD, MPH, FRCP
and Nicole M. Kuderer, MD

CONTENTS

1. INTRODUCTION

1.1. The Economics of Health Care

Health care costs have risen steadily and now exceed US $1 trillion annually, including nearly US $150 billion for cancer care *(1,2)*. By the year 2010, it is projected that health care expenditures in the United States will approach US $3 trillion with US $300 billion spent on cancer care (Fig. 1) *(3)*. Approximately 90% of medical costs for cancer care are associated with five diagnoses: breast cancer (24%), colorectal cancer (24%), lung cancer (18%), prostate cancer (18%), and bladder cancer (8%) *(4,5)*. Hospital care represents the largest single cost component, accounting for 40–50% of total cancer care costs *(2)*. Other major components of health care costs include physician/professional costs and to a lesser extent pharmaceutical and home care costs. The direct medical costs of cancer care are greatest during the period of initial diagnosis and treatment *(6)*. Other illness-related costs in patients with cancer include direct

From: *Cancer Drug Discovery and Development*
Hematopoietic Growth Factors in Oncology: Basic Science and Clinical Therapeutics
Edited by: G. Morstyn, M. A. Foote, and G. J. Lieschke © Humana Press Inc., Totowa, NJ

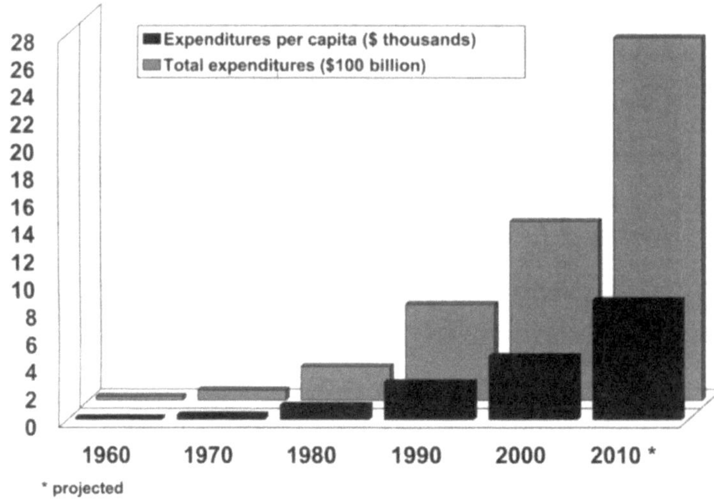

Fig. 1. Bar graph of United States annual total health expenditures in $100 billion (gray shading) and per capita health expenditures in $ thousands (black shading) from 1960 to 2000 and projections for 2010. Data compiled from the United State Healthcare Financing Administration, 2003 Annual Report.

nonmedical costs such as transportation and child care and indirect costs associated with illness-related morbidity and lost earnings owing to premature death from disease. Some intangible costs of illness for the patient and family relate to the impact on quality of life (QOL).

The appropriate costs to consider in any economic analysis depend upon the perspective taken, including the patient and family, the hospital, the physician, the payor, and society. Methods of economic analysis are available for evaluating studies in which either improved outcomes are associated with greater cost or reduced cost is associated with a worsened outcome *(7–9)*. Clinical decision models represent a useful basis for economic analysis incorporating data from the published literature and professional experience, permitting the definition, measurement, and comparison of the relevant positive and negative economic consequences of health care technologies *(10)*. Such models allow the simultaneous consideration of both clinical and economic outcomes in the form of cost-effectiveness and cost-utility analyses (Fig. 2) *(11–13)*.

1.2. Neutropenia and Its Consequences

Myelosuppression continues to represent the major dose-limiting toxicity associated with systemic cancer chemotherapy *(14)*. Fever in the setting of febrile neutropenia (FN) generally prompts immediate hospitalization for evaluation and the administration of empiric broad-spectrum antibiotics *(15)*. The risk of hospitalization for FN varies with the nature and intensity of the treatment regimen and with host-related factors related to age, the type of cancer, and various comorbid conditions. Although episodes of FN clearly add substantial costs to the care of patients with cancer receiving chemotherapy, little systematic study of the actual costs involved has been done *(16)*.

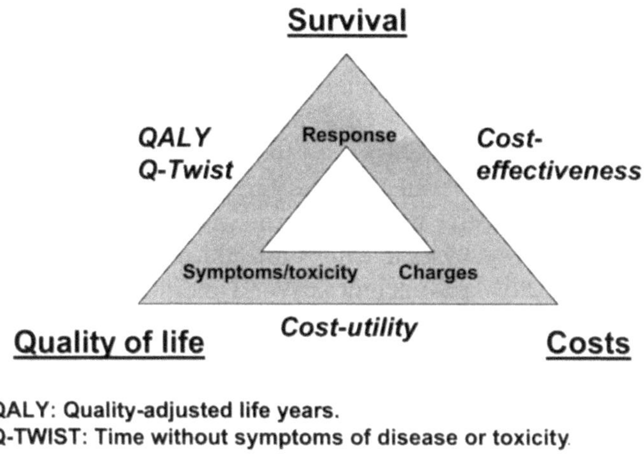

Fig. 2. Triangle representing the dimensions of health care outcome measures including clinical (survival), quality of life, and economic (cost) measures. Combined measures of clinical, quality-of-life, and economic outcome are illustrated on the sides of the triangle including quality-adjusted life-years (QALYs), time without symptoms of disease and toxicity of treatment (Q-TWIST), cost effectiveness (cost per life-year gained), and cost utility (cost per quality-adjusted life-year gained).

1.3. Colony-Stimulating Factors

The recombinant colony-stimulating factors (CSFs) are capable of reducing the severity and duration of neutropenia. CSFs reduce the risk of FN and documented infections and also facilitate the delivery of full dose intensity in patients receiving cancer chemotherapy *(17)*. Although such a use is perhaps more controversial, CSFs given to patients admitted for established FN appear to reduce the duration of neutropenia and the proportion of patients with prolonged hospitalization *(18)*. The decision to use recombinant human granulocyte colony-stimulating factor (rHuG-CSF) involves the clinical efficacy, the impact on patient QOL, and the cost associated with neutropenia and its sequelae. Decision models evaluating the use of CSFs to reduce the risk of FN in patients receiving chemotherapy have been studied *(19,20)*. These models have been used to support the development of clinical practice guidelines for the use of CSFs in cancer therapy *(21,22)*. Such models, however, are highly sensitive to the cost assumptions used. The economics of the hematopoietic growth factors (HGFs) have been found to largely represent the economics of neutropenia and its complications, particularly FN *(23–25)*. An improved understanding of the actual costs associated with the management of FN can provide a more rational basis for evaluating CSFs and further refining of clinical practice guidelines. We summarize the available literature related to the efficacy, cost, and cost effectiveness of CSFs in patients receiving cancer chemotherapy at risk for neutropenia and its consequences.

2. CLINICAL AND ECONOMIC OUTCOMES OF CANCER CARE

2.1. Health Care Outcome Measures

Response and survival often represent the primary clinical endpoints in clinical trials for the assessment of efficacy upon which sample size and power calculations are based.

Alternatively, clinical outcome can be measured in terms of life expectancy or the average number of years of life remaining at a given age. The life-years of an individual can be thought of as representing the area under the corresponding survival curve *(26)*. The gain in life expectancy or life-years saved with treatment represents the marginal efficacy and can be thought of as the area between the survival curves with and without intervention. This method is more powerful for assessing treatment effect than for comparing median survivals or the event-free proportion at a given time. Changes in life expectancy are often used in economic analyses to express the efficacy of treatment.

The assessment of health care outcomes beyond traditional clinical measures of efficacy has become a focus of research. Alternative measures of interest include health-related quality-of-life (HRQOL) and economic outcomes. HRQOL can be assessed either through various health-profile measures or by the global assessment of patient preferences. Health profiles derived from psychosocial theory attempt to assess HRQOL through one of a variety of scales addressing the relevant dimensions, such as functional ability, emotional well-being, sexuality/intimacy, family well-being, treatment satisfaction, and social functioning *(27)*. Alternatively, utility measures derived from economic and decision theory attempt to assess HRQOL by eliciting patient preferences for specific outcome states *(28)*. Patient preferences can be assessed through a time tradeoff method incorporating a standard reference gamble generating a single value of health status along a linear continuum from death to full health.

The major advantage of measures of patient preference or utility is that they can be used to adjust measures of longevity such as life expectancy, e.g., the quality-adjusted life-year (QALY). The QALY represents the time in full health considered by the patient to be equivalent to actual time in the diseased state. Serial measurement of patient preferences over time can be used to estimate the cumulative impact of treatment on HRQOL. The sum over all health care states of the product of the time spent in each state and the utility associated with the state will yield the quality-adjusted time without symptoms of disease or toxicity of treatment (Q-TWIST) described by Gelber et al. *(29)*. The assessment of HRQOL in conjunction with conventional clinical efficacy measures in clinical trials has gained increasing interest over the past few years *(30,31)*.

2.2. Economic Outcome Measures

The most important economic outcome of interest for clinical decision making and health policy formation is cumulative total cost, which considers both the activity level over time and unit costs *(32,33)*. The activity level represents the amount of various resources used and the time expended in providing medical care. Unit costs represent the cost associated with each unit of activity. The major focus of such economic analyses relates to those resources and costs, which might differ between treatment groups. Direct medical costs represent the costs of providing medical services for the prevention, diagnosis, treatment, follow-up, rehabilitation, and palliation of disease. These costs include those associated with hospitalization, professional services, pharmaceuticals, radiologic and laboratory testing, and home health care services. Direct nonmedical costs represent additional expenditures incurred while receiving medical care, such as transportation costs to and from the institution and child care expenses. Indirect costs include those associated with the morbidity of disease and treatment, such as days lost from work, and the economic impact of lost economic output owing to premature death. Intangible costs are those associated with pain and suffering as well as the loss of companionship.

Although it is very difficult to express such concerns in monetary terms, these represent real social and emotional costs to the patient and family.

2.3. Economic Analyses

To facilitate the comparison of different treatment strategies, economic outcome measures are often combined with clinical and HRQOL outcomes into summary measures such as QALY and cost-effectiveness (C/E) and cost-utility (C/U) ratios *(34,35)*. Such combined summary outcome measures reflect the simultaneous difference or change in cost and the change in survival or quality-adjusted survival. When clinical effectiveness is not an issue or is considered equal between therapeutic alternatives, the evaluation may be most reasonably based on differences in resource utilization or cost through a cost-minimization analysis, by which the strategy associated with the lowest total cost is identified. When important differences in both clinical efficacy and cost are anticipated, it is often preferable to combine economic measures with those of clinical efficacy *(36–41)*. In this situation, the measures of interest are generally the additional cost of one strategy over another (marginal cost) and the additional clinical benefit (marginal efficacy) or quality-adjusted clinical benefit (marginal utility).

A cost-effectiveness analysis can be used to define the tradeoff between cost and harm, generally expressed in terms of a C/E ratio. Most commonly, cost-effectiveness analysis compares interventions based on the ratio of the marginal cost and the marginal effectiveness (marginal cost effectiveness) expressed as the added cost per life-year saved. When clinical efficacy is modified to reflect patient preferences, a cost-utility analysis can be performed. Cost-utility analysis compares treatments based on the ratio of the marginal cost and the marginal utility (marginal cost utility) expressed as the added cost per QALY saved. Ultimately, these latter two approaches attempt to identify the most efficient approach, i.e., the least costly strategy associated with the greatest effectiveness or utility. Such combined clinical and economic outcome measures permit more rational comparisons of different clinical strategies for purposes of medical decision making, patient counseling, clinical practice guideline development, and health care policy formulation.

2.4. Limitations of Economic Analyses

The evaluation and interpretation of an economic analysis will often differ substantially depending on the perspective from which it was undertaken, e.g., the patient or family, a health care provider or institution, a third-party payor, or society as a whole. Indirect and intangible costs, although very important to the patient and family, may not be considered in economic analyses from most other perspectives. The analysis of economic outcomes is frequently complicated by the multiple outcomes, skewed distributions, and frequent missing data. In addition, marginal summary measures do not necessarily reflect the absolute benefit or cost of an intervention. A strategy associated with a lower absolute effectiveness may actually appear superior in terms of cost effectiveness or cost utility. It is important, therefore, to measure both the absolute as well as the marginal benefit and cost in such analyses. Nevertheless, when one is faced with new and costly technologies and limited health care resources, economic analyses can be critical to rational clinical and public health decision making. Economic analyses are perhaps most valuable when conducted in association with large randomized clinical trials (RCTs) in which tradeoffs exist between clinical benefit and economic impact

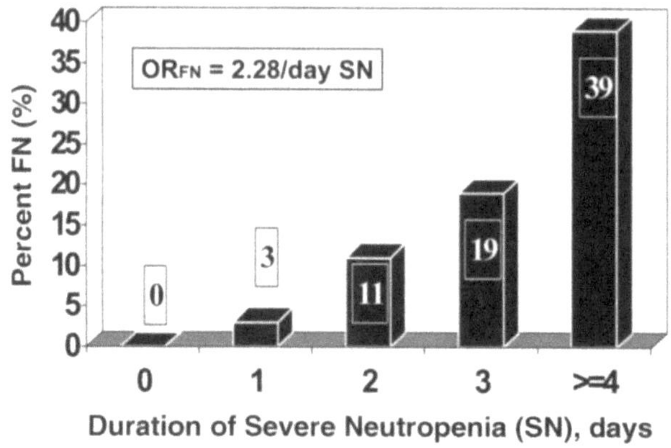

Fig. 3. Graphic representation of the relationship between the duration of severe neutropenia (ANC <500 cells/mm^3) and the incidence of febrile neutropenia (FN). Data were derived from a retrospective analysis of two phase 3 RCTs of breast cancer chemotherapy comparing filgrastim and pegfilgrastim. The odds ratio for FN was 2.28 per day of severe neutropenia *(45)*.

(32,33,42–44). Such analyses are of particular importance in oncology in the evaluation of supportive-care interventions.

3. THE EPIDEMIOLOGY OF NEUTROPENIA AND ITS CONSEQUENCES

3.1. Introduction

The risk of febrile neutropenia increases in direct relationship to both the duration and severity of neutropenia. This fundamental association was originally demonstrated in patients with acute leukemia by the early work of Bodey et al. *(14)*. These observations have been confirmed and extended to solid tumor populations in a review of two phase 3 RCTs (Fig. 3) *(45)*. In logistic regression analysis, the estimated odds ratio for FN was 2.3 per d increase in the duration of severe neutropenia. The clinical impact of neutropenia has been studied on the basis of the reported rates of neutropenic complications including reduced dose intensity in both RCT and in the practice setting through the evaluation of several retrospective databases.

3.2. The Reporting of Risk of FN and Reduced Dose Intensity Reported in RCT

A systematic review of reported hematologic toxicity in RCT conducted over the past decade in early-stage breast cancer (ESBC) and non-Hodgkin's lymphoma (NHL) was recently completed *(46)*. This review showed that many studies fail to report rates entirely, whereas those reporting rates of toxicity did so using varying measures and providing widely varying results for commonly studied regimens. This review also showed that 53% of RCTs reported no data on relative dose intensity (RDI). Of the 18% of ESBC studies and the 34% of NHL studies reporting mean or median RDIs, 32 and 42% of the study cohorts, respectively, received an RDI of <85%. Recent studies of more intensive regimens for both ESBC and NHL suggest that, although such regimens are associated with encouraging results, the risk of FN associated with these treatment schedules is substantial *(47)*.

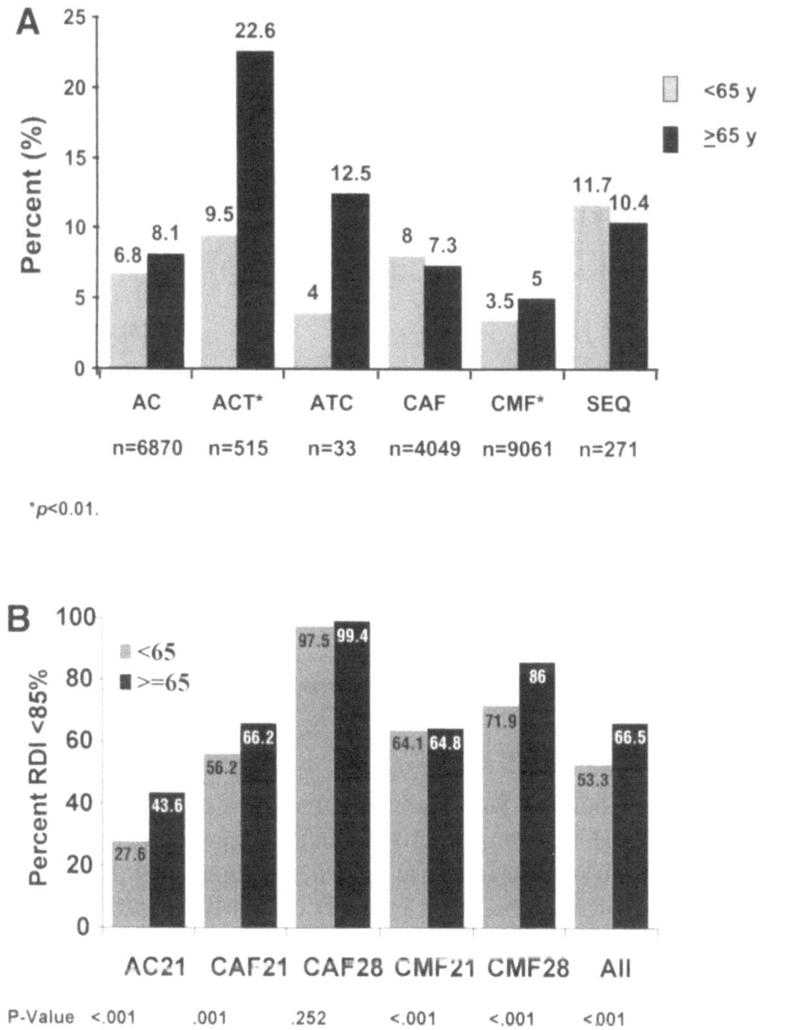

Fig. 4. Bar graphs illustrating the frequency of febrile neutropenia (FN) **(A)** and the frequency of reduced dose intensity <85% of reference standards *(B)* in approx 20,000 women with breast cancer receiving various adjuvant chemotherapy regimens from a large practice-based survey *(48)*. The risk of FN and reduced relative dose intensity (RDI) were generally greater in older women (black shading) than in younger women (gray shading). AC, Adriamycin + cyclophosphamide; ACT, Adriamycin + cyclophosphamide followed by taxol; ATC, Adriamycin + cyclophosphamide + taxotere; CAF, cyclophosphamide + Adriamycin + 5-fluorouracil; CMF, cyclophosphamide + methotrexate + 5-fluorouracil; SEQ, sequential agents. Where appropriate, schedules of every 21 d or every 28 d are indicated. (Figure 4B, data from ref. *48*.)

3.3. The Reported Risk and Timing of FN in Community Practices

The risk of FN and reduced dose intensity in >20,000 women with ESBC treated over the past decade has been reported *(48)*. The risk of FN varies greatly with regimen and age (Fig. 4). In addition, a number of factors are associated with reduced dose intensity including age and high body-surface area. The risk of a neutropenic event including FN is not uniformly distributed across treatment courses. The cumulative

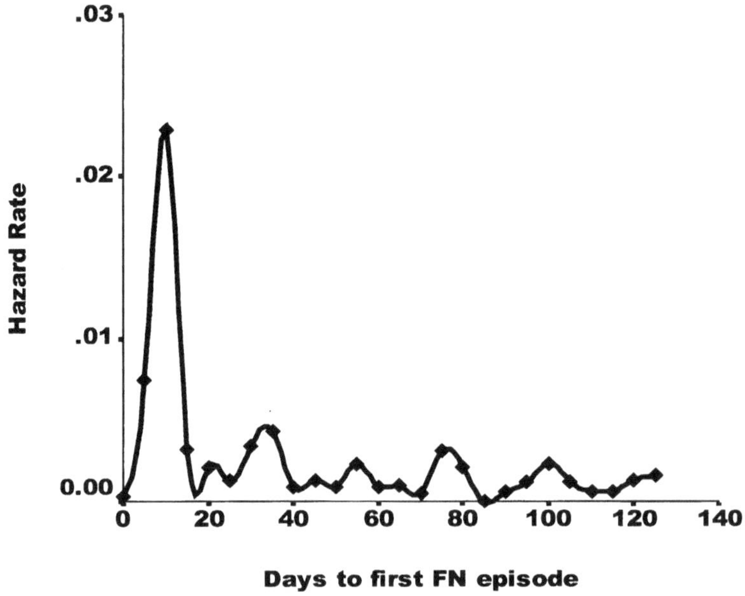

Fig. 5. Hazard plot of the time in days to first episode of febrile neutropenia (FN) in 577 patients with non-Hodgkin's lymphoma treated with CHOP chemotherapy. Data from ref. *49*.

risk of FN appears to increase throughout the treatment course. The risk of FN with each cycle depends on dose intensity, growth factor usage, and prior treatment. Thus, in patients continuing to receive full dose intensity without growth factor support, the risk may increase with each subsequent cycle. It is clearly greatest in those who have experienced FN on a previous cycle. However, the risk of the first FN event appears to be greatest during the first one or two cycles of chemotherapy. The risk of initial FN in 577 patients with NHL receiving chemotherapy with cyclophosphamide, doxorubicin, vincristine, and prednisone (CHOP) showed that 58% of patients destined to experience ≥1 episodes of FN do so during the first cycle of CHOP (Fig. 5) *(49)*. Risk factors for early an FN event included age, low hemoglobin (Hb) concentration, heart or renal disease, planned dose intensity >80%, and failure to provide primary rHuG-CSF prophylaxis. The results of this study have been confirmed in a separate population of 1355 patients with NHL receiving CHOP, CHOP-rituximab, or CNEP *(50)*. A total of 230 patients experienced ≥1 episodes of FN, with >50% experiencing their first episode within the first one or two cycles of treatment. Similar early encounter with the initial FN episode has been observed in patients with ESBC receiving adjuvant chemotherapy.

3.4. Additional Risk Factors for Febrile Neutropenia

A number of efforts to identify risk factors for the occurrence of FN or its consequences in patients with established FN have been reported. A systematic review has been completed of published studies of risk models for FN and its consequences *(51)*. Nearly every study of risk factors for neutropenic complications in patients receiving cancer chemotherapy has identified increasing age as a significant independent predic-

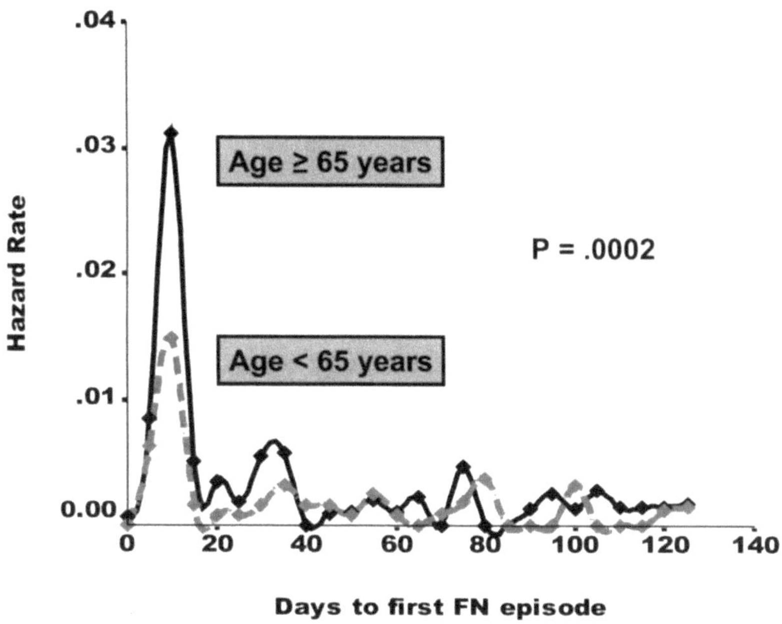

Fig. 6. Hazard plot of the time in days to the first episode of febrile neutropenia (FN) in 577 patients with non-Hodgkin's lymphoma treated with CHOP chemotherapy stratified by age 65 yr and over vs <65 yr ($p = 0.0002$). Modified from ref. *49*.

tor of severe neutropenia or serious medical consequences of FN, including death *(52)*. As noted above, increasing age was a significant independent predictor in a multivariate model of risk of FN across a number of adjuvant breast cancer treatment regimens among approx 20,000 women studied retrospectively in the United States *(48)*. The elderly were more likely to experience significant reductions in dose intensity relative to either target dose intensity or published reference standards with these regimens. Patients aged ≥65 yr experienced nearly twice the rate of reduced dose intensity <85% in multivariate analyses after adjustment for the type of regimen used. In patients receiving CHOP for NHL, the study by Lyman et al. *(49)* reported a doubling of the hazard rate of FN in patients aged ≥65 yr, most of which occurred during the first cycle of therapy (Fig. 6). Similar analyses have been undertaken in women receiving adjuvant chemotherapy for ESBC *(53)*. Silber and colleagues *(54)* previously developed and independently validated a risk model for neutropenic complications in the adjuvant ESBC setting based on a retrospective analysis. The nadir absolute neutrophil count (ANC) during the first cycle was the most predictive factor for future neutropenic events likely to reduce treatment dose intensity.

This approach was studied prospectively in a clinical trial of 729 women started on adjuvant chemotherapy for ESBC with or without growth factor support determined on the basis of the first-cycle ANC nadir *(55)*. If the first-cycle ANC was $\leq 0.5 \times 10^9$/L, women were given prophylactic rHuG-CSF for all subsequent cycles, whereas all other patients received growth factor support only if a neutropenic event actually occurred. In further analysis of these data, Agboola et al. *(56)* found that pretreatment

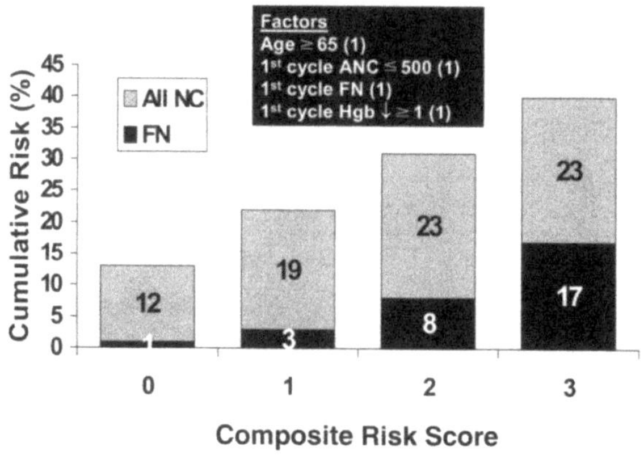

Fig. 7. Bar graph displaying the cumulative proportion of patients with any subsequent neutropenic complication (NC) (febrile neutropenia [FN], dose reduction, or treatment delay) or FN alone based on a composite risk score age ≥65 yr or first cycle events including FN, absolute neutrophil count (ANC) < 5 × 10^9/L or a hemoglobin (Hb) decrease ≥ 1 g/dL ($p < 0.001$) *(56)*.

factors predictive of first-cycle hematologic toxicity included age ≥ 65 yr, white race, use of an anthracycline-containing regimen, body-surface area ≤2 m^2, and low baseline ANC. Significant predictors of subsequent neutropenic complications including FN included age ≥65 yr and first-cycle events including ANC nadir, FN, and a decrease in Hb by ≥1 g/dL (Fig. 7).

3.5. Risk Factors for Serious Medical Complications in Patients With FN

A number of risk factors for serious medical complications including death in patients with FN have been reported. These factors have included the development of FN as an inpatient; hypotension; sepsis; various comorbidities, including cardiovascular and pulmonary disease or leukemia or lymphoma diagnosis; age ≥65 yr; severity and duration of neutropenia; prior fungal infection; visceral organ involvement; organ dysfunction; and uncontrolled malignancy *(57)*. Age was a significant predictor of serious medical complications, including death among patients with FN evaluated by the Multinational Association of Supportive Care of Cancer (MASCC) scoring system *(58)*. In a multinational study of >1100 episodes of FN from 15 countries, analysis of 339 episodes in patients with solid tumors, excluding marrow/stem cell transplants and patients receiving therapeutic CSFs, showed that age >60 yr was a significant risk factor for risk of serious medical complications in multivariate analysis (OR = 4.36, $p < 0.004$). Although the study was retrospective in nature, prophylactic rHuG-CSF use was associated with a non-significant reduction in risk of serious medical complications (OR = 0.24, $p = 0.095$).

4. THE ECONOMIC IMPACT OF HOSPITALIZATION FOR FEBRILE NEUTROPENIA

4.1. Introduction

The major economic impact of neutropenic complications is the cost associated with hospitalization and the ensuing length of stay (LOS). The varying LOS associated with

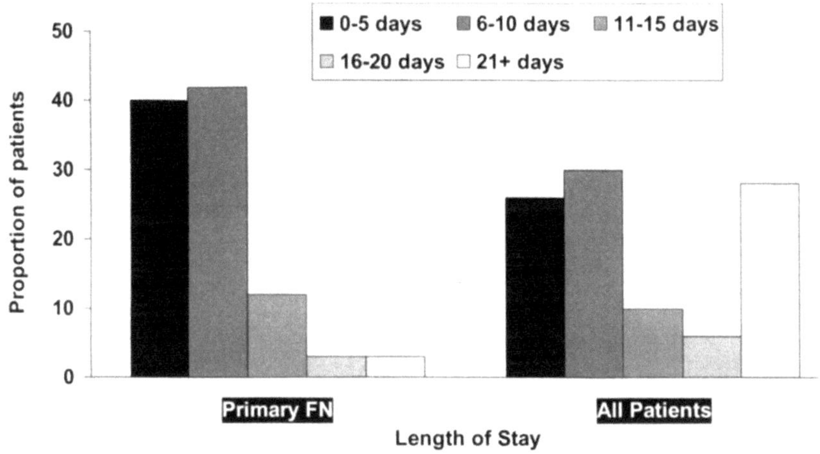

Fig. 8. Frequency distribution of the length of stay for febrile neutropenia (FN) among cancer patients admitted to the H. Lee Moffitt Cancer Center over a 24-mo period *(16)*. The graph on the right shows the length of stay among all patients ($N = 794$), and the graph on the left represents the length of stay among those with FN as the first (primary) diagnosis ($N = 309$).

hospitalization for FN suggests considerable heterogeneity in this patient population and their associated risk factors. Although episodes of FN clearly add substantial costs to the care of patients with cancer receiving systemic chemotherapy, little systematic study has been done of the actual costs involved.

4.2. Single-Institution Studies

Total hospitalization costs associated with admission with FN to the H. Lee Moffitt Cancer Center and Research Institute over a 2-yr period have been reported *(16)*. Data were retrieved on patient demographics, diagnostic and procedure coding, outpatient and inpatient costs, and payor reimbursement. A cost allocation function was used to allocate all fixed and variable direct costs for nonrevenue-generating centers to the revenue-generating centers as indirect costs. In the allocation process, each support center was assigned an allocation statistic based on an appropriate measure of activity such as utilized space, supplies, and work-hours of activity. Each service center was assigned a portion of the overhead center's cost based on its share of the allocation statistic. The total operating expenses for each department represented the sum of direct and indirect institutional costs across all diagnostic and procedure codes assigned to the department. During fiscal years 1994 and 1995, 794 patients were admitted with FN. The primary reasons for admission consisted of neutropenia (39%), malignancy-related conditions (34%), infection-related conditions (11%), vascular complications (4%), and other organ system complications (12%). Approximately one-half of the patients were between 40 and 65 yr of age, and 25% were 65 yr of age or over in both groups. As shown in Fig. 8, patients with FN as the first (primary) diagnosis had relatively short LOS, whereas >25% of patients experienced an LOS of ≥3 wk overall. Patients with solid tumors spent a total of 3279 d in the hospital during the period under study, with an average LOS of 10.4 d. Total operating expenses including both direct and

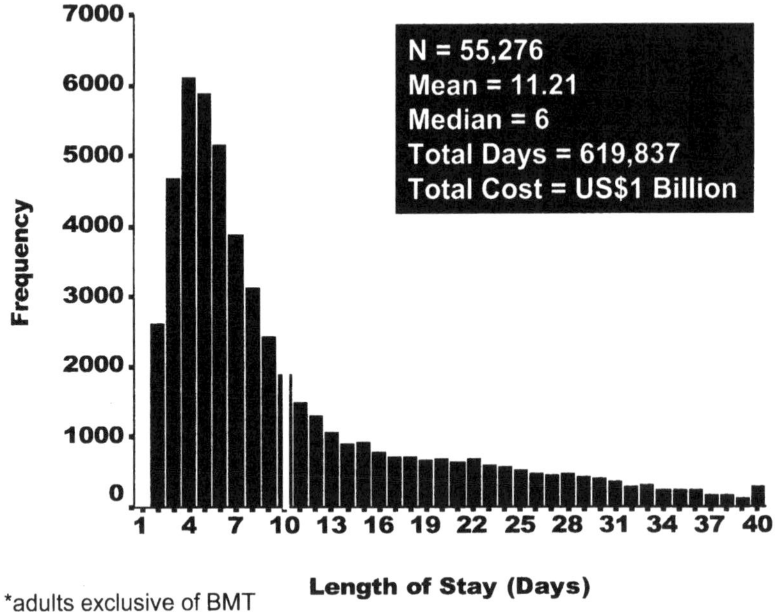

Fig. 9. Frequency distribution of the length of stay in days among adults excluding bone marrow transplantation patients hospitalized for FN in institutions reporting to the University Health System Consortium, 1995–2000 *(59)*.

indirect costs were greatest for the nursing unit (38%), followed by the pharmacy (27%), the blood bank (17%), and the laboratory (6%).

4.3. Multiple Institution Studies

More recently, economic studies of FN in the multiple institutions reporting discharge data to the University Health System Consortium including 115 academic medical centers have been reported *(59)*. In all, 55,276 episodes of FN in 41,779 adult nontransplant patients were reported over a 6-yr period. The average age of the patients was 53.6 yr; 73% were white, 54% were women, and 53% had a solid tumor, whereas 26% had lymphoma and 21% had leukemia. Cost data were available for 52,384 (95%) of the episodes. As shown in Fig. 9, the distributions of LOS, and therefore cost, are skewed to the right, related to a relatively small proportion of patients with more complicated and prolonged hospitalizations. The approx 30% of patients hospitalized for >10 d account for 74% of the hospital days and 78% of the cost. Hospitalization for FN over the 6-yr period totaled 619,837 hospital days and a total cost of approximately US $1 billion.

As shown in Table 1, the LOS and costs are remarkably similar to those reported in studies from clinical trials and the single institutional data discussed above. The average LOS decreased over the 6-yr period by 10%, whereas the cost per day increased by 28%, raising the total cost per episode of FN by 13% (Fig. 10). Significant predictors of long LOS and high cost were admissions associated with other medical conditions, a diagnosis of leukemia, and complications during hospitalization. The mean LOS was

Table 1
Comparison of Outcomes from Studies

Study ref.	*Tumor type*	*Groups*	*No.*	*LOS (d)*	*Cost/day (US $)*	*Cost/episode (US $)*
19, 65	Lung cancer	All	206	10	1000	10,000
16	Solid tumors	All	794	10.4	1488	16,500
		Primary FN	309	6.4	1435	9,345
59	Solid tumor and lymphoma	All	46,099	10.6	1598	18,526
		Primary FN	16,288	5.3	1389	7,493
		Secondary FN	29,811	13.4	1712	24,550

ABBREVIATIONS: FN, febrile neutropenia; LOS, length of stay.

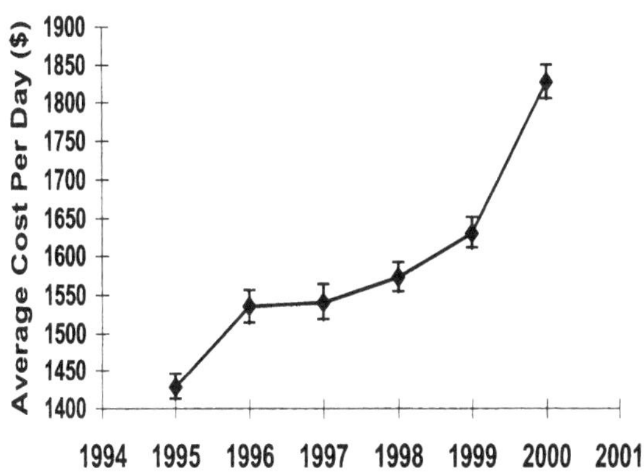

Fig. 10. Distribution of cost per day (mean ± SEM, $) for patients admitted with FN to institutions reporting to the University Health System Consortium, 1995–2000 *(59)*.

longer for patients with leukemia, 19.0 d compared with 10.8 and 8.5 d for patients with lymphoma and solid tumors, respectively. The cost per episode followed a similar pattern, with patients with leukemia having a substantially greater mean cost per episode than patients with lymphomas and patients with solid tumors (Fig. 11). Mortality was greatest in patients with leukemia (18%) compared with patients with lymphomas (10%) and solid tumors (9%). In addition, mortality associated with hospitalization for FN increased progressively with increasing age (Fig. 12).

5. THE IMPACT OF NEUTROPENIA AND ITS COMPLICATIONS ON QUALITY OF LIFE

5.1. Quality of Life and Patient Preferences

The impact of neutropenia and its complications (including FN) on patient QOL has received very little study. Early efforts attempted to evaluate the impact of neutropenia and the HGFs on patient QOL by eliciting patient preferences or utilities for antici-

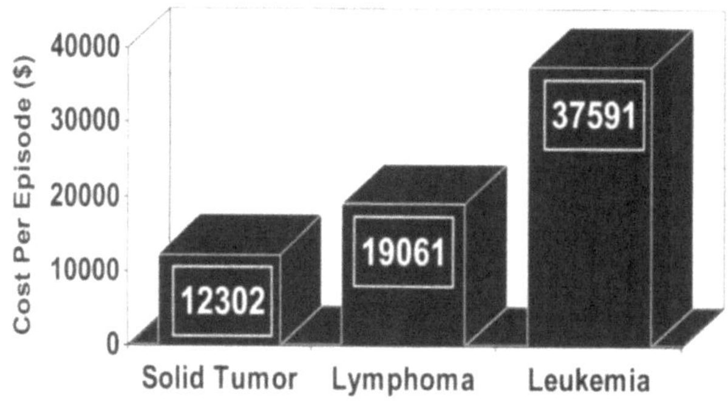

Fig. 11. Bar chart of total cost of hospitalization among patients with solid tumors, lymphoma, and leukemia admitted for FN to institutions reporting to the University Health System Consortium, 1995–2000 *(59)*.

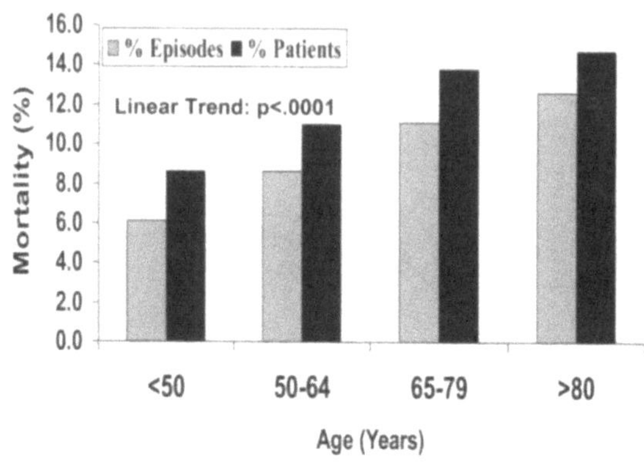

Fig. 12. Bar chart of risk of mortality across age groups based on deaths as a proportion of patients (black shading) or deaths as a proportion of admissions (gray shading) among patients admitted for FN to institutions reporting to the University Health System Consortium, 1995–2000 *(59)*.

pated health states. Using techniques such as a standard reference gamble and time tradeoffs, QOL can be assessed more globally but without detailed information about the impact on the various dimensions of QOL. Preliminary data assessed as willingness to pay to avoid FN corresponded to daily costs ranging from US $0 to US $500. The generated utilities may permit the conduct of useful cost-utility analysis even in the absence of proven effects on patient survival and will extend previous work on the incorporation of QOL measures into cost-minimization risk threshold models *(60)*.

5.2. Quality of Life and Health Profile Measures

More recently, preliminary efforts to study the impact of severe neutropenia on patient QOL have been reported using various health-profile measures. In a series of studies in a practice setting, changes in QOL were measured weekly in patients scheduled to receive myelosuppressive chemotherapy without growth factor support using the Short-Form 36 (SF-36), the Hospital Anxiety and Depression Scale (HADS), and the Psychological Adjustment to Illness Scale (PAIS) *(61,62)*. Significant correlations were observed between changes in neutrophil counts and measures of physical functioning, general health, vitality, and mental health. The greatest decrease in QOL was observed in patients with grade 4 neutropenia. An effort is currently under way to develop a more sensitive and specific measure for detected changes associated with severe or FN in patients receiving cancer chemotherapy. This approach is modeled after the Functional Assessment of Cancer Therapy (FACT) health profile scales and is termed the FACT-N. The current version of the tool consists of 19 questions generated from semistructured interviews and previous studies. The measure has been found to have good construct validity and internal consistency *(63)*. The entire issue of QOL assessment and the impact of rHuG-CSF in patients with cancer and human immunodeficiency virus (HIV) has been reviewed *(64)*.

6. THE EFFICACY AND EFFECTIVENESS OF HEMATOPOIETIC GROWTH FACTORS

6.1. The Efficacy of Prophylactic Colony-Stimulating Factors

Several studies of the efficacy of CSF for prevention of neutropenic complications and the infection risk associated with cancer chemotherapy in a variety of malignancies using different chemotherapy regimens have been reported *(65–72)*. Controlled clinical trials conducted in both Europe and the United States have shown the ability of rHuG-CSF (filgrastim) to reduce the risk of FN associated with systemic chemotherapy in selected patients when it is administered prophylactically before the onset of fever or neutropenia. In the initial clinical trial, Crawford et al. *(65)* randomized patients with small-cell lung cancer (SCLC) in a prospective, double-blind, placebo-controlled trial of rHuG-CSF after treatment with cyclophosphamide, doxorubicin, and etoposide (CAE). During the first cycle of treatment, when all patients were in the double-blind portion of the trial, 27% of filgrastim patients experienced FN compared with 55% of placebo patients ($p < 0.001$). One or more episodes of FN occurred in 77% of the placebo group over the six possible treatment cycles compared with 40% of the filgrastim group ($p < 0.001$). In a nearly identical trial performed by Trillet-Lenoir et al. *(66)*, patients with SCLC were randomized to treatment with CAE with or without filgrastim in a double-blind, placebo-controlled fashion. Over all courses of chemotherapy, 53% of the placebo patients and 26% of the filgrastim patients experienced at least one episode of FN ($p < 0.001$). Significant decreases in the need for treatment delay (47% vs 29%, $p < 0.04$) or dose reduction (61% vs 29%, $p < 0.001$) were observed in patients receiving rHuG-CSF.

6.2. Systematic Review of the Colony-Stimulating Factors

A systematic review with a formal meta-analysis of all RCTs of prophylactically administered rHuG-CSF in patients receiving cancer chemotherapy was reported (Table 2) *(17)*. Treatment dosing and schedules for rHuG-CSF used in these trials are summarized in Table 3. Summary estimates across the eight RCTs confirmed a high level of efficacy and safety across a wide variety of disease entities and treatment regimens (OR = 0.38; $p < 0.001$) (Fig. 13). In addition, patients randomized to receive rHuG-CSF experienced fewer episodes of documented infection (OR = 0.51; $p < 0.001$) and fewer dose reductions and treatment delays (OR = 0.32; $p < 0.001$). The odds ratio for mortality

Table 2
Meta-Analysis of Randomized Controlled Trials of Prophylactic rHuG-CSF

Study ref.	*Chemotherapy*	*Cancer*	*Placebo*	*rHuG-CSF*
65	CAE	Solid	Yes	Filgrastim
66	CAE	Solid	Yes	Filgrastim
68	CEF	Solid	Yes	Lenograstim
72	BEP/EP/BOP/VIP-B	Solid	No	Filgrastim
69	MAID	Solid	Yes	Lenograstim
71	ACVB/NCVB	Lymphoma	Yes	Lenograstim
67	VAPEC-B	Lymphoma	No	Filgrastim
70	VNCOP-B	Lymphoma	No	Filgrastim

ABBREVIATIONS: rHuG-CSF, recombinant human granulocyte colony-stimulating factor; CAE, cyclophosphamide, doxorubicin, and etoposide; BEP/EP, cisplatin, etoposide, bleomycin; CEF, cyclophosphamide, epirubicin, 5-fluorouracil, followed by maintenance regimen; BOP/VIP-B, bleomycin, vincristine, cisplatin, followed by cisplatin, ifosfamide, etoposide, bleomycin; MAID, doxorubicin, ifosfamide, dacarbazine, mesna; ACVB (NCVB), cyclophosphamide, vindesine, bleomycin, prednisone, IT methotrexate, adriamycin or mitoxantrone; VAPEC-B, adriamycin, cyclophosphamide, vincristine, bleomycin, etoposide, prednisolone, cotrimazole, ketoconazole; VNCOP-B, cyclophosphamide, mitoxantrone, vincristine, etoposide, bleomycin, prednisone.

Table 3
Meta-Analysis of Primary Prophylaxis With rHuG-CSF: Administration Schedule

Study ref.	*Start (d after chemo)*	*Dose*	*Frequency*	*Duration (d)*
65	1	230 μg/m^2	Daily	12–14
66	1	230 μg/m^2	Daily	12–14
67	1	230 μg/m^2	Daily	Continuous except for day before and days of chemo
69	1	5 μg/kg	Daily	10–14
68	2	5 μg/kg	Daily	10
70	1–2	5 μg/kg	Daily	5 d/wk
72	1	5 μg/kg	Daily	14
71	2–3	5 μg/kg	Daily	7

was 0.60 (0.30, 1.22) suggesting but not proving a 40% reduction in the odds of mortality ($p = 0.16$). The power to demonstrate a reduction in mortality of this level was only 28% owing to the limited number of events, several studies without mortality information, the availability of only short-term follow-up, and the absence of individual patient data.

6.3. The Efficacy of Therapeutic Colony-Stimulating Factors

Despite the demonstrated efficacy of rHuG-CSF in prevention strategies, it is often administered only after hospitalization for FN. The clinical as well as economic value of these agents administered therapeutically after the onset of FN continues to be debated, however. In a double-blind, placebo-controlled trial, Maher and colleagues *(73)* found that rHuG-CSF reduced the risk of prolonged hospitalization (>11 d) by 50% although the median number of days of hospitalization was unchanged. Mitchel

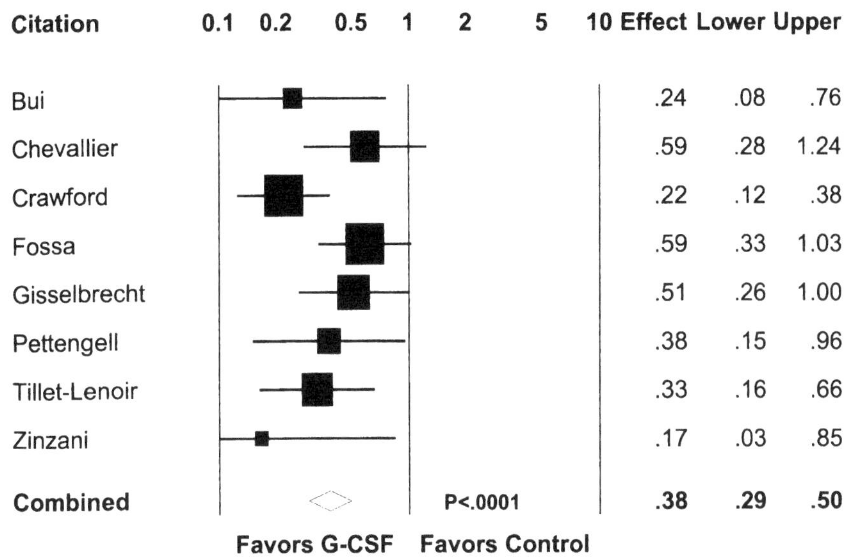

Fig. 13. Forrest plot of the Peto odds ratios for FN among the eight randomized controlled trials of prophylactic recombinant granulocyte colony-stimulating factor (rHuG-CSF) vs control along with a weighted summary measure across trials (OR = 0.38, $p < 0.001$) *(17)*. The size of the point estimate rectangles are in proportion to the weight and inversely proportional to the variance associated with each study. Also shown are the 95% confidence limits for each estimate. All studies demonstrate an effect estimate below 1.0 favoring G-CSF. Data from refs. *65–72* and reported in ref. *17*.

et al. *(74)* presented the results of a double-blind, placebo-controlled, randomized trial of children with established FN. These authors observed fewer d of antibiotics and shorter hospital stays (5 vs 7 d) among patients receiving rHuG-CSF compared with control patients, resulting in a 29% reduction in median bed cost ($p = 0.04$).

In another prospective randomized trial of empiric antibiotics with or without rHuG-CSF in high-risk patients with solid tumors admitted with established FN, those receiving rHuG-CSF experienced short periods of grade 4 neutropenia ($p = 0.0004$), less antibiotic therapy ($p = 0.013$), and shorter hospitalizations ($p = 0.015$) than control patients *(75)*. The median cost of hospital stay was reduced in patients receiving rHuG-CSF by 17% ($p = 0.01$) and total costs by 11% ($p = 0.07$) compared with control patients. Recently, a systematic review of the RCT of hematopoietic growth factors administered therapeutically at the time of hospitalization for FN was conducted under the auspices of the Cochrane Collaboration *(18)*. A significant reduction in the time to neutrophil recovery was observed (OR = 0.36, $p < 0.0001$), with a borderline reduction in the risk of infection-related mortality (Fig. 14) (OR = 0.51, $p = 0.05$).

6.4. The Efficacy of CSF in Elderly Patients

Balducci et al. *(76)* have reviewed the biologic basis for the limited hematopoietic reserve in elderly patients with cancer with the clinical evidence that they are at greater risk for FN while receiving cancer chemotherapy as well as for greater risk of complication from FN if it occurs. A meta-analysis of neutropenic complications and growth factor use in elderly patients with NHL or acute leukemia has been reported *(77,78)*. The

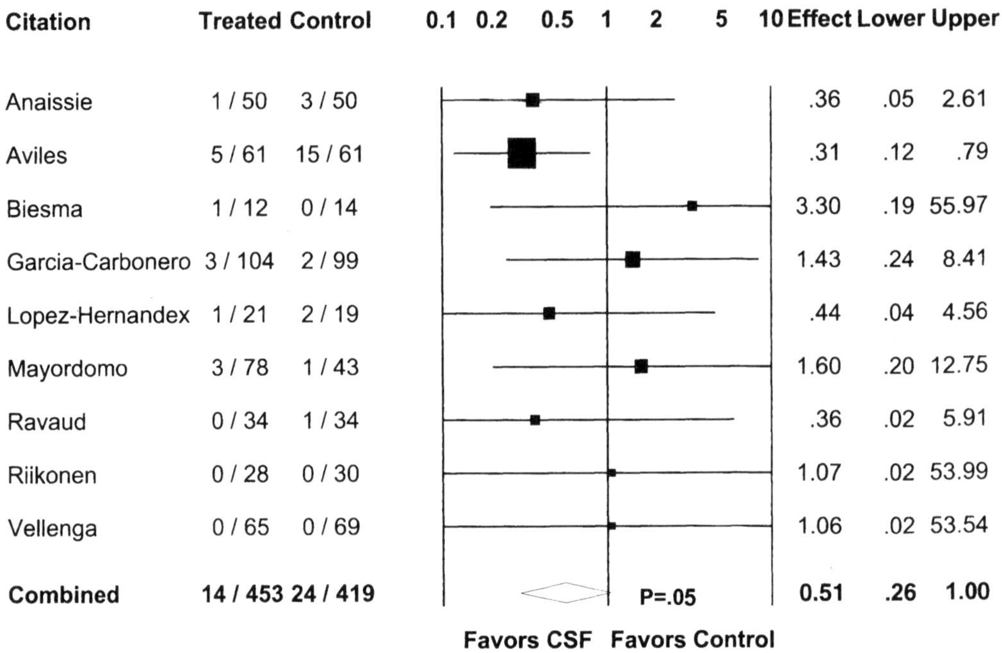

Fig. 14. Forrest plot of the Peto odds ratios for infection-related mortality among the nine randomized controlled trials of therapeutic colony-stimulating factor (CSF) vs control along with a weighted summary measure across trials (OR = 0.51, $p = 0.05$) *(76)*. The sizes of the point estimate rectangles are in proportion to the weight and inversely proportional to the variance associated with each study. Also shown are the 95% confidence limits for each estimate. Point estimates to the left of 1.0 favor rHuG-CSF, and those above 1.0 favor control. Data from refs. *18, 75, 93–99.*

risk of FN in elderly patients with NHL receiving CHOP-like regimens varied from 25 to 40%. Prophylactic growth factor use was associated with a reduction in risk of severe neutropenia (RR = 0.52, $p < 0.001$) and FN (RR = 0.43, $p = 0.036$) in elderly patients with NHL (Fig. 15). Although no difference in complete remission rate was observed in elderly patients with acute myeloid leukemia, the meta-analysis of RCTs revealed a significant increase in disease-free survival at 2 yr (RR = 1.50, $p = 0.025$).

7. THE ECONOMIC IMPACT OF CSF

7.1. Introduction

The cost of the CSFs combined with their wide-scale clinical application has prompted a number of economic analyses along with the development of clinical practice guidelines for their use. As described above, the economics of the CSFs are inseparable from the economics of FN since it is the prevention or alleviation of FN that represents the major cost savings associated with HGF use. However, economic analyses of the CSFs are complicated by a number of factors including the skewed distribution of hospital LOS and cost associated with FN and the unequal variances illustrated by the reduction in overall variability associated with fewer lengthy hospitalizations in those receiving CSFs. Nevertheless, CSFs have been the subject of a number of economic analyses comparing treat-

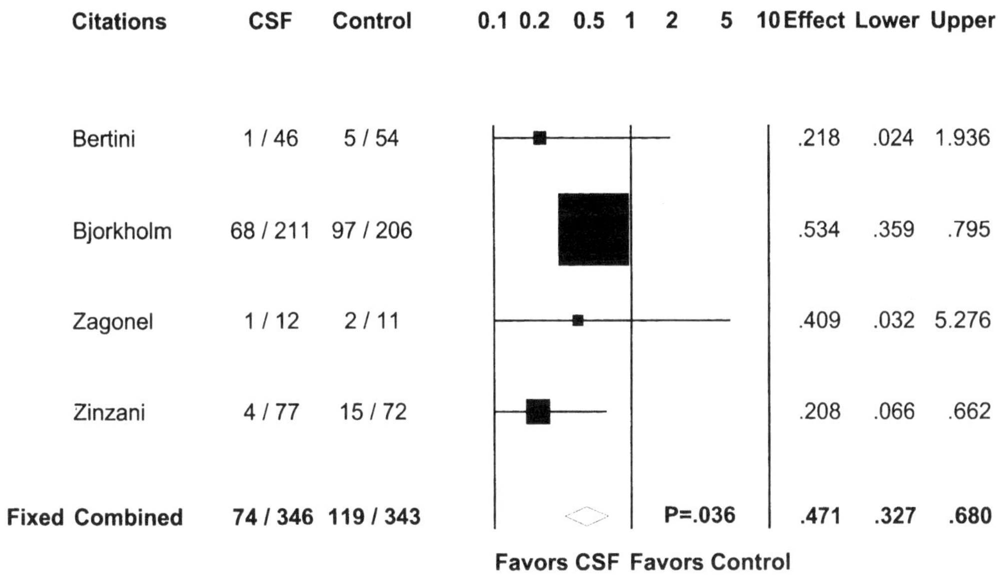

Fig. 15. Forrest plot of the Peto odds ratios for FN among the four controlled trials of prophylactic granulocyte colony-stimulating factor (rHuG-CSF) vs control in elderly patients with non-Hodgkin's lymphoma along with a weighted summary measure across trials (OR = 0.47, p = 0.036) *(78)*. The sizes of the point estimate rectangles are in proportion to the weight and inversely proportional to the variance associated with each study. Also shown are the 95% confidence limits for each estimate. All studies demonstrate an effect estimate below 1.0 favoring rHuG-CSF. Data from refs. 70, 100–102.

ment options based on differences in resource utilization or cost. Clinical decision models have been particularly useful in such analyses for studying the tradeoff between the added cost of growth factor use and any reduction in risk or duration of FN in patients receiving chemotherapy *(16,19,20,23,24)*. These models have been used to support the development of clinical practice guidelines for the use of CSF in support of patients receiving cancer therapy *(21)*. The use of clinical prediction models to select higher risk patients for targeted therapy should further increase the cost efficiency of such interventions and more closely reflect the situation in actual clinical practice *(52,55,79)*.

7.2. Economic Models of Prophylactic CSF

7.2.1. Cost-Minimization Models

The initial economic models of prophylactic CSF administration were based on the results of previously discussed pivotal RCTs and crude estimates of direct medical costs. These cost minimization models using baseline probabilities and resource utilization from the RCT of Crawford et al. *(65)* and local direct institutional cost information generated average risk threshold estimates for cost savings with prophylactic rHuG-CSF use in the range of 40% *(19,20)*. These models assumed that all patients experiencing FN will be hospitalized for empiric parenteral antibiotic therapy (Fig. 16). No impact of CSF on the duration of hospitalization or infection-related mortality was assumed. The expected cost of a specific choice was calculated from the sum of the products of the terminal value or cost and the probability of each branch. The total cost of hospitaliza-

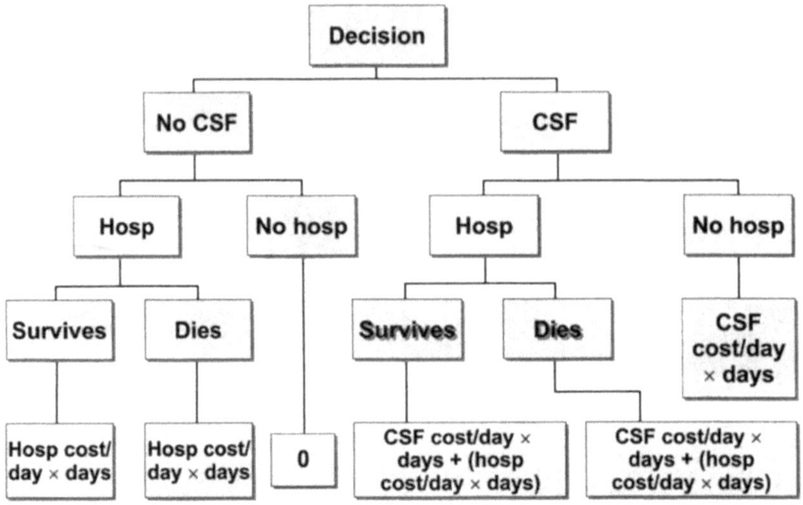

Fig. 16. Decision tree for a cost minimization model of the use of prophylactic granulocyte colony-stimulating factor (rHuG-CSF) or no rHuG-CSF in chemotherapy patients at risk for FN. Model assumes that all patients with FN are hospitalized, that the risk of hospitalization of FN in those receiving prophylactic G-CSF is reduced by 50%, and that there is an equal duration of hospitalization and mortality among those hospitalized for FN in both groups. Cost considerations are limited to those related to hospitalization for FN (average length of stay × average cost/day [$]) and G-CSF (average duration of administration × average cost/day for drug and administration). Patients not hospitalized and not receiving G-CSF have no associated costs. (Data from ref. *19*.)

tion was the product of the average daily cost of hospitalization and the average hospital LOS. The expected cost per treatment cycle represents the marginal or net cost associated with hospitalization for FN and treatment with CSF. The expected cost for each management strategy was calculated as the sum of the products of the costs and probabilities of each outcome.

7.2.2. Sensitivity Analyses

A series of sensitivity analyses were undertaken estimating the expected cost associated with each strategy while varying the assumptions concerning each variable over the range of reasonable values. In a one-way sensitivity analysis, the expected cost was calculated for each value of the variable, forming a curve of cost values for each decision choice. Thresholds were generated for each variable at which the expected costs were equal for management with and without CSFs. The relationship between the threshold risk of hospitalization for FN while varying the cost associated with hospitalization was studied in a two-way sensitivity analysis. A family of threshold curves was generated on the basis of multivariate sensitivity analyses for a combination of two or more variables.

Under baseline assumptions, a threshold risk for FN of 40% was estimated where the added cost of CSF was offset by the reduction in cost associated with hospitalization for FN (Fig. 17). As the daily cost increases, the threshold risk of hospitalization favoring the use of CSF decreases. Likewise, the longer the expected LOS, the lower the threshold favoring the use of CSF. Above this risk threshold, the overall costs of treatment are less when a CSF is used, whereas below it the use of a CSF actually

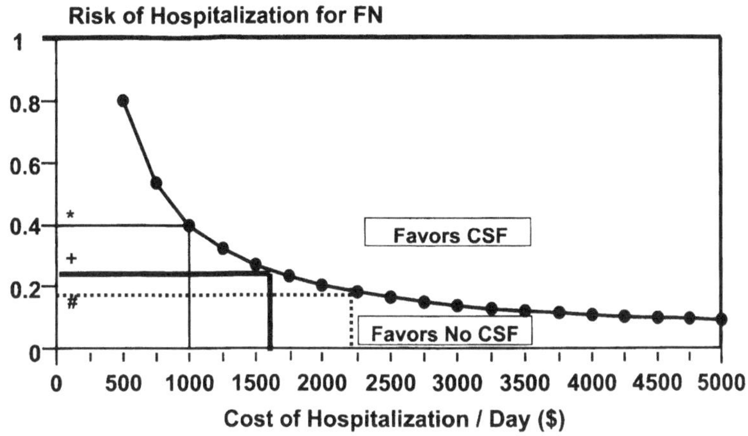

Fig. 17. Two-way sensitivity analysis of the threshold for cost associated with FN hospitalization and granulocyte colony-stimulating factor (rHuG-CSF) use based on the decision model shown in Fig. 16. The horizontal axis varies the cost/day ($) for hospitalization, and the vertical axis varies the risk of FN hospitalization. The threshold curve demonstrates lower thresholds for cost saving use of rHuG-CSF with increasing cost of hospitalization. Combinations of risk and cost above the threshold curve are associated with a reduction in cost with the use of prophylactic G-CSF, whereas those below the threshold curve are associated with greater cost with the use of rHuG-CSF. Illustrated are three sequential cost estimates and the accompanying risk threshold based on the original study using crude direct medical costs, * (Threshold = 40% *[19]*), the updated total hospital cost estimate, + (Threshold = 23% *[16]*), and the recent addition of indirect and out-of-pocket cost estimates, # (Threshold = 18% *[81]*).

increases the costs of treatment, although the added cost of the CSFs is partially offset by the reduction in cost of hospitalization. As the daily cost of hospitalization or the LOS increase, the FN risk threshold favoring the use of these agents decreases. The American Society of Clinical Oncology (ASCO) used the early results to support its clinical practice guidelines for the use of CSFs. The original risk threshold estimates were subsequently updated using the single-institution estimates of total costs for FN hospitalization described above *(16)*. Incorporation of total hospital costs into the new FN cost estimates and their use in the previously reported cost-minimization models, generated FN risk threshold estimates for CSF use of 20–25% (Fig. 17).

7.2.3. Model Extensions

Additional efforts to refine risk threshold estimates further for the prophylactic use of the CSF have included the addition of indirect and out-of-pocket cost estimates, a study of the impact of incorporating an option to treat selected low-risk patients with FN in the ambulatory setting, consideration of special high-risk populations such as the elderly, and the use of predictive models permitting individualization of risk estimation and the study of other practice changes that might influence threshold estimates.

7.3. Economic Models Incorporating Indirect and Out-of-Pocket Costs

Limited information is available pertaining to direct nonmedical and indirect costs, which would provide a more societal perspective on the economic impact of neutropenia and CSF. A survey reported on 26 women with ovarian cancer experiencing severe or FN, including time lost from work for patients and caregivers and out-of-pocket expenses *(80)*. All patients were recruited within 1 mo after the occurrence of grade 3 or 4 neutropenia. Resource utilization was tracked through a detailed questionnaire administered at study entry and at least twice more during the episode. Estimates of indirect costs (e.g., productivity loss) were based on modified Labor Force, Employment, and Earnings data. Totals of the indirect and patient out-of-pocket costs per episode of severe neutropenia were calculated for each patient.

Mean indirect and out-of-pocket expenses for an episode of severe or FN were estimated to be US $5176 per patient. This total does not include any of the direct costs of hospitalization, which are accounted for in the existing threshold model. These additional indirect and patient out-of-pocket costs were incorporated into the cost minimization model discussed above. These costs were added to the direct costs of hospitalization for FN as well as those of the growth factor and its administration. The additional costs in the branches for patients treated with prophylactic CSFs were adjusted based on the assumption that the incidence of severe neutropenia would be 50% less with prophylactic CSFs. A sensitivity analysis was then conducted across a range of potential indirect cost estimates from US $0 to US $5000 per inpatient FN episode. With no indirect costs being considered, the risk threshold based on total direct medical costs discussed above was 23%. As the estimates for indirect costs increase, the threshold favoring the use of CSF decreases. When the indirect and patient out-of-pocket costs attributable to severe neutropenia approach the figure estimated from the survey data, the risk threshold is reduced to 18% (Fig. 18) *(81)*.

7.4. Economic Models Incorporating an Ambulatory Treatment Option

7.4.1. Risk Models for Patient Selection

With the identification of several risk factors for serious medical complications and prolonged hospitalization associated with FN, it has become possible to identify a population of patients at lower risk for these serious outcomes *(82,83)*. In these studies, Talcott stratified patients with FN into three high-risk groups. Group 1 comprised patients with hematologic malignancy or after bone-marrow transplant (BMT), already hospitalized at the onset of FN. Group 2 comprised outpatients with comorbidities, such as pulmonary or cardiovascular disease. Group 3 comprised outpatients with uncontrolled cancer. All these patients have high and unacceptable rates of morbidity and mortality and should be treated according to standard inpatient procedures for the entire duration of FN. Group 4 represented low-risk patients, stable outpatients with responsive tumors and no comorbidities. It has been suggested that such an approach will reduce the costs associated with episodes of FN based on the reduced need for hospitalization of a proportion of these patients *(83,84)*. MASCC has developed a formal scoring system for evaluating cancer patients with FN for possible outpatient management, including age, burden of illness, dehydration, hypotension, lung disease, tumor type, and admission status *(85)*. A number of institutions have developed strategies for treating some patients in the ambulatory setting generally after 1 or 2 d of evaluation and initiation of antibiotics in the hospital with early discharge to complete therapy as an outpatient.

7.4.2. Limitations of Ambulatory Treatment of FN

The limitations of this approach have been extensively discussed, including the need for a very low predictive value negative, and the need for a substantial (and costly)

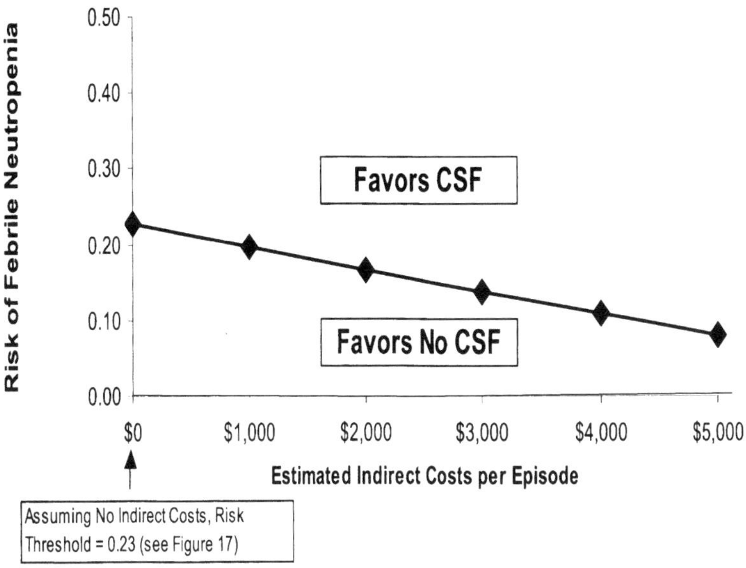

Fig. 18. Two-way sensitivity analysis of the threshold for cost associated with FN hospitalization and granulocyte colony-stimulating factor (rHuG-CSF) use based on the decision model shown in Fig. 16. The horizontal axis varies the estimated indirect and out-of-pocket costs per episode of FN, and the vertical axis varies the risk of FN hospitalization. The threshold curve demonstrates a lower threshold for cost saving use of rHuG-CSF with increasing estimates of indirect and out-of-pocket costs. Combinations of risk and cost above the threshold are associated with a reduction in cost with the use of prophylactic rHuG-CSF, whereas those below the threshold curve are associated with greater cost with the use of rHuG-CSF. The indirect cost estimates were based on the estimates in women with ovarian cancer receiving cancer chemotherapy *(80)* and modifications of the original cost minimization model shown in Fig. 17 *(81)*.

infrastructure and organization to manage patients with FN as outpatients, the large number of logistical and social issues that must be addressed including proximity to the health care facility, availability of a full-time caretaker, as well as sufficient awareness and education concerning the seriousness of the condition. Nevertheless, it has been suggested that reduced hospitalization costs will have a direct impact on cost-minimization thresholds and, by increasing those thresholds, will lessen the economic basis for the use of CSFs.

A number of additional economic factors must be considered in an analysis of the economic impact of the ambulatory management of selected patients with FN in the ambulatory setting even when patient selection, as well as institutional, logistical, and social issues, have been satisfactorily addressed. It is very likely that such a shift will result in some increase in indirect and out-of-pocket expenses to the family and other caretakers. Indirect medical as well as direct medical expenses to the patient and family may increase because of more restrictive reimbursement for outpatient care. Nevertheless, the issue remains whether total direct medical costs for the care of FN can be reduced by an ambulatory care strategy. Fundamental to a full understanding of this approach is the recognition that patients with FN are a heterogeneous population with considerable variation in the potential risk for serious medical complications including death. We have seen that it is this recognized variation in patients that also accounts for the enormous variation in observed LOS and cost for inpatient care. Clearly, it is the proportion of high-risk patients with often long hospitalizations that drives most of the overall cost. The population of low-risk patients generally has relatively short hospitalizations and accounts for a correspondingly small proportion of the overall costs associated with FN.

7.4.3. Cost-Minimization Model Incorporating Outpatient Treatment Option

An analysis of an economic model for the use of CSFs incorporating an ambulatory treatment strategy for low-risk FN patients demonstrated that such an approach has minimal impact on risk thresholds for CSF use independent of shifts in nonmedical and indirect expenses and the costs of putting a substantial institutional infrastructure in place *(86)*. This result appears to be primarily owing to the continued need for hospitalization of high-risk individuals, generating longer hospitalizations and greater cost. Risk stratification of patients was based on the method of Talcott *(14)* and applied to a population of 82 patients admitted to the Albany Medical Center between 1998 and 1999. In this model, low-risk patients are admitted for a short inpatient stay of 48 h to obtain initial laboratory studies, including cultures, and to commence empiric antibiotics. They then continue subsequent management as outpatients. Baseline probabilities for risk of hospitalization for FN, duration of hospitalization, and proportional hospitalization risk with prophylactic CSFs were based on previously reported models *(19,20)*. The expected total treatment costs for FN without prophylactic rHuG-CSF were US $9625; with prophylactic rHuG-CSF but without an outpatient option for FN, they were US $6812, and with rHuG-CSF but with stratification into a low-risk group and treatment with an outpatient option, they were US $6449. Comparison with a standard inpatient approach and a strategy incorporating an outpatient treatment option for low-risk patients revealed nearly identical risk threshold estimates (Fig. 19).

7.5. Economic Models of CSF in High-Risk Populations

7.5.1. Clinical Prediction (Risk) Models

The use of CSFs in all patients at risk for severe neutropenia or its complications has been considered cost-prohibitive. Selecting patients for CSF use has generally been based on the previous occurrence of such complications, the intensity of the chemotherapy regimen selected, or the clinical perception of risk. Several investigators have attempted to complement such considerations to improve the ability to predict those at greatest risk of neutropenia. Clinical prediction or risk models capable of identifying patients at high risk for FN or its consequences for the targeted application of CSF mimics decision making in actual clinical practice and should improve the cost efficiency of these agents. Such models may allow patients to be divided into high- and low-risk categories for neutropenic complications, with rHuG-CSF selectively applied to the high-risk group. In addition to further reducing risk thresholds for the cost-saving use of CSFs, such models can be extended to cost-effectiveness studies in which treatment impacts on clinical outcome as well as cost and is discussed for patients receiving standard adjuvant chemotherapy for ESBC. The value of cost-effectiveness analysis of

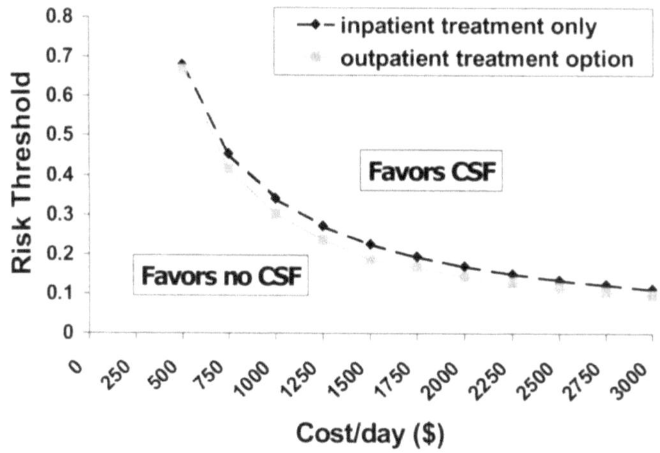

Fig. 19. Two-way sensitivity analysis based on the original cost model but incorporating a third option with stratification into low-risk and high-risk patients based on Talcott et al. *(82)*. After an initial 48 h of observation and evaluation, low-risk patients are then discharged to complete their antibiotic course as outpatients. Length of stay estimates for low-risk and high-risk patients were based on a study of 82 cancer patients hospitalized with FN at the Albany Medical Center *(86)*. Risk threshold estimates are seen to vary little across a range of estimated hospital costs/day, as most of the cost is associated with the longer length of stay observed in the high-risk patients. CSF, colony-stimulating factor.

rHuG-CSF support based on sustaining dose intensity and translating into prolonged disease-free and overall survival has only recently gained attention. Nevertheless, rHuG-CSF is considered integral to efforts to sustain dose intensity or deliver dose-dense therapy in both ESBC and NHL (87–90).

7.5.2. Retrospective Risk Models of FN and Its Complications

A systematic review was undertaken of previous published efforts to develop risk models for the development of severe FN and serious medical consequences including death in those hospitalized with FN *(91)*. Nineteen studies were identified providing enough information about design and analysis to assess the risk factors reported adequately. All of these studies were retrospective in design. Shown in Fig. 20 are those characteristics reported in two or more studies to be significant independent risk factors in multivariate analysis. Those shown at the top were predictive of severe neutropenia or FN and those at the bottom were predictive of serious medical complications, long LOS, or mortality for established FN.

7.5.3. Early-Stage Breast Cancer

In the study of adjuvant breast cancer patients discussed above, a clinical prediction model incorporating baseline and first-cycle hematologic data was capable of discriminating high-risk women for future neutropenic complications that might compromise dose intensity and long-term outcome *(54)*. Based on the importance of sustained dose intensity on disease-free survival reported in patients with ESBC, Silber et al. *(79)* studied a strategy of targeted rHuG-CSF support in the 50% of women at greatest risk

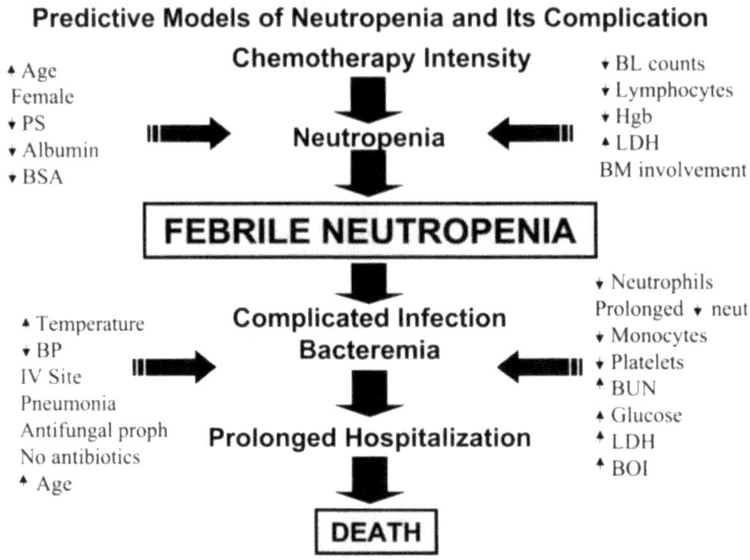

Fig. 20. Diagram summarizing the results of a systematic review of 19 prognostic or risk factor studies for severe or febrile neutropenia (top) as well as serious medical consequences including bacteremia, prolonged hospitalization, or death (bottom). Shown are those factors associated with these outcomes in multivariate analysis in two or more reported studies *(87)*. BSA, bovine serum albumin; Hgb, hemoglobin; LDH, lactate dehydrogenase; BM, bone marrow; BP, blood pressure; BUN, blood urea nitrogen, BOI, burden of illness; BL, baseline; PS, performance status.

in order to sustain dose intensity compared with a standard dose-reduction strategy. The estimated cost effectiveness for the rHuG-CSF support strategy for high-risk patients of US $34,000 per life-year gained was reasonably robust across a range of baseline assumptions (Fig. 21). In Fig. 22, the C/E ratio for targeted rHuG-CSF support is compared with the cost effectiveness attributed to other therapeutic strategies in oncology. The value of such a simple prediction tool for reducing the risk of neutropenic complications with targeted use of CSF has been validated prospectively *(55)*. Women receiving adjuvant breast cancer chemotherapy ($N = 614$) who were assigned to rHuG-CSF using a simple risk model consisting of the first-cycle ANC nadir experienced significantly fewer episodes of hospitalization for FN ($p < 0.001$) and greater dose intensity ($p = 0.003$) than historical controls without such a strategy. It has been shown in this same population that consideration of age and first-cycle events such as FN, a decrease in Hb concentration >1 g/dL, and ANC nadir $< 0.5 \times 10^9$/L permits more accurate risk prediction providing potentially better cost effectiveness *(56)*.

7.5.4. Non-Hodgkin's Lymphoma

Similarly, a number of important predictive factors for the risk and time to occurrence of FN have been identified in patients with NHL receiving CHOP *(49,50)*. These pretreatment or unconditional models incorporate age, planned dose intensity, low baseline Hb concentration, and comorbidities such as heart and renal disease and are

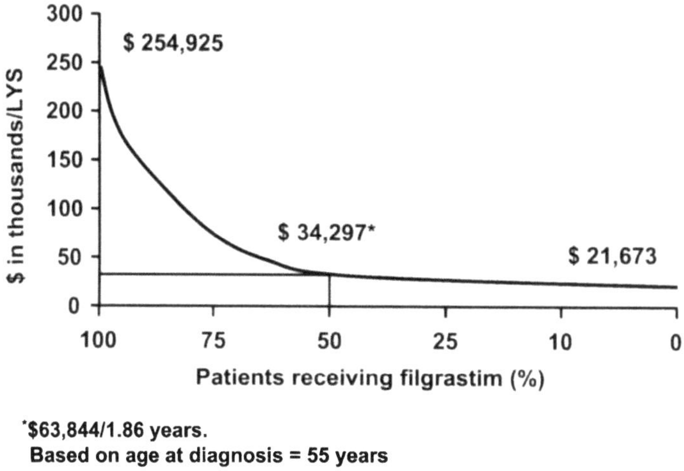

Fig. 21. Two-way sensitivity analysis of a decision model comparing a strategy of targeted rHuG-CSF for the one-half of breast cancer adjuvant chemotherapy patients at greatest risk for future dose-limiting neutropenic complications based on a conditional risk model compared with a strategy of standard dose reduction without rHuG-CSF support. The horizontal axis varies the proportion of patients planned to receive rHuG-CSF (50% at baseline). The vertical axis presents the associated cost effectiveness ratio in terms of cost per life-year saved by avoiding decreased dose intensity with the targeted use of G-CSF in high-risk women *(54,80)*. LYS, life-year saved.

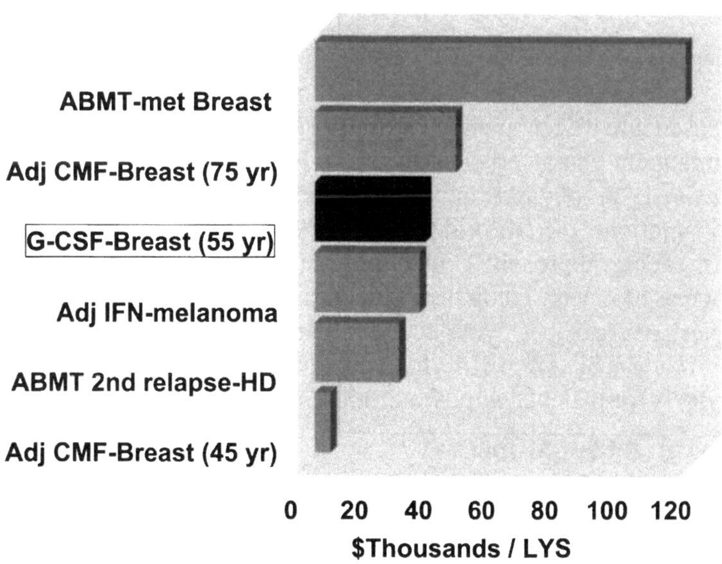

Fig. 22. Bar graph illustrating estimates of cost-effectiveness ratios for targeted granulocyte colony-stimulating factor (rHuG-CSF) support based on the conditional risk model reported by Silber et al. *(54,80)*. These are compared with cost effectiveness reported for other therapeutic approaches in oncology *(32)*. LYS, life-year saved; ABMT, autologous bone marrow transplant; Adj CMF, adjuvant cyclophosphamide, methotrexate, and 5-fluorouracil; Adj IFN, adjuvant interferon; HD, Hodgkin's disease.

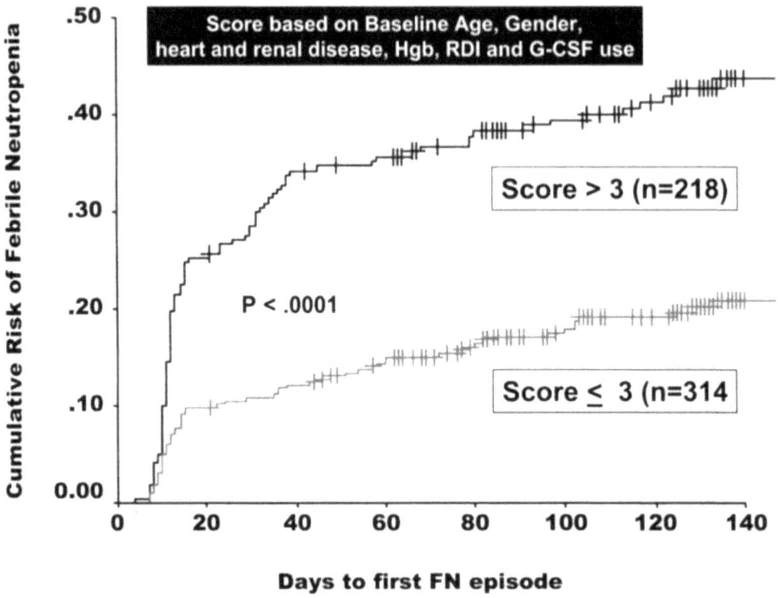

Fig. 23. Actuarial plot of the time to first febrile neutropenia (FN) event in patients with non-Hodgkin's lymphoma receiving CHOP chemotherapy based on the method of Kaplan and Meier *(49)*. Patients were stratified into high risk (>3 factors, $n = 218$) or low risk (≤3 factors, $n = 314$) based on an unconditional model for increased risk based on older age, female gender, heart or renal disease, pretreatment hemoglobin < 12 g/dL, intended dose intensity > 80% and the absence of rHuG-CSF prophylaxis. High-risk patients had a significantly greater cumulative risk of FN than patients in the low-risk group ($p < 0.0001$).

capable of reasonable discrimination of high-risk from low-risk patients for FN based on such pretreatment characteristics (Fig. 23). Incorporation of a risk model-targeted strategy for primary prophylaxis in NHL into an economic model demonstrates that in higher risk populations, e.g., the elderly, primary prophylaxis of all patients represents the most cost-saving approach. Under most other situations, targeting CSF toward patients at increased risk based on the model is associated with lower overall costs than other strategies. Average per cycle cost per patient under baseline conditions is US $3149 for no rHuG-CSF, US $3148 for universal prophylaxis, and US $2794 for targeted prophylaxis for patients with two or more risk factors.

7.5.5. Prospective Risk Models

Efforts are under way to develop more accurate risk models and to validate them based on prospectively collected data, to assist clinicians in the selection of high-risk patients and the targeting of supportive care measures such as CSFs *(92)*. Such models must explicitly state both the dependent variables or outcomes and the independent variables or predictors of interest. The economic impact of incorporation of a risk or clinical prediction model into a treatment decision pathway for the management of patients at risk for FN depends on the risk of FN in the population and the performance characteristics of the model. The net cost advantage of targeted rHuG-CSF increases as model predictive performance increases. As more accurate risk models are developed that are independently validated in a variety of clinical settings, their value to clinicians in providing optimal care to patients receiving cancer chemotherapy and to society in terms of obtaining the most value with limited resources cannot be overstated.

8. SUMMARY AND CONCLUSIONS

8.1. The Problem

Health care costs have risen dramatically, with hospital care representing a substantial portion of this burden. Although it is under-reported, myelosuppression with associated neutropenia still represents the most important dose-limiting toxicity of systemic cancer chemotherapy, often compromising dose intensity in treatable and potentially curable malignancies. The development of fever in the setting of neutropenia represents a life-threatening condition generally prompting hospitalization for evaluation and administration of broad-spectrum antibiotics. FN often occurs early in the course of chemotherapy and is associated not only with treatment intensity but also with age and a number of additional patient- and disease-related factors. The economics of CSFs are largely determined by the cost associated with the management of FN and its consequences. The length of hospitalization and the accompanying cost associated with FN vary greatly. Most of the cost associated with hospitalization for FN is associated with prolonged and complicated hospitalizations in high-risk patients.

8.2. The Solution

CSFs have demonstrated efficacy when used prophylactically in numerous randomized controlled trials by reducing the risk of FN, the risk of documented infections, and the need for dose reductions and treatment delays. The efficacy of CSFs is evident in elderly patients with cancer and across a number of disease entities and treatment regimens. Although apparently less effective, CSFs appear to be active when administered therapeutically to patients with established FN by shortening the duration of neutropenia and reducing the proportion of patients requiring prolonged hospitalization. More controversial emerging data from controlled clinical trials suggest a possible impact of rHuG-CSFs on both short-term survival (by reducing infection-related mortality) and long-term survival (by sustaining dose intensity and the impact of full-dose or dose-intensified chemotherapy on disease-free and overall survival). Although improved survival provides an opportunity for the performance of cost-effectiveness and cost-utility analyses, economic studies of CSF have largely focused on cost minimization and the tradeoffs between the cost of these interventions and the reduced cost of hospitalization for FN.

8.3. The Cost

Decision models represent a valuable method of economic analysis permitting the simultaneous consideration of benefit (decreased risk of hospitalization for FN) and harm (cost of hospitalization for FN and cost of CSF). Cost-minimization studies have demonstrated that rHuG-CSF use reduces cost in many specific clinical situations. Consideration of direct medical costs based on estimated total hospital expenses yields FN risk thresholds for the cost-saving use of rHuG-CSF in the range of 20–25%. The addition of an ambulatory treatment option for the management of FN has minimal impact on cost and risk thresholds, as most of the cost of FN is associated with high-

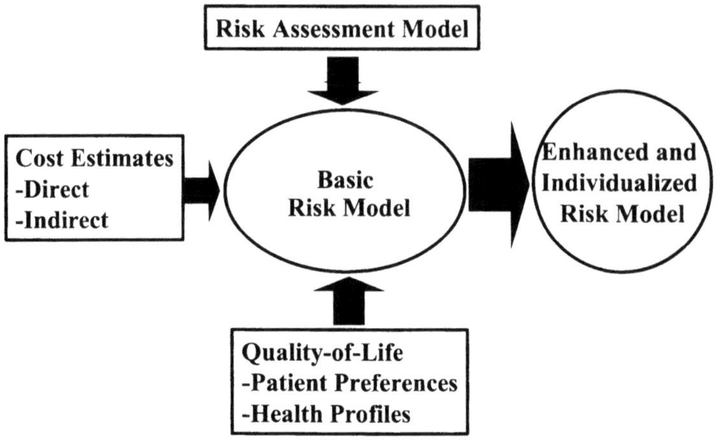

Fig. 24. Schema illustrating the relationship between the basic risk model and enhanced risk modeling based on more accurate and validated risk models, enhanced cost estimates including direct and indirect costs, and information on quality of life from both health profiles and utility measures.

risk patients experiencing complicated and often prolonged hospitalizations. Incorporation of indirect and out-of-pocket expenses as well as QOL considerations in the form of intangible costs further reduces risk thresholds from a societal perspective.

8.4. Clinical Prediction Models

Clinical prediction models represent a tool for improving patient selection for the targeting of rHuG-CSF treatment toward high-risk patients, potentially reducing costs further and improving cost effectiveness. Factors of importance in predicting FN include treatment intensity, disease stage, age, performance status, and both baseline and first-cycle nadir blood counts. Such risk models have been extended to a cost-effectiveness evaluation of rHuG-CSF use in women receiving adjuvant chemotherapy for breast cancer. Based on the apparent impact of reduced dose intensity on disease-free survival, the strategy of selecting women for filgrastim use who are at high risk for neutropenic complications using a valid risk model considering first-cycle blood counts has been shown to be cost-effective compared with other accepted technologies. Improved predictive models based on high-quality prospective data and validated on independent sets of patients are under development. As illustrated in Fig. 24, early basic efforts to develop risk models for FN based largely on retrospective datasets will soon give way to powerful and individualized interactive models based on prospectively developed and validated risk models enhanced by improved information on the QOL and economic impact of FN on patients, facilitating the rational and effective targeting of CSF to those in need.

8.5. Clinical Practice Guidelines

Clinical practice guidelines have been developed using both evidence-based (ASCO) and consensus-based (National Comprehensive Cancer Network) methodologies. Recommendations provided in these guidelines vary and have changed over time owing to rapidly expanding information about the clinical, QOL, and economic impact of neutropenic complications and the recent introduction of longer acting agents capable of improving convenience and compliance with cancer treatment. Because of these rapid advances, it is essential that these practice guidelines be continually re-evaluated in the light of rapidly emerging data that are expanding awareness of the impact of neutropenia and its consequences on patients and their disease course as well as the ability of CSFs to improve short-term and long-term clinical, QOL, and economic outcomes in patients.

The proper decision on whether to use CSF support should consider the total clinical and economic impact of FN on the patient and society as well as the importance of chemotherapy dose intensity on disease outcomes. Prophylactic use of CSFs should be considered in patients at any risk level when it is considered necessary to sustain dose intensity in responsive and potentially curable malignancies. Routine use of CSFs administered prophylactically should be considered in patients at 20% or greater risk of FN by virtue of either the intensity of chemotherapy or treatment with the same dose and schedule of chemotherapy, which previously resulted in hospitalization for FN and perhaps even at a risk as low as 10% when an unusually complicated and prolonged course of management is anticipated, as in elderly patients.

REFERENCES

1. Vincenzino JV. Health care costs: market forces and reform. *Oncology* 1995; 9:367–374.
2. Schuette HL, Tucker TC, Brown ML, Potosky AC, Samuel T. The costs of cancer care in the United States: implications for action. *Oncology* 1995; 11:19–22.
3. Centers for Medicare and Medicaid Services, 2002 Annual Report. US Washington, DC: Government Printing Office. 2003.
4. Brown ML. The national economic burden of cancer: an update. *J Natl Cancer Inst* 1990; 82:1811–1814.
5. Baker MS, Kessler LC. Site-specific treatment costs in cancer. In: *Cancer Care and Cost.* Health Administration Press Washington, DC, 1989, pp. 140–163.
6. Gaumer GL, Stavins J. Medicare use in the last 90 days of life. *Med Care* 1991; 29:725–742.
7. Task Force on Principles for Economic Analysis of Health Care Technology. Economic analyses of health care technology: a report on principles. *Ann Intern Med* 1995; 122:61–70.
8. Schulman KA, Yabroff KR. Measuring the cost effectiveness of cancer care. *Oncology* 1995; 9:523–533.
9. American Society of Clinical Oncology. Outcomes of cancer treatment for technology assessment and cancer treatment guidelines. *J Clin Oncol* 1996; 14:671–679.
10. Smith TJ, Hillner BE, Desch CE. Efficacy and cost-effectiveness of cancer treatment: rational allocation of resources based on decision analysis. *J Natl Cancer Inst* 1993; 85:1460–1474.
11. Russell LB, Gold MR, Siegel JE, Daniels N, Weinstein MC. The role of cost-effectiveness analysis in health and medicine. *JAMA* 1996; 276:1172–1177.
12. Weinstein MC, Siegel JE, Gold MR, Kamiet MS, Russell LB. Recommendations of the panel on cost-effectiveness in health and medicine. *JAMA* 1996; 276:1253–1258.
13. Siegel JE, Weinstein MC, Russell LB, Gold MR. Recommendations for reporting cost-effectiveness analysis. *JAMA* 1996; 276:1330–1341.
14. Bodey GP, Buckley M, Sathe YS, et al. Quantitative relationships between circulating leukocytes and infection in patients with acute leukemia. *Ann Intern Med* 1966; 64:328–340.
15. Infectious Diseases Society of America. 2002 guidelines for the use of antimicrobial agents in neutropenic patients with cancer. *Clin Infect Dis* 2002; 34:730–751.
16. Lyman GH, Kuderer N, Greene J, Balducci L. The economics of febrile neutropenia: iImplications for the use of colony-stimulating factors. *Eur J Cancer* 1998; 34:1857–1864.
17. Lyman GH, Kuderer NM, Djulbegovic B. Prophylactic granulocyte colony-stimulating factor in patients receiving dose intensive cancer chemotherapy: a meta-analysis. *Am J Med* 2002; 112:406–411.
18. Clark O, Lyman G, Castro AA, Clark LGO, Djulbegovic B. Colony stimulating factors for the treatment of chemotherapy induced febrile neutropenia. *Cochrane Database Systematic Rev* 2003; 3:1–12 (CD 00 3039).

19. Lyman GH, Lyman CG, Sanderson RA, Balducci L. Decision analysis of hematopoietic growth factor use in patients receiving cancer chemotherapy. *J Natl Cancer Inst* 1993; 85:488–493.
20. Lyman GH, Balducci L. A cost analysis of hematopoietic colony-stimulating factors. *Oncology* 1995; 9:85–91.
21. Ozer H, Armitage JO, Bennett CL, et al. 2000 update of recommendations for the use of hematopoietic colony-stimulating factors: evidence-based clinical practice guidelines. *J Clin Oncol* 2000; 18:3558–3585.
22. Balducci L, Lyman GH, Ozer H. Patients aged >70 are at high risk of neutropenic infection and should receive hemopoietic growth factors when treated with moderately toxic chemotherapy. *J Clin Oncol* 2001; 19:1583–1585.
23. Lyman GH, Kuderer NM, Balducci L. Granulopoiesis stimulating agents: economic impact on the management of febrile neutropenia. *Curr Opin Oncol* 1998; 10:291–298.
24. Lyman GH, Kuderer NM, Balducci L. Economic analyses of the use of the colony-stimulating factors: an update. *Curr Opin Hematol* 1999; 6:145–151.
25. Lyman GH, Kuderer NM, Balducci L. Cost-benefit analysis of G-CSF in the management of elderly cancer patients. *Curr Opin Hematol* 2002; 9:207–214.
26. Wright JC, Weinstein MC. Gains in life expectancy from medical interventions—standardizing data on outcomes. *N Engl J Med* 1998; 330:380–404.
27. Cella DF, Bonomi AE. Measuring quality of life: 1995 update. *Oncology* 1995; 9:47–60.
28. Weeks J. Measurement of utilities and quality-adjusted survival. *Oncology* 1995; 9:67–70.
29. Gelber RD, Goldhirsch A, Cavelli F. Quality-of-life-adjusted evaluation of adjuvant therapy for operable breast cancer. *Ann Intern Med* 1991; 114:621–628.
30. Gotay CC, Korn EL, McCabe MS, Moore TD, Cheson BD. Quality-of-life assessment in cancer treatment protocols: research issues in protocol development. *J Natl Cancer Inst* 1992; 84:575–579.
31. Bottomley A, Vanvoorden V, Fletchner H, et al. The challenges and achievements involved in implementing quality of life research in cancer clinical trials. *Eur J Cancer* 2003; 39:275–285.
32. Lyman GH. Methodological issues related to health economic analysis in controlled clinical trials. In: Crowley J, ed. *Handbook of Statistics in Clinical Oncology.* New York: Marcel Dekker. 2001:291–320.
33. Lyman GH. The economics of randomized controlled trials. *Curr Oncol Rep* 2001; 3:396–403.
34. Djulbegovic B, Cantor A, Lyman GH, Ruckdeschel. Understanding treatment benefits and harms, evidence-based *Oncology* 2000; 1:66–68.
35. Lyman GH, Djulbegovic B. Understanding economic analyses: evidence-based. *Oncology* 2001; 2:2–5.
36. Detsky AS, Naglie IG. A clinician's guide to cost-effectiveness analysis. *Ann Intern Med* 1990; 113:147–154.
37. Task Force on Principles for Economic Analyses of Health Care Technology. Economic analyses of health care technology: a report on principles. *Ann Intern Med* 1995; 122:61–70.
38. American Society of Clinical Oncology. Outcomes of cancer treatment for technology assessment and cancer treatment guidelines. *J Clin Oncol* 1996; 14:671–679.
39. Russell LB, Gold MR, Siegel JE, Daniels N, Weinstein MC. The role of cost-effectiveness analysis in health and medicine. *JAMA* 1996; 276:1172–1177.
40. Weinstein MC, Siegel JE, Gold MR, Kamiet MS, Russell LB. Recommendations of the panel on cost-effectiveness in health and medicine. *JAMA* 1996; 276:1253–1258.
41. Siegel JE, Weinstein MC, Russell LB, Gold MR. Recommendations for reporting cost-effectiveness analysis. *JAMA* 1996; 276:1330–1341.
42. Brown M, Glick HA, Harrell F, et al. Integrating economic analysis into cancer clinical trials: the National Cancer Institute-American Society of Clinical Oncology Economics Workbook. *J Natl Cancer Inst* 1998; 24:1–28.
43. Coyle D, Davies L , Drummond MF. Trials and tribulations: emerging issues in designing economic evaluations alongside clinical trials. *Int J Technol Assess Health Care* 1998; 14:135–144.
44. Barber JA, Thompson SG. Analysis and interpretation of cost data in randomized controlled trials: review of published studies. *BMJ* 1998; 317:1195–1200.
45. Meza L, Baselga J, Holmes FA, et al. Incidence of febrile neutropenia is directly related to duration of severe neutropenia after myelosuppressive chemotherapy. *Proc ASCO* 2002; 21:255b.
46. Myelotoxicity and dose intensity of chemotherapy: Reporting practices from randomized clinical trials. *J Natl Comprehensive Cancer Network* 2003; 1:440–454.
47. Ellis GK, Livingston RB, Gralow JR, et al. Dose-dense anthracycline-based chemotherapy for node-positive breast cancer. *J Clin Oncol* 2002; 20:3637–3643.

48. Lyman GH, Crawford J, Dale D, et al. Incidence, practice patterns, and predictors of low dose intensity in adjuvant breast cancer chemotherapy: results of a nationwide survey of community oncology practices. *J Clin Oncol* 2003 (in press).
49. Lyman GH, Morrison VA, Dale DC, et al. Risk of febrile neutropenia among patients with intermediate-grade non-Hodgkin's lymphoma receiving CHOP chemotherapy. *Leuk Lymphoma* 2003; 44:2069–2076.
50. Lyman GH, Delgado D. Risk and timing of hospitalization for febrile neutropenia in patients receiving CHOP, CHOP-R, or CNOP chemotherapy for intermediate grades of non-Hodgkin's lymphoma. *Cancer* 2003 (in press).
51. Lyman GH, Lyman C, Ogboola Y. Risk models for the prediction of chemotherapy-induced neutropenia. *Neutropenia Oncol* 2001:1; 2–7.
52. Lyman GH. Risk assessment in oncology practice: from risk factors to risk models. *Oncology* 2003 (in press).
53. Lyman GH. A predictive model for neutropenia associated with cancer chemotherapy. *Pharmacotherapy* 2000; 20:1045–1115.
54. Silber JH, Fridman M, DiPaola RS, et al. First-cycle blood counts and subsequent neutropenia dose reduction or delay in early-stage breast cancer therapy. *J Clin Oncol* 1998; 16:2392–2400.
55. Rivera E, Erder MH, Moore TD, et al. Targeted filgrastim support in patients with early-stage breast carcinoma: toward the implementation of a risk model. *Cancer* 2003; 98:222–228.
56. Agboola O, Crawford J, Dale DC, et al. Risk models for neutropenic complications associated with breast cancer adjuvant chemotherapy. *Proc ASCO* 2002; 21:66a.
57. Talcott JA, Siegel RD, Finberg R, Goldman L. Risk assessment in cancer patients with fever and neutropenia: a prospective, two-center validation of a prediction rule. *J Clin Oncol* 1992; 10:316–322.
58. Kim YJ, Rubenstein EB, Rolston KV, et al. Colony-stimulating factors may reduce complications and death in solid tumor patients with fever and neutropenia. *Proc Am Soc Clin Oncol* 2000; 19:612a.
59. Lyman GH, Kuderer NM. Cost effectiveness of myeloid growth factors in cancer chemotherapy. *Curr Hematol Rep* 2003; 2:471–479.
60. Lyman GH, Kuderer NM. Incorporation of quality of life considerations into decision models for the use of colony stimulating factors in chemotherapy patients at risk for febrile neutropenia. In: Klastersky JA, ed., *Febrile Neutropenia.* New York: Springer-Verlag. 1997:17–22.
61. Fortner BV, Stolshek B, Schwartzberg LS, et al. Decline in absolute neutrophil count (ANC) is associated with lower quality of life (QOL) in cancer patients receiving docetaxel. *Proc ASCO* 2002; 21:2808a.
62. Okon TA, Fortner BV, Schwartzberg L, et al. Quality of life (QOL) in patients with grade IV chemotherapy-induced neutropenia (CIN). *Proc ASCO* 2002; 21:2920a.
63. Calhoun EA, Chang C-H, Welshman EE, Cella D. A neutropenia-specific quality of life instrument: rationale for the development of the FACT-N. *Proc ASCO* 2002; 21:1498a.
64. Lyman GH, Kuderer NM. Filgrastim in patients with neutropenia: potential effects on quality of life. *Drugs* 2002; 62:65–78.
65. Crawford J, Ozer H, Stoller R, Johnson D, et al. Reduction by granulocyte colony-stimulating factor of fever and neutropenia induced by chemotherapy in patients with small-cell lung cancer. *N Engl J Med* 1991; 325:164–170.
66. Trillet-Lenoir V, Green J, Manegold C, et al. Recombinant granulocyte colony stimulating factor reduces the infectious complications of cytotoxic chemotherapy. *Eur J Cancer* 1993; 29A:319–324.
67. Pettengell R, Gurney H, Radford JA, et al. Granulocyte colony-stimulating factor to prevent dose-limiting neutropenia in non-Hodgkin's lymphoma: a randomized controlled trial. *Blood* 1992; 80:1430–1436.
68. Chevallier B, Chollet P, Merrouche Y, et al. Lenograstim prevents morbidity from intensive induction chemotherapy in the treatment of inflammatory breast cancer. *J Clin Oncol* 1995; 13:1564–1571.
69. Bui BN, Chevallier B, Chevreau C, et al. Efficacy of lenograstim on hematologic tolerance to MAID chemotherapy in patients with advanced soft tissue sarcoma and consequences on treatment dose-intensity. *J Clin Oncol* 1995; 13:2629–2636.
70. Zinzani PL, Pavone E, Storti S, et al. Randomized trial with or without granulocyte colony-stimulating factor as adjunct to induction VNCOP-B treatment of elderly high-grade non-Hodgkin's lymphoma. *Blood* 1997; 89:3974–3979.
71. Gisselbrecht C, Haioun C, LePage E, et al. Placebo-controlled phase III study of lenograstim (glycosylated recombinant human granulocyte colony-stimulating factor) in aggressive non-Hodgkin's lymphoma: factors influencing chemotherapy administration. *Leuk Lymphoma* 1997; 25:289–300.

72. Fossa SD, Kaye SB, Mead GM, et al. Filgrastim during combination chemotherapy of patients with poor-prognosis metastatic germ cell malignancy. *J Clin Oncol* 1998; 16:716–724.
73. Maher DW, Graham JL, Green M, et al. Filgrastim in patients with chemotherapy-induced febrile neutropenia: a double blind, placebo-controlled trial. *Ann Intern Med* 1994; 121:492–501.
74. Mitchell PLR, Morland B, Stevens MCG, et al. Granulocyte colony-stimulating factor in established febrile neutropenia: a randomized study of pediatric patients. *J Clin Oncol* 1997; 15:1163–1170.
75. Garcia-Carbonero R, Mayordomo JI, Tornamira MV, et al. Granulocyte colony-stimulating factor in the treatment of high-risk febrile neutropenia: a multicenter randomized trial. *J Natl Cancer Inst* 2001; 93:31–38.
76. Balducci L, Hardy CL, Lyman GH. Hematopoietic growth factors in the older cancer patient. *Curr Opin Hematol* 2001; 8:170–187.
77. Lyman GH, Balducci L, Agboola Y. Use of hematopoietic growth factors in the older cancer patient. *Oncol Spectrums* 2001; 2:414–421.
78. Lyman GH, Kuderer NM. Epidemiology of febrile neutropenia. *Supp Cancer Ther* 2003 (in press).
79. Silber JH, Fridman, Shpilsky A, et al. Modeling the cost-effectiveness of granulocyte colony-stimulating factor use in early-stage breast cancer. *J Clin Oncol* 1998; 16:2435–2444.
80. Calhoun EA, Chang CH, Welshman EE, Fishman DA, Lurain JR, Bennett CL. Evaluating the total costs of chemotherapy-induced toxicity: results from a pilot study with ovarian cancer patients. *Oncologist* 2001; 6:441–445.
81. Cosler L, Calhoun E, Agboda O, Lyman GH. Impact of indirect and out-of-pocket costs on the risk threshold for prophylaxis with colony-stimulating factors in patients at risk for neutropenia complications. *Pharmacotherapy* 2003 (in press).
82. Talcott JA, Siegel RD, Finberg R, Goldman L. Risk assessment in cancer patients with fever and neutropenia: a prospective, two-center validation of a prediction rule. *J Clin Oncol* 1992; 10:316–322.
83. Talcott JA, Whalen A, Clark J, et al. Home antibiotic therapy for low-risk cancer patients with fever and neutropenia: a pilot study of 30 patients based on a validated prediction rule. *J Clin Oncol* 1994; 12:107–114.
84. Rubenstein EB, Rolston KVI, Benjamin RS, et al. Outpatient treatment of febrile episodes in low-risk neutropenic patients with cancer. *Cancer* 1993; 71:3640–3646.
85. Klastersky J, Paesmans M, Rubenstein EB, et al. The multinational association for supportive care in cancer risk-index: a multinational scoring system for identifying low-risk febrile neutropenic cancer patients. *J Clin Oncol* 2000; 18:3038–3051.
86. Sivasubramaniam V, Dale D, Crawford J, et al. Impact of outpatient treatment of febrile neutropenia on risk thresholds for G-CSF prophylaxis in cancer chemotherapy. *Proc Am Soc Clin Oncol* 2001; 20:392a.
87. Thatcher NT, Girling DJ, Hopwood P, et al. Improving survival without reducing quality of life in small-cell lung cancer patients by increasing the dose intensity of chemotherapy with granulocyte colony-stimulating factor support: results of a British Medical Research Council Multicenter Randomized Trial. *J Clin Oncol* 2000; 18:395–404.
88. Ellis GK, Livingston RB, Gralow JR, et al. Dose-dense anthracycline-based chemotherapy for node-positive breast cancer. *J Clin Oncol* 2002; 20:3637–3643.
89. Citron M, Berry D, Cirrincione C, et al. Superiority of dose-dense over conventional scheduling and equivalence of sequential vs combination adjuvant chemotherapy for node-positive breast cancer. *Breast Cancer Res Treat* 2002.
90. Nabholtz J-M, Cantin J, Chang J, et al. Phase III trial comparing granulocyte colony-stimulating factor to leridistim in the prevention of neutropenic complications in breast cancer patients treated with docetaxel/doxorubicin/cyclophosphamide: results of the BCIRG 004 Trial. *Clin Breast Cancer* 2002; 3:268–275.
91. Lyman GH, Lyman C, Agboola Y. Risk models for the prediction of chemotherapy-induced neutropenia. *Neutropenia Oncol* 2001; 1:2–7.
92. Lyman GH, Crawford J, Dale D, Wolf D. Predicting the risk of chemotherapy-induced neutropenia (CIN) in patients with breast cancer: rationale for prospective risk model development. *Breast Cancer Res Treat* 2002; 76:S537.
93. Anaissie EJ, Vartivarian S, Bodey GP, et al. Randomized comparison between antibiotics alone and antibiotics plus granulocyte-macrophage colony-stimulating factor (*Escherichia coli*-derived in cancer patients with fever and neutropenia. *Am J Med* 1996; 100:17–23.

94. Aviles A, Guzman R, Garcia EL, Talavera A, Diaz-Maqueo JC. Results of a randomized trial of granulocyte colony-stimulating factor in patients with infection and severe granulocytopenia. *Anticancer Drugs* 1996; 7:392–397.
95. Biesma B, de Vries EG, Willemse PH, et al. Efficacy and tolerability of recombinant human granulocyte-macrophage colony-stimulating factor in patients with chemotherapy-related leukopenia and fever. *Eur J Cancer* 1990; 26:932–936.
96. Lopez-Hernandez MA, Jimenez-Alvarado R, Borbolla-Escoboza R, et al. Granulocyte colony-stimulating factor in the treatment of febrile neutropenia]. *Gaceta Medica Mexicana* 2000; 136:99–105.
97. Mayordomo Jl, Rivera F, Diaz-Puente MT,, et al. Improving treatment of chemotherapy-induced neutropenic fever by administration of colony-stimulating factors. *J Natl Cancer Inst* 1995; 87:803–808.
98. Ravaud A, Chevreau C, Cany L, et al. Granulocyte-macrophage colony-stimulating factor in patients with neutropenic fever is potent after low-risk but not after high-risk neutropenic chemotherapy regimens: results of a randomized phase III trial. *J Clin Oncol* 1998; 16:2930–2936.
98. Riikonen P, Saarinen UM, Makipernaa A, et al. Recombinant human granulocyte-macrophage colony-stimulating factor in the treatment of febrile neutropenia: a double blind placebo-controlled study in children. *Pediatr Infect Dis J* 1994; 13:197–202.
99. Vellenga E, Uyl-de Groot CA, de Wit R, et al. Randomized placebo-controlled trial of granulocyte-macrophage colony-stimulating factor in patients with chemotherapy-related febrile neutropenia. *J Clin Oncol* 1996; 14:619–627.
100. Bertini M, Freilone R, Vitolo U, et al. The treatment of elderly patients with aggressive non-Hodgkin's lymphomas: Feasiblity and efficacy of an intensive multidrug regimen. *Leukemia Lymphoma* 1996; 22:483–493.
101. Osby E, Hagberg H, Kvaloy S, et al. CHOP is superior to CNOP in elderly patients with aggressive lymphoma while outcome is unaffected by filgrastim treatment: results of a Nordic Lymphoma Group randomized trial. *Blood* 2003; 101:3840–3848.
102. Zagonel V, Bagare R, Merola MC, et al. Cost-benefit of granulocyte colony-stimulating factor administration in older patients with non-Hodgkin's lymphoma treated with combination chemotherapy. *Ann Oncol* 1994; 5(suppl2): 127–132.

V FUTURE DIRECTIONS

22

Potential for Hematopoietic Growth Factor Antagonists in Oncology

Hayley S. Ramshaw, PhD, *Timothy R. Hercus*, PhD, *Ian N. Olver*, MD, PhD, *and Angel F. Lopez*, MD, PhD

CONTENTS

1. INTRODUCTION

Hematopoietic growth factors (HGFs) have long been implicated in the development and progression of malignancies. Their pleiotropic effect on cells of different tissues means that in principle they have the capacity to stimulate a wide variety of functions that can contribute to a malignant phenotype. Stimulation of cell proliferation can accelerate tumor cell growth and mass, whereas inhibition of apoptosis may give a malignant clone a distinct survival advantage over normal cells. Similarly, certain growth factors can influence angiogenesis, potentially regulating tumor neovascularization, and effects on adhesion phenomena may facilitate tumor-cell migration and metastases.

A role for HGFs in oncogenesis has received support from observations that abnormal production of HGFs, either in an autocrine or paracrine manner, can occur in certain malignancies such as leukemias. In addition, some HGF receptors normally expressed on the cell surface at very low levels are known to be overexpressed in certain solid tumors. This potential for excessive cell stimulation, whether it is from ligand or receptor origin, has strengthened the concept that some HGFs and their

From: *Cancer Drug Discovery and Development*
Hematopoietic Growth Factors in Oncology: Basic Science and Clinical Therapeutics
Edited by: G. Morstyn, M. A. Foote, and G. J. Lieschke © Humana Press Inc., Totowa, NJ

receptors participate in the oncogenic process. It is not surprising that significant efforts have been directed toward developing antagonists of growth factors.

In this review, we focus on antagonists of HGF that are being used clinically or are on the verge of entering clinical trials. We have taken a less strict view of what an antagonist is to encompass a variety of molecules that, although they may work at different levels on the ligand-receptor complex, all have as a common thread the inhibition of receptor-initiated signaling and cellular function. In the concluding section, current limitations with the use of HGF antagonists are discussed, as well as the potential and opportunities to improve their use in oncology.

2. HEMATOPOIETIC GROWTH FACTORS AND MECHANISM OF ACTION

Before expanding on HGF antagonists, it is important to comment briefly on the native HGFs themselves and on how many of them work. HGFs are small glycosylated peptides of about 25,000–30,000 MW, many of which are also called cytokines or interleukins (ILs). They are produced by a variety of cells in the body and can act either locally or at a distance. In this review, we refer largely to antagonists of growth factors that operate on the hematopoietic system but also discuss those antagonists of related growth factors that exhibit similar mechanism of action and are beginning to show clinical promise in oncology.

HGFs exert their activity by binding to cell surface receptors normally present in very low numbers. The receptors may be single polypeptide chains that bind ligand and also signal, as is the case for the macrophage colony-stimulating factor (M-CSF) or granulocyte-CSF (G-CSF) or comprise two or more chains. The receptors for granulocyte-macrophage-CSF (GM-CSF) and IL-3, on the other hand, have two subunits, a cytokine-binding subunit (α-chain) and a β-subunit, the major signaling subunit of the receptor.

A feature common to many HGFs is the use of receptor subunits that are shared by multiple HGFs. The IL-3, IL-5, and GM-CSF family of HGFs bind through ligand-specific receptor α-chains, but all use the β-common (β_c) receptor chain for signal transduction. Similarly, the receptors for the IL-6 family, which includes IL-6, IL-11, leukemia inhibitory factor (LIF), oncostatin M (OSM), ciliary neurotrophic factor (CNTF), and cardiotrophin (CT), all share and use the gp130 signaling chain. The epidermal growth factor (EGF) receptor (EGFR) is bound by several ligands other than EGF, including transforming growth factor-α (TGF-α), amphiregulin, heparin-binding EGF, epiregulin, and betacellulin. Members of the EGFR family of receptor tyrosine kinases, including EGF receptor (HER1/ErbB1), ErbB2 (Her2/Neu), ErbB3 (Her3), and ErbB4 (Her4), are capable of homo- and heterodimerization. The ErbB2 receptor that has no known natural ligand appears to act as the preferred heterodimerization and signaling partner for other ErbB receptors *(1)*, including ErbB3, which binds neuregulins and heregulins but lacks tyrosine kinase activity.

HGFs and related growth factors activate their receptors by inducing homo- or heterodimerization of cell surface-receptor chains, leading to receptor phosphorylation by intrinsic or associated kinases and recruitment of accessory signaling molecules. The receptors for some growth factors have intrinsic tyrosine kinase activity, typified by EGF, whereas certain HGF receptors, such as those for GM-CSF and IL-6, have receptor-associated kinases such as those of the JAK family of tyrosine kinases. Receptor dimerization brings into close proximity these tyrosine kinases that transphosphorylate the receptors, creating docking sites on which adaptor molecules can bind and initiate a cascade of biochemical events. This signaling downstream of the receptor involves multiple biochemical pathways that, although integrated, may be dissected into modules, and that in some cases can be ascribed to specific biologic responses. This process offers the potential to provide targets for the inhibition of specific HGF-mediated responses such as cell survival, proliferation, or other functions involved in oncogenesis.

3. CATEGORIES OF ANTAGONISTS BASED ON MODE OF ACTION

Strategies to block biologic signals arising from HGF receptors generally attempt to prevent the assembly of an active ligand-receptor complex or to perturb the transduction of intracellular signaling events from an activated ligand-receptor complex (Fig. 1). Different types of receptor antagonists have been generated, depending on their target in the ligand-receptor complex, their mechanism of action, or their molecular nature.

One type of HGF antagonist is represented by soluble receptors. Soluble HGF receptors arise in vivo as a result of alternative splicing or proteolytic cleavage (reviewed in ref. *2*) and antagonize growth factor function by sequestering their ligand in solution, thereby preventing HGF-mediated dimerization and activation of cell-associated receptors. Recombinant soluble HGF receptors have shown antagonist activity for several HGF and related growth factors including GM-CSF *(3)*, vascular endothelial growth factor (VEGF) *(4)*, and TNF-α *(5)*. Of these, the soluble TNF receptor antagonist is being used clinically, albeit largely in inflammatory conditions *(6)*.

A second type of HGF antagonist involves specific monoclonal antibodies (MAbs). These MAbs may be directed against either the HGF itself or against receptor components and are becoming a common method of antagonizing HGF function in vivo. In the case of antibodies (Abs) to the HGF, their effect is believed to extend from simply blocking their interaction with the appropriate receptor to promoting clearance of the HGF from the circulation. Abs directed toward the receptor may be directed against the specific cytokine-binding subunit *(7)* or the signaling subunit shared by two or more receptors *(8)*. Antagonistic Abs have been generated against ligand and receptor components of many HGFs, including GM-CSF receptor *(7,8)*, EGF receptor *(9,10)*, VEGF *(11)*, IL-6 *(12)*, IL-6R *(13)*, and TNF-α *(14)*. An interesting variation of the antagonistic Ab approach involved vaccination with an IL-6 antagonist to elicit a polyclonal Ab response, with at least some of the Abs possessing IL-6-neutralizing activity *(15)*.

Alternative strategies have been explored to discover novel inhibitors of HGF-receptor activation, with peptide phage display being a common example. Small peptides that are able to bind HGFs or their receptors, thereby preventing the assembly of an active ligand-receptor complex, have been reported for IL-1 *(16)* and VEGF *(17,18)*.

A third type of receptor antagonist involves the engineering of natural ligands so that they can bind the natural receptor but are unable to induce receptor oligomerization and signal transduction. Antagonistic analogs have been reported for many HGFs including IL-6 *(19)*, GM-CSF *(20)*, and VEGF *(21–23)*. The antagonists for GM-CSF and IL-6

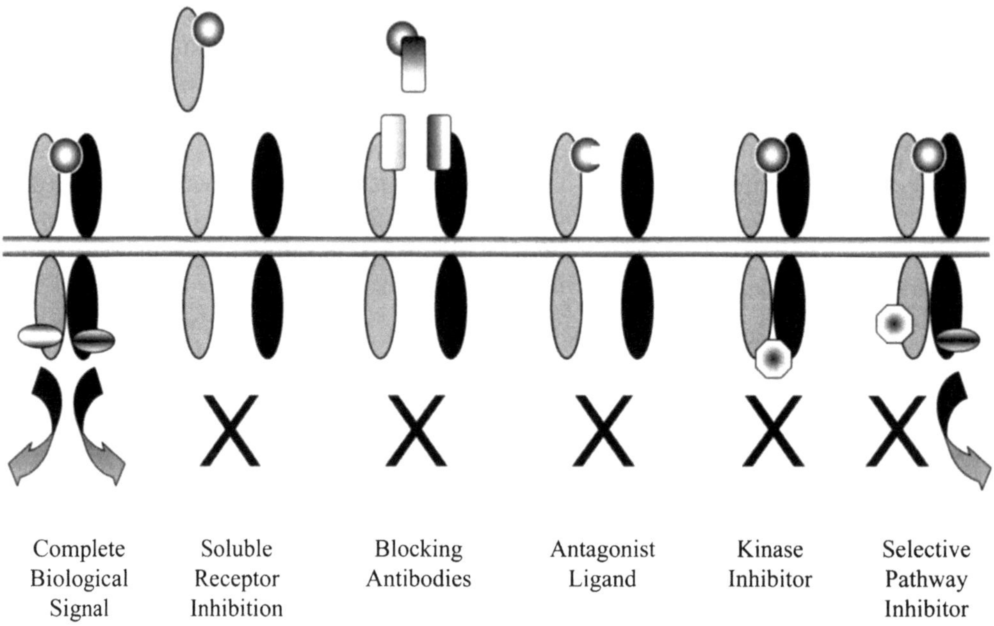

Fig. 1. The activation of hematopoietic growth factor (HGF) receptors is mediated by the ligand-induced homo- or heterodimerization of cell surface receptor chains, resulting in receptor phosphorylation by intrinsic or associated kinases and the recruitment of a raft of accessory signaling molecules. A number of strategies have been devised that are able to perturb the receptor activation process and, as a consequence, inhibit signaling from the HGF receptors. The presence of HGF binding soluble receptors sequesters HGF into a soluble complex that is unable to activate cell surface receptors. Neutralizing antibodies act to block the formation of an active HGF-receptor complex by preventing HGF association with receptor or by interfering with receptor dimerization. Antagonist ligands bind specific HGF receptor chains through the HGF binding site but lack an active second receptor binding site so are unable to induce receptor dimerization. The intrinsic tyrosine kinase activity typical of some HGF receptors and required for signaling can be targeted by enzyme inhibitors that bind to cytoplasmic regions of the receptor associated with tyrosine kinase activity. Specific motifs in the cytoplasmic regions of HGF receptors, used for the binding of accessory signaling molecules, may be amenable to blockade by cell-permeable inhibitors leading to the inhibition of specific signaling pathways associated with cell survival or proliferation.

involved discrete mutations that abolished HGF interaction with the receptor-signaling subunit while preserving or enhancing the interaction with the major binding subunits, thus behaving as classical competitive antagonists. HGF antagonists exist in nature, as illustrated by the IL-1 antagonist IL-1Ra *(24,25)*.

A fourth and exciting modality of blocking HGF action involves targeting critical cytoplasmic regions of the receptor rather than the extracellular ligand binding sites of HGF receptors. Small molecules are being designed and developed that do just this, as exemplified by low-molecular-weight, selective inhibitors of HGF receptor tyrosine kinase activity. The drug STI-571 binds to the ATP binding site of tyrosine kinase domains, thereby blocking tyrosine kinase function *(26)*. Kinase inhibitors have been developed for use against EGF receptor (reviewed in ref. *27*) and VEGF-R2 *(28)*.

The next generation of HGF blockers awaits the identification of specific functional motifs in the cytoplasmic region of HGF receptors coupled to specific functions, which may provide an opportunity to develop small molecules able to target the relevant motif, thereby preventing the recruitment of proteins required for activation of a specific signal-transduction pathway *(29)*.

4. USE OF ANTAGONISTS IN MYELOID LEUKEMIAS

Human leukemias are a complex and heterogeneous group of diseases, which until recently had very few therapeutic options. The role of HGFs in leukemia is well documented, so directing therapies against HGFs, either themselves or their receptors, may provide a therapeutic alternative to chemotherapy or bone marrow transplantation (BMT). Each of these two treatments has toxicity problems. For BMT, mortality rates are between 10 and 40% depending on donor source and patient age *(30,31)*. GM-CSF is a pleiotropic cytokine that stimulates the production of a wide variety of cell types including macrophages, eosinophils, and neutrophils. Receptors capable of binding GM-CSF with high affinity have been detected on a several hematopoietic cell types including bone marrow cells, primary myeloid leukemias, a variety of hematopoietic cell lines, neutrophils, monocytes, eosinophils, and basophils. Autocrine or paracrine production of GM-CSF is believed to play a role in at least some cases of acute myeloid leukemia (AML), chronic myelogenous leukemia (CML), chronic myelomonocytic leukemia (CMML), and juvenile myelomonocytic leukemia (JMML); blocking the interaction of this cytokine with its receptor may provide a therapeutic option for some of these diseases.

Other cytokines are able to compensate for the lack of GM-CSF, as evidenced by GM-CSF knockout mice and mice that lack the β_c of the GM-CSF receptor. These animals have no reduction or abnormalities in their hematopoietic compartment *(32)*. Thus, the disruption of the interaction between GM-CSF and its receptor may provide a therapy with potentially few effects on normal cells. The ability to inhibit the action of GM-CSF specifically has become possible with the discovery of a specific antagonist, E21R.

A group of leukemias is characterized by the expression of molecular abnormalities that result in dysfunctional signaling from cytokines and their receptors. Examples of such abnormalities are seen across a wide spectrum of diseases including CML, AML, and acute promyelocytic leukemia (APL). The most commonly described of these is a translocation of chromosomes 9 and 22 in CML, leading to the generation of the Philadelphia chromosome. The *abl* oncogene (from chromosome 9) becomes fused head to tail with the *bcr* (breakpoint cluster region) gene on chromosome 22 to produce an abnormal protein with an enhanced tyrosine kinase activity relative to p145, the normal *abl* gene product *(33)*. This 210-kDa bcr/abl fusion protein ($p210^{bcr\text{-}abl}$) leads to induction of inappropriate mitosis in target cells *(34)*. Mice reconstituted with cells that express $p210^{bcr\text{-}abl}$ develop a CML-like disease, which is transplantable to secondary recipient animals *(35,36)*. Engraftment of these $p210^{bcr\text{-}abl}$-expressing cells results in unusually high concentrations of IL-3 and GM-CSF in the diseased mice, similar to the condition of patients with CML *(36,37)*.

Patients with AML exhibit a range of molecular abnormalities, but the most common are within the N-*ras* proto-oncogene, which is seen in AML, with a frequency of almost 25%. Ras proteins cycle between an active guanosine triphosphate (GTP)-bound state (GTP-Ras) and an inactive guanosine diphosphate (GDP)-bound state (GDP-Ras). The mutated N-*ras* in AML is thought to deregulate the pathway that normally controls the growth and differentiation of the immature myeloid cells. These point mutations lead to an accumulation of the activated GTP-bound N-*ras* owing to a decreased GTPase activity of N-*ras*. Activation of Ras is an essential component of the proliferative response seen when cytokines bind to their receptors. Additionally, children with JMML frequently exhibit dysregulation of the Ras pathway. They have either activating point mutations in their *Ras* genes or lose the neurofibromin gene (NF1) *(38)*. *NF1* is a tumor-suppressor gene that also acts as a Ras GTPase-activating protein *(39)* and plays a role in the aberrant response of leukemic cells to growth factors. The lack of the neurofibromin gene leads to a hyper-response to GM-CSF, as shown by in vitro assays such as semisolid colony cultures *(38–40)*. The mechanism of this hypersensitivity has not been fully elucidated, but it is generally considered that the hyper-response to GM-CSF results from the deregulated signaling through the Ras pathway.

Another subset of leukemias and other malignancies exhibit several mutations in class 3 receptor tyrosine kinases, including Flt3, kit (stem cell factor [SCF] receptor), FMS (M-CSF receptor), and the platelet-derived growth factor (PDGF) receptor. The binding of ligand to the extracellular domain of receptor tyrosine kinase leads to receptor dimerization and stabilizes the catalytic intracellular domain leading to phosphorylation of tyrosine residues. Greater than 20% of cases of AML have mutations in the Flt3 receptor, which exhibit an internal tandem duplication of the membrane proximal domain and lead to constitutive dimerization and autophosphorylation. Additionally, point mutations in the intracellular activation domain of Flt3 that lead to autophosphorylation of the receptor have been identified in 7% of all patients with AML *(41)*. One other receptor tyrosine kinase mutation seen in leukemia involves a subgroup of CMML patients with a t(5;12) translocation. This translocation fuses the tyrosine kinase domain of the PDGF receptor with the *tel* gene (an *ets*-like transcription factor that is mutated in several myeloid leukemias) *(42)* and constitutively activates the PDGF receptor tyrosine kinase domain, leading to transformation of cells *(43)*.

Although these examples confirm the importance of alterations in cytokine receptors and signaling molecules in leukemogenesis, the role of dysregulation of cytokine production is less clear.

Serum-free culture conditions have been used to illustrate the fact that SCF can stimulate the Philadelphia chromosome-positive cells from patients with CML while not affecting the normal cells *(44)*. This situation is thought to be owing to a complex formation between the SCF receptor $p145^{c\text{-}kit}$ and the $p210^{bcr\text{-}abl}$, a complex that is unable to form in normal cells due to lack of $p210^{bcr\text{-}abl}$. Using fluorescence-activated cell sorting (FACS), primitive cells from patients with CML were isolated and shown by reverse-transcription polymerase chain reaction (RT-PCR) to have transcripts for both IL-3 and G-CSF *(37)*. In the primitive state, these cells possess high potential for autonomous growth, but as they mature they lose the expression of these cytokines and become factor-dependent. Additionally, SCF from serum of patients may synergize with IL-3 or G-CSF to enable the high level of proliferation of the leukemic clone seen in CML.

In the pediatric disorder JMML, dysregulation of the *Ras* signaling pathway leads to a marked hypersensitivity to GM-CSF *(45)*. Unlike those of normal subjects, bone marrow cells from patients with JMML form colonies in the absence of added cytokines *(46)*. Additionally, patients with JMML have suppressed hematopoiesis, giving a competitive advantage to the diseased clone of cells. The adult disorder CMML also produces the phenomenon of spontaneous colony growth. GM-CSF is thought to be the primary stimulant, but this cytokine may stimulate the action of IL-6 *(47)*. Inhibition of GM-CSF leads to negative growth effects on in vitro colony formation, possibly through IL-10 *(48,49)*. Additionally, studies in our laboratory have shown a direct role for GM-CSF in the pathogenesis of CMML *(50)*. Spontaneous colonies formed from bone marrow mononuclear cells from patients with CMML are reduced by up to 98% by the addition of the GM-CSF antagonist E21R (*see* Subheading 4.5. for details of E21R action). AML cells have been shown to have reduced colony growth from neutralizing antiserum to GM-CSF *(51)*. Therefore, therapies targeting key cytokines such as GM-CSF may have the capacity to decrease their proliferative capacity in vivo.

Advances in the understanding of the molecular basis of these disorders are continuously leading to the development of more targeted therapies, with HGF antagonists being at its forefront. Autocrine and paracrine stimulation of leukemic cells in vitro by growth factors has been shown for several leukemias, including AML *(52,53)*, CML *(37)*, JMML *(46,54)*, CMML *(55,56)*, and polycythemia vera *(57)*, raising the possibility that these HGFs have an oncogenic role in vivo.

4.1. TNF Antagonists

Several TNF-α antagonists have been developed for a variety of conditions, generally for inflammatory disorders *(6)*. However, growth of AML cells in vitro can be regulated by TNF-α. Amounts of TNF-α are increased in the serum of patients with chronic and acute leukemia, especially with advanced forms of disease *(58)*, and in some patients with myelodysplastic syndromes (MDS) *(59)*. TNF-α enhances GM-CSF/IL-3-induced growth but suppresses G-CSF-stimulated cell proliferation *(58)*. Spontaneous growth of JMML cells is reduced by the addition of Abs to TNF-α, although this is thought to be indirect since the action of TNF-α can be overcome by Abs to GM-CSF *(60)*. Exploitation of this phenomenon could identify TNF-α as a therapeutic target in a number of leukemias *(61)*.

4.2. IL-1 Antagonists

IL-1 is composed of three separate proteins, IL-1α, IL-1β, and IL-1ra. These proteins cause secretion of other cytokines including G-CSF and IL-6, and act as mediators of inflammation and immune modulation *(62)*. IL-1ra acts as an antagonist by binding to the receptor without inducing signals in vitro. It is unclear, however, whether IL-1ra actually acts as an antagonist in vivo since it is found in high concentration at sites of inflammation in patients with rheumatoid arthritis *(62)*. Patients with advanced CML and AML have increased amounts of IL-1β *(52,63,64)*, with patients with CML often exhibiting reduced expression of IL-1ra *(65)*. The potential for IL-1 inhibitors to be used as therapies for leukemia has been investigated, and research has shown that the presence of IL-1ra reduces colony formation and suppresses growth of progenitor cells in colony assays *(66)*. Although these in vitro studies have implied a potential clinical role for IL-1ra in AML, to date no clinical studies have been described.

4.3. IL-6 Antagonists

The IL-6 family of proteins includes LIF, OSM, CNTF, CT, IL-11, and IL-6. All these proteins use the common signaling chain gp130. Binding of IL-6 to thc IL-6 receptor α-chain (IL6-Rα) enables oligomerization with gp130, leading to signaling. Several agents for antagonizing IL-6 function have been described and efficacy demonstrated in vitro or in vivo. These include IL-6 antagonist ligands, an IL-6 vaccine, and neutralizing MAbs specific for IL-6 or IL-6-Rα. A family of IL-6 antagonists has been developed by introducing multiple amino acid substitutions into IL-6 that abolish or perturb IL-6-gp130 interactions while maintaining or enhancing the binding affinity of the IL-6-IL-6Rα interaction *(19,67)*.

Hyper-IL-6 (H-IL-6) is a designed, generated antagonist formed by the combination of an IL-6 antagonist defective in site II or site III interactions fused together with the soluble IL-6 receptor (sIL-6Rα) through a protein linker *(68)*. H-IL-6 acts on cells that express the IL-6 receptor, including hematopoietic cells, but, unlike IL-6, it is able to bind to all cells that express gp130 *(69)*, which means that it can completely neutralize not only IL-6 action, but also that of other family members that act by gp130. The neutralization of gp130, however, may not prove to be a useful therapeutic option owing to drastic consequences, which is implied by the data from gp130 homozygous knockout mice who are not viable *(69)*. The IL-6 vaccine strategy uses an antagonist analog of IL-6 (Sant1) as an antigen to elicit a polyclonal Ab response able to neutralize endogenous IL-6 function. In a human IL-6-transgenic mouse model, immunization with Sant1 was shown to correct fully the clinical and biologic effects associated with chronic overproduction of IL-6 *(15)*. Abs that block IL-6 function have been generated against both IL-6 *(12,70)* and IL-6Rα *(71)*. Additionally, the proteolytic cleavage form of gp130, soluble gp130 (sgp130), which is secreted by melanoma cell lines, may be a natural antagonist for members of this family *(72)*.

4.4. Imatinib in Chronic Myelogenous Leukemia

For CML, the tyrosine kinase inhibitor STI-571 has recently shown remission potential even for patients in blast crisis *(73,74)*. Imatinib inhibits the constitutively active tyrosine kinase product of the Bcr-Abl fusion gene and inhibits the Abl tyrosine kinase *(75)*. Using a variety of in vitro assays, imatinib has been shown to inhibit autophosphorylation of v-abl, PDGFR, and Kit receptor at submicromolar concentrations and also to block both mitogen-activated protein (MAP) kinase activation and c-fos mRNA expression *(76)*. Imatinib can reduce proliferation of Bcr-Abl-expressing cells and reduce colony formation from only the Bcr-Abl-positive cells while leaving the chromosomally normal cells unaffected *(77)*.

Phase 1 and 2 studies using this drug have shown dramatic early responses (within 3 wk), with a high incidence of complete hematologic and molecular responses in patients receiving daily doses *(76,78)*. High response rates have been reported in patients with CML myeloid blast crisis, which is generally considered to be a highly resistant form of the disease *(74)*. Current research is focusing on combination therapies with imatinib being used with chemotherapeutic agents or with interferon-γ (IFN-γ) *(79)*.

Despite the remarkable efficacy of imatinib in the treatment of CML, primary (no initial response) and secondary (developed after an initial response) resistance has been observed, particularly in patients with acute leukemia. Patients with chronic-phase disease show a favorable and durable response to imatinib, but when tested by PCR, most retain some level of Philadelphia chromosome-positive leukemic cells *(80)*. In at least some situations, the activity of GM-CSF and IL-3 may protect Bcr-Abl^{+} leukemic cells from the effects of imatinib. The activity of imatinib on leukemic cells isolated from patients with chronic-phase CML was shown to be significantly reduced (median inhibitory concentration [IC_{50}] = 0.46 μM –0.12 SE vs 2.57 μM –0.42 SE) in the presence of 500 U/mL exogenous GM-CSF *(81)*. The IL-3-responsive, p210$^{Bcr\text{-}Abl}$ transformed cell lines 32Dp210$^{Bcr\text{-}Abl}$, and Baf3p210$^{Bcr\text{-}Abl}$ undergo apoptosis when incubated with Bcr-Abl tyrosine kinase inhibitors such as imatinib but the effects of these inhibitors on cell viability were blocked when the cells were cultured in 10 ng/mL exogenous recombinant IL-3 *(82)*. These observations suggest that inhibition of GM-CSF and IL-3 may enhance the effectiveness of imatinib treatment in CML.

4.5. The GM-CSF Antagonist E21R

The GM-CSF antagonist E21R was generated following directed substitution of residues along the GM-CSF molecule. Examination of regions of interaction between the cytokine and receptor suggested the appropriate region for mutagenesis. Substitution of the Glu^{21} of wild-type GM-CSF with an arginine highlighted the essential role of this residue for binding to the high-affinity receptor (β_c) but not the low-affinity receptor (β alone), indicating that Glu_{21} must be a critical β_c contact residue. Additionally, mutations at this position exhibited a variety of activities, with the most striking seen by a charge reversal at this position. Introduction of the basic amino acids arginine or lysine eliminated all typical GM-CSF agonistic activity. Importantly, since the two charge reversal mutants (E21R and E21K) are able to retain essentially unaltered binding to the α-chain of the receptor, they can act as competitive antagonists *(20)*. We have shown in vitro a direct interaction between GM-CSF and a soluble form of β_c that is abolished in the GM-CSF antagonist E21R *(83)*, providing further evidence of the key role played by Glu_{21} in the action of GM-CSF. Experiments have shown that E21R is able both to inhibit the in vitro proliferation of JMML and to induce apoptosis in those cells that express the GM-CSF receptor *(84)*. Additionally, injection of the antagonist into NOD/SCID mice transplanted with human JMML cells can both prevent the engraftment and development of the leukemia and eradicate an established leukemia in animals *(85)*.

Formal preclinical toxicology and dose-finding studies were done in two baboon studies. For the first trial, nine animals received daily subcutaneous injections of E21R for 21 d, 3 at each dose level: 10, 100, and 1000 μg/kg/d. Two control animals received saline injections. Clinical, biochemical, and hematologic variables were measured. The second trial was an extension of the first in which six animals (three male, three female) received daily sc injections of E21R for 21 d, at 1000 μg/kg/d. Four control animals (two male, two female) received saline injections. Clinical, biochemical, and hematologic variables were measured. All animals were euthanized 1 d after the last injection, and histopathologic analysis was undertaken on a range of organs and tissues. The only biologic effects observed in the treated baboons were transient, non-dose-related increases in the circulating eosinophil and neutrophil numbers seen in some animals. No other significant biologic effects were noted. In the second study, peak serum E21R concentrations varied in the six treated baboons, ranging from approx 180 to 1800 ng/mL. The studies in baboons confirmed that significant circulating amounts of E21R could be achieved in vivo without significant toxicity. No consistent hematologic effects (apart from the mild eosinophilia and neutrophilia) were noted, and nothing suggested pulmonary toxicity.

This later effect was a concern given the syndrome of pulmonary alveolar proteinosis seen in the GM-CSF knockout mouse model *(86)*.

Based on preclinical baboon studies, a phase 1 toxicity and dose-escalation study was done at the Royal Adelaide Hospital. The phase 1 study of E21R enrolled patients with terminal solid organ malignancies *(87)*. Cohorts of three patients received doses of 10, 30, 100, 300, 600, and 1000 μg/kg/d given sc, daily for 10 d. Eligible patients had solid tumors known to express GM-CSF receptors (breast, prostate, colon, lung cancer, and melanoma). No bone marrow involvement or concomitant steroids were permitted. Twenty-two patients (18 men and 4 women, median age 60 yr) received doses ranging from 10 to 1000 μg/kg/d. Ten patients with colon cancer, four with prostate, three with lung, three with melanoma, and two with breast cancer were enrolled.

E21R was well tolerated with, the most severe toxicities being World Health Organization grade 3 injection site erythema ($n = 1$), grade 2 lethargy ($n = 3$), grade 2 muscle aches and soreness ($n = 1$), grade 2 joint pains ($n = 1$), and grade 2 thirst ($n = 1$). Dose-dependent transient mild eosinophilia was noted from d 3. Serum from patients treated at 600 μg/kg/d or higher antagonized GM-CSF-mediated TF-1 cell proliferation in vitro. No evidence of pulmonary toxicity was seen based on symptoms, examination findings, or changes in circulating surfactant concentrations. In 10 of these patients with solid tumors, stable disease was the best response. A further hint of activity was observed in two of the four patients with prostate cancer, one at the initial and one at the final dose level who had decreases in their prostate-specific antigen concentration and received a second cycle of E21R. This study confirmed that E21R could be administered safely for 10 d. It further confirmed that levels of up to 1 μg/mL E21R could be achieved in vivo in serum. These concentrations are comparable to the concentrations required to inhibit GM-CSF activity in vitro.

E21R has been administered on compassionate grounds to a few children with JMML. The first was an 8-yr-old patient who was considered to be at a very late stage of the disease. He received two 10-d courses and one 14-d course of E21R at 1 mg/kg/d administered as daily sc infusions. After the first two courses of treatment, his white blood cell count decreased from 51.7×10^9/L to 6.2×10^9/L (normal range: 4–10×10^9/L), and monocyte count was reduced from 21.2×10^9/L to 1.6×10^9/L (normal range: 0.1–1.0×10^9/L). The patient's general condition improved, with reduced pain and greater activity. No adverse effects were associated with the treatment. Between the second and third courses of treatment, the patient underwent a blast crisis, his condition worsened, and, despite a third course of E21R, he died. Although the patient did not survive after E21R treatment, the treating clinician considered that he would have died sooner if that treatment had not been given. It was felt that the response to E21R indicated that the agent could act in vivo in patients, in a way consistent with its in vitro actions *(88)*.

5. HEMATOPOIETIC GROWTH FACTOR ANTAGONISTS IN MULTIPLE MYELOMA

The therapeutic use of antagonists of IL-6 in patients with AML *(89)* or multiple myeloma has been described. IL-6 has a major role in the pathogenesis of multiple myeloma by promoting tumor survival and preventing dexamethasone-induced apoptosis *(12,90)*. Inhibition of IL-6 activity has been shown to induce apoptosis in a

Table 1
Summary of Existing Hemopoietic Growth Factor Antagonists and Their Molecular and Oncologic Targets

Agent	*Target and/or mode of action*	*Diseases*	*Ref.*
Trastuzumab	Anti-HER2 MAb	Breast cancer	*95,96*
Bevacizumab	Anti-VEGF MAb	Breast, prostate, and colorectal cancers	*11*
CLB IL6/8	Anti-IL-6 MAb	Multiple myeloma, breast cancer	*70*
Cetuximab	Anti-EGFR MAb	Head and neck, colorectal cancers	*99*
Sant7	IL-6 antagonist	Prostate cancer, Castleman's disease	*15*
E21R	GM-CSF antagonist	AML, JMML, breast and prostate cancers	*83–88*
Imatinib	TK inhibitor	CML, gastrointestinal stromal tumour	*73–77*
Gefitinib	EGFR TK	Ovarian, pancreatic, and prostate cancers	*94,100,101*
Semaxanib	VEGF-R2 TK	Colon cancer	*102*

ABBREVIATIONS: VEGF, vascular endothelial growth factor; IL, interleukin; EGFR, epidermal growth factor receptor; GM-CSF, granulocyte-macrophage colony-stimulating factor; TK, tyrosine kinase; AML, acute myeloid leukemia; JMML, juvenile myelomonocytic leukemia; CML, chronic myelogenous leukemia.

myeloma cell line and freshly isolated myeloma cells *(13)*. Blockade of IL-6 function may not be sufficient to inhibit myeloma proliferation or survival in the presence of bone marrow stromal cells *(91)* but may enhance the antiproliferative and proapoptotic effects of cytotoxic drugs *(12,92,93)*. Clinical studies in patients with advanced multiple myeloma support the idea that anti-IL-6 therapy enhances the action of cytotoxic drugs. A phase 1 study using a chimeric anti-IL-6 MAb as a single agent found no evidence of efficacy *(70)*. In contrast, a phase 2 study using a murine anti-IL-6 MAb in combination with dexamethasone and high-dose melphalan induced a high complete response rate *(12)*.

6. SOLID TUMORS

A major initiative in the control of solid tumors has been the advent of therapies targeted specifically to cancer cells. This succeeds the strategy of developing cytotoxic drugs that disrupt the DNA of any dividing cells, resulting in widespread normal tissue toxicity. New targets include proteins involved in cell-signaling pathways, antigens, or growth factor receptors on the cell surface. Targeted therapies already used in the treatment of solid tumors include the MAb trastuzumab in breast cancer, imatinib for patients with gastrointestinal stromal tumors, and the tyrosine kinase inhibitor gefitinib, which targets the tyrosine kinase associated with EGF commonly expressed in squamous cell carcinomas (Table 1) *(94)*.

6.1. Breast Cancer Treatment With MAb Anti-HER2

Trastuzumab targets a HER-2, a member of the EGF receptor/erbB family. This MAb is effective when the *Her2* gene is overexpressed, as seen in 25–30% of breast cancers *(95)*. In a study of 108 assessable women whose metastatic breast cancer overexpressed HER2, an objective response rate of 34% was reported *(96)*.

6.2. Gastrointestinal Stromal Tumors Treated With Imatinib

The success of the small molecule imatinib in gastrointestinal stromal tumors provides an outstanding example that the strategy of targeted therapies can be useful in solid tumors *(97)*. Conventional systemic chemotherapy is ineffective in gastrointestinal stromal tumors. For example, the intense DMAP (dacarbazine, mitomycin, doxorubicin, and cisplatin) regimen plus rHuGM-CSF achieved a 1.8% objective response compared with a 61% response in other leiomyosarcomas in one comparative study *(98)*. A response rate of 54% has been reported in patients with advanced gastrointestinal stromal tumors treated with imantinib, with an estimated 1-yr survival of 88% *(97)*.

6.3. Lung Cancer Treatment

EGF receptor regulates the growth of many types of cells. EGF receptor overexpression is common in lung cancer. The EGF receptor can be blocked by an Ab such as the human-chimeric MAb cetuximab that binds to its extracellular domain or by small molecules such as gefitinib, a reversible inhibitor of EGF receptor tyrosine kinase *(94,99)*. In two large phase 2 trials of patients previously treated with chemotherapy for nonsmall-cell lung cancer (NSCLC), response rates of up to 19% were reported for gefitinib *(100,101)*.

6.4. Other Solid Tumors

VEGF is a potent endothelial cell growth and survival factor, essential for normal vascularization and tumor angiogenesis. Inhibition of VEGF activity with the small molecule tyrosine kinase inhibitor semaxanib in a phase 1 study of 22 patients with a range of solid tumors was found to produce a clinical benefit in 4/19 eligible patients *(102)*.

6.5. Prostate Cancer

Considerable evidence indicates that IL-6 is a pathologic agent in prostate cancer, with serum IL-6 concentrations correlating with tumor burden and patient morbidity *(103)*. The growth of prostate cancer cells in vitro can be regulated by exogenous IL-6 in a paracrine or an autocrine manner *(104,105)*, whereas chronic exposure to IL-6 may facilitate prostate tumor growth *(106)*. Inhibition of IL-6 signaling through the gp130 subunit blocks IL-6-mediated proliferation of the PC-3 prostate cancer cell line and sensitizes the cells to cytotoxic drugs *(107)*. In vitro studies with prostate cancer cell lines has shown that IL-6 is able to increase androgen receptor expression and induce an androgen receptor response in prostate cancer cell lines *(108,109)*. Aromatase has a pivotal role in controlling estrogen synthesis, and aromatase inhibitors have been used to treat hormone-dependent breast cancer in postmenopausal women *(110)*. Exogenous IL-6 can stimulate aromatase activity in cultured fibroblasts from normal or malignant breast tissue.

GM-CSF receptors are known to be expressed on certain solid tumors, including breast cancer, NSCLC, small-cell lung cancer, prostate cancer, colorectal cancer, and melanoma, but their importance in promoting cell growth is not well defined *(87)*. Exogenous GM-CSF has been shown to stimulate cell proliferation in small-cell carcinoma lines *(111)* and the LNCaP prostate cancer cell line *(112)*; however, the potential therapeutic usefulness of blocking GM-CSF action in these diseases is not known.

7. FUTURE DIRECTIONS

As we gather more experience in the use of HGF antagonists in clinical medicine and learn more about the mechanism of action of HGF receptors and the fundamental processes underlying oncogenesis, a few options for improvement are beginning to emerge.

In observing the biologic response of certain malignancies to HGFs, it is clear that redundancy exists. For example, some cases of AML may respond similarly to GM-CSF and IL-3 mainly because the receptors for this HGF share the signaling subunit β_c. In CML too, both GM-CSF and IL-3 have been implicated in promoting the expansion of leukemic clones. In some conditions, therefore, it would be advantageous, if not necessary, to block two or more HGFs, which may be possible by targeting receptor subunits such as β_c that are shared by two or more receptors. Proof of principle for this approach has been obtained with the MAb BION-1, which, by binding to the common binding site in β_c used by GM-CSF, IL-3, and IL-5, can simultaneously antagonize the effect of these three HGFs.

As it is becoming clear that several signaling pathways are being triggered by HGFs binding to their receptors and that at least some of them can be linked to certain functions, it may be possible in the future to design drugs with selective HGF antagonist properties that tackle only a biologically relevant pathway, for example, one that leads to proliferation or cell survival.

As part of their clinical development, HGF antagonists have been used largely as single agents. The expectation that a single HGF would be solely responsible for malignancy may be seen as too high, with the exception of a few diseases in which the malignant cells are completely HGF-dependent. An alternative strategy would be to use HGF antagonists together with other anticancer agents such as cytotoxic drugs, a combination that may lead to wider therapeutic effects while allowing a lowering of cytotoxic dosage, thus minimizing side effects.

The next step for targeted therapies in solid tumors is to consider combination therapies. Combinations with conventional cytotoxics have, thus far, yielded mixed results. Combining trastuzumab with taxanes in breast cancer, for example, has proved to be beneficial in both preclinical and clinical trials *(113)*; however, the combination of gefitinib with chemotherapy in NSCLC showed no benefit *(114)*. In vitro studies using human tumor xenografts indicate that VEGF blockade is able to enhance the tumoricidal effect of vinblastine in neuroblastoma *(115)*, pacliataxel in transitional cell carcinoma of the bladder *(116)*, doxorubicin in soft tissue sarcoma *(117)*, and gemcitabine in pancreatic cancer *(118)*. Another positive example is in breast cancer. Treating HER2-overexpressing cells with both trastuzumab and gefitinib results in additive efficacy of these agents. This efficacy was predicted from studies suggesting that gefitinib dephosphorylates both HER1 and HER2 and that combining EGF receptor (HER1) and HER2 blockade may improve antitumor efficacy *(119)*. Similarly, in HER2-overexpressing breast cancer cell lines cotargeting the HER2 and insulin-like growth factor-1 receptor causes synergistic inhibition *(120)*. Simultaneous blockade of VEGF and EGF receptors appears to be more effective than single-agent therapies in mouse models of human colon cancer carcinomatosis *(121)* and gastric cancer *(122)*. Finally, the advent of genomics and proteomics may herald a new era in oncology when the role of HGF and signaling pathways may be more precisely defined for better application of HGF antagonists.

ACKNOWLEDGMENTS

This work was supported by grants from the NH and MRC of Australia, The Anti-Cancer Foundation of South Australia, and the National Institutes of Health (grant 1-RO1-AI50744-01A1).

REFERENCES

1. Sundaresan S, Roberts PE, King KL, Sliwkowski MX, Mather JP. Biological response to ErbB ligands in nontransformed cell lines correlates with a specific pattern of receptor expression. *Endocrinology* 1998; 139:4756–4764.
2. Heaney ML, Golde DW. Soluble cytokine receptors. *Blood* 1996; 87:847–857.
3. Brown CB, Beaudry P, Dickinson Laing T, Shoemaker S, Kaushansky K. In vitro characterization of the human recombinant soluble granulocyte-macrophage colony-stimulating factor receptor. *Blood* 1995; 85:1488–1495.
4. Aiello LP, Pierce EA, Foley ED, et al. Suppression of retinal neovascularization in vitro by inhibition of vascular endothelial growth factor (VEGF) using soluble VEGF-receptor chimeric proteins. *Proc Natl Acad Sci USA* 1995; 92:10457–10461.
5. Aderka D. The potential biological and clinical significance of the soluble tumor necrosis factor receptors. *Cytokine Growth Factor Rev* 1996; 7:231–240.
6. Standiford TJ. Anti-inflammatory cytokines and cytokine antagonists. *Curr Pharm Des* 2000; 6:633–649.
7. Nicola NA, Wycherley K, Boyd AW, Layton JE, Cary D, Metcalf D. Neutralizing and nonneutralizing monoclonal antibodies to the human granulocyte-macrophage colony-stimulating factor receptor a-chain. *Blood* 1993; 82:1724–1731.
8. Sun Q, Jones K, McClure B, et al. Simultaneous antagonism of interleukin-5, granulocyte-macrophage colony-stimulating factor, and interleukin-3 stimulation of human eosinophils by targetting the common cytokines binding site of their receptors. *Blood* 1999; 94:1943–1951.
9. Goldstein NI, Prewett M, Zuklys K, Rockwell P, Mendelson J. Biological efficacy if a chimeric antibody to the epidermal growth factor receptor in a human tumor xenograft model. *Clin Cancer Res* 1995; 1:1311–1318.
10. Ciardello F. An update of new targets for cancer treatment: receptor-mediated signals. *Ann Oncol* 2002; 13:29–38.
11. Presta L, Chen H, O'Connor SJ, et al. Humanization of an anti-vascular endothelial growth factor monoclonal antibody for the therapy of solid tumours and other disorders. *Cancer Res* 1997; 57:4593–4599.
12. Moreau P, Harousseau J-L, Wijdenes J, Morineau N, Milpied N, Bataille R. A combination of anti-interleukin 6 murine monoclonal antibody with dexamethasone and high-dose melphalan induces high complete response rates in advanced multiple myeloma. *Br J Haematol* 2000; 109:661–664.
13. Hirata T, Shimazaki C, Sumikuma T, et al. Humanized anti-interleukin-6 receptor monoclonal antibody induced apoptosis of fresh and cloned human myeloma cells in vitro. *Leuk Res* 2003; 27:343–349.
14. Cohen RB, Dittrich KA. Anti-TNF therapy and malignancy—a critical review. *Can J Gastroenterol* 2001; 15:376–384.
15. De Benedetti F, Pignatti P, Vivarelli M, et al. In vivo neutralization of human IL-6 (hIL-6) achieved by immunization of hIL-6-transgenic mice with a hIL-6 receptor antagonist. *J Immunol* 2001; 166:4334–4340.
16. Yanofsky SD, Baldwin DN, Butler JH, et al. High affinity type I interleukin 1 receptor antagonists discovered by screening recombinant peptide libraries. *Proc Natl Acad Sci USA* 1996; 93:7381–7386.
17. Fairbrother WJ, Christinger HW, Cochran AG, et al. Novel peptides selected to bind vascular endothelial growth factor target the receptor-binding site. *Biochemistry* 1998; 37:17754–17764.
18. Binetruy-Tournaire R, Demangel C, Malavaud B, et al. Identification of a peptide blocking vascular endothelial growth factor (VEGF)-mediated angiogenesis. *EMBO J* 2000; 19:1525–1533.
19. Sporeno E, Savino R, Ciapponi L, et al. Human interleukin-6 receptor super-antagonists with high potency and wide spectrum on multiple myeloma cells. *Blood* 1996; 87:4510–4519.
20. Hercus TR, Bagley CJ, Cambareri B, et al. Specific human granulocyte-macrophage colony-stimulating factor antagonists. *Proc Natl Acad Sci USA* 1994; 91:5838–5842.

21. Siemeister G, Schirner M, Reusch P, Barleon B, Marme D, Martiny-Baron G. An antagonistic vascular endothelial growth factor (VEGF) variant inhibits VEGF-stimulated receptor autophosphorylation and proliferation of human endothelial cells. *Proc Natl Acad Sci USA* 1998; 95:4625–4629.
22. Leenders W, Lubsen N, van Altena M, et al. Design of a variant of vascular endothelial growth factor-A (VEGF-A) antagonizing KDR/Flk-1 and Flt-1. *Lab Invest* 2002; 82:473–481.
23. Boesen TP, Soni B, Schwartz TW, Halkier T. Single-chain vascular endothelial growth factor variant with antagonist activity. *J Biol Chem* 2002; 277:40335–40341.
24. Arend WP, Malyak M, Guthridge CJ, Gabay C. Interleukin-1 receptor antagonist: role in biology. *Annu Rev Immunol* 1998; 16:27–55.
25. Arend WP. The balance between IL-1 and IL-1Ra in disease. *Cytokine Growth Factor Rev* 2002; 13:323–340.
26. Hao D, Rowinsky EK. Inhibiting signal transduction: recent advances in the development of receptor tyrosine kinase and Ras inhibitors. *Cancer Invest* 2002; 20:387–404.
27. Baselga J. Why the epidermal growth factor receptor? The rationale for cancer therapy. *Oncologist* 2002; 7:4:2–8.
28. Fong TA, Shawver LK, Sun L, et al. SU5416 is a potent and selective inhibitor of the vascular endothelial growth factor receptor (Flk-1/KDR) that inhibits tyrosine kinase catalysis, tumor vascularization, and growth of multiple tumor types. *Cancer Res* 1999; 59:99–106.
29. Guthridge MA, Stomski FC, Barry EF, et al. Site specific serine phosphorylation of the IL-3 receptor is required for hemopoietic cell survival. *Mol Cell* 2000; 6:99–108.
30. Guglielmi C, Arcese W, Hermans J, et al. Risk assessment in patients with Ph+ chronic myelogenous leukemia at first relapse after allogeneic stem cell transplant: an EBMT retrospective analysis. The Chronic Leukemia Working Party of the European Group for Blood and Marrow Transplantation. *Blood* 2000; 95:3328–3334.
31. Hansen JA, Gooley TA, Martin PJ, et al. Bone marrow transplants from unrelated donors for patients with chronic myeloid leukemia. *N Engl J Med* 1998; 338:962–968.
32. Scott CL, Hughes DA, Cary D, Nicola NA, Begley CG, Robb L. Functional analysis of mature hematopoietic cells from mice lacking the bc chain of the granulocyte-macrophage colony-stimulating factor receptor. *Blood* 1998; 92:4119–4127.
33. Ben Neriah Y, Daley GQ, Mes-Masson AM, Witte ON, Baltimore D. The chronic myelogenous leukemia-specific P210 protein is the product of the bcr/abl hybrid gene. *Science* 1986; 233:212–214.
34. Pendergast AM, Quilliam LA, Cripe LD, et al. BCR-ABL-induced oncogenesis is mediated by direct interaction with the SH2 domain of the GRB-2 adaptor protein. *Cell* 1993; 75:175–185.
35. Pear WS, Miller JP, Xu L, et al. Efficient and rapid induction of a chronic myelogenous leukemia-like myeloproliferative disease in mice receiving P210 bcr/abl-transduced bone marrow. *Blood* 1998; 92:3780–3792.
36. Zhang X, Ren R. Bcr-Abl efficiently induces a myeloproliferative disease and production of excess interleukin-3 and granulocyte-macrophage colony-stimulating factor in mice: a novel model for chronic myelogenous leukemia. *Blood* 1998; 92:3829–2840.
37. Jiang X, Lopez A, Holyoake T, Eaves A, Eaves C. Autocrine production and action of IL-3 and G-CSF in chronic myeloid leukaemia. *Proc Natl Acad Sci USA* 1999; 96:12804–12809.
38. Bollag G, Clapp DW, Shih S, et al. Loss of Nf1 results in activation of the Ras signalling pathway and leads to aberrant growth in haemopoietic cells. *Nat Genet* 1996; 12:144–148.
39. Zhang Y-Y, Vik TA, Ryder JW, et al. Nf1 regulates hematopoietic progenitor cell growth and Ras signalling in response to multiple cytokines. *J Exp Med* 1998; 187:1893–1902.
40. Largaespada DA, Shaughnessy JD, Jenkins NA, Copeland NG. Retroviral integration at the Evi-2 locus in BXH-2 myeloid leukemia cell lines disrupts Nf1 expression without changes in steady-state Ras-GTP levels. *J Virol* 1995; 69:5095–5102.
41. Yamamoto Y, Kiyoi H, Nakano Y, et al. Activating mutation of D835 within the activation loop of FLT3 in human hematologic malignancies. *Blood* 2001; 97:2434–2439.
42. Golub TR, Barker GF, Lovett M, Gilliland DG. Fusion of PDGF receptor β to a novel ets-like gene, tel, in chronic myelomonocytic leukemia with t(5;12) chromosomal translocation. *Cell* 1994; 77:307–316.
43. Carroll M, Tomasson MH, Barker GF, Golub TR, Gilliland DG. The TEL/platelet-derived growth factor β receptor (PDGFβR) fusion in chronic myelomonocytic leukemia is a transforming protein that self-associates and activates PDGFbR kinase-dependent signaling pathways. *Proc Natl Acad Sci USA* 1996; 93:14845–14850.

44. Moore S, Haylock DN, Levesque JP, et al. Stem cell factor as a single agent induces selective proliferation of the Philadelphia chromosome positive fraction of chronic myeloid leukemia CD34+ cells. *Blood* 1998; 92:2461–2470.
45. Emanuel PD, Bates LJ, Castleberry RP, Gualtieri RJ, Zuckerman KS. Selective hypersensitivity to granulocyte-macrophage colony-stimulating factor by juvenile chronic myeloid leukemia hematopoietic progenitors. *Blood* 1991; 77:925–929.
46. Estrov Z, Grunberger T, Chan HSL, Freedman MH. Juvenile chronic myelogenous leukemia: characterization of the disease using cell cultures. *Blood* 1986; 67:1382–1387.
47. Everson MP, Brown CB, Lilly MB. Interleukin-6 and granulocyte-macrophage colony-stimulating factor are candidate growth factors for chronic myelomonocytic leukemia cells. *Blood* 1989; 74:1472–1476.
48. Geissler K, Ohler L, Födinger M, et al. Interleukin 10 inhibits growth and granulocyte/macrophage colony-stimulating factor production in chronic myelomonocytic leukemia cells. *J Exp Med* 1996; 184:1377–1384.
49. Oehler L, Foedinger M, Koeller M, et al. Interleukin-10 inhibits spontaneous colony-forming unit growth from human peripheral blood mononuclear cells by suppression of endogenous granulocyte-macrophage colony-stimulating factor release. *Blood* 1997; 89:1147–1153.
50. Ramshaw H, Bardy P, Lee M, Lopez A. Chronic myelomonocytic leukemia requires granulocyte-macrophage colony-stimulating factor for growth in vitro and in vivo. *Exp Hematol* 2002; 30:1124.
51. Young DC, Griffin JD. Autocrine secretion of GM-CSF in acute myeloblastic leukemia. *Blood* 1986; 68:1178–1181.
52. Oster W, Cicco NA, Klein H, et al. Participation of the cytokines interleukin 6, tumor necrosis factor-alpha, and interleukin 1-beta secreted by acute myelogenous leukemia blasts in autocrine and paracrine leukemia growth control. *J Clin Invest* 1989; 84:451–457.
53. Lowenberg B, van Putten WL, Touw IP, Delwel R, Santini V. Autonomous proliferation of leukemic cells in vitro as a determinant of prognosis in adult acute myeloid leukemia. *N Engl J Med* 1993; 328:614–619.
54. Emanuel PD, Bates LJ, Zhu S-W, Castleberry RP, Gualtieri RJ, Zuckerman KS. The role of monocyte-derived hemopoietic growth factors in the regulation of myeloproliferation in juvenile chronic myelogenous leukemia. *Exp Hematol* 1991; 19:1017–1024.
55. Geissler K, Hinterberger W, Bettelheim P, Haas O, Lechner K. Colony growth characteristics in chronic myelomonocytic leukemia. *Leuk Res* 1988; 12:373–377.
56. Seymour JF, Cortes JE. Chronic myelomonocytic leukemia. In: Talpaz M, Kantarjian HM, eds., *Medical Management of Chronic Myelogenous Leukemia.* New York, NY: Dekker, 1998:43–76.
57. Butcher C, D'Andrea RJ. Molecular aspects of polycythemia vera (review). *Int J Mol Med* 2000; 6:243–252.
58. Elbaz O, Mahmoud LA. Tumor necrosis factor and human acute leukemia. *Leuk Lymphoma* 1994; 12:191–195.
59. Raza A, Mundle S, Shetty V, et al. Novel insights into the biology of myelodysplastic syndromes: excessive apoptosis and the role of cytokines. *Int J Hematol* 1996; 63:265–278.
60. Freedman MH, Cohen A, Grunberger T, et al. Central role of tumour necrosis factor, GM-CSF, and interleukin-1 in the pathogenesis of juvenile chronic myelogenous leukaemia. *Br J Haematol* 1992; 80:40–48.
61. Raza A. Anti-TNF therapies in rheumatoid arthritis, Crohn's disease, sepsis, and myelodysplastic syndromes. *Microsc Res Tech* 2000; 50:229–235.
62. Dinarello CA. Interleukin-1 and interleukin-1 antagonism. *Blood* 1991; 77:1627–1652.
63. Wetzler M, Kurzrock R, Estrov Z, et al. Altered levels of interleukin-1 beta and interleukin-1 receptor antagonist in chronic myelogenous leukemia: clinical and prognostic correlates. *Blood* 1994; 84:3142–3147.
64. Sakai K, Hattori T, Matsuoka M, et al. Autocrine stimulation of interleukin 1 beta in acute myelogenous leukemia cells. *J Exp Med* 1987; 166:1597–1602.
65. Kurzrock R. Cytokine deregulation in cancer. *Biomed Pharmacother* 2001; 55:543–547.
66. Estrov Z, Kurzrock R, Talpaz M. Role of interleukin-1 inhibitory molecules in therapy of acute and chronic myelogenous leukemia. *Leuk Lymphoma* 1993; 10:407–418.
67. de Hon FD, Ehlers M, Rose-John S, et al. Development of an interleukin (IL) 6 receptor antagonist that inhibits IL-6-dependent growth of human myeloma cells. *J Exp Med* 1994; 180:2395–2400.

68. Renne C, Kallen KJ, Mullberg J, Jostock T, Grotzinger J, Rose-John S. A new type of cytokine receptor antagonist directly targeting gp130. *J Biol Chem* 1998; 273:27213–27219.
69. Yoshida K, Taga T, Saito M, et al. Targeted disruption of gp130, a common signal transducer for the interleukin 6 family of cytokines, leads to myocardial and hematological disorders. *Proc Natl Acad Sci USA* 1996; 93:407–411.
70. Van Zaanen HC, Lokhorst HM, Aarden LA, et al. Chimaeric anti-interleukin 6 monoclonal antibodies in the treatment of advanced multiple myeloma: a phase I dose-escalating study. *Br J Haematol* 1998; 102:783–790.
71. Nishimoto N, Sasai M, Shima Y, et al. Improvement in Castleman's disease by humanized anti-interleukin-6 receptor antibody therapy. *Blood* 2000; 95:56–61.
72. Montero-Julian FA, Brailly H, Sautes C, et al. Characterization of soluble gp130 released by melanoma cell lines: a polyvalent antagonist of cytokines from the interleukin 6 family. *Clin Cancer Res* 1997; 3:1443–1451.
73. Druker BJ, Sawyers CL, Kantarjian H, et al. Activity of a specific inhibitor of the BCR-ABL tyrosine kinase in the blast crisis of chronic myeloid leukemia and acute lymphoblastic leukemia with the Philadelphia chromosome. *N Engl J Med* 2001; 344:1038–1042.
74. Sawyers CL, Hochhaus A, Feldman E, et al. Imatinib induces hematologic and cytogenetic responses in patients with chronic myelogenous leukemia in myeloid blast crisis: results of a phase II study. *Blood* 2002; 99:3530–3539.
75. Schindler T, Bornmann W, Pellicena P, Miller WT, Clarkson B, Kuriyan J. Structural mechanism for STI-571 inhibition of abelson tyrosine kinase. *Science* 2000; 289:1938–1942.
76. Druker BJ, Lydon NB. Lessons learned from the development of an abl tyrosine kinase inhibitor for chronic myelogenous leukemia. *J Clin Invest* 2000; 105:3–7.
77. Druker BJ, Tamura S, Buchdunger E, et al. Effects of a selective inhibitor of the Abl tyrosine kinase on the growth of Bcr-Abl positive cells. *Nat Med* 1996; 2:561–566.
78. Thiesing JT, Ohno-Jones S, Kolibaba KS, Druker BJ. Efficacy of STI571, an abl tyrosine kinase inhibitor, in conjunction with other antileukemic agents against bcr-abl-positive cells. *Blood* 2000; 96:3195–3199.
79. Capdeville R, Silberman S, Dimitrijevic S. Imatinib: the first 3 years. *Eur J Cancer* 2002; 38:S77–S82.
80. Gambacorti-Passerini CB, Gunby RH, Piazza R, Galietta A, Rostagno R, Scapozza L. Molecular mechanisms of resistance to imatinib in Philadelphia-chromosome-positive leukaemias. *Lancet Oncol* 2003; 4:75–85.
81. Gambacorti-Passerini C, le Coutre P, Mologni L, et al. Inhibition of the ABL kinase activity blocks the proliferation of BCR/ABL+ leukemic cells and induces apoptosis. *Blood Cells Mol Dis* 1997; 23:380–394.
82. Dorsey JF, Cunnick JM, Lanehart R, et al. Interleukin-3 protects Bcr-Abl-transformed hematopoietic progenitor cells from apoptosis induced by Bcr-Abl tyrosine kinase inhibitors. *Leukemia* 2002; 16:1589–1595.
83. McClure BJ, Hercus TR, Cambareri BA, et al. Molecular assembly of the ternary granulocyte-macrophage colony-stimulating factor receptor complex. *Blood* 2003; 101:1308–1315.
84. Iversen PO, Rodwell RL, Pitcher L, Taylor KM, Lopez AF. Inhibition of proliferation and induction of apoptosis in juvenile myelomonocytic leukemic cells by the granulocyte-macrophage colony-stimulating factor analogue E21R. *Blood* 1996; 88:2634–2639.
85. Iversen PO, Lewis ID, Turczynowicz S, et al. Inhibition of granulocyte-macrophage colony-stimulating factor prevents dissemination and induces remission of juvenile myelomonocytic leukemia in engrafted immunodeficient mice. *Blood* 1997; 90:4910–4917.
86. Nishinakamura R, Nakayama N, Hirabayashi Y, et al. Mice deficient for the IL-3/GM-CSF/IL-5 bc receptor exhibit lung pathology and impaired immune response, while bIL3 receptor-deficient mice are normal. *Immunity* 1995; 2:211–222.
87. Olver IN, Hercus T, Lopez A, et al. A phase I study of the GM-CSF antagonist E21R. *Cancer Chemother Pharmacol* 2002; 50:171–178.
88. Bernard F, Thomas C, Emile JF, et al. Transient hematologic and clinical effect of E21R in a child with end-stage juvenile myelomonocytic leukemia. *Blood* 2002; 99:2615–2616.
89. Saily M, Koistinen P, Zheng A, Savolainen E-R. Signaling through interleukin-6 receptor supports blast cell proliferation in acute myeloblastic leukemia. *Eur J Haematol* 1998; 61:190–196.
90. Chauhan D, Pandey P, Hideshima T, et al. SHP2 mediates the protective effect of interleukin-6 against dexamethasone-induced apoptosis in multiple myeloma cells. *J Biol Chem* 2000; 275:27845–27850.

91. Chatterjee M, Honemann D, Lentzsch S, et al. In the presence of bone marrow stromal cells human multiple myeloma cells become independent of the IL-6/gp130/STAT3 pathway. *Blood* 2002; 100:3311–3318.
92. Honemann D, Chatterjee M, Savino R, et al. The IL-6 receptor antagonist SANT-7 overcomes bone marrow stromal cell-mediated drug resistance of multiple myeloma cells. *Int J Cancer* 2001; 93:674–680.
93. Tassone P, Galea E, Forciniti S, Tagliaferri P, Venuta S. The IL-6 receptor super-antagonist Sant7 enhances antiproliferative and apoptotic effects induced by dexamethasone and zoledronic acid on multiple myeloma cells. *Int J Oncol* 2002; 21:867–873.
94. Ranson M, Hammond LA, Ferry D, et al. ZD1839, a selective oral epidermal growth factor receptor-tyrosine kinase inhibitor, is well tolerated and active in patients with solid, malignant tumors: results of a phase I trial. *J Clin Oncol* 2002; 20:2240–2250.
95. Hainsworth JD, Litchy S, Burris HA, et al. Rituximab as first-line and maintenance therapy for patients with indolent non-hodgkin's lymphoma. *J Clin Oncol* 2002; 20:4261–4267.
96. Vogel CL, Cobleigh MA, Tripathy D, et al. Efficacy and safety of trastuzumab as a single agent in first-line treatment of HER2-overexpressing metastatic breast cancer. *J Clin Oncol* 2002; 20:719–726.
97. Croom KF, Perry CM. Imatinib mesylate: in the treatment of gastrointestinal stromal tumours. *Drugs* 2003; 63:513–522.
98. Edmonson JH, Marks RS, Buckner JC, Mahoney MR. Contrast of response to dacarbazine, mitomycin, doxorubicin, and cisplatin (DMAP) plus GM-CSF between patients with advanced malignant gastrointestinal stromal tumors and patients with other advanced leiomyosarcomas. *Cancer Invest* 2002; 20:605–612.
99. Herbst RS, Langer CJ. Epidermal growth factor receptors as a target for cancer treatment: the emerging role of IMC-C225 in the treatment of lung and head and neck cancers. *Semin Oncol* 2002; 29:27–36.
100. Baselga J, Yano K, Giaccone G, et al. Initial results from a phase II trial of ZD 1839 (Iressa), as second- and third-line monotherapy for patients with advanced non-small cell lung cancer (IDEAL1). *Clin Cancer Res* 2001; 7:3780S (abstract 630A).
101. Natale RB, Skarin A, Maddox A-M, et al. Improvement in symptoms and quality of life for advanced non-small cell lung cancer patients recieving ZD 1839 ('Iressa') in IDEAL2. *Proc Am Soc Clin Oncol* 2002; 21:292a (abstract 1167).
102. Stopeck A, Sheldon M, Vahedian M, Cropp G, Gosalia R, Hannah A. Results of a phase I dose-escalating study of the antiangiogenic agent, SU5416, in patients with advanced malignancies. *Clin Cancer Res* 2002; 8:2798–2805.
103. Smith PC, Hobisch A, Lin DL, Culig Z, Keller ET. Interleukin-6 and prostate cancer progression. *Cytokine Growth Factor Rev* 2001; 12:33–40.
104. Okamoto M, Lee C, Oyasu R. Autocrine effect of androgen on proliferation of an androgen responsive prostatic carcinoma cell line, LNCAP: role of interleukin-6. *Endocrinology* 1997; 138:5071–5074.
105. Okamoto M, Lee C, Oyasu R. Interleukin-6 as a paracrine and autocrine growth factor in human prostatic carcinoma cells in vitro. *Cancer Res* 1997; 57:141–146.
106. Steiner H, Godoy-Tundidor S, Rogatsch H, et al. Accelerated in vivo growth of prostate tumors that up-regulate interleukin-6 is associated with reduced retinoblastoma protein expression and activation of the mitogen-activated protein kinase pathway. *Am J Pathol* 2003; 162:655–663.
107. Borsellino N, Bonavida B, Ciliberto G, Toniatti C, Travali S, D'Alessandro N. Blocking signaling through the Gp130 receptor chain by interleukin-6 and oncostatin M inhibits PC-3 cell growth and sensitizes the tumor cells to etoposide and cisplatin-mediated cytotoxicity. *Cancer* 1999; 85:134–144.
108. Chen T, Wang LH, Farrar WL. Interleukin 6 activates androgen receptor-mediated gene expression through a signal transducer and activator of transcription 3-dependent pathway in LNCaP prostate cancer cells. *Cancer Res* 2000; 60:2132–2135.
109. Lin DL, Whitney MC, Yao Z, Keller ET. Interleukin-6 induces androgen responsiveness in prostate cancer cells through up-regulation of androgen receptor expression. *Clin Cancer Res* 2001; 7:1773–1781.
110. Purohit A, Singh A, Ghilchik MW, Serlupi-Crescenzi O, Reed MJ. Inhibition of IL-6+IL-6 soluble receptor-stimulated aromatase activity by the IL-6 antagonist, Sant 7, in breast tissue-derived fibroblasts. *Br J Cancer* 2003; 88:630–635.

111. Baldwin GC, Gasson JC, Kaufman SE, et al. Nonhematopoietic tumor cells express functional GM-CSF receptors. *Blood* 1989; 73:1033–1037.
112. Rivas CI, Vera JC, Delgado-Lopez F, et al. Expression of granulocyte-macrophage colony-stimulating factor receptors in human prostate cancer. *Blood* 1998; 91:1037–1043.
113. Dieras V, Beuzeboc P, Laurence V, Pierga JY, Pouillart P. Interaction between Herceptin and taxanes. *Oncology* 2001; 61:43–49.
114. Giaconne G, Johnson DH, Maegold C, et al. A phase III clinical trial of ZD 1839 ('Iressa') in combination with gemcitabine and cisplatin in chemotherapy-naive patients with advanced non-small cell lung cancer (INTACT 1). *Ann Oncol* 2003; 13:3 (abstract 40).
115. Klement G, Baruchel S, Rak J, et al. Continuous low-dose therapy with vinblastine and VEGF receptor-2 antibody induces sustained tumor regression without overt toxicity. *J Clin Invest* 2000; 105:R15–R24.
116. Inoue K, Slaton JW, Davis DW, et al. Treatment of human metastatic transitional cell carcinoma of the bladder in a murine model with the anti-vascular endothelial growth factor receptor monoclonal antibody DC101 and paclitaxel. *Clin Cancer Res* 2000; 6:2635–2643.
117. Zhang L, Yu D, Hicklin DJ, Hannay JA, Ellis LM, Pollock RE. Combined anti-fetal liver kinase 1 monoclonal antibody and continuous low-dose doxorubicin inhibits angiogenesis and growth of human soft tissue sarcoma xenografts by induction of endothelial cell apoptosis. *Cancer Res* 2002; 62:2034–2042.
118. Bruns CJ, Shrader M, Harbison MT, et al. Effect of the vascular endothelial growth factor receptor-2 antibody DC101 plus gemcitabine on growth, metastasis and angiogenesis of human pancreatic cancer growing orthotopically in nude mice. *Int J Cancer* 2002; 102:101–108.
119. Moasser MM, Basso A, Averbuch SD, Rosen N. The tyrosine kinase inhibitor ZD1839 ("Iressa") inhibits HER2-driven signaling and suppresses the growth of HER2-overexpressing tumor cells. *Cancer Res* 2001; 61:7184–7188.
120. Camirand A, Lu Y, Pollak M. Co-targeting HER2/ErbB2 and insulin-like growth factor-1 receptors causes synergistic inhibition of growth in HER2-overexpressing breast cancer cells. *Med Sci Monit* 2002; 8:BR521–BR526.
121. Shaheen RM, Ahmad SA, Liu W, et al. Inhibited growth of colon cancer carcinomatosis by antibodies to vascular endothelial and epidermal growth factor receptors. *Br J Cancer* 2001; 85:584–589.
122. Jung YD, Mansfield PF, Akagi M, et al. Effects of combination anti-vascular endothelial growth factor receptor and anti-epidermal growth factor receptor therapies on the growth of gastric cancer in a nude mouse model. *Eur J Cancer* 2002; 38:1133–1140.

Acronyms and Selected Abbreviations

5-FU	5-fluorouracil

AA	aplastic anemia
Ab	antibody
ABV	chemotherapy with doxorubicin, bleomycin, and vincristine
ABVD	chemotherapy with doxorubicin, bleomycin, vincristine, and dacarbazine
AC	chemotherapy with doxorubicin and cyclophosphamide
ACD	anemia of chronic disease
ACE	angiotensin-converting enzyme
ACNU	nimustine
ADCC	antibody-dependent cell-mediated cytotoxicity
ADP	adenosine diphosphate
Ag	antigen
AGC	absolute granulocyte count
AIDS	acquired immunodeficiency syndrome
ALG	antilymphocyte globulin
ALL	acute lymphoblastic/lymphocytic leukemia
AlloBMT	allogeneic bone marrow transplantation
ALT	alanine aminotransferase
AML	acute myeloid/myelogenous leukemia
ANC	absolute neutrophil count
APL	acute promyelocytic leukemia
ASCO	American Society of Clinical Oncology
ATG	antithymocyte globulin
AuBMT	autologous bone marrow transplantation
AUC	area under the curve

β_c	beta common
BEACOPP	chemotherapy with bleomycin, etoposide, Adriamycin, cyclophosphamide, vincristine, procarbazine, and prednisone
BFU-E	erythroid blast-forming unit
bid	twice a day
BMT	bone marrow transplantation

BSA	bovine serum albumin
BSF	B-cell stimulating factor-3
CAE	chemotherapy with cyclophosphamide, doxorubicin, and etoposide
CALGB	The Cancer and Leukemia Group B
CBC	complete blood count
CDE	chemotherapy with cyclophosphamide, doxorubicin, and etoposide
CDE-C	chemotherapy with cyclophosphamide, doxorubicin, etoposide, and cisplatin
C/E	cost-effectiveness ratio
CFC-G	granulocyte colony-forming cell
CFU	colony-forming unit(s)
CFU-E	erythroid colony-forming unit
CFU-Mix	mixed colony-forming unit
CHO	Chinese hamster ovary
CHOP	chemotherapy with cyclosphosphamide, doxorubicin, vincristine, and prednisone
CHOPE	chemotherapy with cyclosphosphamide, doxorubicin, vincristine, prednisone, and etoposide
CHVmP + VP	chemotherapy with cyclophosphamide, doxorubicin, teniposide, vincristine, bleomycin, and prednisone
CI	confidence interval
CIS	cytokine-induced SRC homology; cytokine-inducible SH2-containing protein
CLL	chronic lymphocytic leukemia
CMF	chemotherapy with cyclophosphamide, methotrexate, and 5-fluorouracil
CML	chronic myelogenous leukemia
CMML	chronic myelomonocytic leukemia
CMV	cytomegalovirus
CNEP	chemotherapy with cyclophosphamide, doxorubicin, etoposide, and prednisone
CNOP	chemotherapy with cyclophosphamide doxorubicin, vincritine, and prednisone
CNTF	ciliary neurotrophic factor
CODE	chemotherapy with cisplatin, oncovin, doxorubicin, and etoposide
COP-BLAM	chemotherapy with cyclophosphamide, vincristine, prednisolone, bleomycin, doxorubicin, and procarbazine
COPP/ABVD	chemotherapy with cyclophosphamide, vincristine, procarbazine, prednisone, doxorubicin, bleomycin, vinblastine, and dacarbazine
CSF	colony-stimulating factor
CSF-1	colony-stimulating factor-1 (*or* macrophage colony-stimulating factor)

CT	computed tomography *or* cardiotrophin
CTL	cytotoxic T lymphocyte
C/U	cost-utility ratio
Dexa-BOM	chemotherapy with dexamethasone, carmustine, melphalan, cytarabine, and etoposide
DHAP	chemotherapy with cisplatin, cytarabine, and dexamethasone
DMAP	chemotherapy with dacarbazine, mitomycin, doxorubicin, and cisplatin
DSN	days of severe neutropenia
E-BFC	erythroid blast-forming cell
EBMT	European Group for Blood and Marrow Transplantation
EC_{50}	median effective concentration
ECOG	Eastern Cooperative Oncology Group
ED_{50}	median effective dose
EGF	epidermal growth factor
ELISA	enzyme-linked immunosorbent assay
E-LTC-IC	extended leukotriene cysteinyl initiating cell
EMP1	EPO mimetic peptide 1
EPO	erythropoietin
EPOR	erythropoietin receptor
ESBC	early-stage breast cancer
ESHAP	chemotherapy with etoposide, solumedrol, cytarabine, and cisplatin
ESMO	European Society for Medical Oncology
EVI	chemotherapy with epirubicin, vindensine, and ifosfamide
FAC	chemotherapy with 5-fluorouracil, doxorubicin, and cyclophosphamide
FACS	fluorescence-activated cell sorting
FACT	Functional Assessment of Cancer Therapy
FACT-An	FACT dealing with anemia
FACT-F	FACT dealing with fatigue
FACT-N	FACT dealing with neutropenia
FATR	febrile-associated transfusion reaction
FDA	Food and Drug Administration
FGF	fibroblast growth factor
FIH	factor inhibiting hypoxia-inducible factor
FISH	fluorescence *in situ* hybridization

FLICE	caspase-activating enzyme
FN	febrile neutropenia
G-CSF	granulocyte colony-stimulating factor
GDP	guanosine diphosphate
GEF	guanine nucleotide exchange factor
GH	growth hormone
GI	gastrointestinal
GIST	gastrointestinal stromal tumor
GM-CFC	granulocyte-macrophage colony-forming cell
GM-CSF	granulocyte-macrophage colony-stimulating factor
GTP	guanosine triphosphate
GvHD	graft-vs-host disease
GvL	graft-vs-leukemia
HAART	highly active antiretroviral therapy
HADS	Hospital Anxiety and Depression Scale
Hb	hemoglobin
HCL	hairy cell leukemia
HCP	hematopoietic cell phosphatase
Hct	hematocrit
HD	Hodgkin's disease
HGF	hematopoietic growth factor
HIF	hypoxia-inducible factor
HIF-PH	hypoxia-inducible factor prolyl hydroxylase
H-IL-6	hyper-IL-6
HIV	human immunodeficiency virus
HLA	human leukocyte antigen
HMO	health maintenance organization
HPP-CFC	high proliferative-potential colony-forming cell
HRQOL	health-related quality of life
HSA	human serum albumin
HSC	hematopoetic stem cell
HTS	high-throughput screening
IC_{50}	mean inhibitory concentration, 50%
IEL	intraepithelial lymphoctye

IFN	interferon
IGF	insulin-like growth factor
IGF-1R	insulin-like growth factor-1 receptor
IL	interleukin
ip	intraperitoneal or intraperitoneally
IPSS	International Prognostic Scoring System
iv	intravenous, intravenously
Jak or JAK	Janus kinase
JH	Jak or JAK homology
JMML	juvenile myelomonocytic leukemia
kDa	kilodalton
KGF	keratinocyte growth factor
KIR	kinase inhibitory region
LDH	lactate dehydrogenase
LGL	large granular lymphocyte
LIF	leukemia inhibitory factor
LNH84	chemotherapy with cyclophosphamide, doxorubicin, vindesine, bleomycin, methylprednisolone, and methotrexate
LOS	length of stay
LPS	lipopolysaccharide
LTBMC	long term bone marrow culture
LTC	cysteinyl leukotriene
LTC-IC	cysteinyl leukotriene initiating cell
LTR	long-term multilineage reconstitution
MAb	monoclonal antibody
MAP	mitogen-activated protein
MAPK	mitogen-activated protein kinase
MASCC	Multinational Asociation of Supportive Care of Cancer
M-CSF	macrophage colony-stimulating factor or CSF-1; monocyte colony-stimulating factor
MDR	multidrug resistance
MDS	myelodysplastic syndromes
Meg-CFC	megakaryocyte colony-forming cell
MGDF	megakaryocyte growth and development factor

MIP	macrophage inflammatory protein
MOPP	chemotherapy with mechlorethamine, vincristine, procarbazine, and prednisone
MOPP/ABVD	chemotherapy with mechlorethamine, vincristine, procarbazine, prednisone, doxorubicin, bleomycin, vinblastine, and dacarbazine
MRT	mean residence time
MTD	maximum tolerated dose
MVAC	chemotherapy with methotrexate, vinblastine, doxorubicin, and cisplatin
MVP	chemotherapy with mitocycin C, vindestine, and cisplatin
NASBP	The National Surgical Adjuvant Breast and Bowel Project
NGF	nerve growth factor
NHL	non-Hodgkin's lymphoma
NK	natural killer
NNT	novel neutrophin-1
NSCLC	nonsmall-cell lung cancer
ODD	oxygen-dependent domain
O/P	observed to predicted values
OSM	oncostatin M
PAIS	Psychological Adjustment to Illness Scale
PBPC	peripheral blood progenitor cell
PDGF	platelet-derived growth factor
PEG	polyethylene glycol
PEG-rHuMGDF	pegylated recombinant human megakaryocyte growth and development factor
PI3K	phosphatidylinositol 3 kinase
PIAS	protein inhibitor of activated Stat
PLC	phospholipase C
PLL	prolymphocytic leukemia
PMEF	primary mouse embryonic fibroblast
PMP	promegapoietin
PRL	prolactin
ProGP	progenipoietin
ProMACE-CytaBOM	chemotherapy with cyclophosphamide, doxorubicin, etoposide, prednisone, cytarabine, bleomycin, vincristine, methotrexate, and leucovorin

PSA	prostate-specific antigen
QALY	quality-adjusted life-year
qd	twice a day
QOL	quality of life
Q-TWIST	quality-adjusted time without symptoms of disease or toxicity of treatment
RA	refractory anemia
RAEB	refractory anemia with excess blasts
RAEB-T	refractory anemia with excess blasts in transformation
RARα	retinoic acid receptor
RARE	retinoic acid response element
RARS	refractory anemia with ring sideroblasts
RBC	red blood cell
RCT	randomized clinical trial
RDI	relative dose intensity
rEBP	recombinant EPO binding protein
rHu	recombinant human
rHuEPO	recombinant human erythropoietin
rHuG-CSF	recombinant human granulocyte colony-stimulating factor
rHuGM-CSF	recombinant human granulocyte-macrophage colony-stimulating factor
rHuIL	recombinant human interleukin
rHuMGDF	recombinant human megakaryocyte growth and development factor
rHuTPO	recombinant human thrmbopoietin
r-methHUG-CSF	filgrastim
rMuTPO	recombinant murine thrombopoietin
RT-PCR	reverse transcriptase polymerase chain reaction
sc	subcutaneous, subcutaneously
SCF	stem cell factor
SCID/Hu	human severe combined immunodeficiency
SCLC	small-cell lung cancer
SCN	severe chronic neutropenia
SCNIR	Severe Chronic Neutropenia International Registry
SDS-PAGE	sodium dodecyl sulfate-polyacrylamide gel electrophoresis
SF-36	Short-Form 36

SOCS	supressor of cytokine signaling
STAT or Stat	signal transducer and activator of transcription
sTfR	serum transferrin receptor
STR	short-term radioprotection
TBI	total body irradiation
TCR	T-cell receptor or transcription-coupled repair
TGF	transforming growth factor
TNF	tumor necrosis factor
TPO	thrombopoietin
TRAP	transfusion-related alloimmunization
TRIM	transfusion-related immunomodulation
UV	ultraviolet
VEGF	vascular endothelial growth factor
VICE	chemotherapy with vincristine, ifosfamde, carboplatin, and etoposide
WBC	white blood cell
WHO	World Health Organization

Index

I

MIX
Papier aus verantwortungsvollen Quellen
Paper from responsible sources
FSC® C105338

If you have any concerns about our products,
you can contact us on
ProductSafety@springernature.com

In case Publisher is established outside the EU,
the EU authorized representative is:
Springer Nature Customer Service Center GmbH
Europaplatz 3, 69115 Heidelberg, Germany

Printed by Libri Plureos GmbH
in Hamburg, Germany